FUNDAMENTALS OF
ANORECTAL
SURGERY

FUNDAMENTALS OF ANORECTAL SURGERY

EDITORS

David E. Beck, M.D.

Chairman and Program Director, Department of General Surgery
Wilford Hall U.S.A.F. Medical Center, Lackland AFB, Texas
Associate Professor of Surgery
Uniformed Services University of Health Sciences
Bethesda, Maryland
Chief Consultant to the U.S.A.F. Surgeon General in Colorectal Surgery

Steven D. Wexner, M.D.

Staff Colorectal Surgeon and Residency Program Director
Department of Colorectal Surgery
Director, Anorectal Physiology Laboratory
Cleveland Clinic Florida
Fort Lauderdale, Florida

McGRAW-HILL, INC.
Health Professions Division
New York   St. Louis   San Francisco   Auckland   Bogotá   Caracas
Lisbon   London   Madrid   Mexico   Milan   Montreal   New Delhi
Paris   San Juan   Singapore   Sydney   Tokyo   Toronto

FUNDAMENTALS OF ANORECTAL SURGERY

1234567890 HAL HAL 98765432

ISBN 0-07-105436-7

This book was set in Bembo by Better Graphics, Inc.

The editors were Michael J. Houston and Peter McCurdy.

The production supervisor was Clare Stanley.

The text and cover were designed and the project
was supervised by M 'N O Production Services, Inc.

Arcata Graphics/Halliday was the printer and binder.

Library of Congress Cataloging-in-Publication Data

Fundamentals of anorectal surgery / edited by David E. Beck, Steven D.
 Wexner.
     p.   cm.
   Includes bibliographical references and index.
   ISBN 0-07-105436-7
   1. Anus—Surgery. 2. Rectum—Surgery. I. Beck, David E.
 II. Wexner, Steven D.
   [DNLM: 1. Anus Diseases—surgery. 2. Rectal Diseases—surgery.
 WI 650 F981]
 RD544.F86   1992
 617.5'55059—dc20
 DNLM/DLC   92-2983
 for Library of Congress   CIP

CONTENTS

CONTRIBUTORS

David C. C. Bartolo, M.S., F.R.C.S.
Consultant Surgeon
Royal Infirmary of Edinburgh
Edinburgh, Scotland

David E. Beck, Lt. Col., USAF, MC
Chairman and Program Director, Department of
  General Surgery
Wilford Hall USAF Medical Center, Lackland AFB,
  Texas
Associate Professor of Surgery
Uniformed Services University of Health Sciences
Bethesda, Maryland
Chief Consultant to the USAF Surgeon General in
  Colorectal Surgery

Garnet J. Blatchford, M.D.
Assistant Professor of Surgery and Director
Colon and Rectal Physiology Laboratory
Creighton University School of Medicine
Clinical Assistant Professor of Surgery
University of Nebraska College of Medicine
Omaha, Nebraska

Ronald Bleday, M.D.
Department of Surgery
New England Deaconess Hospital
Boston, Massachusetts

John D. Cheape, M.D.
Alabama Colon and Rectal Surgery Institute
Birmingham, Alabama

David A. Cherry, M.D., F.R.C.S.(C)
Assistant Clinical Professor of Surgery
University of Connecticut Medical School and
  St. Francis Hospital
Hartford, Connecticut

Mark A. Christensen, M.D., F.A.C.S.
Chief of Section of Colon and Rectal Surgery
Department of Surgery
Creighton University School of Medicine
Omaha, Nebraska

Phillip Dean, M.D.
Department of Surgery
St. Louis University School of Medicine
St. Louis, Missouri

Graeme S. Duthie, F.R.C.S. (Ed)
Royal Infirmary of Edinburgh
Edinburgh, Scotland

Ridzuan Farouk, F.R.C.S. (Glas), F.R.C.S. (Ed)
Royal Infirmary of Edinburgh
Edinburgh, Scotland

James W. Fleshman, M.D.
Assistant Professor of Surgery
The Jewish Hospital of St. Louis
Washington University Medical Center
St. Louis, Missouri

**Stanley M. Goldberg, M.D., F.A.C.S.,
  F.R.A.C.S. (Hon)**
Clinical Professor of Surgery
Director Division of Colon and Rectal Surgery
Department of Surgery
University of Minnesota Medical School
Minneapolis, Minnesota

Lester Gottesman, M.D.
Division of Colon and Rectal Surgery
St. Luke's Roosevelt Hospital Center
New York, New York

Marc L. Greenwald, M.D.
Colorectal Surgeon
North Shore University Hospital
Manhasset, New York

Frank J. Harford, M.D., F.A.C.S.
Associate Professor of Surgery
Loyola University Medical Center
Maywood, Illinois

Terry C. Hicks, M.D., F.A.C.S.
Vice-Chairman
Department of Colon and Rectal Surgery
Ochsner Clinic Foundation
New Orleans, Louisiana

David G. Jagelman, M.S., F.R.C.S. (Eng)
Chairman, Department of Colorectal Surgery
Cleveland Clinic Florida
Ft. Lauderdale, Florida

Richard E. Karulf, Major, USAF, MC
Assistant Chief, Colorectal Surgery Service
Wilford Hall USAF Medical Center
Lackland AFB, Texas

Kevin P. Lally, M.D., F.A.C.S., F.A.A.P.
Associate Professor
Division of Pediatric Surgery
University of Texas Health Science Center at Houston
Houston, Texas

Ann C. Lowry, M.D.
Clinical Assistant Professor
Division of Colon and Rectal Surgery
University of Minnesota
Minneapolis, Minnesota

Robert D. Madoff, M.D.
Clinical Assistant Professor of Surgery
Division of Colon and Rectal Surgery
University of Minnesota Medical School
Chief, Colon and Rectal Section
Veterans Administration Medical Center
Minneapolis, Minnesota

Jorge E. Marcet, M.D.
Assistant Professor of Surgery
University of South Florida
Tampa, Florida

Jeffrey W. Milsom, M.D.
Staff Surgeon, Department of Colorectal Surgery
Head, Section of Colorectal Surgery Research
The Cleveland Clinic Foundation
Cleveland, Ohio

Gregory C. Oliver, M.D., F.A.C.S.
Assistant Clinical Professor of Surgery
Division of Colon and Rectal Surgery
The Robert Wood Johnson School of Medicine
Plainfield, New Jersey

Frank G. Opelka, M.D.
Department of Colon and Rectal Surgery
Ochsner Clinic Foundation
New Orleans, Louisiana

Bruce A. Orkin, M.D.
Assistant Professor of Surgery
Division of Colorectal Surgery
George Washington University
Washington, D.C.

John H. Pemberton, M.D., F.A.C.S.
Associate Professor of Surgery, Mayo Medical School
Consultant, Section of General and Colon and Rectal Surgery
Mayo Clinic
Rochester, Minnesota

Neil W. Randall, M.D.
Staff Gastroenterologist
Cleveland Clinic Florida
Ft. Lauderdale, Florida

Patricia L. Roberts, M.D., F.A.C.S.
Staff Surgeon, Department of Colon and Rectal Surgery
Lahey Clinic Medical Center
Burlington, Massachusetts

Alan G. Thorson, M.D., F.A.C.S.
Assistant Professor of Surgery and Program Director
Section of Colon and Rectal Surgery
Creighton University School of Medicine
Clinical Assistant Professor of Surgery
University of Nebraska College of Medicine
Omaha, Nebraska

Carol-Ann Vasilevsky, M.D., C.M., F.R.C.S.C., F.A.C.S.
Assistant Professor of Surgery, McGill University
Attending Surgeon, Department of Colorectal Surgery
Sir Mortimer B. Davis Jewish General Hospital
Montreal, Canada

Anthony M. Vernava III, M.D.
Assistant Professor of Surgery
Chief, Section of Colon and Rectal Surgery
Department of Surgery
St. Louis University School of Medicine
St. Louis, Missouri

Steven D. Wexner, M.D., F.A.C.S.
Residency Program Director
Director, Anorectal Physiology Laboratory
Department of Colorectal Surgery
Cleveland Clinic Florida
Ft. Lauderdale, Florida

W. Douglas Wong, M.D., F.A.C.S.
Clinical Assistant Professor
Division of Colon and Rectal Surgery
University of Minnesota
St. Paul, Minnesota

Richard L. Whelan, M.D.
Assistant Professor of Surgery
Columbia University Medical Center
College of Physicians and Surgeons
New York, New York

FOREWORD

I am sure it will be a pleasure for all readers, as it was for me, to be instructed by this remarkable book on anorectal surgery. Anorectal disorders are within the interest and clinical practice of many clinicians, ranging from generalists to those with a special interest or subspecialty in coloproctology.

It has been over fifty years since the initial text entitled *Practical Proctology* was edited by Dr. Louis A. Buie. Much has happened in the field of coloproctology and medicine since that original tome was published. In the past few years major advances have been made in the understanding and assessment of pelvic floor physiology in normal and abnormal conditions. The chapters on anatomy, physiology, and physiologic assessment of pelvic floor function provide the reader with current concepts that will assist in a better understanding of these principles.

The current surgical techniques for hemorrhoids, fistula, and fissure are well illustrated, and the fine points of technique are beautifully outlined. The newer operations for anal incontinence and prolapse are discussed with particular attention to functional and anatomic results.

For those who teach and study in the field of coloproctology as a specialty, the most prominent focus of practice is the anorectum. Few current textbooks have covered the difficult problems of the anorectum associated with AIDS. This book very thoroughly handles some of these most pressing, difficult, and life-threatening problems.

To Drs. Wexner and Beck, my congratulations for bringing together a star-studded array of young, energetic teachers of coloproctology. They have succeeded in providing us with an excellent, readable text on surgical problems of the anorectum.

STANLEY M. GOLDBERG, M.D.

PREFACE

Numerous excellent textbooks of colon and rectal surgery exist, and many more are published each year. By definition, these books focus largely upon the diagnosis and surgical management of diseases of the colon. Unfortunately, anorectal rather than colonic pathology is what usually poses the greatest difficulty to most practitioners. For this reason, *Fundamentals of Anorectal Surgery* was written. This textbook is a complete, comprehensive, and current compendium of the diagnosis and treatment of the entire spectrum of anorectal diseases. Colonic diseases have been specifically excluded because this book is not intended to duplicate the efforts of the many excellent works alluded to above.

Specifically, 26 chapters have been written to cover the gamut of problems with which the surgeon must be familiar. Chapters 1 to 3 review applied clinical anorectal anatomy, physiology, and embryology. Chapters 4 and 5 discuss general preoperative, intraoperative, and postoperative patient management. Chapters 6 to 8 present functional anorectal disorders including constipation and incontinence. Chapters 9 to 15 provide a comprehensive review of specific commonly seen benign anorectal disorders. Chapters 16 to 20 examine the presentation, evaluation, and treatment of patients with anorectal neoplasms. These include coverage of both rectal adenocarcinoma and anal squamous carcinoma as well as challenging lesions such as carcinoid and melanoma. Chapters 21 and 22 provide thorough detailed evaluation of anorectal sexually transmitted and infectious diseases and the anorectal manifestations of AIDS. Chapters 23 to 26 evaluate other important anorectal conditions that frequently demand surgical evaluation including trauma, ulcerative proctitis, and Crohn's disease.

Chapters have been carefully crafted neither to stand independent nor to duplicate each other. One of the marked and immediately obvious advantages of a multiauthored textbook is the skillfully executed interplay among authors. These authors have deftly intertwined their chapters to provide the reader with all of the current concepts, theories, and practices relative to anorectal surgery. Clearly, enunciation of this ideal and execution of the concept to fruition are not necessarily synonymous. This goal was realized only through the outstanding, indefatigable efforts of the 33 actively practicing clinicians who authored the chapters contained herein. Specifically, *Fundamentals of Anorectal Surgery* has been authored exclusively by energetic young colorectal surgeons and gastroenterologists. This has enabled the textbook to impart a uniquely current perspective on the evaluation and management of anorectal disorders. The chapters have been well written, amply illustrated, and comprehensively referenced. As such, this book provides an excellent resource for both the practicing surgeon and the resident.

ACKNOWLEDGMENTS

This text owes its existence to the efforts of many individuals. The editors are indebted to our talented contributors for their superlative efforts and to Stanley M. Goldberg, M.D., for his kind foreword to this text. It is appropriate that he was chosen for this project as he was the senior editor of *Essentials of Anorectal Surgery,* the excellent but unfortunately out of print text that inspired this textbook. In addition, we thank our publishers for their continued support, our teachers and mentors who kept us on our paths of learning, and our residents, fellows, and students who daily challenge us. The persistent efforts of our secretaries Liz Arzola and Kathy McGee allowed us to complete the multiple tasks required to produce this text and to them we are also indebted. Finally we owe much to our families. Our wives, Sharon and Pam, and children, Allison, Lauren, and John, have freely given their understanding, love, and support essential to the completion of this text.

The opinions expressed in this text are those of the authors and do not reflect the opinions of the United States Air Force or the Department of Defense.

CHAPTER 1

ANATOMY AND PHYSIOLOGY OF THE ANUS AND RECTUM

John H. Pemberton

The anatomy of the anorectum, although researched thoroughly, continues to be debated; several dogmatic versions of anatomy have been modified as a result of newer research that quantifies function of the pelvic floor muscles. The goals of this chapter are to describe the functional anatomy of the anus, pelvic floor, and rectum and to detail recent changes in our understanding of anal, rectal, and pelvic floor physiology.

Anatomy

Anal Canal

The anal canal extends from the hairy skin of the anal verge to the anorectal ring (Fig. 1-1). At rest, the lateral walls of the anal canal are opposed so that an anteroposterior slit is formed.[1] The anal canal is related to the internal and external anal sphincters. The anal canal is also related posteriorly to the coccyx, laterally to the ischiorectal fossa and its contents, and anteriorly to the urethra in men and to the lower vagina and perineal body in women.

Anal Canal Epithelium

Approximately 2 cm proximal to the anal verge is a line of anal valves (Fig. 1-1). This landmark, the dentate line, is located a the junction of the middle and distal two thirds of the internal sphincter. Above each valve is an anal crypt; connected to the crypts are a variable number of glands (4 to 10) that traverse the submucosa to terminate either in the submucosa, the internal anal sphincter, or the intersphincteric plane (Fig. 1-2). These

glands are the source of perianal abscesses and fistulas if they become obstructed and suppurate.

Proximal to the anal valves, but still in the anal canal, the mucosa becomes pleated into columns (columns of Morgagni) (see Fig. 1-1). The mucosa above the valves in the area of the columns consists of several layers of cuboidal cells. At variable distances around the anal canal (0.5 cm–1 cm) this transitional mucosa becomes a single layer of cuboidal columnar epithelium characteristic of the rectum. The color of the mucosa changes as well; at 1 cm above the dentate line the mucosa is deep purple, whereas the rectal mucosa is pink.[2] This variegated area above the dentate line is the *anal transition zone* (ATZ): the transition from continuous rectal epithelium above to uninterrupted squamous epithelium (dentate line) below.

Distal to the dentate line, the anal canal is lined by modified squamous epithelium without hair and glands, which appears smooth and thin.[2] Farther caudally, this changes to squamous epithelium with hair and glands at the anal verge. It is important to remember that none of the mucosal boundaries described here are absolute, nor are they located at the same level about the circumference of the anal canal.[3]

Anal Canal Musculature

Smooth Muscle (Fig. 1-3)

The internal anal sphincter is the continuation of the inner circular muscle of the rectum and ends with a rounded edge about 1 cm caudal to the dentate line, but cranial to the terminus of the external anal sphincter.[2] The internal anal sphincter is 2.5 to 4 cm in length and about 0.5 cm thick.

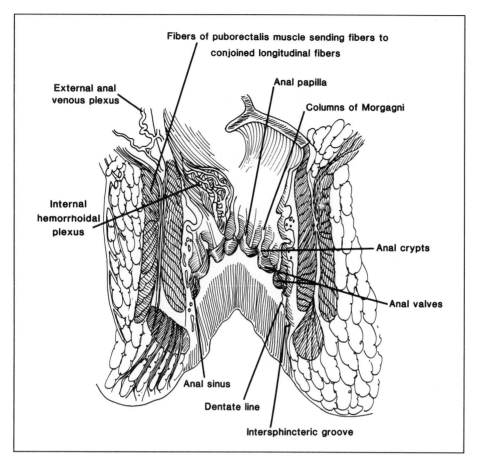

Figure 1-1. The anal canal. (*From*: Pemberton JH. Anatomy and physiology of the anus and rectum. In: Condon RE, ed. *Shackelford's Surgery of the Alimentary Tract*. 3rd ed. Philadelphia: WB Saunders; 1991:vol 4.)

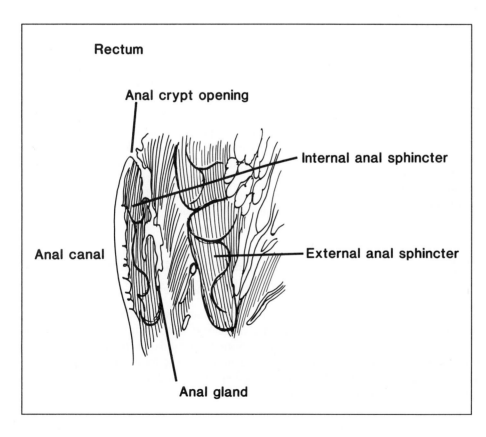

Figure 1-2. Connection between an anal gland and an anal crypt. (*From*: Pemberton JH. Anatomy and physiology of the anus and rectum. In: Condon RE, ed. *Shackelford's Surgery of the Alimentary Tract*. 3rd ed. Philadelphia: WB Saunders; 1991:vol 4.)

Longitudinal muscle fibers lie between the internal anal sphincter and the external anal sphincter. Superiorly, they are continuous with the outer longitudinal muscle of the rectal wall and pubococcygeus muscle,[4] whereas inferiorly, fibers course through the internal and external anal sphincters to the perianal skin (corrugator cutis ani).

Striated Muscle

The external anal sphincter is slightly longer than the internal anal sphincter and occupies a position outside the internal anal sphincter, enveloping it completely (see Fig. 1-3). The external anal sphincter is continuous with the puborectalis muscle superiorly and becomes subcutaneous inferiorly. The external anal sphincter is divided into deep and superficial compartments. Posteriorly, the external anal sphincter is attached to the skin superficially and to the sacrococcygeal raphe and coccyx more deeply and is continuous with the puborectalis muscle at the level of the anorectal ring. Anteriorly, the external anal sphincter is attached to the skin superficially and to the transverse perineus muscle more deeply. It proceeds with the puborectalis muscle toward the pubis at the level of the anorectal ring.

The Pelvic Floor

The levator ani plate consists of three muscles that form the posterior pelvic diaphragm (Fig. 1-4). The iliococ-

cygeus originates from the ischial spine and obturator fascia and is inserted on the sacrum (at S-4 and S-5) and on the anococcygeal raphe. The pubococcygeus muscle originates from the obturator fascia and the pubis and passes posteriorly, caudally, and medially to decussate with fibers from the contralateral side.

The puborectalis muscle (Figs. 1-4 and 1-5) arises with the pubococcygeus from the pubis and urogenital diaphragm to proceed posteriorly alongside the anorectal junction. Fibers from one side join with fibers from the other to form a sling behind the rectum at the anorectal ring (Fig. 1-6). This ring is an important landmark because incising it almost always leads to fecal incontinence.

An interesting anatomic controversy is whether the puborectalis muscle and external anal sphincter should be considered as one anatomic muscle group; the best evidence that the two are of the same striated muscle complex is provided by Wendell-Smith[5] and Wood.[4]

The pelvic diaphragm fixes the pelvic viscera and provides a firm wall against which increased abdominal pressure is exerted during defecation, coughing, and laughing. The bilateral involuntary rectococcygeus muscles tether the rectum to the coccyx. The coccygeus muscles are also bilateral but are voluntary. They arise from the ischial spine and insert into the fifth sacral vertebra and the coccyx. These muscles support the rectum and bring the coccyx forward during squeezing. The superficial transverse perineus muscle (see Fig. 1-4)

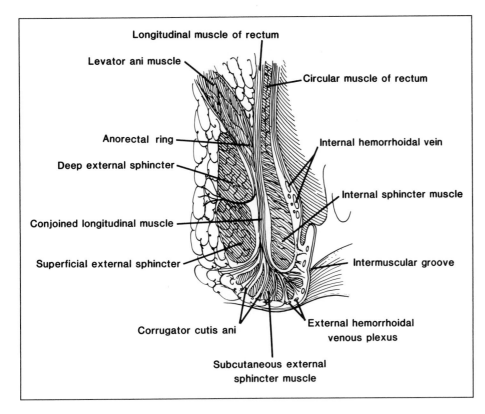

Figure 1-3. The voluntary and involuntary muscles of the anorectum and their relationships to the topography of the anal canal. (*From:* Pemberton JH. Anatomy and physiology of the anus and rectum. In: Condon RE, ed. *Shackelford's Surgery of the Alimentary Tract.* 3rd ed. Philadelphia: WB Saunders; 1991:vol. 4.)

Longitudinal muscle of rectum

Levator ani muscle

Circular muscle of rectum

Anorectal ring

Deep external sphincter

Internal hemorrhoidal vein

Internal sphincter muscle

Conjoined longitudinal muscle

Superficial external sphincter

Intermuscular groove

Corrugator cutis ani

External hemorrhoidal venous plexus

Subcutaneous external sphincter muscle

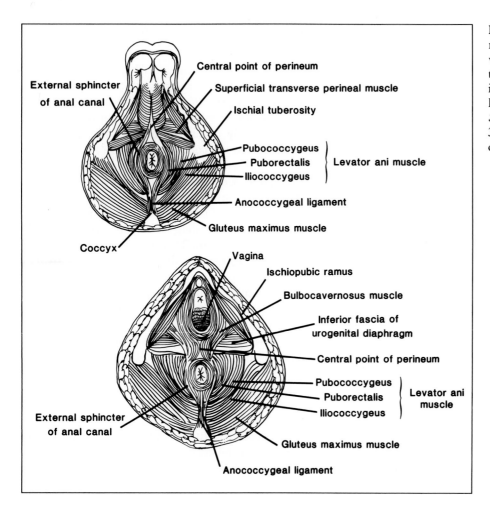

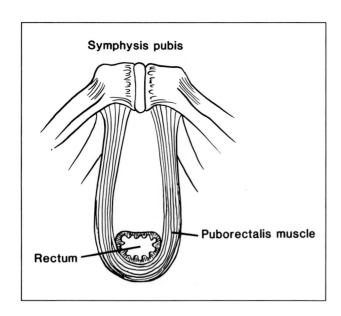

Figure 1-4. The levator ani muscles in men (*above*) and in women (*below*). (*From:* Pemberton JH. Anatomy and physiology of the anus and rectum. In: Condon RE, ed. *Shackelford's Surgery of the Alimentary Tract.* 3rd ed. Philadelphia: WB Saunders; 1991:vol 4.)

Figure 1-5. The puborectalis muscle viewed from above. This muscle is adjacent to the anorectal junction laterally, indeed forming it, and swings around to encircle the sphincter posteriorly. (*From:* Pemberton JH. Anatomy and physiology of the anus and rectum. In: Condon RE, ed. *Shackelford's Surgery of the Alimentary Tract.* 3rd ed. Philadelphia: WB Saunders; 1991:vol 4.)

arises from the pubis and inserts into the central perineal raphe. The function of this muscle is to fix the central tendon. The deep transverse perineus muscle (see Fig. 1-4) arises from the ischium bilaterally. In men, these muscles merge with the external urinary sphincter and act to voluntarily terminate urination.

Para-anal and Pararectal spaces

Several potential spaces in the anorectal anorectum have surgical importance (Figs. 1-7, 1-8, and 1-9).[6]

Ischiorectal Space (Figs. 1-7 and 1-9). The apex is at the origin of the levator ani muscles from the obturator fascia (Figs. 1-7 and 1-9). This space is bounded inferiorly by the perineal skin, anteriorly by the transverse muscles of the perineum, posteriorly by the sacrotuberous ligament and gluteus maximus muscle, medially by the external anal sphincter and levator ani, and laterally by the external obturator muscle. In the lateral wall of this space is Alcock's canal, through which course the pudendal vessels and nerves. There is a potential extension of this space anteriorly, *above* the urogenital diaphragm. The contents of this space include fat, the inferior hemorrhoidal vessels and nerves, and the scrotal or labial vessels.

4

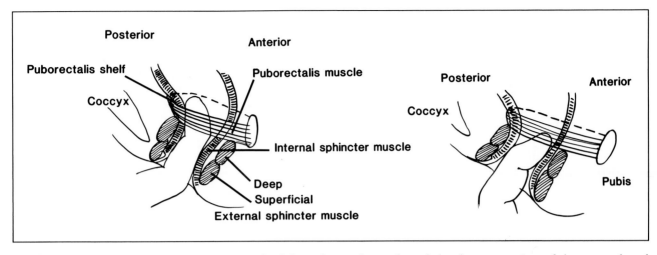

Figure 1-6. The anorectal ring is composed of the puborectal muscle and the deepest portion of the external anal sphincter. The ring is most easily palpated *posteriorly* as the puborectalis "shelf." (*From:* Pemberton JH. Anatomy and physiology of the anus and rectum. In: Condon RE, ed. *Shackelford's Surgery of the Alimentary Tract.* 3rd ed. Philadelphia: WB Saunders; 1991:vol 4.)

Perianal Space (Figs. 1-7 and 1-9). This potential space surrounds the anal verge, is continuous with the fat of the buttocks laterally, and extends into the intersphincteric space. Its contents are the most caudal part of the external anal sphincter, the external hemorrhoidal plexus, and the inferior hemorrhoidal vessels. This space is bound down tightly by the corrugator cutis.

Intersphincteric Space (Fig. 1-9). The intersphincteric space is a potential space between the sphincteric muscles and is continuous with the perianal space.

Supralevator Spaces (Figs. 1-7, 1-8, and 1-9). The supralevator space is bounded superiorly by the peritoneum, laterally by the obturator fascia, medially by the rectum, and inferiorly by the levator plate. These spaces may connect to each other posteriorly behind the rectum, deep to the anococcygeal raphe but superficial to the rectosacral fascia.

Submucous Space. The submucous space likely begins at the dentate line and extends cranially to join the submucosa of the rectum proper. The internal hemorrhoidal plexus is in this space.

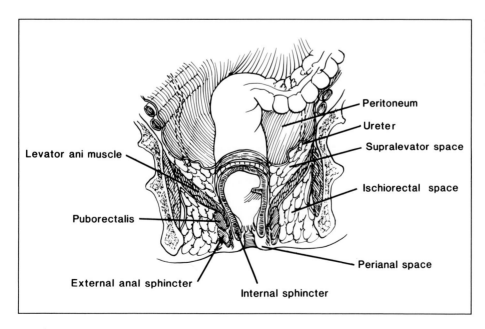

Figure 1-7. The para-anal and pararectal spaces (coronal view). (*From:* Pemberton JH. Anatomy and physiology of the anus and rectum. In: Condon RE, ed. *Shackelford's Surgery of the Alimentary Tract.* 3rd ed. WB Saunders; 1991:vol 4.)

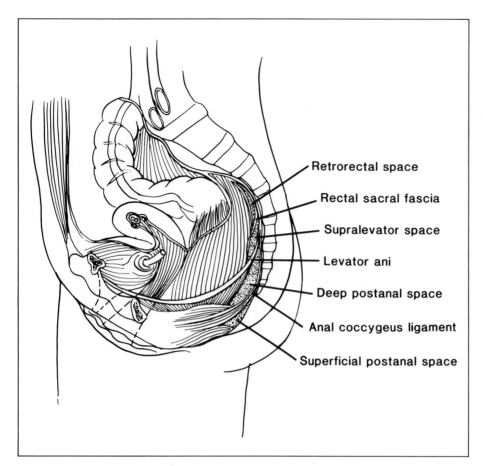

Retrorectal space

Rectal sacral fascia

Supralevator space

Levator ani

Deep postanal space

Anal coccygeus ligament

Superficial postanal space

Figure 1-8. The posterior pararectal spaces seen in lateral projection. (*From:* Pemberton JH. Anatomy and physiology of the anus and rectum. In: Condon RE, ed. *Shackelford's Surgery of the Alimentary Tract.* 3rd ed. Philadelphia: WB Saunders; 1991:vol 4.)

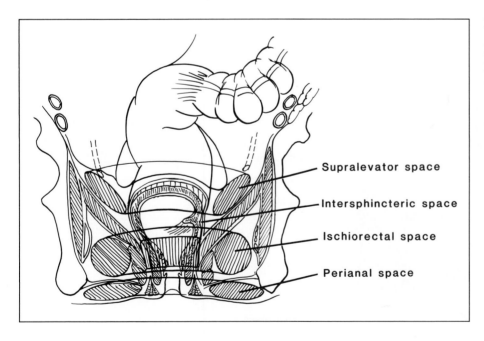

Supralevator space

Intersphincteric space

Ischiorectal space

Perianal space

Figure 1-9. Pararectal and para-anal spaces. Abscesses form tracts posteriorly from one lateral space to gain access to the contralateral space. The view is coronal. (*From:* Pemberton JH. Anatomy and physiology of the anus and rectum. In: Condon RE, ed. *Shackelford's Surgery of the Alimentary Tract.* 3rd ed. Philadelphia: WB Saunders; 1991:vol 4.)

Superficial Postanal Space (Fig. 1-8). The superficial postanal space is continuous with the superficial ischiorectal fossa posteriorly, deep to the skin but superficial to the anococcygeal ligament.

Deep Postanal Space (Fig. 1-8). The deep postanal space, in contrast, connects the deeper parts of the ischiorectal fossa posteriorly behind the anal canal, deep to the anal coccygeal ligament but superficial to the anococcygeal raphe. Horseshoe abscesses usually occur through this space but also may occur in the superficial postanal space (Fig. 1-8).

Retrorectal Space (Fig. 1-8). The retrorectal space begins cranial to the rectosacral ligament between the rectum and the sacrum and is continuous with the retroperitoneum above. Its boundaries are the fascia propria of the rectum anteriorly, the presacral fascia posteriorly, and the lateral rectal ligaments. This plane is avascular. The fascia propria protects the mesorectal vessels, and the presacral fascia invests the presacral vessels.

Rectum

The rectum is described by anatomists as beginning at S-3, but surgeons describe it as beginning at the sacral promontary.[2] The rectum descends caudally, following the curve of the sacrum first downward and then forward for a distance of 13 to 15 cm to end at the anorectal ring (Fig. 1-10). This ring is formed by the pelvic floor muscles (the puborectalis muscle, in particular) and the external and internal anal sphincters (see Fig. 1-6). The anal canal continues below the anorectal ring by turning abruptly downward and backward to terminate at the anal verge.

The rectum has three lateral curves (Fig. 1-11). The upper and lower curves are concave and toward the right; the middle one is convex and to the left. The valves of Houston are located at the intraluminal aspects of the rectum. These infoldings incorporate all layers of the rectal wall except the outer longitudinal muscle layer. The middle valve is the most consistent and usually marks the level of the anterior peritoneal reflection.[6] Importantly for surgeons, when the curves are straightened by rectal mobilization the rectum elongates by about 5 cm.

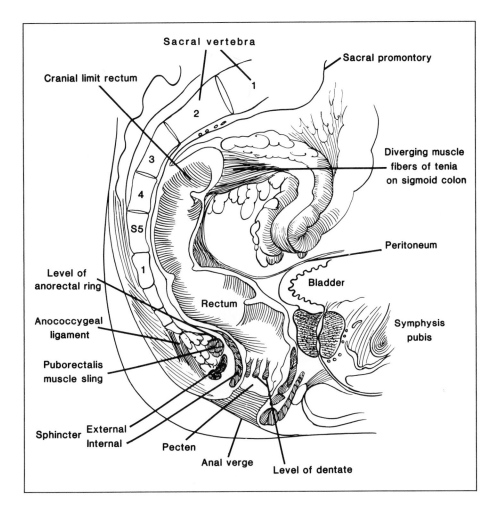

Figure 1-10. The rectum as it courses through the pelvis. The rectum descends downward from S-3 to the level of the coccyx, then downward and forward to end at the anorectal ring. The tenia diverge at the level of S-2 to S-3, providing a visual landmark distinguishing sigmoid from rectum. (*From:* Pemberton JH. Anatomy and physiology of the anus and rectum. In: Condon RE, ed. *Shackelford's Surgery of the Alimentary Tract.* 3rd ed. Philadelphia: WB Saunders; 1991:vol 4.)

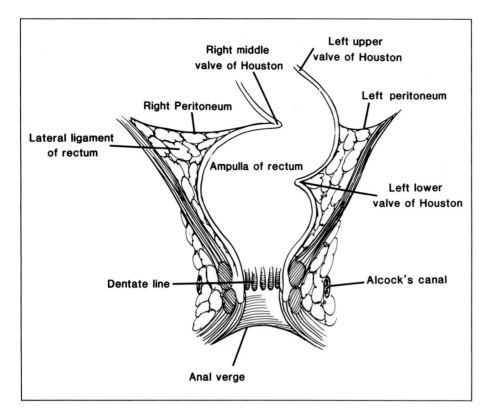

Figure 1-11. The curves of the rectum. The uppermost and lowermost curves are convex to the right whereas the middle curve is convex to the left. The three valves of Houston are also seen. The peritoneum is reflected off the rectum at the level of the middle valve. (*From:* Pemberton JH. Anatomy and physiology of the anus and rectum. In: Condon RE, ed. *Shackelford's Surgery of the Alimentary Tract.* 3rd ed. Philadelphia: WB Saunders; 1991:vol 4.)

At the rectosigmoid junction, the transverse folds characteristic of the sigmoid colon give way to the smoother rectal mucosa (Fig. 1-12).[4] Externally at this same junction, the three taeniae coli disappear as they spread to encircle the rectum as the longitudinal muscle layer (see Fig. 1-10). Although this is sometimes difficult to appreciate, the rectum can also be identified because it has no epiploic tags, sacculations, or obvious posterior mesentery.[2] In addition the rectal lumen is usually larger in diameter than the sigmoid.

Peritoneum covers the exterior surface of the rectum on the anterior and lateral sides in the upper one third (see Figs. 1-10 and 1-11), wrapping around to encircle the rectum except for the short mesorectum. In the middle third, only the anterior aspect of the rectum is covered by peritoneum; the rectum is devoid of peritoneum in its lower portion. The level of the anterior peritonal reflection is variable: it is about 7 to 9 cm above the anal verge in men, and between 5 and 7.5 cm in women.[6] The peritoneum is reflected from the rectum onto the pelvic sidewalls to form the perirectal fossa. In males the anterior peritoneum reflects onto the seminal vesicles and bladder, and in females it reflects onto the vagina and uterus.

Anatomic Relationships of the Rectum

Posteriorly, the rectum is related to the sacrum, coccyx, levator ani muscles, medial sacral vessels, and roots of the sacral nerve plexus. Anteriorly, in males, the extra-

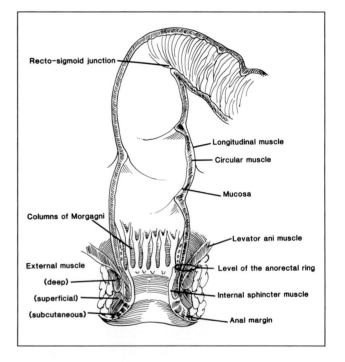

Figure 1-12. Level at which the "rough" mucosa of the sigmoid colon gives way to the smooth mucosa of the rectum. As compared with Figure 1-11, the rectum has been "stretched" and the curves straightened. Finally, note the diagram's depiction of the layers of the rectal wall. (*From:* Pemberton JH. Anatomy and physiology of the anus and rectum. In: Condon RE, ed. *Shackelford's Surgery of the Alimentary Tract.* 3rd ed. Philadelphia: WB Saunders; 1991:vol 4.)

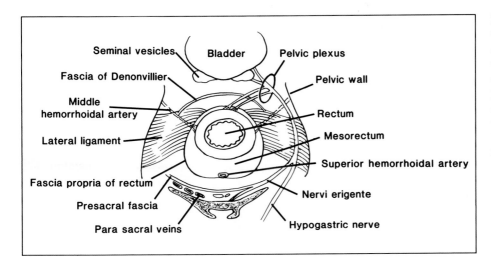

Figure 1-13. The pelvis viewed from above, drawn quite diagrammatically to show the major fascial, nervous, and arterial structures. Note that the pelvic plexus is located far laterally, nearly on the pelvic sidewall *under* the enveloping pelvic fascia. It is also evident that the nerves going to the prostate and bladder are easily spared in benign disease by staying on the rectal side of Denovillier's fascia. (*From:* Pemberton JH. Anatomy and physiology of the anus and rectum. In: Condon RE, ed. *Shackelford's Surgery of the Alimentary Tract.* 3rd ed. Philadelphia: WB Saunders; 1991:vol 4.)

peritoneal rectum is related to the prostate, seminal vesicles, vas deferens, and urinary bladder. In females, the extraperitoneal rectum lies behind the posterior vaginal wall.

Fascial Relationships and Attachments (Fig. 1-13)

The fascia propria envelops the rectal vessels. Below the anterior peritoneal reflection, the condensations of this fascia on each side of the rectum are the lateral ligaments attaching the rectum to the pelvic side walls. These ligaments support the rectum, and dividing them facilitates rectal mobilization. The accessory branches of the middle hemorrhoidal artery, but not the main arteries, sometimes traverse these lateral ligaments.

From the S-4 level, the retrosacral fascia (fascia of Waldeyer), a portion of the parietal pelvic fascia, runs downward and forward to reflect onto the fascia propria above the anorectal ring (Fig. 1-14A). This is a very thick fascial layer, and safe posterior rectal mobilization necessitates that it be incised with a scissors or by electrocautery (Fig. 1-14B).

Anteriorly, the extraperitoneal rectum is also covered by the visceral pelvic fascia (Denonvilliers' fascia), which extends from the peritoneal reflection downward to the urogenital diaphragm, *parallel to the rectum* and dorsal to the urogenital structures (Fig. 1-15). This fascia separates the rectum from the prostate gland and seminal vesicles in males or from the vagina in females.

Blood Supply

The major arterial blood supply to the rectum and anal canal is from the superior and inferior hemorrhoidal

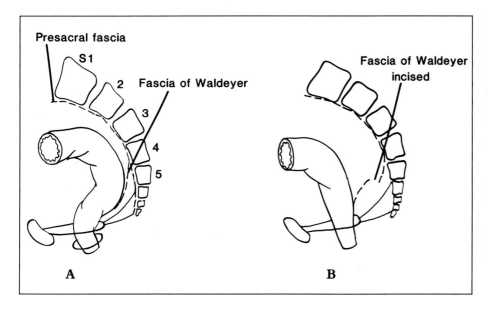

Figure 1-14. The presacral fascia and the fascia of Waldeyer. (A) Waldeyer's fascia reflects off the presacral fascia *above* the anorectal ring. Sharply incising the fascia (B) frees the rectum *posteriorly*, facilitating complete mobilization. Blunt dissection of Waldeyer's fascia at this level may tear the rectum. (*From:* Pemberton JH. Anatomy and physiology of the anus and rectum. In: Condon RE, ed. *Shackelford's Surgery of the Alimentary Tract.* 3rd ed. Philadelphia: WB Saunders, 1991:vol 4.)

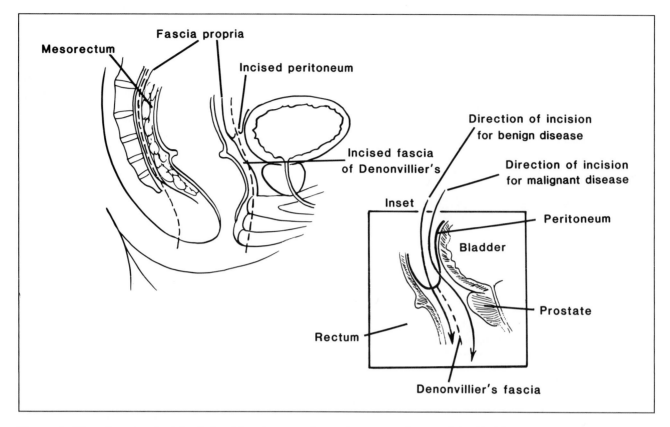

Figure 1-15. Anterior fascial relationships. In men, the peritoneum reflects off the bladder onto the rectum. Denonvillier's fascia runs *parallel* to the rectum separating the rectum from anterior structures. For benign disease, *anterior* mobilization is accomplished by incising the peritoneum at its reflection and *then* incising posteriorly through Denonvillier's fascia; the "correct" plane can be bluntly developed readily. (*From:* Pemberton JH. Anatomy and physiology of the anus and rectum. In: Condon RE, ed. *Shackelford's Surgery of the Alimentary Tract.* 3rd ed. Philadelphia: WB Saunders; 1991:vol 4.)

arteries, whereas the middle hemorrhoidal artery has a variable contribution (Fig. 1-16).

The superior hemorrhoidal artery is a direct continuation of the inferior mesenteric artery. It descends in the sigmoid mesocolon to the level of S-3, at which point it bifurcates into right and left branches and then further bifurcates into anterior and posterior branches.[7] These branches enter the rectal wall, penetrate to the submucosa, and then descend in that plane to the level of the columns of Morgagni.

The inferior hemorrhoidal arteries are branches of the internal pudendal artery, which in turn is a branch of the internal iliac artery. The inferior hemorrhoidal artery traverses the external anal sphincter to reach the submucosa of the anal canal and then ascend in this plane.

A substantial middle hemorrhoidal artery is present if the superior hemorrhoidal artery is small.[8] The middle hemorrhoidal artery arises from the internal iliac artery and reaches the rectum by traversing the supralevator space on top of the levator ani musculature but deep to the levator fascia. The artery does not itself traverse

through the lateral stalks but sends minor branches through them.

These three major vessels contribute to an intramural anterial anastomotic network.[4] This anatomic finding supports the clinical observation that division of both the superior hemorrhoidal and middle hemorrohoidal arteries does not cause necrosis of the rectum.

Venous drainage of the rectum and anal canal runs with the arterial supply. Drainage through the superior hemorrhoidal vein is into the portal system, whereas drainage through the middle and inferior hemorrhoidal veins is into the caval system.

Lymphatic drainage likewise follows the vascular supply (Fig. 1-17). Drainage from the upper two thirds of the rectum reaches the inferior mesenteric nodes. The lower third of the rectum drains not only into the inferior mesenteric nodes but also into the internal iliac nodes. Lymphatic drainage from the anal canal above the dentate line courses to the inferior mesenteric nodes and internal iliac nodes. Drainage below the dentate line is usually to the inguinal lymph nodes but can be to the

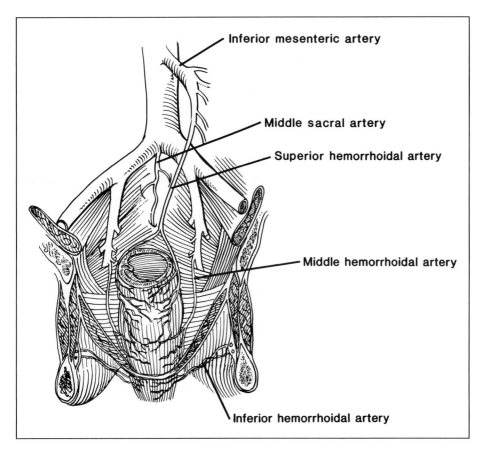

Figure 1-16. The vasculature of the rectal and anal canals. Note that the middle hemorrhoidal artery, if present, is small and lies immediately atop the levator ani musculature, *not* in the lateral rectal stalks. (*From:* Pemberton JH. Anatomy and physiology of the anus and rectum. In: Condon RE, ed. *Shackelford's Surgery of the Alimentary Tract.* 3rd ed. Philadelphia: WB Saunders; 1991:vol 4.)

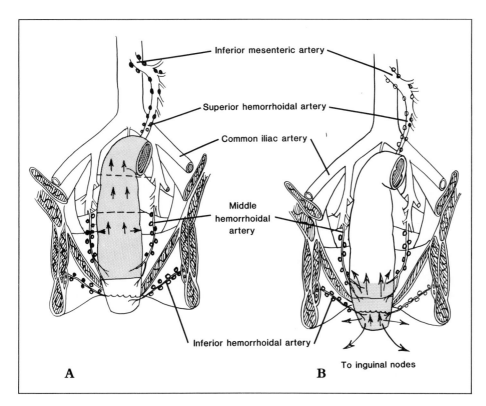

Figure 1-17. The lymphatic drainage of the rectum and anal canal. The "watershed" area is the dentate line. (A) Tumors above the dentate line metastasize to the internal iliac and inferior mesenteric nodes. (B) Tumors below the dentate may metastasize to the inguinal lymph node chain. (*From:* Pemberton JH. Anatomy and physiology of the anus and rectum. In: Condon RE, ed. *Shackelford's Surgery of the Alimentary Tract.* 3rd ed. Philadelphia: WB Saunders; 1991:vol 4.)

inferior mesenteric nodes and to nodes along the course of the inferior hemorrhoidal artery. Usually, retrograde lymphatic spread below the level of a rectal cancer occurs only if extensive involvement of proximally draining lymphatic and venous channels has occurred.[9] Injection studies have shown that lymphatic drainage in females spreads to the posterior vaginal wall, uterus, broad ligament, ovaries, and cul-de-sac.[10]

Innervation of the Rectum

Extrinsic innervation of the rectum and anal canal is both sympathetic and parasympathetic in origin. In general, the sympathetic response inhibits contraction of smooth muscle of the rectum when the internal anal sphincter contracts, whereas the *parasympathetic response* contracts the rectal wall but relaxes the internal sphincter.

Sympathetic Innervation. The sympathetic supply to the upper rectum arises from L-1 to L-3, exiting as lumbar sympathetics to join the aortic plexus (superior hypogastric plexus, hypogastric plexus) (Fig. 1-18). The lumbar sympathetics also run along the inferior mesenteric artery to the inferior mesenteric plexus. From

there, postganglionic fibers follow branches of the inferior mesenteric artery and superior hemorrhoidal artery terminating in the upper rectum. The lower rectum is innervated by the presacral nerves, which are formed by fusion of the terminal branches of the aortic plexus and lumbar splanchnics. The presacral nerves extend over the bifurcation of the aorta and divide below the sacral promontory and adjacent to the posterolateral aspect of the rectum to form the right and left hypogastric nerves. The right and left hypogastric nerves each pass to a pelvic plexus, located deep to the peritoneum but superficial to the endopelvic fascia on each pelvic side wall, at about the level of the lower third of the rectum and *lateral to the lateral stalks* (see Fig. 1-13). Branches from the pelvic plexus innervate the lower rectum, upper anal canal, bladder, and sexual organs.

Parasympathetic Innervation. The parasympathetic innervation originates from the anterior roots of S-2, S-3, and S-4 (Fig. 1-18). Fibers from S-3 and S-4 are termed the *nervi erigentes.* These nerves join with the hypogastric nerves (sympathetic) in the pelvic plexus. Parasympathetics then pass upward to the inferior mesenteric plexus to be distributed to the superior hemor-

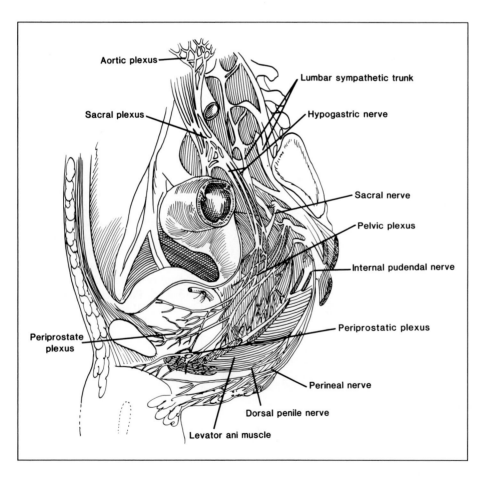

Aortic plexus

Sacral plexus

Lumbar sympathetic trunk

Hypogastric nerve

Sacral nerve

Pelvic plexus

Internal pudendal nerve

Periprostatic plexus

Periprostate plexus

Perineal nerve

Dorsal penile nerve

Levator ani muscle

Figure 1-18. Innervation of the rectum, anal canal, and anterior structures. (*From:* Pemberton JH. Anatomy and physiology of the anus and rectum. In: Condon RE, ed. *Shackelford's Surgery of the Alimentary Tract.* 3rd ed. Philadelphia: WB Saunders; 1991:vol 4.)

rhoidal artery and the sigmoidal and left colonic arteries. Other parasympathetics are distributed from the pelvic plexus to the bladder, genitals, and internal anal sphincter. An important subdivision of the pelvic plexus (inferior hypogastric plexus) is the periprostatic plexus, which is adjacent to the rectum and prostate and supplies parasympathetic and sympathetic input via anterolateral connections to the prostate, seminal vesicles, corpora cavernosum, vas deferens, urethra, ejaculatory ducts, and bulbourethral glands (Fig. 1-18). Fortunately, these fibers terminate *above* Denonvilliers' fascia and thus they can be protected by careful dissection below it.[11] Erection of the penis is controlled by parasympathetic input (sympathetic input does inhibit vasoconstriction, thereby increasing vascular engorgement), whereas sympathetic inflow causes emission and parasympathetic inflow causes ejaculation.

The somatic pelvic nerves arise from S-3, S-4, and S-5 and cross the pelvic floor under the facia covering the levator ani. The levator muscles are supplied by these nerves, as is the anal canal. The pudendal nerve arises from S-2, S-3, and S-4 and enters the perineum from Alcock's canal. Branches of the pudendal nerves are the inferior hemorrhoidal, perianal, and dorsal penile or clitoral nerves (Fig. 1-18).

Innervation of the Anal Canal

Internal Anal Sphincter. The motor supply to the internal anal sphincter is sympathetic (L-5) and parasympathetic (S-2, S-3, and S-4). The tone of the internal anal sphincter is mediated by both sympathetic and parasympathetic fibers;[4] contraction of the internal anal sphincter, however, is for the most part sympathetically mediated.[12] Relaxation of the internal anal sphincter occurs as part of an intramural (intrinsic) reflex called the *rectoanal sphincter inhibitory response* mediated by noncholinergic, nonadrenergic nerves. Distention of the rectal wall above the anorectal ring leads to relaxation of the internal anal sphincter.

External Anal Sphincter (Fig. 1-18). Motor supply to the external anal sphincter travels in the pudendal nerve (S-2 and S-3) and the perineal branch of S-4. The fibers cross over at the cord level in such a way that unilateral transection of a pudendal nerve does not abolish function of the external anal sphincter.[13]

Levator Ani. The motor supply of the puborectalis muscle is controversial. It consists of the pudendal nerve alone, direct pelvic branches of S-3 and S-4 alone, or a combination of the two. The pubococcygeus and iliococcygeus muscles are supplied on their superior aspects by S-4 and on their inferior aspects by perineal branches of pudendal nerves.

Anorectal Sensation

Rectum. Although many nonmyelinated nerve fibers exist in the rectum, organized endings are generally lacking in the rectal mucosa. Receptors for rectal distention likely lie outside the rectal wall itself.[11,14,15] Sensation from the rectum is carried in parasympathetic nerves S-2, S-3, and S-4.

Anal Canal. From 1 to 1.5 cm above the anal valves to the anal verge, the anal canal epithelium contains free nerve endings, Meissner's corpuscles (touch), Krause's bulbs (cold), Golgi-Mazzoni bodies (pressure), and genital corpuscles (friction).[16,17] Sensation is carried in the inferior hemorrhoidal branch of the pudendal nerve.

Physiology

A clearer understanding of anorectal physiology has been made possible by the introduction of several techniques for **quantitating** anorectal motility. The pathophysiologic basis of fecal incontinence, constipation, expulsion disorders, rectal intussusception, rectal prolapse, solitary rectal ulcer, rectocele, posterior rectal hernia, and obstructed defecation are undergoing intense investigation.

Factors Maintaining Fecal Continence

Continence depends on the ability to defer the "call to stool" to a socially convenient time and place. Table 1-1 details the factors that maintain fecal continence and facilitate defecation.

Anal Canal High Pressure Zone

The mean length of the anal canal high pressure zone is 4 cm. Women have a shorter anal canal than do men (mean 3.7 cm versus 4.6 cm).[18] During anal sphincter squeeze, the anal canal lengthens, whereas during straining it shortens.[19]

Table 1-1 Factors Maintaining Fecal Continence

Anal canal high pressure zone
Anorectal angle (puborectal muscle)
Anorectal sensory and reflex mechanism
Distensibility, tone, and capacity of the rectum
Motility and evacuability of the rectum
Motility of the anal canal
Colon transit
Small bowel transit
Stool volume and consistency

Resting Pressure. The external anal sphincter and internal anal sphincter envelop the anal canal. They are responsible for maintaining resting pressures and generating squeeze pressures. There is a graduated increase in pressure from proximal to distal in the anal canal (Fig. 1-19); highest pressures are 1 to 2 cm proximal to the anal verge. The mean anal canal resting pressure is approximately 90 cm H_2O ($\pm$ SEM).[20] Resting pressure is lower in women than in men[21,22] and may be lower in older subjects.

It is likely that resting pressures are distributed unequally around the circumference of the anal canal because of the anatomic arrangement of the anal sphincter and pubococcygeus muscles. Posteriorly, resting pressure is highest proximally and lowest near the anal verge.[23,24] McHugh and Diamant[21] showed that anterior resting pressures were highest distally in the anal canal in women but were highest proximally in men. The internal anal sphincter contributes about 85 percent of the resting tone of the anal canal.[25] Dividing the internal anal sphincter *in the presence of a normal external anal sphincter* weakens tone but does not entirely abolish it.

Anal canal tone is maintained day and night.[26]

Coughing and the Valsalva maneuver increase external anal sphincter activity;[19,27] this tone is mediated by a low sacral reflex. Straining to defecate, however, usually renders the external anal sphincter electrically silent.

Squeeze Pressure. Squeeze pressure is generated by contraction of the external anal sphincter *and* the puborectalis muscle. During maximal effort intra-anal canal pressures are increased to more than twice the normal resting level.[19]

Squeeze pressure may also be distributed unequally around the anal canal. Taylor and associates[24] found that squeeze pressures in the proximal anal canal were highest posteriorly and lowest anteriorly. In the midanal canal, squeeze pressure was distributed equally. In the distal anal canal, squeeze pressure was highest anteriorly and lowest posteriorly.

Maximum squeeze pressure elevation lasts less than 1 minute because the sphincter fatigues rapidly after that time (Fig. 1-20).[1,19] Because squeeze efforts generate high pressure briefly, the squeeze mechanism is probably effective only in preventing immediate leakage. This mechanism then is likely not responsible for maintaining fecal continence from hour to hour.

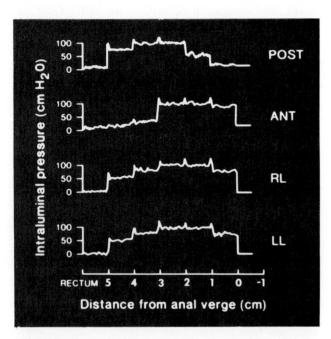

Figure 1-19. Perfused four-channel recordings of resting anal canal pressure (*upper*—posterior; next—right lateral; next—left lateral; *bottom*—anterior). A stepped pullthrough technique was used. Note that upon pulling the probe into the anal canal, pressures are recorded posteriorly first and anteriorly last because the puborectal muscle is present high in the anal canal and absent low in the canal.

Anorectal Angle

A mechanism that probably helps maintain hour-to-hour fecal continence, particularly of solid content, is the configuration of the pelvic floor, namely the *anorectal angle*. This angle is formed by the anteriorly directed pull of the puborectal muscle as it envelops the anorectum at the level of the anorectal ring (Fig. 1-21). Barkel and associates[28] found that the mean ($\pm$ SD) angle was 102 ± 18 degrees at rest in the left lateral position. Standing changed the angle slightly, but sitting widened the angle significantly to 119 ± 17 degrees. Sphincter squeeze, a maneuver that augments anorectal continence, and the Valsalva maneuver, which stresses continence, sharpened the angle to 81 ± 19 degrees and 87 ± 23 degrees, respectively ($p < .05$, lying position).

The puborectalis muscle has the property of *continuous* resting electrical activity. Although it may act as a flap valve, more likely its sphincterlike function at the level of the anorectal ring is more important.[29]

The anorectal angulation must be overcome to evacuate solid enteric content. This is accomplished by squatting; the angle is straightened to greater than 110 degrees by hip flexion. Straightening of the anorectal angle is augmented by straining, which usually but not invariably causes the puborectalis muscle and external anal sphincter to become electrically silent.[19] With the angle overcome, content passes into the anal canal.

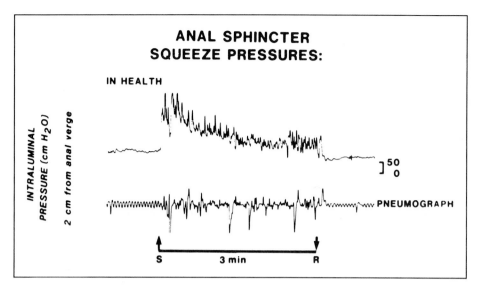

ANAL SPHINCTER SQUEEZE PRESSURES:

IN HEALTH

INTRALUMINAL PRESSURE (cm H₂O)
2 cm from anal verge

PNEUMOGRAPH

S   3 min   R

Figure 1-20. Anal canal squeeze pressure recorded by a perfused probe positioned about 2 cm proximal to the anal verge. This is a single-channel recording. The overall duration of elevated pressure was 3 minutes, but the duration of maximal pressure was less than 1 minute. (*From:* Pemberton JH. Anatomy and physiology of the anus and rectum. In: Condon RE, ed. *Shackelford's Surgery of the Alimentary Tract.* 3rd ed. Philadelphia: WB Saunders; 1991:vol 4.)

Anorectal Sensation

Sensory mechanisms allow discrimination of the character of enteric content (gas, liquid, or solid stool) and detection of the need to pass that content. The site of these sensory receptors is either in the rectal muscularis or in the surrounding pelvic floor musculature.[30] More-over, the ability to detect interrectal pressure differentials was hypothesized by Goligher and Hughes[20] to be important in discriminating content character; flatus generated a lower perceived intrarectal pressure than did solid stool.

Duthie and Bennett[31] found that acute sensation resided only in the mucosa of the proximal anal canal. Their observations have been confirmed by others who determined that sensation was most acute in the region of the anal valves.[29] In order to be distinguished, enteric content, therefore, would have to gain access to the anal canal. This occurs if the internal sphincter relaxes just enough to allow content to bathe the anal canal mucosa, but not enough to cause leakage.

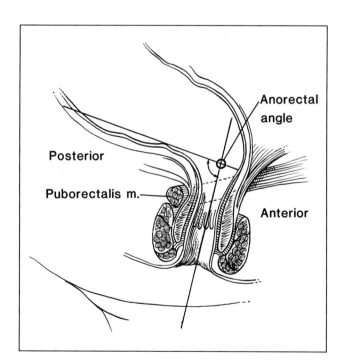

Anorectal angle

Posterior

Puborectalis m.

Anterior

Figure 1-21. Angulation between the rectum and anal canal. This angle is formed by the pull of the puborectalis muscle, which is directed anteriorly. (*From:* Pemberton JH. Anatomy and physiology of the anus and rectum. In: Condon RE, ed. *Shackelford's Surgery of the Alimentary Tract.* 3rd ed. Philadelphia: WB Saunders; 1991:vol 4.)

Rectal Anal Sphincter Inhibitory Response

With acute rectal distention, the rectal wall contracts slightly, the proximal portion of the anal canal relaxes (presumably, the internal anal sphincter), and the distal portion contracts (external anal sphincter). This is the rectal anal sphincter inhibitory response (RASIR) (Fig. 1-22). Sensory receptors for this response are located in the rectum, and the response is mediated by noncholinergic, nonadrenergic intramural nervevs.[12]

The role of the rectoanal sphincter inhibitory response is not fully understood. It was hypothesized that relaxation of the internal anal sphincter would allow the enteric content to come into contact with the sensitive mucosa of the proximal anal canal; its character could then be recognized. If rectal distention continued unabated, however, the external anal sphincter was inhibited and the perceived need to evacuate became urgent. In an interesting study, Miller and colleagues[32] documented that this sampling response occurred in healthy

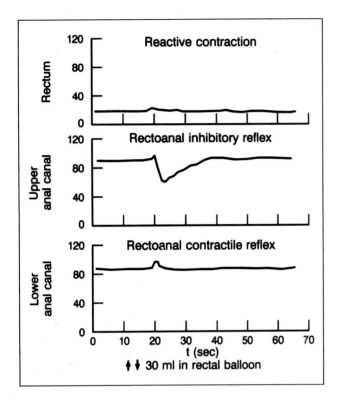

Figure 1-22. The rectal anal sphincter inhibitory response (RASIR) is composed of three parts: (1) reactive rectal contraction, (2) decreased anal canal pressure proximally, and (3) increased anal canal pressure distally. The decrease in resting pressure lasts approximately 20 seconds and is thought to be caused by relaxation of the internal anal sphincter. The brief increase in pressure distally may be caused by reactive contraction of the external anal sphincter. (*From:* Pemberton JH. Anatomy and physiology of the anus and rectum. In: Condon RE, ed. *Shackelford's Surgery of the Alimentary Tract.* 3rd ed. Philadelphia: WB Saunders; 1991:vol 4.)

ambulatory patients between four and ten times per hour. These observations confirm those of Ihre,[33] who found that each passage of enteric content into the rectum is accompanied by internal sphincter relaxation and external anal sphincter and puborectalis muscle contraction.

Although this is an attractive hypothesis, its importance is disputed by findings that after ileoanal anastomosis, the response often cannot be recorded,[34] yet continence is not seemingly affected.[35] Moreover, if enteric content comes in contact only with the tissues of the anal canal, *distinction between gas and stool could not be made.*[33] Finally, continence to large volumes of saline infused into the rectum was unaffected when local anesthesia was applied to the mucosa of the anal canal.[36]

Rectal Distensibility ("Compliance") and Capacity

The rectum accommodates passively to distention: intraluminal pressure remains low, whereas intraluminal volume increases (Fig. 1-23). The maximal tolerable volume in healthy individuals approximates 400 ml, yet intraluminal pressure remains less than 20 mm Hg. By plotting the slope of $\Delta V/\Delta^{-1}$, the distensibility of the rectum in seven healthy volunteers[34] was calculated to be 16.8 ± 2 ml/cm H_2O (mean $\pm$ SEM).

These characteristics of rectal compliance appear to be very similar to those of the fundus of the stomach; that is, they entail passive accommodation to volume. Azpiroz and Malagelada (1985)[37] found that this characteristic of the gastric fundus made interpretation of intraluminal contractile events confusing. They therefore developed a novel technique to study gastric motility, and this technique has been adapted to the study of rectal motility.

Bell and colleagues,[38] using an electromechanical air barostat, studied changes in rectal tone. The tone of a viscus is defined as resistance to stretch of the muscular wall, which in turn is related to its contractile state. An increase in contractility increases resistance to stretch and thereby tone. The air barostat used by Bell measured changes in tone indirectly by measuring changes in the volume of the air within a bag placed inside the rectum. The device maintains a constant intraluminal pressure by injecting or withdrawing air from the bag (Fig. 1-24). The lag time for injecting or withdrawing

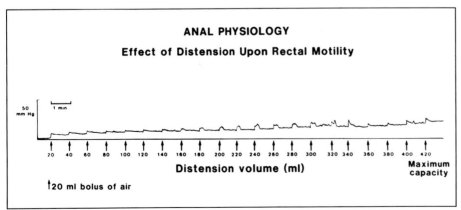

Figure 1-23. Effect of distention of an intrarectal balloon upon rectal pressure. Rectal accommodation assures little rise in intraluminal pressure even at 420 ml of inflation. (*From:* Pemberton JH. Anatomy and physiology of the anus and rectum. In: Condon RE, ed. *Shackelford's Surgery of the Alimentary Tract.* 3rd ed. Philadelphia: WB Saunders; 1991:vol 4.)

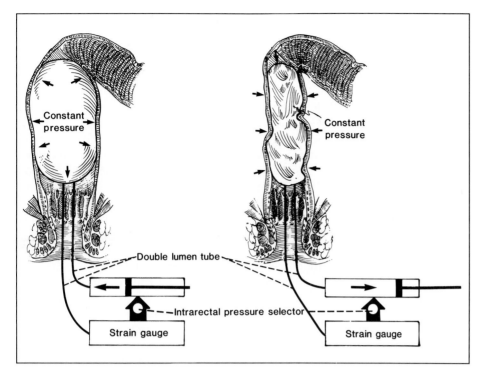

Figure 1-24. Barostat balloon within the rectum. The device acts to maintain a constant preselected pressure within the intrarectal bag. When the rectum relaxes, the system injects air (*left*); when it contracts, air is aspirated (*right*). (*From:* Bell AM, Pemberton JH, Hanson RB, Zinsmeister AR. Variations in muscle tone of the human rectum: recordings with an electromechanical barostat. *Am J Physiol.* 1991;260:G17–G25.)

air was 5 ms and the flow of air was 22 ml/s. The bag could be filled with air to a volume of about 900 ml before any intrabag pressure was recorded; hence, within its operating range of less than 200 ml, the bag was infinitely compliant. A conventional perfused manometric recording catheter was placed alongside the barostat bag in the rectum.

We used Bell's device to study fourteen healthy volunteers. During fasting, two patterns of volume changes (volume waves; decreases in intraluminal vol-ume equals an increase in rectal tone) occurred; "rapid" volume waves (RVWs) and slow volume waves (SVWs). During fasting, 20 ± 10 RVWs and 2 ± 0.8 SVWs occurred.

After eating, there was no change in the frequency of RVWs. However, there was a prompt and significant reduction in bag volume (increase in rectal tone) in response to the meal (Fig. 1-25). Neostigmine (a smooth muscle stimulant) increased the frequency of RVWs and caused a prompt and steady reduction in the

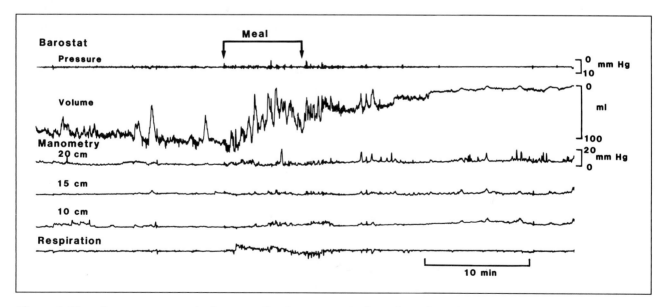

Figure 1-25. Barostat pressure (volume, perfused manometric channels, and respiratory recording) in a healthy control subject before, during, and after feeding. The volume trace shows a progressive reduction in barostat bag volume in response to a meal. This begins at the onset of the meal and continued until bag volume was 0. (*From:* Bell AM, Pemberton JH, Hanson RB, Zinsmeister AR. Variations in muscle tone of the human rectum: recordings with an electromechanical barostat. *Am J Physiol.* 1991;260:G17–G25.)

mean bag volume (SVWs). Glucagon (a relaxor of smooth muscle) given after neostigmine, terminated the neostigmine-induced RVW activity and caused an increase in bag volume (decrease of rectal wall tone).

We concluded that rectal motor activity is complex and not adequately characterized by conventional intraluminal manometric recording techniques alone. A meal increases rectal tone. Increased tone may act to make the rectum more sensitive to distention, inducing the RASIR promptly and thus acting to clear the rectum to make space for the next fecal bolus. This increased tone after eating renders the rectum *less* compliant; rectal compliance therefore is a *variable* phenomenon, characterized by slow volume changes that reflect changes in muscular tone, which in turn are controlled by extrarectal cofactors. Clearly, these changes cannot be quantitated by manometric studies. Disturbed function, which often correlates poorly with anorectal manometry, may instead be mediated by changes in the contractile state (tone of the rectal wall).

In other studies, the barostat recorded changes in rectal tone while a Dent sleeve was placed in the anal canal to determine changes in anal canal pressure in response to acute stress (cold, pain, and dichotomous listening tasks).[39] We found that stress increased rectal tone, but had no effect on the anal canal pressures.

Motility of the Rectum and Anal Canal

Rectum

Resting intraluminal rectal pressure approximates 5 mm Hg. Infrequent, small-amplitude contractions have been recorded in the rectum; these do not change in frequency or amplitude as intraluminal volume increases. The mean ($\pm$ SEM) amplitude of these waves is about 10 ± 3 cm H_2O, which is very low. There are three types of rectal contractile activity: (1) simple contractions at a frequency of 5 to 10 cycles/min, (2) contractions (about 3 cycles/min) but with amplitudes of up to 100 cm H_2O, and (3) slow contractions of high amplitude, which appeared to propagate.[40]

In an interesting study by Kumar and colleagues,[41] prolonged (19 h) recordings of rectal motility using microtransducers were performed in healthy volunteers during fasting, after feeding, and during sleep. Three types of motor activity were seen: isolated prolonged contractions (10–20 s duration) while awake; 1-minute to 2-minute clustered contractions (frequency 5–6/min, periodicity 20–30 min) after feeding; and powerful phasic contractions (frequency 2 min, duration 3–10 s, periodicity 90 min) termed *rectal motor complexes* (RMCs). These complexes were more regular and had a shorter periodicity during sleep.

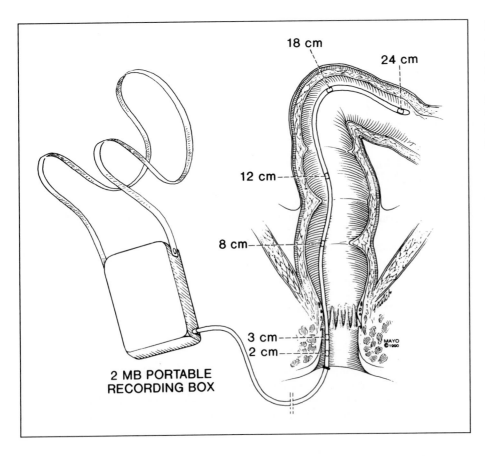

18 cm

24 cm

12 cm

8 cm

3 cm
2 cm

2 MB PORTABLE
RECORDING BOX

Figure 1-26. Recording device and catheter used to study sigmoid, rectal, and anal canal motility. The sensors at 24 and 18 cm were positioned in the sigmoid, those at 12 and 8 cm were in the rectum, and those at 3 and 2 cm were in the anal canal.

Recent studies support and extend these observations. We recently reported on a modification of Kumar's technique which recorded motility from the sigmoid colon, rectum, and anal canal *concurrently* using a six-channel microtransducer and a 2-megabite digital recorder (Fig. 1-26).[26,42,43] Sigmoid and rectal motility index (MI = mmtg/h 10^2) was calculated. We observed that feeding increased sigmoid and rectal motor activity significantly as compared with that recorded during fasting (Fig. 1-26). Moreover, awakening increased motor activity significantly as compared with sleep (Fig. 1-27). Motor complexes were present in the nor-mal rectum; we confirmed that RMCs were particularly evident during sleep (Fig. 1-27). A mean of 16 RMCs was identified in each subject; 35 percent of the RMCs appeared to propagate aborally whereas 11 percent propagated orally.

Anal Canal

The anal canal exhibits a unique motility pattern: small oscillations of pressure occur at frequencies of about 15 cycles/min with an amplitude of about 10 cm H_2O superimposed on the resting tone (Fig. 1-28). An ultra-slow wave also can be recorded in 40 percent of normal subjects,[44] the mean duration of which is 33 seconds with an amplitude of 30 to 100 cm H_2O.[19] There is also a slow wave gradient in the anal canal; the frequency of the slow wave is highest distally.[19,45,46] This would tend to propel the content back into the rectum, keeping the canal itself clean and assuring continence.

The effect of pharmocologic agents on anal sphincter motility varies. Lomotil® has no effect on anal canal pressures, phenoxybenzamine (an alpha blocker) relaxes the internal anal sphincter, Loperamide® increases the maximum basal anal canal pressure, and glucagon decreases resting pressure.

Characteristics of Rectal Filling and Emptying

Instilling large volumes of material (saline, artificial stool) into the rectum causes progressive accommodation to increasing volume. The ability of the rectal wall to relax leads to a decrease in intrarectal pressure as the rectum fills.[47] This response, in turn, maintains the rectal pressure lower than anal canal pressure. Approximately 10 to 15 seconds after rectal distention has occurred, the rapid decrease in pressure reverses and there is a transient increase in anal canal tone.[48] This may explain why infused material does not remain solely in the rectum; recent studies have shown that about one third promptly refluxes into the sigmoid colon and remains there. When evacuation occurs, the sigmoid colon empties first into the rectum and *then* the rectal volume is evacuated (Fig. 1-29). These results suggest that the sigmoid colon in health plays an active role in maintaining overall enteric continence. Moreover, these findings support the clinical impression that in healthy people, the rectum is sometimes found to be empty of feces;[49] only just prior to evacuation does the rectum fill. Ihre has shown that perception of content presence occurs at about 25 percent of maximal tolerable rectal volume.[50] Therefore, hour-to-hour continence may also depend to some extent upon the more proximal bowel; only when sufficiently filled would the sigmoid and more proximal colon empty a portion of their contents into the rectum and the events described above

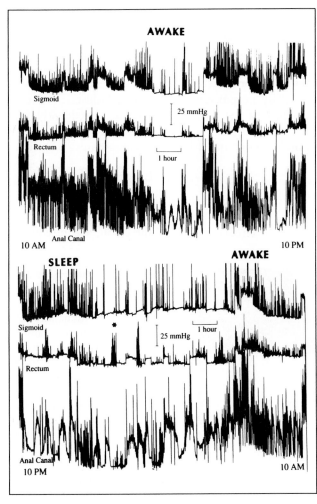

Figure 1-27. (*Top*) A 12-hour daytime recording of contractions of the sigmoid colon, rectum, and anal canal. (*Bottom*) A 12-hour nighttime recording of contractions from the sigmoid colon, rectum, and anal canal. There is a readily apparent *decrease* of activity in the sigmoid and rectum and an easily identifiable cyclical pattern of relaxation of the anal canal during sleep as compared with the awake recordings. Note that the rectal motor complexes (RMCs) (one is denoted by an asterisk) are most readily evident at night. Upon awakening, contractile activity increased across all channels.

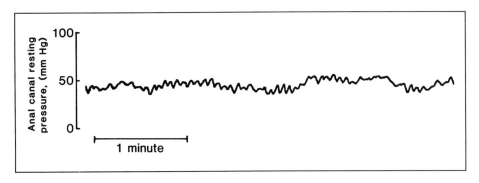

Figure 1-28. Single-channel recording from the anal canal. Superimposed on the resting pressure are small oscillations of pressure which occur at a frequency of 15 per minute with an amplitude of about 10 mm Hg. (*From:* Pemberton JH. Anatomy and physiology of the anus and rectum. In: Condon RE, ed. *Shackelford's Surgery of the Alimentary Tract.* 3rd ed. Philadelphia: WB Saunders; 1991:vol 4.)

occur. This observation is supported by scintigraphic studies which have determined that the transverse colon plays a role in storage of content.[51] Moreover, the interplay between the more proximal bowel and the rectum was investigated by Kellow and associates[52]: upon distention of the rectum with a balloon, duodenal–cecal transit time was increased both during fasting and after feeding, as compared with control values. Gastric emptying was also delayed by rectal distention in studies performed by Youle and Read.[53]

Radiographically Detectable Movements

Retrograde Propulsion. These contractions originate in the transverse colon, migrate toward the cecum, and may retard the aboral progression of feces.

Segmental, Nonpropulsive Motility. These movements are composed of retrograde and anterograde contractions in a single colon segment and are not responsible for aboral progression. Transit through the distal colon is faster than through the right colon.

Mass Movements. These movements are characterized by propulsion of large fecal boluses over long segments of the colon. They occur infrequently and have also been seen during defecation; the entire rectum, sigmoid colon, and descending colon empty together.

Electrical Events

Two types of activity have been observed in the human colon—slow waves and spike bursts. *Slow waves* originate in the circular muscle of the colon, are infrequent,

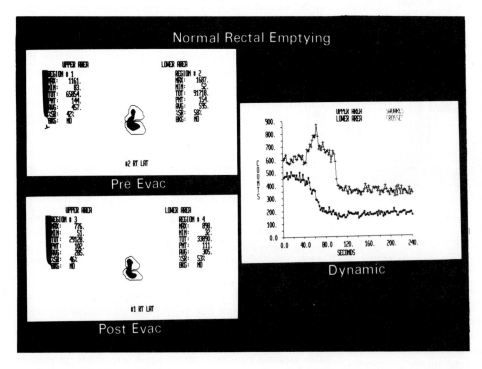

Figure 1-29. Patterns of rectal filling and emptying recorded from a healthy volunteer. Evacuation dynamics are obtained by gamma camera imaging of ^{99m}Tc-labeled artificial stool. (*Upper left*) The infused artificial stool distributes into the sigmoid colon and rectum. (*Lower left*) A postevacuation scan. (*Right*) A dynamic record of evacuation from the sigmoid colon (*boxes*) and rectum (*triangles*). Note that the sigmoid colon empties into the rectum first (counts decrease in the sigmoid and rise in the rectum), and then both evacuate together. The mean percentage of evacuation among healthy volunteers is approximately 75 to 85%. (*From:* Pemberton JH. Anatomy and physiology of the anus and rectum. In: Condon RE, ed. *Shackelford's Surgery of the Alimentary Tract.* 3rd ed. Philadelphia: WB Saunders; 1991:vol 4.)

and may produce contractions. The longitudinal muscle exhibits a distinctly different slow wave frequency than does the circular muscle, but activity of both is linked.[54] These properties of the colonic slow wave differ from the slow wave of the stomach and small bowel. In general, the slow wave frequency is 11 cycles/min proximally, decreasing to about 6 cycles/min in the sigmoid. The site of a possible colonic pacemaker is in the transverse colon.[55] Torsoli and colleagues[56] found that the transverse and left colon generate pressure waves at greater frequencies than does the right colon; the higher the frequency of contraction, the greater the impediment to aboral flow. The rectal slow wave frequency is about 20 cycles/min; a gradient is thus observed between colon and rectum.

The canine colon demonstrates cyclical activity, as does the small intestine, but this is incompletely understood.[57] The ascending and transverse colon store solid material. Proano and coworkers recently showed that the ascending colon has variable patterns of emptying into the more distal colon; constant, intermittent, or mass movement.[58] They also found that the descending colon behaved like a conduit and that the sigmoid colon acted as a terminal reservoir.[58]

Interestingly, recordings of intraluminal pressure from the "rectosigmoid" have shown an area of elevated pressure[59] and high frequency of phasic contraction.[60] Such specialized motility could help prevent aboral progression of stool from the sigmoid colon to the rectum. Although it is doubtful that a true sphincter (O'Beirne) exists at the rectosigmoid junction, storage in the sigmoid colon is probably facilitated by the firm nature of the stools.[61]

Spike bursts are associated with contractions. Two patterns of colonic spike burst activity have been recorded in humans: short bursts of a few seconds and long bursts that last approximately 30 seconds. Reliable correlations between these electrical events and the organized movements well recognized radiographically are difficult to make.

Coordination of Rectal and Anal Canal Motility

In what manner anal canal motility might be related to contractile events occurring proximally in the rectum and sigmoid colon, and how this is related to fecal continence, are unknown. Our aim in recent experiments was therefore to determine whether anal canal pressures and motility were associated with contractile activity of the more proximal bowel.[26,43] A fully ambulatory system for 24-hour motility reading was used. A microtransducer catheter was placed so that sensors were located 2, 3, 8, 10, 12, and 24 cm from the anal verge. Mean anal canal pressure was calculated and rectal motor complexes (RMCs) were characterized.

During sleep, mean resting anal canal pressures were 72 ± 12 (SD) mm Hg. Canal pressure showed cyclic relaxations (periodicity 95 ± 11 min), during which the mean pressure trough was 15 ± 4 mm Hg. During sleep, a mean of 6 RMCs was identified (range 3–9). Importantly, an RMC was *always* accompanied by rapid return of anal canal pressure from trough to basal values *and* increased contractile activity (Fig. 1-30) such that mean anal canal pressure was always greater than anal rectal pressure (Figs. 1-30 and 1-31).

We concluded that motor activity of the rectum was associated with changes in pressure and contractile activity of the anal canal; the onset of rectal contractions was accompanied invariably by increased resting pressure and contractile activity of the anal canal so that a rectal anal canal pressure gradient, and in turn fecal continence, was preserved.

Stool Volume and Consistency

Absorption of water primarily by the proximal colon reduces the 1500 ml of small bowel content emptied into the cecum each day to about 150 ml.[62] This volume is passed with a frequency of three stools per day to three stools per week. The consistency of the stools is usually firm.

If the consistency or volume of the stool changes suddenly, the continence mechanism is stressed. For example, if small pellets of hard stool are introduced slowly into the rectum, rectal distention and, in turn,

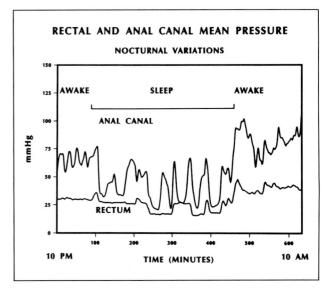

Figure 1-30. Nocturnal variations in rectal and anal canal mean pressure in a healthy subject. Cyclical decreases in pressure in the anal canal occurred several times with lowest pressures approximating 15 to 20 mm Hg. However, a rectal:anal canal pressure differential was always present.

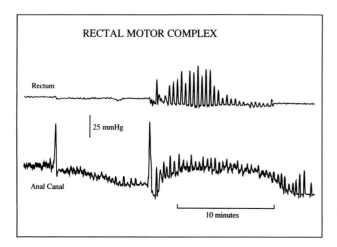

RECTAL MOTOR COMPLEX

Rectum

25 mmHg

Anal Canal

10 minutes

Figure 1-31. Recording from one rectal (*above*) and one anal canal transducer (*below*) in a control subject. The rectal transducer recorded a typical rectal motor complex (RMC). Note that the anal canal began to contract *before* the start of the RMC. Throughout the RMC, the anal canal maintained an increased basal pressure and contractile activity was likewise increased. As the RMC disappeared, contractile activity in the anal canal decreased, as did the baseline pressure.

perception of the presence of enteric content likely does not occur. Indeed, Bannister and colleagues[63] showed that volunteers defecated large deformable stools more readily and with less strain than small hard pellets. Ambroze[64] demonstrated that semisolid stool is more completely evacuated than either solid or liquid stool.

Conversely, liquid stool presented to the rectum suddenly in large volumes quickly overcomes the continence mechanism, causing incontinence even in healthy individuals.

The influence of stool volume and consistency in maintaining continence is great; by simply changing the character of the stool in some incontinent patients with low resting and squeeze pressures and an obtuse anorectal angle, *continence can be restored.*

Sequence of Defecation

Figure 1-32 illustrates a possible model of defecation. Importantly, defecation may occur in one of two ways—either with or without straining. The arbiter of which path is taken is probably stool consistency, as the pattern of defecation changes from day to day in the same individual.

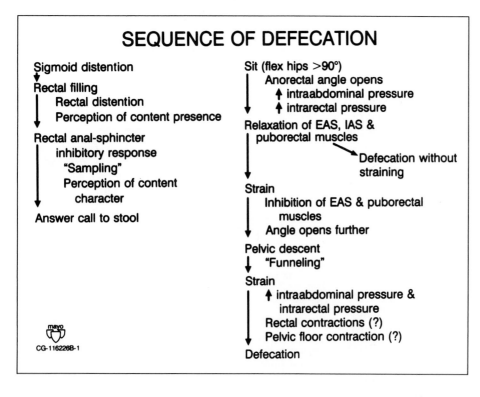

SEQUENCE OF DEFECATION

Sigmoid distention
Rectal filling
    Rectal distention
    Perception of content presence
Rectal anal-sphincter
    inhibitory response
    "Sampling"
    Perception of content
        character
Answer call to stool

Sit (flex hips >90°)
    Anorectal angle opens
        ↑ intraabdominal pressure
        ↑ intrarectal pressure
Relaxation of EAS, IAS &
    puborectal muscles
                        Defecation without
                            straining
Strain
    Inhibition of EAS & puborectal
        muscles
    Angle opens further
Pelvic descent
    "Funneling"
Strain
    ↑ intraabdominal pressure &
        intrarectal pressure
    Rectal contractions (?)
    Pelvic floor contraction (?)
Defecation

mayo

CG-116226B-1

Figure 1-32. A hypothesis proposed for the sequence of normal defecation. (*From:* Pemberton JH: Anatomy and physiology of the anus and rectum. In: Condon RE, ed. *Shackelford's Surgery of the Alimentary Tract.* 3rd ed. Philadelphia: WB Saunders;1991:vol 4.)

References

1. Phillips SF, Edwards DAW. Some aspects of anal continence and defecation. *Gut* 1965;6:396–406.
2. Goligher JC. *Surgery of the Anus, Rectum and Colon.* 5th ed. London: Bailliere Tindall; 1984.
3. Walls EW. Observations of the microscopic anatomy of the human anal canal. *Br J Surg.* 1958;45:504–512.
4. Wood B. Anatomy of the anal sphincters and pelvic floor. In: Henry MM, Swash M, eds. *Coloproctology and the Pelvic Floor: Pathophysiology and Management.* London: Butterworths; 1985:3–21.
5. Wendell-Smith CP. Quoted in Wood BA. Anatomy of the anal sphincters and pelvic floor. In: Henry MM, Swash M, eds. *Coloproctology and the Pelvic Floor: Pathophysiology and Management.* London: Butterworths; 1985.
6. Goldberg SM, Gordon PH, Nivatvongs S. *Essentials of Anorectal Surgery.* Philadelphia: JB Lippincott; 1980.
7. Foster ME, Lancaster JB, Leaper DJ. Leakage of low rectal anastomosis: an anatomic explanation? *Dis Colon Rectum.* 1984;27:157–158.
8. Ayoub SE. Arterial supply to the human rectum. *Acta Anat* (Basel). 1978;100:317–327.
9. Quer EA, Daklin DC, Mayo CW. Retrograde intramural spread of carcinoma of the rectum and rectosigmoid: a microscopic study. *Surg Gynecol Obstet.* 1953;96:24–30.
10. Block IR, Enquist IF. Studies pertaining to local spread of carcinoma of the rectum in females. *Surg Gynecol Obstet.* 1961;112:41–46.
11. Lane RHS, Parks AG. Function of the anal sphincters following colo-anal anastomosis. *Br J Surg.* 1977;64:596–599.
12. Burleigh DE, D'Mello A. Neural and pharmacologic factors affecting motility of the internal anal sphincter. *Gastroenterology.* 1983;84:409–417.
13. Wunderlich M, Swash M. The overlapping innervation of the two sides of the external anal sphincter by the pudendal nerves. *J Neurol Sci.* 1983;59:97–109.
14. Scharli AF, Kiesewetter WB. Defecation and continence: some new concepts. *Dis Colon Rectum.* 1970;13:81–107.
15. Stephens ED, Smith ED. *Ano-rectal Malformation in Children.* Chicago: Year Book Medical Publishers; 1971.
16. Duthie HL, Gairns FN. Sensory nerve-endings and sensation in the anal region of man. *Br J Surg.* 1960;47:585–595.
17. Schuster MM. Motor action of rectum and anal sphincters in continence and defecation. In: Cade CF, Heidel W, eds. *Handbook of Physiology, Section 6: Alimentary Canal.* Washington, DC: American Physiological Society; 1968;vol 4:2121–2140.
18. Nivatvongs S, Stern HS, Fryd DS. The length of the anal canal. *Dis Colon Rectum,* 1981;24:600–601.
19. Kerremans R. Morphological and physiological aspects of anal continence and defecation. Arscia, Ultgavin, Brussels, 1969.
20. Goligher JR, Hughes ESR. Sensibility of the rectum and colon: its role in the mechanism of anal continence. *Lancet.* 1951;1:543–548.
21. McHugh SM, Diamant NE. Anal canal pressure profile: a reappraisal as determined by rapid pullthrough technique. *Gut.* 1987;28:1234–1241.
22. Read NW, Harford WV, Schmulen AC, et al. A clinical study of patients with fecal incontinence and diarrhea. *Gastroenterology.* 1979;76:747–756.
23. Coller JA. Clinical application of anorectal manometry. *Gastroenterol Clin North Am.* 1987;16:17–33.
24. Taylor BM, Beart RW Jr, Phillips SF. Longitudinal and radial variations of pressure in the human anal sphincter. *Gastroenterology.* 1984;86:693–697.
25. Frenckner B, Euler CV. Influence of pudendal block on the function of the anal sphincters. *Gut.* 1975;16:482–489.
26. Ferrara A, Pemberton JH, Hanson RB. Coordination between ileal pouch and anal canal motor activity preserves continence after ileo-anal anastomosis. *Am J Surg.* In press.
27. Floyd WF, Walls EW. Electromyography of the sphincter ani externus in man. *J Physiol.* 1953;122:599–609.
28. Barkel DC, Pemberton JH, Pezim ME, et al. Effect of stool size and consistency on defecation. *Gut.* 1987;28:1246–1250.
29. Bartolo DCC, Roe AM, Locke-Edmunds JC, et al. Flapvalve theory of anorectal continence. *Br J Surg.* 1986;73:1012–1014.
30. Winckler G. Remarques sur la morphologie et l'innervation du muscle releveur de l'anus. *Arch Anat Histol Embryol* (Strasb) 1958;41:77–95.
31. Duthie HL, Bennett RC. The relation of sensation in the anal canal to the functional anal sphincter: a possible factor in anal continence. *Gut* 1963;4:179–182.
32. Miller R, Bartolo DCC, Cervero F, Mortensen NJ. Anorectal temperature sensation: a comparison of normal and incontinent patients. *Br J Surg.* 1987;74:511–515.
33. Ihre T. Studies on anal function in continent and incontinent patients. *Scand J Gastroenterol.* 1974;25(suppl):1–64.

34. Heppell J, Kelly KA, Phillips SF, et al. Physiologic aspects of continence after colectomy, mucosal proctectomy, and endorectal ileo-anal anastomosis. *Ann Surg.* 1982;195:435–443.

35. Beart RW Jr, Dozois RR, Wolff BG, Pemberton JH. Mechanisms of rectal continence: lessons from the ileoanal procedure. *Am J Surg.* 1985;149:31–34.

36. Read MG, Read NW. The role of anorectal sensation in preserving continence. *Gut.* 1982;23:345–347.

37. Azpiroz F, Malagelada JR. Intestinal control of gastric tone. *Am J Physiol.* 1985;249:G501–G509.

38. Bell AM, Pemberton JH, Hanson RB, Zinsmeister AR. Variations in muscle tone of the human rectum: recordings with an electromechanical barostat. *Am J Physiol.* 1991;260:G17–G25.

39. Bell AM, Pemberton JH, Camillerri M, Hanson RB, Zimsmeister AR. The effect of acute stress on rectal tone and anal sphincter pressure. *Gastroenterology.* 1989;96A:38.

40. Whitehead WE, Engel BT, Schuster MM. Irritable bowel syndrome: physiological and psychological differences between diarrhea-predominant and constipation-predominant patients. *Dig Dis Sci.* 1980;25:404–413.

41. Kumar D, Waldron D, Williams NS, Browning C, Hutton MRE, Wingate DL. Prolonged anorectal manometry and external anal sphincter electromyography in ambulant human subjects. *Dig Dis Sci* 1990;35:641–648.

42. Ferrara A, Pemberton JH, Levin KE, Hanson RB. A new ambulatory recording system for sigmoid, rectal, and anal canal motor activity. *Gastroenterology.* 1991;100:A442.

43. Ferrara A, Pemberton JH, Hanson RB. Relationship between anal canal tone and rectal motor activity. *Dis Colon Rectum* 1991;34:P5.

44. Haynes WG, Read NW. Ano-rectal activity in man during rectal infusion of saline: a dynamic assessment of the anal continence mechanism. *J Physiol.* 1982;330:45–56.

45. Hancock BD. Measurement of anal pressure and motility. *Gut.* 1976;17:645–651.

46. Penninckx F, Kerremans R, Beckers J. Pharmacological characteristics of the nonstriated anorectal musculature in cats. *Gut.* 1973;14:393–398.

47. Arhan P, Devoroede G, Persoz B, Verdin FA, Dornic C, Pellerin D. Response of the anal canal to repeated distention of the rectum. *Clin Invest Med.* 1979;2:83–88.

48. Akervall S, Fasth S, Nordgren S, Oresland T, Hulton L. Rectal reservoir and sensory function studied by graded isobasic distension in normal man. *Gut.* 1989;30:496–502.

49. McNeil NI, Rapton DS. Is the rectum usually empty? A quantitative study in subjects with and without diarrhea. *Dis Colon Rectum.* 1981;24:590–599.

50. Ihre T. Studies on anal function in continent and incontinent patients. *Scand J Gastroenterol.* 1974;25:1–64.

51. Moreno-Osset E, Bazzocchi G, et al. Association between postprandial changes in colonic intraluminal pressure and transit. *Gastroenterology.* 1989;96:1265–1273.

52. Kellow JE, Gill RC, Wingate DL. Modulation of human upper gastrointestinal motility by rectal distension. *Gut.* 1987;28:864–868.

53. Toule MS, Read NW. Effect of painless rectal distension on gastrointestinal transit of solid meal. *Dig Dis Sci.* 1984;29:902–906.

54. Huizinga JD, Chow E, Diamant NW, El-Sharkawy TY. Coordination of electrical activities in muscle layers of the pig colon. *Am J Physiol.* 1987;252:G136–G142.

55. Christensen J. Motility of the colon. In: Johnson LR, ed. *Physiology of the Gastrointestinal Tract.* New York: Raven Press; 1987:665–693.

56. Torsoli A, Ramorino ML, Crucioli V. The relationships between anatomy and motor activity of the colon. *Am J Dig Dis.* 1968;13:462–467.

57. Sarna SH, Condon R, Cowles V. Colonic migrating and nonmigrating motor caplets in days. *Am J Physiol.* 1984;246:G355–G360.

58. Proano M, Camilleri M, Phillips SF, Brown MC, Thomforde GM. Transit of solids through the human colon: region qualification in the unprepared bowel. *Am J Physiol.* 1990;258:G856–G862.

59. Hardcastle JD, Mann CV. Study of large bowel peristalsis. *Gut.* 1968;9:512–520.

60. Connell AM. The motility of the pelvic colon: motility in normals and in patients with asymptomatic duodenal ulcers. *Gut.* 1961;2:175–186.

61. Pemberton JH, Phillips SF. Colonic absorption. In: Schrock TR, ed. *Prospectives in Colon and Rectal Surgery.* St. Louis: Quality Medical Publishing 1988;89–103.

62. Phillips SF, Giller J. The contribution of the colon to electrolyte and water conservation in man. *J Lab Clin Med.* 1973;81:733–746.

63. Bannister JJ, Davison P, Timms JM, et al. Effect of stool size and consistency on defecation. *Gut.* 1987;28:1246–1250.

64. Ambroze WL, Pemberton JH, Bell AM, et al. The effect of stool consistency on rectal and neorectal emptying. *Dis Colon Rectum.* 1991;341–347.

CHAPTER 2

PATIENT EVALUATION

Patricia L. Roberts

The surgeon frequently evaluates a wide range of ano-rectal conditions from carcinomas and inflammatory conditions to incontinence, constipation, and disorders of evacuation. The cornerstone of any evaluation of the anorectum is a detailed and thorough history and physical examination. A variety of diagnostic and physiologic tests can further assist the clinician in establishing the diagnosis and treating the problem.

History

The diagnosis of anorectal disease can often be made on the basis of the history and can be confirmed by physical examination.

Bleeding

Rectal bleeding of varying degrees is often the predominant reason the patient consults a physician. The duration, severity, and relation of bleeding to stool is important to elicit. Bright red rectal bleeding that drips into the bowl, streaks the stool, and appears on the toilet tissue is frequently caused by bleeding internal hemorrhoids. Blood on the toilet tissue associated with a painful bowel movement is often a result of an anal fissure or abrasion. Small amounts of blood on the toilet tissue are also seen in patients with pruritus ani. Melena is commonly the result of a more proximal source of bleeding and should be evaluated accordingly. Blood mixed with the stool may indicate a proximal lesion and warrants total colonic evaluation. Blood with mucus is found in patients with inflammatory bowel disease, and carcinoma and should be investigated accordingly. Inges-

tion of certain foods, such as beets, may spuriously give the appearance of blood in the stool.

Pain

Anorectal pain is most commonly caused by an anal fissure, an abscess, or a thrombosed external hemorrhoid. Anal fissure often occurs after passage of a large or constipated stool and is associated with pain that is severe during defecation. An abscess is associated with continuous throbbing pain, and the patient may also complain of a fever and the presence of a tender mass or swelling. Severe pain, especially in the posterior aspect of the anus, in the absence of external signs of a mass or swelling is typical of an abscess in the postanal space. Sudden onset of throbbing pain sometimes associated with straining or heavy lifting is seen in patients with a thrombosed external hemorrhoid. The pain is typically severe for 1 or 2 days and gradually resolves. Sharp rectal pain frequently described by the patient as knifelike or resembling rectal spasm is more consistent with levator muscle spasm or proctalgia fugax. Such pain is often misdiagnosed as hemorrhoidal in origin. Coccygeal pain, often a vexing problem for both patient and clinician, is infrequently a result of anorectal disease. A small number of patients may have a history of trauma, but the cause of such pain is often obscure.

Abdominal pain may also be present. A distended right colon caused by an obstructing rectosigmoid lesion may cause pain in the right lower quadrant.

Mucus or Discharge

Mucus is produced by the goblet cells of the colon. Large villous adenomas may be associated with production of appreciable quantities of mucus. The presence of mucus may also be a prominent complaint of patients with irritable bowel syndrome. The presence of blood associated with mucus is usually the result of inflammatory bowel disease or colorectal carcinoma.

Altered Bowel Habits

Although great variation exists in "normal" bowel habits, any change in the usual pattern should be investigated. The patient should be questioned about change in the number, consistency, and relative ease of passing a stool. A sensation of incomplete evacuation or tenesmus is associated with distal lesions or with colitis. A change in medications, especially antihypertensive medications, can cause a change in bowel habits, particularly constipation. Various dietary habits can also produce a similar change. Operations, such as vagotomy, cholecystectomy, or small bowel resection, can also alter bowel habits.

Incontinence

Anal incontinence is the inability to control the passage of stool or flatus and is a frequent complaint evaluated by the clinician. The degree, duration, and onset of incontinence should be investigated carefully. Patients may have minor degrees of fecal incontinence for liquid stool only or major incontinence (loss of control of a formed stool). The frequency and onset of episodes of incontinence should be ascertained. A history of surgery and potential sphincter injury should be obtained, particularly with reference to anorectal surgery, obstetric injuries, and anal trauma. A history of back surgery, intestinal surgery, inflammatory bowel disease, and radiation therapy should be noted.

Lumps, Masses, or Perianal Swelling

The subjective complaint of a perianal lump or swelling may be the result of a thrombosed external hemorrhoid, abscess, anal wart, prolapsing rectal polyp, hypertrophied anal papilla, or tumor. With adequate inspection and palpation, the diagnosis is relatively easy to establish.

Protrusion or Prolapse

The most common condition that causes protrusion or prolapse of rectal tissue is hemorrhoids. Large anal papillae, polyps, and rectal prolapse can also cause protrusion of various degrees. The sulci between folds in full-thickness rectal prolapse are circumferential, whereas the sulci between prolapsing hemorrhoids are radially oriented.

Pruritus Ani

Pruritus ani is a common symptom associated with a variety of anorectal conditions. Itching is associated with Bowen's disease and Paget's disease. Varying degrees of pruritus may occur in the perianal area in patients with systemic skin conditions, such as psoriasis. Pruritus is associated with healing of an anal condition, such as a healing anal fissure or hemorrhoidectomy incision. Patients with seepage of loose stools may experience pruritus. Pruritus ani is discussed in depth in Chapter 11.

Associated Conditions

A history of anorectal surgery should be elicited. A previous anorectal surgery, such as hemorrhoidectomy or fistulotomy, may alert the clinician to the presence of specific defects of the sphincter contributing to alteration of continence.

Patients with a long-standing history of inflammatory bowel disease, familial adenomatous polyposis; a history of neoplastic polyps; or a history of breast, endometrial, or ovarian carcinoma are at increased risk for the development of colorectal carcinoma. Such patients require total colonic evaluation with either colonoscopy or sigmoidoscopy and air contrast barium enema.

The presence of concomitant medical disease, including cardiac disease, which may necessitate the use of prophylactic antibiotics before diagnostic endoscopic procedures, should be sought. In the most recent recommendations of the American Heart Association by Dajani and associates,[1] gastrointestinal endoscopy with or without biopsy was considered a low-risk procedure for the development of endocarditis. Although prophylaxis is not usually recommended for such procedures, it may be considered for patients with high-risk cardiac conditions, such as the presence of a prosthetic heart valve, a history of bacterial endocarditis, congenital cardiac malformations, rheumatic and acquired valvular dysfunction, hypertrophic cardiomyopathy, and mitral valve prolapse with valvular regurgitation. A standard prophylactic regimen is 1 g ampicillin and 1.5 mg/kg gentamycin given intravenously immediately before the colonoscopy. An alternative is 1.0 g cephalosporin administered intravenously. Numerous alternatives exist.[1] A medication history should be obtained, particularly with reference to ingestion of warfarin (Coumadin) or aspirin, or a history of bleeding tendencies may make biopsy or polypectomy hazardous. If possible, aspirin, aspirin-containing compounds, and anticoagulants should be discontinued 10 to 14 days before planned excision, polypectomy, or rubber band ligation.

Physical Examination

The anticipation of examination of the anorectal area causes apprehension and embarrassment to the patient. Simple explanation and reassurance about planned examinations ensure cooperation of the patient and minimize discomfort. Examination can be performed in the prone jackknife, knee-chest, or left lateral decubitus position (Fig. 2-1). Some patients, particularly older patients or patients with conditions that make kneeling difficult (such as osteoarthritis), may find the prone jackknife position uncomfortable. The knee-chest position is usually uncomfortable for both patient and examiner and should be avoided. When the patient is examined in the left lateral decubitus (Sims') position, it is helpful to position the buttocks slightly over the side of the examination table and the patient's head near the opposite side of the table. Instruments should be within easy reach of the examiner (Fig. 2-2). Keeping such instruments covered and out of view of the patient allays apprehension. Adequate lighting, suction apparatus, and an electrocautery unit are essential (Table 2-1).

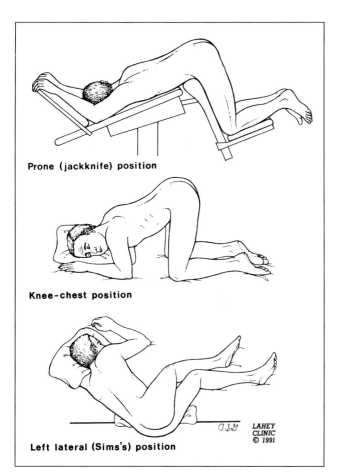

Prone (jackknife) position

Knee-chest position

Left lateral (Sims's) position

LAHEY CLINIC © 1991

Figure 2-1. Positions of patient for anorectal examination. The prone jackknife or left lateral position is preferred for sigmoidoscopy. (By permission of the Lahey Clinic.)

Digital Examination

Inspection

Inspection is a much neglected yet essential part of the digital examination. Examination of the anorectum begins with gentle retraction of the buttocks close to the anal verge. The perianal skin, in addition to the sacrococcygeal area, is examined visually. Superficial fissuring or excoriation may be found in patients with pruritus ani. Rarely, perianal tumors may be encountered. Draining sinuses are seen in patients with fistulas, furuncles, or hidradenitis. An asymmetric area of redness, swelling, and tenderness suggests the presence of an abscess. Anal warts are frequently found in young patients who complain of lumps. The anus is examined for evidence of skin tags, external hemorrhoids, scarring, or prolapsing anal papillae. A patulous anus may be seen in patients with rectal prolapse. Most anal fissures are easily seen with gentle traction applied on the anus. Asking the patient to strain may also identify perineal descent or prolapse.

Palpation

Digital rectal examination is undertaken with a well-lubricated gloved index finger. The patient should not experience pain during the examination. The tone of the anus is evaluated in the resting state, particularly in the evaluation of a patient with incontinence. Asking the patient to squeeze will provide further information with respect to the integrity of the external sphincter and puborectalis muscle. When the resting and squeeze pressures are low, the clinician should search for a palpable sphincteric defect. In men, the prostate is palpated, and in women, the cervix and uterus are felt. The examining finger is swept circumferentially, and a conscious effort is made to appreciate any nodularity, masses, or abnormalities.

Anoscopy

Anoscopy permits evaluation of the distal several centimeters of the anal canal. Several anoscopes are available, including beveled and bivalved types. An advantage of the beveled anoscope is that it does not require repeated insertions, and therefore examination can be performed by rotating the anoscope around the anal canal circumferentially. An anoscope of sufficient length is used to permit evaluation of the entire anal canal. An anoscope can be used before insertion of a rigid proctoscope or flexible sigmoidoscope. Use of an anoscope after insufflation of the distal gastrointestinal tract with air after flexible sigmoidoscopy is not recommended.

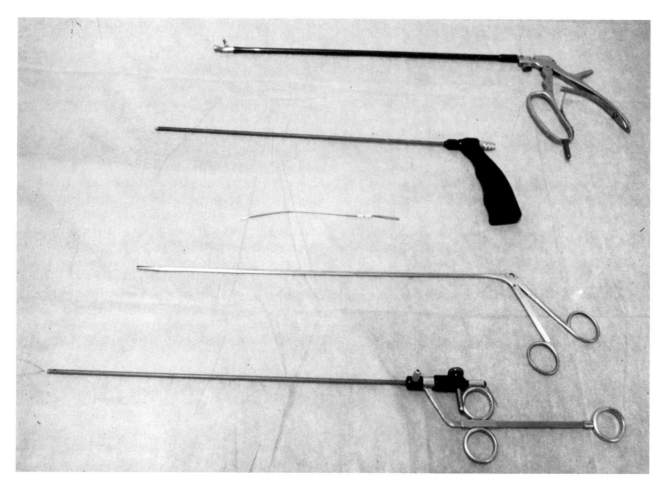

Figure 2-2. Various probes, biopsy forceps, and snares should be accessible. Rectal lesions (polyps or carcinomas) are usually excised or biopsied more readily through a rigid sigmoidoscope.

A lighted anoscope, such as the Hirschmann ano-scope, is ideal for evaluation of the anal canal (Fig. 2-3). A well-lubricated anoscope is introduced slowly to its full length, the obturator is withdrawn, and the instrument is supported with the left hand. The right hand is used for suctioning, use of a probe, obtaining biopsy specimens, or swabbing. The entire circumference of the anal canal is visualized.

The patient is asked to strain, and the degree of protrusion of internal hemorrhoids is assessed and graded (see Chapter 14). In patients with a fistula, a probe can be placed in the external opening and guided to the anal canal to determine the site of the internal opening. Distal rectal tumors can be seen in addition to polyps and hypertrophied anal papillae. Fissures can also be seen; however, it is often impossible to insert an anoscope in a patient with an acute fissure and resultant spasm.

Rigid Sigmoidoscopy

Use of a rigid sigmoidoscope is largely being replaced by the use of the flexible sigmoidoscope. However,

sometimes the rigid type is preferable. Accurate measurement of the distance between the anal verge and a carcinoma is best obtained with the rigid sigmoidoscope and has important therapeutic implications when planning operative strategy, particularly when the carcinoma is at the midrectal level. Excision of rectal polyps is often easily performed with the use a snare through the rigid sigmoidoscope.

Preparation

A single Fleet enema is given before rigid sigmoidoscopy. Premedication is not necessary.

Technique

After examination of the rectum, the lubricated instrument is inserted, the obturator is removed, and the instrument is advanced with the lumen of the bowel continuously in view. A suction wand is helpful to remove retained fluid or stool. Air is insufflated only to aid in visualization of the lumen and should be minimized to avoid discomfort. Although anesthesia is not

Table 2-1 Instruments and Equipment for Anorectal Evaluation

Disposable equipment
  Disinfectants
  Enemas
  Gauze pads
  Gloves
  Gowns
  Lubricants
  Swabs

Diagnostic equipment
  Anoscopes
  Rigid sigmoidoscopes
  Flexible sigmoidoscopes
  Vaginal speculum
  Electrocautery machine
  Suction apparatus

Lighting
  Good room lighting
  Gooseneck lamp or headlight for perianal inspection
  Light source for endoscopes

Other
  Probes
  Specimen containers
  Scalpels
  Biopsy forceps
  Snares

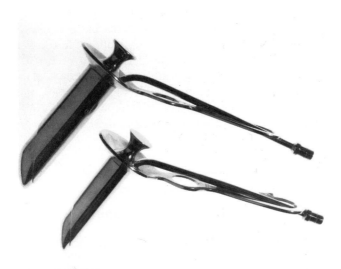

Figure 2-3. Different sized Hirschmann anoscopes with obturators are useful for evaluation of the anal canal and may be inserted before examination with the rigid or flexible sigmoidoscope.

necessary, "verbal anesthesia" is helpful. The patient must be reassured continually about what to expect. The patient is told that a bowel movement will not occur during the examination and that minor amounts of cramping and discomfort are normal.

Although the rigid sigmoidoscope is 25 cm long, insertion to this depth is not always possible, the average depth of insertion being 17 to 20 cm. The goal is to perform an adequate examination without hurting the patient. The depth of insertion is often less in women because of fixation from gynecologic disease or acute angulation.[2,3] At 14 to 16 cm, the rectosigmoid junction is encountered and negotiated. Pathologic findings are noted on intubation although most of the inspection is accomplished on removal of the instrument. Particular attention should be paid to examining behind the valves of Houston, which are frequently blind areas. Vascularity, inflammation, ulceration, and the presence of polyps or tumors are noted. Biopsy of abnormal areas is carried out. The safest place to obtain a specimen for biopsy in the presence of diffuse disease is posteriorly because a swab can be used to tamponade bleeding against the sacrum.

Complications

Complications associated with sigmoidoscopy with the rigid instrument are rare. The incidence of perforation is 0.005 to 0.01 percent of such procedures.[4] By keeping the lumen in view and not advancing the instrument blindly, complications should be avoided. Bleeding is also uncommon after the procedure and is usually self-limited. Persistent bleeding is usually treated by pressure and coagulation. Bacteremia may occur after rigid sigmoidoscopy in up to 9.6 percent of patients.[5] Patients with certain cardiac conditions may need prophylactic antibiotics before such procedures according to the guidelines of the American Heart Association[1] or as described previously.

Flexible Sigmoidoscopy

Flexible sigmoidoscopes are available in short lengths (30–35 cm) and long lengths (60–65 cm). Although the shorter instrument is usually easier to use, the longer sigmoidoscope is preferred by most surgeons because it provides examination of a longer length of bowel. Studies[6-8] have demonstrated that a flexible sigmoidoscope is better tolerated than a rigid sigmoidoscope. In addition, a much larger number of lesions are visualized with use of the flexible instrument.[6-12] Flexible sigmoidoscopy is an office procedure and requires no special anesthesia.

Indications for flexible sigmoidoscopy are listed in Table 2-2.

Table 2-2 Indications for Flexible Sigmoidoscopy

Screening for colorectal carcinoma or polyps

Evaluation of
    Rectal bleeding
    Anorectal complaints
    Sigmoid neoplasm or sigmoid diverticular disease
    Ischemic colitis

Follow-up study for carcinoma of the colon

Reduction of sigmoid volvulus

Preparation

The several preparations used before flexible sigmoidoscopy consist of a single Fleet enema before examination, two Fleet enemas before examination, and a laxative followed by an enema before the examination. Although use of two Fleet enemas before examination is preferred, some studies[6,9,10,13] have found administration of a single enema to be more effective in adequately cleansing the colon before flexible sigmoidoscopy, presumably because the second enema may wash fecal debris from the more proximal colon into the rectosigmoid.

Technique

After rectal examination, the lubricated flexible sigmoidoscope is introduced into the rectum. The instrument is introduced for several centimeters before deflection of the tip of the instrument is attempted. When a "red out" is detected, the tip of the instrument is against the mucosa of the bowel and is withdrawn slowly until the lumen comes into view. The instrument is gently advanced, keeping the lumen in view at all times. Overdistention of the bowel with air should be avoided because this increases the patient's discomfort and accentuates the acute angles and bends of the colon, making intubation more difficult. Several methods have been described[14] for insertion of the flexible sigmoidoscope, including elongation, looping, and accordionization. Intubation by elongation involves insertion of the sigmoidoscope while the lumen is kept in view. Intubation is useful in a sigmoid colon that is straight and is not usually successful in a redundant colon because intubation only stretches the sigmoid colon on its mesenteric attachments. Increasing angulation of the sigmoid prevents further advancement. Intubation by formation of a sigmoid loop, performed by application of counterclockwise torque on the sigmoidoscope, is an effective method of intubating a redundant sigmoid colon. The accordionization method is a successful technique whereby the endoscopist attempts to pull the bowel down onto the instrument versus pushing the instrument through the colon. In all techniques, the endoscopist should attempt to insert the flexible sigmoidoscope as far as possible while minimizing discomfort to the patient.

Lesions are usually looked for and visualized on withdrawal of the instrument. Biopsy of a polyp, a carcinoma, or an abnormal area is possible, but use of the electrocautery is avoided because the risk of an explosion is appreciable in the patient with a minimally prepared colon.

Several additional reasons support deferring biopsy or polypectomy during screening flexible endoscopy. First, many lesions identified in the distal bowel (e.g., polyps or cancers) are associated with synchronous lesions. When a patient requires a subsequent colonoscopy, it makes sense to wait until the bowel is completely prepared. Second, if a complication were to occur during sigmoidoscopy (i.e., perforation or hemorrhage), the patient might require emergency surgery. The patient's management would be complicated if the proximal colon had not been cleared adequately before the examination.

Great care is taken in examination of the distal rectum, a potential blind spot when performing flexible sigmoidoscopy. Retroflexion of the instrument is often helpful. As previously mentioned, an anoscopic examination is necessary for adequate evaluation of the anal canal.

Complications

Flexible sigmoidoscopy is a well-tolerated procedure in which relatively few complications occur. Perforation of the colon is rare. In a series by Marks and associates,[9] 1 perforation occurred in 1012 examinations. In another series[15] of 5000 procedures, no perforations occurred.

Bleeding is rare after flexible sigmoidoscopy. Bacteremia may be caused by flexible sigmoidoscopy, and rare cases of endocarditis have been reported.[16,17] Antibiotic prophylaxis should be used as indicated.[1]

Radiologic Tests

Computed Tomography

The main use of computed tomography (CT) in the evaluation of anorectal disease is in the staging of colorectal carcinoma and in follow-up study of patients with colorectal carcinoma. Computed tomography may also be helpful in defining the extent of retrorectal tumors (Fig. 2-4). In the staging of carcinoma of the rectum, CT may offer information regarding the extent of tumor into the perirectal fat, adjacent organs, and lymph

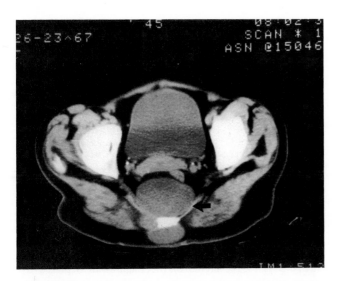

Figure 2-4. Retrorectal cysts are rare lesions. Computed tomography is helpful to define the extent of such lesions with respect to the sacrum and may modify the operative approach. A retrorectal (*arrow*) cyst is shown; at surgery, a benign epidermal cyst was excised through a posterior York-Mason approach.

nodes. Unfortunately, the bony pelvis limits its accuracy, and CT is not reliable in detection of the extent of bowel wall invasion or in detection of tumor involvement in normal-sized lymph nodes. Although initial reports[18-21] of the use of CT for preoperative staging of colorectal carcinoma showed an accuracy of 90 percent or greater, subsequent reports[22-24] have shown the accuracy to be only 48 to 74 percent with an accuracy of the detection of lymph node metastases of 25 to 73 percent.

Recurrence of a pelvic tumor after resection for rectal carcinoma is notoriously difficult to detect. Often, by the time symptoms have developed, the most common symptom being pain in the sacral area, buttock, or perineum, the lesion is advanced. Computed tomography may detect a recurrent pelvic tumor before the patient has symptoms. One difficulty associated with use of CT is in the differentiation between normal postoperative changes and recurrent carcinoma. A "presacral mass" or density is present in most patients who have undergone abdominoperineal resection for carcinoma of the rectum.[25] This "presacral mass" may be caused by the presence of the uterus in the presacral space, an enlarged prostate gland, unopacified bowel loops, or granulation of fibrous tissue.[25] Therefore, when a patient is to undergo follow-up studies by CT after resection for rectal carcinoma, it is important to obtain a baseline CT study of the pelvis within 2 to 4 months after resection and serial CT on an interval basis thereafter. The stable presence of a presacral mass suggests a benign cause. Presacral cysts and tumors are discussed fully in Chapter 20.

Magnetic Resonance Imaging

As is true of CT, magnetic resonance imaging (MRI) is mainly used in the staging of rectal carcinoma and in follow-up study of patients with rectal carcinoma. Magnetic resonance imaging provides good resolution of soft tissues and may therefore be of some theoretical benefit in distinguishing fat from tumor. Before use of MRI, the bowel is cleansed because stool may be difficult to distinguish from tumor. Introduction of air into the rectum by a small catheter is helpful. Air distends the bowel but has no effect on MRI, and air is believed by some examiners[26] to be an ideal contrast agent.

Magnetic resonance imaging can demonstrate perirectal extension of tumor in addition to invasion of adjacent organs. Perirectal extension is better seen with MRI than with CT.[26] Although lymph nodes can be detected by MRI, the study cannot differentiate between normal-sized nodes that are found to contain tumor and enlarged nodes that may show only benign reactive hyperplasia (Fig. 2-5). The overall accuracy of MRI with respect to preoperative staging is 68 to 73 percent.[27,28] Magnetic resonance imaging is often accurate in preoperative staging of advanced tumors (Fig. 2-6). It is precisely these tumors that are often easy to stage on clinical examination. The role of MRI in staging rectal carcinoma remains to be determined. The accuracy of preoperative staging, cost, and whether staging has an

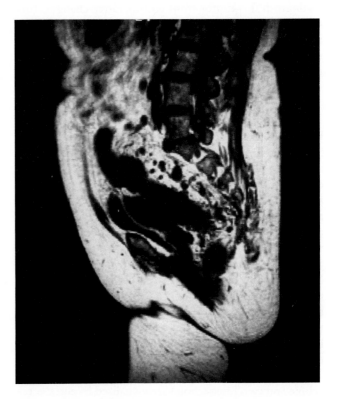

Figure 2-5. Advanced rectal lesion shown on MRI, with extensive pelvic and lymph node involvement.

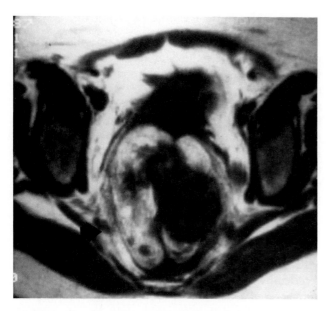

Figure 2-6.   Large rectal tumor with extensive involvement of the pararectal tissues (*arrow*).

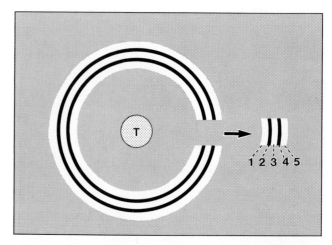

Figure 2-7.   Five layers of the rectal wall depicted by intrarectal ultrasonography include *1*, the interface between the balloon, the water contained in the balloon, and the mucosa (first hyperechoic layer); *2*, the interface between the mucosa and muscularis mucosa (second hypoechoic layer); *3*, submucosa (third hyperechoic layer); *4*, muscularis propria (fourth hypoechoic layer); and *5*, interface between the muscularis propria and perirectal fat or serosa when present (fifth hyperechoic layer). The transducer (T) is shown in the center of the rectal lumen. (By permission of the Lahey Clinic.)

impact on clinical decision making must be taken into account.

In terms of its use in the detection of recurrent colorectal carcinoma, MRI has the same inherent problems as CT. It is difficult to detect recurrent tumor and to distinguish this tumor from postoperative changes. Initial promising reports[29-31] of a difference in the signal intensity of radiation-induced fibrosis compared with recurrent tumor have unfortunately not been conclusive.

Intrarectal Ultrasonography

Intrarectal ultrasonography has been used with increasing frequency to stage distal and midrectal carcinomas, in follow-up study of patients who have undergone operation for rectal carcinoma, and to diagnose complex anorectal abscesses and fistulas in selected patients. The technique involves transrectal introduction of a transducer covered with a latex balloon that is inflated with water. A variety of ultrasonographic scanners are available. The probe, which is mounted to a 5.5- or 7.0-MHz transducer, can be inserted directly into the rectum or introduced through a sigmoidoscope that has been inserted to 20 to 25 cm. Insertion of the probe through a sigmoidoscope may increase the distance from the anal verge that the probe can scan. In women, transvaginal examinations can be performed.

Five distinct layers of the rectal wall (three hyperechoic and two hypoechoic) are visualized by intrarectal ultrasonography (Figs. 2-7 and 2-8). Hildebrandt and

Fiefel[32] suggested that the TNM system by UICC (Union Internationale Contre le Cancer) standards be used for staging tumors seen by intrarectal ultrasonography, with the initial "U" to denote ultrasonic staging.

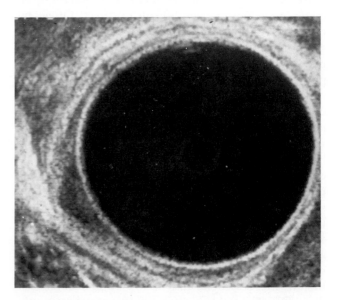

Figure 2-8.   Actual intrarectal ultrasound view showing three hyperechoic layers and two hypoechoic layers.

The accuracy of preoperative staging with use of intrarectal ultrasonography has varied. In a reported series,[33-36] an accuracy of 84 to 93 percent was found with respect to accurate detection of penetration of the bowel wall by tumor. The technique of intrarectal ultrasonography takes time to master; the performance of many examinations is necessary to get past the learning curve. With respect to involved mesorectal lymph nodes, the accuracy of detection is much less (73 to 88%).[33-36] Detection of involved small nodes is difficult as is distinguishing between large inflammatory nodes and nodes involved with tumor (Fig. 2-9).

Intrarectal ultrasonography can also be used for follow-up study of patients treated for carcinoma of the rectum. Beynon[33] reported 85 patients examined by digital examination, rigid sigmoidoscopy, and intrarectal ultrasonography for local recurrence of rectal carcinoma. Of the patients, 22 were found to have a recurrent tumor, and 3 of these 22 patients had a recurrent tumor diagnosed by intrarectal ultrasonography only. Ultrasonography may have a role in the detection of recurrence of extrarectal pelvic carcinoma at an early stage when it cannot be diagnosed by digital examination or any other technology. This recurrent tumor often appears as an echo-poor area in the pelvic tissues adjacent to the anastomosis.

Intrarectal ultrasonography appears to be fairly accurate in determining the degree of local invasiveness of carcinoma of the rectum but is less accurate in determining involvement of the lymph nodes. Intrarectal ultrasonography is a relatively new diagnostic technique, and its role in the staging of rectal carcinoma is still evolving. Its use is discussed further in Chapter 17.

Fistulography

Contrast studies are rarely needed in patients with an anal fistula. In instances of a complex anal fistula, particularly the extrasphincteric or recurrent fistula,[37] injection of the external opening with contrast media is helpful to define both the tract of the fistula and the internal opening (Fig. 2-10). Fistulography is discussed further in Chapter 9.

Physiologic Examination

Anal continence and defecation are complex bodily functions for which no specific test can provide an all-encompassing evaluation. Such tests as anal manometry, defecography, and electromyography are being used with increasing frequency for evaluation of anorectal function, particularly in patients with fecal incontinence, chronic constipation, and pelvic floor disorders. These diagnostic modalities are described fully in Chapter 6.

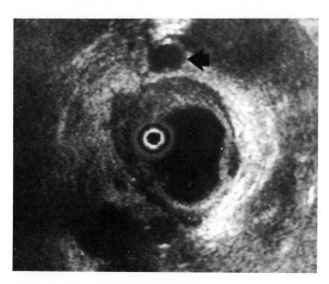

Figure 2-9.   Intrarectal ultrasound of an advanced rectal lesion with lymph node involvement (*arrow*).

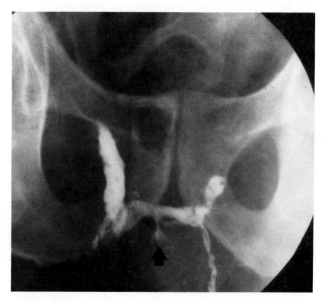

Figure 2-10.   Fistulogram through the external opening shows bilateral horseshoe extension of the fistulous tracts and an internal opening in the posterior midline (*arrow*).

References

1. Dajani AS, Bisno AL, Chung KJ, et al. Prevention of bacterial endocarditis: recommendations by the American Heart Association. *JAMA*. 1990;264: 2919–2922.

2. Salazar M, Jackson RJ. Reasons for incomplete proctoscopy. *Dis Colon Rectum*. 1969;12:19–21.

3. Nicholls RJ, Dubé S. The extent of examination by rigid sigmoidoscopy. *Br J Surg*. 1982;69:438.

4. Shrock TR. Complications of gastointestinal endoscopy. In: Sleisenger MH, Fordtran JS, eds. *Gastrointestinal Disease: Pathophysiology, Diagnosis, Management*. 4th ed. Philadelphia: WB Saunders; 1989;vol 1:216–222.

5. LeFrock JL, Ellis CA, Turchik JB, Weinstein L. Transient bacteremia associated with sigmoidoscopy. *N Engl J Med*. 1973;289:467–469.

6. Bohlman TW, Katon RW, Lipshutz GR, McCool MS, Smith FW, Melnyx CS. Fiberoptic pansigmoidoscopy: an evaluation and comparison with rigid sigmoidoscopy.*Gastroenterology*. 1977;72: 644–649.

7. Leicester RJ, Hawley PR, Pollett WG, Nicholls RJ. Flexible fiberoptic sigmoidoscopy as an outpatient procedure. *Lancet*. 1982;1:34–35.

8. Manier JW. Fiberoptic pansigmoidoscopy: an evaluation of its use in office practice. *Gastrointest Endosc*. 1978;24:119–120.

9. Marks G, Boggs HW, Castro AF, Gathright JB, Ray JE, Salvati E. Sigmoidoscopic examinations with rigid and flexible fiberoptic sigmoidoscopes in the surgeon's office: a comparative prospective study of effectiveness in 1,012 cases. *Dis Colon Rectum*. 1979;22:162–168.

10. Vellacott KD, Hardcastle JD. An evaluation of flexible fibreoptic sigmoidoscopy. *Br Med J*. 1981;283: 1583–1586.

11. Winawer SJ, Leidner SD, Boyl C, Kurtz RC. Comparison of flexible sigmoidoscopy with other diagnostic techniques in the diagnosis of rectocolon neoplasia. *Dig Dis Sci*. 1979;24:277–281.

12. Winnan G, Berci G, Panish J, Talbot TM, Overholt BF, McCallum RW. Superiority of the flexible to the rigid sigmoidoscope in routine proctosigmoidoscopy. *N Engl J Med*. 1980;302:1011–1012.

13. Crespi M, Casale V, Grassi A. Flexible sigmoidoscopy: a potential advance in cancer control. *Gastrointest Endosc*. 1978;24:291–292.

14. Coller JA. Technique of flexible fiberoptic sigmoidoscopy. *Surg Clin North Am*. 1980;60:465–479.

15. Traul DG, Davis CB, Pollack JC, Scudamore HH. Flexible fiberoptic sigmoidoscopy—the Monroe Clinic experience: a prospective study of 5000 examinations. *Dis Colon Rectum*. 1983;26:161–166.

16. Rodriguez W, Levine JS. Enterococcal endocarditis following flexible sigmoidoscopy. *West J Med*. 1984;140:951–953.

17. Rigiliano J, Mahapatra R, Barnhill J, Gutierrez J. Enterococcal endocarditis following sigmoidoscopy and mitral valve prolapse. *Arch Intern Med*. 1984; 144:850–851.

18. Thoeni RF, Moss AA, Schnyder P, Margulis AR. Detection and staging of primary rectal and rectosigmoid cancer by computed tomography. *Radiology*. 1981;141:135–138.

19. van Waes PF, Koehler RP, Feldberg MA. Management of rectal carcinoma: impact of computed tomography. *AJR*. 1983;140:1137–1142.

20. Mayes GB, Zornoza J. Computed tomography of colon carcinoma. *AJR*. 1980;134:43–46.

21. Zaunbauer W, Haertel M, Fuchs WA. Computed tomography in carcinoma of the rectum. *Gastrointest Radiol*. 1981;6:79–84.

22. Thompson WM, Halvorsen RA, Foster WL Jr, Roberts L, Gibbons R. Preoperative and postoperative CT staging of rectosigmoid carcinoma. *AJR*. 1986;146:703–710.

23. Balthazar EJ, Megibow AJ, Hulnick D, Naidich DP. Carcinoma of the colon: detection and preoperative staging by CT. *AJR*. 1988;150:301–306.

24. Freeny PC, Marks WM, Ryan JA, Bolen JW. Colorectal carcinoma evaluation with CT: preoperative staging and detection of postoperative recurrence. *Radiology*. 1986;158:347–353.

25. Kelvin FM, Korobkin M, Heaston DK, Grant JP, Akwari O. The pelvis after surgery for rectal carcinoma: serial CT observations with emphasis on nonneoplastic features. *AJR*. 1983;141:959–964.

26. Butch RJ, Stark DD, Wittenberg J, et al. Staging rectal cancer by MR and CT. *AJR*. 1986;146: 1155–1160.

27. Guinet C, Buy J-N, Sézeur A, et al. Preoperative assessment of the extension of rectal carcinoma: correlation of MR, surgical, and histopathologic findings. *J Comput Assist Tomogr*. 1988;12:209–214.

28. Guinet C, Buy J-N, Ghossain MA, et al. Comparison of magnetic resonance imaging and computed tomography in the preoperative staging of rectal cancer. *Arch Surg*. 1990;125:385–388.

29. Glazer HS, Levitt RG, Lee JK, Emami B, Gronemeyer S, Murphy WA. Differentiation of radiation fibrosis from recurrent pulmonary neoplasms by magnetic resonance imaging. *AJR*. 1984;143;729–730.

30. Glazer HS, Lee JK, Levitt RG, et al. Radiation fibroses: differentiation from recurrent tumor by MR imaging. *Radiology*. 1985;156:721–726.

31. de Lange EE, Fechner RE, Wanebo HJ. Suspected recurrent rectosigmoid carcinoma after abdomino-perineal resection: MR imaging and histopathologic findings. *Radiology*. 1989;170:323–328.

32. Hildebrandt U, Fiefel G. Preoperative staging of rectal cancer by intrarectal ultrasound. *Dis Colon Rectum*. 1985;28:342–346.

33. Beynon J. An evaluation of the role of rectal endo-sonography in rectal cancer. *Ann R Coll Surg Engl*. 1989;71:131–139.

34. Saitoh N, Okui K, Sarashina H, Suzuki M, Arai T, Nunomura M. Evaluation of echographic diagnosis of rectal cancer using intrarectal ultrasonic examination. *Dis Colon Rectum*. 1986;29:234–242.

35. Hildebrandt U, Fiefel G, Schwarz HP, Scherr O. Endorectal ultrasound: instrumentation and clinical aspects. *Int J Colorectal Dis* 1986;1:203–207.

36. Rifkin MD, Wechsler RJ. A comparison of computed tomography and endorectal ultrasound in staging rectal cancer. *Int J Colorectal Dis*. 1986;1:219–223.

37. Parks AG, Gordon PH. Fistula-in-ano: perineal fistula of intra-abdominal or intrapelvic origin simulating fistula-in-ano. Report of seven cases. *Dis Colon Rectum*. 1976;19:500–506.

CHAPTER 3

CONGENITAL AND PEDIATRIC ANORECTAL CONDITIONS

Kevin P. Lally

An understanding of the common pediatric anorectal problems is important for the practicing surgeon. Although some adult conditions such as anal fissure and prolapse occur in children, the presentation and management may be quite different. Patients with the more unusual problems such as Hirschsprung's disease and imperforate anus may have difficulties well into adulthood. Indeed, some patients with Hirschsprung's disease may not present until adulthood. Awareness of these problems assists in appropriate management.

This chapter briefly reviews the embryologic development of the colon and rectum. Some of the more common congenital lesions as well as pediatric anorectal problems are also discussed.

Embryology

The proximal colon including the cecum, appendix, ascending colon, and most of the transverse colon originates from the midgut. It is supplied by the artery to the midgut, the superior mesenteric artery. The hindgut is formed after development of the tail fold and gives rise to the left third of the transverse colon, the descending colon, the sigmoid colon, the rectum, and the upper part of the anal canal.[1] At the end of week 2 of gestation, the hindgut gives off a ventral bud, the allantois, which gives rise to most of the genitourinary system.[2] The arterial supply to most of the hindgut comes from fused branches of the ventral aorta which form the

inferior mesenteric artery. Segmented somatic arteries from the iliac trunk supply the lower rectum. The cloaca is formed by the junction of the hindgut, the tailgut (the blind termination of the hindgut), and the allantois (Fig. 3-1). The cloacal membrane is formed by fusion of ectoderm and endoderm, with no mesoderm in between, at approximately week 5 of gestation. A wedge of mesoderm, the urorectal septum, gradually separates the cloaca into the urogenital sinus anteriorly and the hindgut posteriorly. Before the eighth week of gestation, the urorectal septum fuses with the cloacal membrane to form the urogenital membrane ventrally and the anal membrane caudally. These two separate further, forming the perineal body. The anal membrane lies in the floor of a small depression, the anal pit. This membrane ruptures during the eighth week of gestation. The site of the anal membrane becomes the pectinate line in the newborn.

The external sphincters form around the cloacal area from the mesoderm of the lower sacral and coccygeal myotomes. Should the rectum end blindly, development of this voluntary muscle is unaffected.[3] The smooth muscle of the internal sphincter forms from the hindgut.

Ganglion cells to the alimentary tract originate from the neural crest and migrate to the upper intestine. The cells then follow vagal nerve fibers and migrate the entire length of the bowel. Ganglion cells reach the proximal colon by 7 weeks and the distal rectum by 12 weeks.[4] The point of arrested migration determines the length of the aganglionic segment seen in Hirschsprung's disease.

Around the 10th week of gestation, the midgut extends beyond the abdominal cavity as it elongates from a straight tube. The distal part of the midgut, the cecocolic portion, undergoes a counterclockwise rota-

The opinions expressed herein are those of the author and do not necessarily represent the Department of Defense or the United States Air Force.

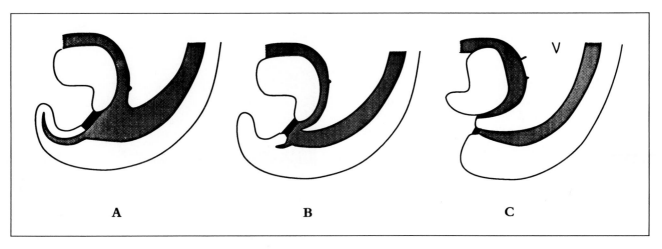

Figure 3-1.   Development of the anus and rectum. (A) The hindgut, tailgut, and allantois form the cloaca. (B) The urorectal septum separates the hindgut posteriorly and the allantois anteriorly. (C) The rectum with the persistent anal membrane has separated from the urogenital structures.

tion around the superior mesenteric artery. As the bowel returns to the abdomen, the cecum and appendix lie near the liver. With further development, the cecum migrates caudally, coming to rest in the iliac fossa. Failure of rotation or fixation can lead to partial or complete volvulus of the midgut.

Congenital Problems

Hirschsprung's Disease

Isolated reports of patients with congenital megacolon appeared in the literature as early as the late 17th century. However, it was not until 1886 at the Berlin Pediatric Congress that Harald Hirschsprung, a Danish pediatrician, described two patients who had died with massively dilated intestines.[5,6] Originally, it was thought that the disorder involved an abnormality in the dilated colon, but in the late 1940s it was recognized that the problem actually lay in the normal-appearing distal bowel. Surgical options for these patients initially were ineffective and included segmental bowel resection, total abdominal colectomy, and lumbar sympathectomy.[7] Swenson and Bill's description of a curative operation in 1948 ushered in a new era in the treatment of Hirschsprung's disease.[8] Although there have been a number of important modifications in the operative approach, the fundamental basis for treatment has not changed.[9]

The incidence of Hirschsprung's disease is approximately 1 in 5000 live births, which is similar for other common pediatric gastrointestinal anomalies. There have been increasing reports of a familial occurrence of

Hirschsprung's disease. The exact mode of inheritance is not known, but Hirschsprung's disease is believed to be a multifactorial sex-linked trait.[10] There is a significantly greater risk to siblings of patients with Hirschsprung's disease; the greatest risk is for family members of patients with total colonic aganglionosis.[11] There is a male predominance of between 2:1 to 5:1 except in cases of total colonic disease, for which the sex ratio is equal.

Hirschsprung's disease is found with greater frequency in patients with Down's syndrome and from 5 to 10 percent of patients with Hirschsprung's disease have Down's syndrome.[12] Other associations include Waardenberg syndrome, a rare syndrome comprised of Hirschsprung's disease and congenital deafness probably reflecting a defect in neural crest migration.[13] Hirschsprung's disease is also occasionally reported in patients with intestinal atresia.[14,15]

Most patients with Hirschsprung's disease present before 1 year of age.[16] Acute intestinal obstruction in the newborn is often seen. Hirschsprung's disease must be considered in any infant who fails to pass meconium during the first 48 hours of life. If not diagnosed in the neonatal period, Hirschsprung's disease can present with acute enterocolitis manifested by diarrhea, fever, and occasionally by overwhelming sepsis. Enterocolitis associated with Hirschsprung's disease is potentially fatal. Patients in whom the diagnosis has been delayed and those with Down's syndrome are at increased risk of developing enterocolitis.[17] The child may have vomiting with foul-smelling bloody stools, sometimes progressing to shock. The role of *Clostridium difficile* in Hirschsprung enterocolitis is controversial.[18,19] Early recognition and appropriate treatment with fluids, antibiotics, and bowel decompression are essential. Patients with unrecognized Hirschsprung's disease will present at a later age with lifelong constipation. These children do not have the soiling and overflow incontinence often seen in children with functional constipation.

Physical findings in the newborn are characterized by a distended, tympanitic abdomen. The older child with Hirschsprung's disease will usually have abdominal distention from retained stool. Palpation reveals large loops of distended colon filled with feces. Rectal examination demonstrates a tight anal sphincter. Importantly, there is usually no stool in the rectal vault and there is often a characteristic explosive passage of stool after removal of the examining finger. Patients with functional constipation will usually have stool palpable on digital examination. The older child with Hirschsprung's disease often has wasted extremities from severe malnutrition, although this presentation is uncommon in developed countries. Occasionally, the disorder will remain undiagnosed until adulthood although all of these individuals will have severe constipation.[20,21]

In the overwhelming majority of patients, a good history and physical examination will exclude other diagnoses. The definitive diagnosis of Hirschsprung's disease is achieved with a rectal biopsy, although other studies can prove helpful. Imaging studies in patients with suspected Hirschsprung's disease include a plain abdominal radiograph and a barium enema. The plain film in the newborn shows several dilated loops of bowel consistent with obstruction. In the older child, large amounts of stool are visible. A barium enema without preparation is often obtained in patients with suspected Hirschsprung's disease. In the newborn, a normal diameter colon may be present and the transition zone may not be readily apparent.[22] After the first few weeks of life, a transition from normal caliber distal bowel to dilated proximal bowel is visible. A lateral view is very helpful in demonstrating this transition zone (Fig. 3-2). A sawtooth appearance of the mucosa may be present in patients with enterocolitis. Finally, delayed passage of the barium beyond 24 to 48 hours should raise a suspicion of Hirschsprung's disease.[23] Other contrast studies such as an upper GI series are of little benefit.

Anorectal manometry can be helpful in evaluation of the patient with constipation. Children with Hirschsprung's disease will not demonstrate relaxation of the internal sphincter with rectal balloon inflation (rectal inhibitory reflex)[24,25] (Chapters 1, 2, and 6). The presence of a relaxation response to balloon inflation effectively excludes Hirschsprung's disease, but the lack of relaxation does not establish the diagnosis. Some children with documented presence of ganglion cells will have manometric findings similar to those of patients with Hirschsprung's disease.[26]

The definitive diagnosis of Hirschsprung's disease requires demonstrating an absence of ganglion cells in

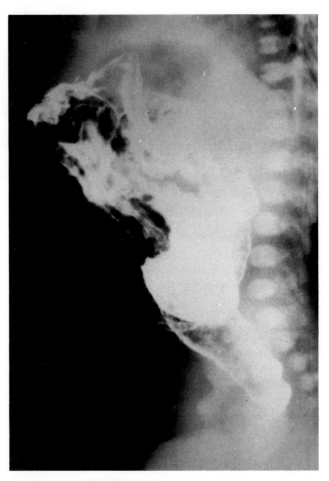

Figure 3-2.   Lateral view of barium enema in patient with Hirschsprung's disease. Note the transition zone from the relatively normal diameter of the distal rectum to the dilated proximal bowel.

the bowel. A normal biopsy of the distal rectum excludes Hirschsprung's disease. In the newborn, biopsy can be easily performed using a suction biopsy kit and should be obtained on any infant in whom Hirschsprung's disease cannot be excluded. The biopsy should be obtained from the posterior rectal wall several centimeters above the dentate line. This procedure is easily performed at the bedside or in the clinic with a very low complication rate.[27] With an experienced pathologist, the diagnosis can be established with the suction biopsy alone and a treatment plan can be initiated. Interpretation of the suction rectal biopsy can occasionally be difficult. In these cases, acetylcholinesterase staining of the specimen can be helpful.[28,29] The increased parasympathetic activity and nerve fibers allows a characteristic dark staining of the biopsy specimen. This technique does require special reagents but can be performed in most laboratories.

In summary, a thorough history and physical examination can exclude most patients with functional constipation. In instances where the diagnosis is not clear, anorectal manometry and barium enema may be helpful. In the small group of patients whose diagnosis is still uncertain, a rectal biopsy should be performed.

Treatment

Treatment of the patient with Hirschsprung's disease depends on the patient's age and presentation. The initial treatment in the newborn is supportive with intravenous fluids and gastric decompression. Patients with enterocolitis should receive broad spectrum antibiotics as well. The goal is to relieve the obstruction. In the newborn, a simple digital rectal exam may be helpful. The patient then receives daily or twice-daily rectal irrigations using normal saline. This is essential in the patient with severe enterocolitis. A colostomy in the newborn is established in conjunction with an intraoperative biopsy of the muscular layer of the bowel which is examined for the presence of ganglion cells. The colostomy is then positioned at the level where the normal bowel begins. The stoma should not be fashioned in the transition zone but rather several centimeters proximally. Use of a leveling colostomy avoids the need for obtaining multiple biopsies at the time of pullthrough and identifies functioning bowel for the pullthrough. Authors have reported success performing a primary pullthrough procedure in the first 3 months of life.[30] The advantage is that a colostomy can be avoided; however, others believe the technical difficulty of performing a pullthrough in a newborn warrants delaying.[31] Although there is no standard age, many surgeons, including the author, will perform the definitive procedure when the child is between 8 and 10 kg or approximately 1 year of age.[32]

In the older patient with newly diagnosed Hirschsprung's disease, dramatic improvement in the patient's nutritional status and well-being can be obtained by daily saline rectal irrigations. The irrigations can be continued for several months or until the patient is clearly well. When the bowel has returned to normal size, a pullthrough procedure can be performed. Should irrigations fail or if the parents and family refuse this treatment, a staged procedure can be performed.

The aim of definitive operation for Hirschsprung's disease is to bring normal intestine to the perineum. This can be accomplished with or without resection of the involved rectum. The rectal resection with pullthrough as described by Swenson and Bill was the first successful operation for Hirschsprung's disease.[8] Soave and Duhamel introduced operations that have also proved reliable although the primary principle is the same.[33,34] The anterior resection used by Rehbein is not widely used in the United States. As mentioned, most

children weigh between 8 and 10 kg before undergoing operative correction of Hirschsprung's disease.

A preoperative bowel preparation should be performed; the author uses a room temperature electrolyte lavage solution at 30 ml/kg per hour via nasogastric tube until the effluent is clear. Cathartics are an effective alternative. Small children should receive intravenous fluids overnight to prevent significant dehydration. If luminal antibiotics are used, neomycin and erythromycin base can be given in three doses the day prior to operation. The author uses a single dose of perioperative intravenous broad spectrum antibiotic. Patients with a diverting colostomy should have several weeks of routine preoperative rectal dilations to assure adequate room for the pullthrough.

The **Swenson procedure** involves a full-thickness dissection of the rectum. The dissection is carried out to within 1.5 cm of the dentate line anteriorly and close to the dentate line posteriorly (Fig. 3-3). At this point, the rectum is everted through the anus. An incision is made in the rectum and the proximal colon segment is delivered transanally. A two-layer anastomosis is performed which is then returned through the anus to the pelvis. A meticulous dissection of the rectum on the rectal wall is an essential component of this procedure to avoid damage to surrounding pelvic structures. Use of the circular stapling instrument has been described but is difficult in the small child. As with the other operations, the decision to perform a proximal colostomy is up to the individual surgeon. A proximal stoma does not decrease the chance of anastomotic leakage, but it can prevent life-threatening pelvic sepsis should a leak occur.

Following the original description of the Swenson procedure, inexperienced surgeons performed wide pelvic dissections that led to a high complication rate. Soave, in 1964, described an endorectal procedure to avoid these complications. The **Soave procedure** involves a dissection of the mucosa and submucosa, leaving a muscular cuff. The proximal pullthrough segment is then brought through the muscular cuff and an anastomosis is made 1 to 2 cm above the dentate line (Fig. 3-4).

A drain is left in the muscular cuff for 1 or 2 days to avoid hematoma formation. The original procedure left the pullthrough segment extending beyond the anus, which was then revised several weeks later. Boley modified this by performing a primary anastomosis at the time of pullthrough.[35]

The **Duhamel procedure** was originally described in 1964 and was later modified by Martin.[36] The procedure involves dissection posterior to the rectum in the relatively avascular space. The pullthrough segment is then anastomosed to the rectum anteriorly. The posterior rectal wall and anterior wall of the pullthrough

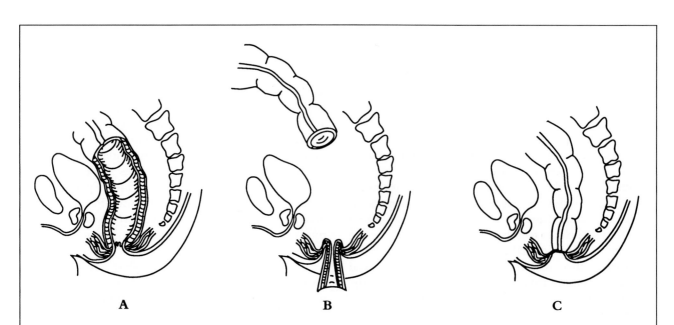

Figure 3-3.   Swenson pullthrough procedure. The entire rectum is dissected (A), the anastomosis is performed outside the anus (B), and then returned into the pelvis (C).

segment are then anastomosed using the linear cutting–stapling device (Fig. 3-5). This operation can be performed quickly and with minimal pelvic dissection. This is advantageous in patients who require a repeat pullthrough following a Soave or Swenson procedure, because a previously undissected plane is available.

Postoperatively, many patients will have problems with intermittent soiling and incontinence. Although this may last for years in a few children, it appears to resolve by adolescence.[37] The patient who had enterocolitis prior to operation is at increased risk for postoperative recurrence. Young patients initially may

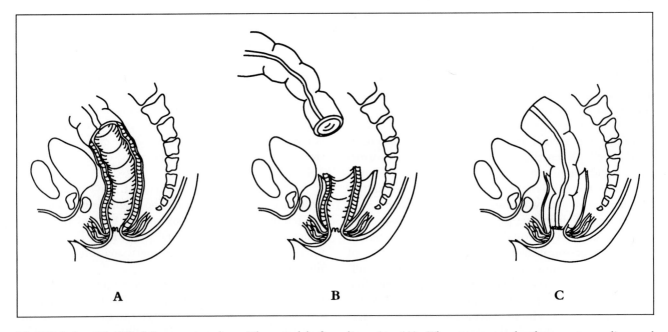

Figure 3-4.   Modified Soave procedure. The rectal before dissection (A). The mucosa and submucosa are dissected leaving a muscular cuff (B). The pullthrough segment is anastomosed just proximal to the dentate line (C).

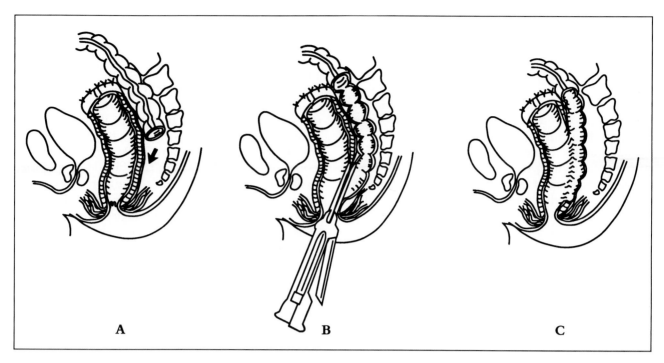

Figure 3-5.   Modified Duhamel procedure. (A) The pullthrough segment is brought to the perineum in the presacral space. (B) and (C) An anastomosis is performed and the septum separating the two segments is divided with the stapling device.

have difficulty with intermittent distention which is probably related to the small amount of residual disease left after operation. This can be managed by rectal irrigations for several months to years and is usually self-limited. In patients with recurrent enterocolitis or obstruction in whom medical management fails a posterior anal myomectomy can be considered.

The longest follow-up available is for patients who have undergone the Swenson procedure.[37,38] The operative mortality is 1% in recent years; 50% of patients have no postoperative complications or enterocolitis after operation. In experienced hands, pelvic nerve injury should not occur and the long-term morbidity rate is low. Follow-up on the Soave and Duhamel procedures shows similar results to the Swenson pull-through.[39,40]

Special Considerations

The patient with Down's syndrome and Hirschsprung's disease may be more difficult to manage. These patients are usually slower to toilet train even if normal intestinal function exists. The addition of a pullthrough can make continence problematic. Indeed, some series exclude patients with Down's syndrome from long-term follow-up reports. Although acceptable continence can be achieved in most patients, a discussion with the family

regarding a pullthrough or permanent colostomy is advisable.[41]

Long-segment Hirschsprung's disease (involvement of the entire colon or more proximal bowel) occurs in 5 to 10 percent of patients with intestinal aganglionosis.[42] The diagnosis may be difficult to establish with barium enema as there is no transition zone in the colon. Although rectal biopsy will confirm angglionosis, at laparotomy, a lack of ganglion cells will be found throughout the colon. Operative management is varied. Kimura and others have described a colon onlay patch to the pullthrough segment which may help increase water absorption.[43] Follow-up of four patients over 5 years shows a range of 1 to 4 bowel movements per day with only one patient having episodes of soiling. Others have used an endorectal pullthrough with an intestinal patch graft or an extended type of Duhamel with reported good results.[44,45]

Ultra-short-segment Hirschsprung's disease may also be difficult to diagnose. The barium enema is often normal, but manometry shows a classic absence of internal sphincter relaxation with balloon inflation. These patients will have ganglion cells if the rectal biopsy is performed too high in the rectum. Appropriate treatment is a transanal rectal myectomy.

If the patient with Hirschsprung's disease is diagnosed early and appropriately managed with decompression and a technically adequate pullthrough, the long-term outlook is excellent.

Imperforate Anus

The earliest attempts at correction of imperforate anus date back to the seventh century. Previously infants succumbed to either uncorrected obstruction or postoperative sepsis. More aggressive approaches to repair were attempted in the late 19th century. In 1897, Matas reviewed the literature to that date and recommended a posterior approach with partial sacral resection.[46] This was often performed in malnourished, critically ill newborns without the availability of ventilatory or intravenous volume support. With advanced neonatal care, the death of an infant with imperforate anus is rarely due to the obstruction but rather to associated anomalies. A recognition of the importance of placing the bowel within the levator ani was an important advance in achieving continence. Despite these advances, and the ability to create an anatomically correct position for the anus, the long-term success rate in patients with high lesions is far from ideal.

The incidence of imperforate anus is about 1 in 5000 births. The covered anus most likely represents failure of the anal membrane to regress. Higher degrees of anorectal agenesis are probably caused by an abnormal development of the urorectal septum, which would also account for the high incidence of rectourinary fistulas.

Although there are many variations, anorectal malformations may be generally classified as high, intermediate, or low, depending on the relation of the rectum to the levator ani (Fig. 3-6).[47] A high lesion is present if the end of the rectum is above the levator ani.

In intermediate lesions it is translevator, and in low lesions the rectum has descended through the levators. A persistent cloaca, where the rectum and the genital, and urinary systems have one external opening, is a separate variant in the female (Fig. 3-7).

Children with imperforate anus have a high incidence of associated congenital anomalies. The incidence of genitourinary anomalies ranges from 5 to 20 percent with low lesions and from 60 to 90 percent with high lesions; therefore the urinary tract should be evaluated in all patients.[48,49] The most common finding is a fistula from the rectum to the urinary tract. This occurs in over 80 percent of males with high imperforate anus. Other genitourinary anomalies include duplicated or ectopic ureters, vesicoureteral reflux, solitary kidney, and renal agenesis. The VACTERL (formerly VATER) association is a constellation of anomalies occurring in greater frequency in patients with imperforate anus. The acronym stands for **v**ertebral defects, **a**nal atresia, **c**ardiac anomalies, **t**racheo**e**sophageal fistula, esophageal atresia **r**enal anomalies, and **l**imb anomalies. VACTERL is not a true syndrome, but one should be aware of the possibility of associated problems in these patients. Recognition of sacral anomalies is important as the child with a high sacral deformity (absent below S-2) has a very high incidence of associated urinary tract anomalies.[50] These children also have a much worse prognosis for a good functional outcome. Additionally, some infants with anorectal anomalies may have spinal cord anomalies such as a tethered cord or lipomeningocele.[51]

The diagnosis of imperforate anus is usually clinically obvious. Occasionally, an imperforate anus with a rectoperineal fistula may be confused with an anterior

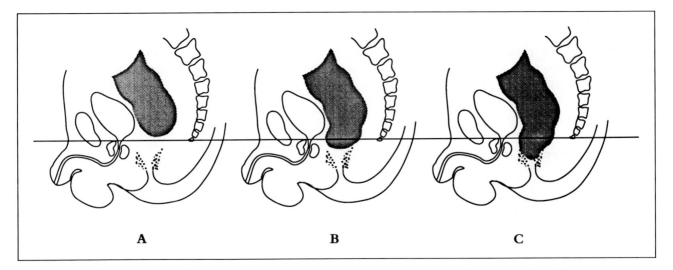

Figure 3-6.   Variants of imperforate anus. (A) The "high" lesion ends above the pubococcygeal line. (B) The "intermediate" lesion ends between the pubococcygeal line and the ischium. (C) The low lesion ends below the ischium.

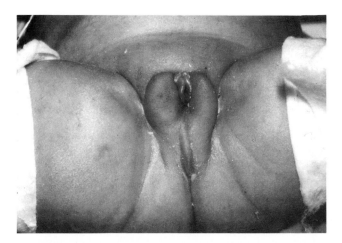

Figure 3-7. Persistent cloaca in a newborn. Note the single perineal opening.

anus. The fistula is usually small, will not admit an examining finger, and lacks sphincter contraction with cutaneous stimulation. It is occasionally difficult to determine by physical examination whether the patient has a high or low lesion. An obvious meconium-filled fistula on the perineum indicates a low lesion (Fig. 3-8). Meconium at the tip of the urethra, however, is due to a rectourinary fistula and is not helpful in determining the extent of the lesion. Fistulae within the vagina usually indicate a higher anomaly.

Diagnostic studies in infants with imperforate anus are helpful in locating the level of the blind ending rectum and in determining associated anomalies. A plain radiograph of the abdomen should be obtained in all infants. This will demonstrate the sacrum and any lower vertebral anomalies. An orogastric tube in the stomach rules out esophageal atresia. The inverted cross table radiograph was described by Wangensteen and

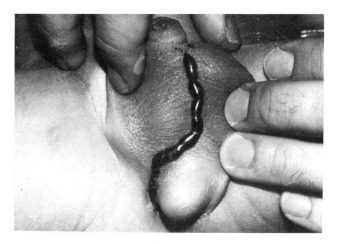

Figure 3-8. "Low" imperforate anus in an infant. The fistula can be followed to the rectum and an anoplasty performed in the neonatal period.

Rice.[52] This is performed by holding the infant inverted for at least 3 minutes and obtaining a radiograph laterally with the knees flexed. A radiopaque marker on the perineal skin is helpful to measure the level of the atresia. The difficulties with this study are several: Infants can desaturate with prolonged inversion, impacted meconium in the distal rectum may give a false reading, and the rectum may move some with crying. Ultrasonography is an extremely useful diagnostic study in infants with anorectal malformations. Ultrasound of the perineum can demonstrate the distance between the meconium-filled distal rectum and a finger on the perineum. This distance can then be easily measured. A pouch to perineal distance of less than 1 cm is indicative of a low lesion and a distance of over 1.5 cm indicates a high lesion.[53] Ultrasonography is also helpful in determining associated urogenital anomalies.

Although not widely used in the neonate, a sacral MRI can be helpful in patients with imperforate anus.[54,55] The MRI demonstrates the location of the blind rectum and the surrounding pelvic musculature as well as any associated spinal lesions. The CT scan is useful to delineate presence of muscle structures which can be helpful prior to definitive operation. Finally, a needle contrast study obtained through the perineum into the blind rectal pouch has been described to help locate the rectum.[56]

Treatment

Initial management of infants with imperforate anus depends upon the location of the blind-ending rectum. Low lesions can be repaired in the neonatal period by either a perineal anoplasty or a fistula transfer operation. If one is unsure of the location of the rectal pouch, the safest course is to perform a diverting colostomy. Most pediatric surgeons will routinely perform a colostomy in the neonate with a high lesion, although neonatal repair of imperforate anus has been described.[57] The primary reason to delay operative repair is to allow the infant time to grow, which facilitates the definitive repair.

The colostomy in infants with imperforate anus can be placed in either the sigmoid or the transverse colon. The author prefers a divided, proximal sigmoid colostomy for several reasons. Occasionally, absorption of urine through a large rectourinary fistula can cause hyperchloremic acidosis.[58] This complication is worsened if a long bowel segment is available for absorption as is found with a transverse colostomy. A divided stoma is preferable to avoid spillover and build-up of material in the blind distal bowel. The stoma, however, should not be placed too distally as this could interfere with achieving adequate length at the subsequent pullthrough. In general, stomas in infants should be sutured with a relatively large number of sutures as there is a risk of prolapse and of bowel extruding around the stoma.

Once the child has reached an acceptable size (6–10 kg), a primary pullthrough is performed. The sacroperineal pullthrough as described by Stephens has been widely used in children with imperforate anus.[59,60] More recently, the posterior sagittal anorectoplasty (PSARP) as originally described by DeVries and Pena and popularized by Pena has gained widespread acceptance.[61,62] With the PSARP, fibers are split in the midsagittal plane. The levators are also divided and the rectal pouch is identified. The pouch is opened and dissected, and the rectourinary fistula closed. The dilated rectum usually requires tapering to fit within the muscles and the muscles are then closed around the bowel. Routine anal dilations are begun several weeks postoperatively and are continued for 6 to 7 months postoperatively until a soft, mature scar is obtained. The colostomy is usually closed a few months after operation.

Outcome

Many factors determine the outcome after correction of imperforate anus, the most important being whether the lesion is high or low and whether or not severe sacral anomalies are present.[63] Absence of the sacrum below S-2, a high lesion, and a flat perineum with no intergluteal fold portend a bad outcome. Less than two thirds of patients with high lesions obtain a "good" result (Table 3-1), although the rate of continence improves significantly with longer follow-up. The results from different studies must be examined carefully, however, because definitions of a good or fair outcome vary. A poor result, defined as frequent accidents or poor control occurs in 5 to 23 percent of patients.[63–66] This group is the most difficult to manage. Bowel training regimens with stimulant cathartics and daily enemas, if necessary, may be helpful. Dietary counseling can also be valuable. Reoperation should be approached cautiously as many patients will have some improvement with time. Reoperation should usually be postponed until the child is of preschool age, unless the initial procedure was clearly inadequate. Pelvic CT

scanning and MRI are extremely valuable adjuncts prior to reoperation.[67] A relatively normal-appearing gluteal crease and perineum should be present. A permanent colostomy may be required in the occasional patient who continues to have socially unacceptable incontinence.

Other Congenital Problems

Small Left Colon Syndrome

The small left colon syndrome (SLCS) is usually seen in infants of diabetic mothers.[68,69] The infant presents with evidence of intestinal obstruction in the first days of life with vomiting and abdominal distention. Plain radiographs of the abdomen reveal dilated loops of bowel. A barium enema reveals a small colon with a change in caliber at the splenic flexure (Fig. 3-9). The differential diagnosis is primarily between SLCS and Hirschsprung's disease.

Factors that suggest to SLCS include maternal diabetes, a normal-sized rectum, and the fact that Hirschsprung's disease usually does not have a splenic flexure transition zone. In an infant where there remains a question as to diagnosis, a suction rectal biopsy can exclude Hirschsprung's disease.

Treatment for SLCS is supportive, since the problem is usually self-limited. A gastrograffin enema may be helpful in infants who have persistent symptoms. The patient can be started on feeding as soon as the obstruction has clinically resolved. There appear to be no long-term sequelae and most authorities believe the SLCS represents a delay in maturation of the descending colon.

Duplications

Duplications of the colon and rectum are rare and can be either cystic or tubular.[70] They are usually found along the mesenteric border of the bowel. Duplications can present as an intestinal obstruction, gastrointestinal bleeding, or an abdominal mass. Rectal duplications

Table 3-1   Outcome Following Repair of High Imperforate Anus

Series	No. Patients	Good, %	Fair, %	Poor, %	Follow-up, yr.
Ditesheim and Templeton[63]	61	72	23	5	2.5–24
Ong and Beasley[64]	37	35	45	20	5–32
Kiesewetter and Chang[65]	78	51	26	23	5–30
Swenson and Donnellan[66]	22	64	23	13	2–6

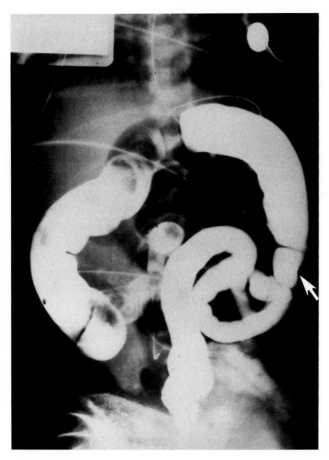

Figure 3-9. Neonatal small left colon syndrome. The transition zone (arrow) is located at the splenic flexure.

often present as a presacral mass. Evaluation includes a contrast study and an ultrasound. The diagnosis is suspected if a cystic mass is found, but the diagnosis is occasionally made at operation.

Duplications should be excised when discovered since they may cause obstruction or continue to enlarge. Complete excision may require segmental colonic resection. The rare total duplication can be opened into the lumen of the bowel if excision is not feasible. Most rectal duplications can be excised with good results.[71]

Sacral Dimples

The congenital sacral dimple or sinus is often confused with a pilonidal sinus tract. The congenital sinus is present at birth and is relatively common. Most are small dimples and need no further attention. These are not pilonidal sinuses (Chapter 13) since they are present at birth. Occasionally a deep sacral sinus may drain or get infected. In these patients, close attention must be paid to the location of the sinus. Sinus tracts over the lower lumbar and upper sacral area are associated with

spinal dysraphism and intraspinal anomalies.[72] Evaluation of the spine should be performed prior to excision to rule out these problems.

Pediatric Anorectal Problems

Children can develop many of the common anorectal problems seen in adults. Hemorrhoidal disease is infrequently seen in children and if so, usually in the older adolescent. Clinical procedures and diagnostic studies are more difficult to perform in children and often require sedation or general anesthesia.

Constipation

Constipation is a very common problem in infants and children and can account for 5 to 10 percent of outpatient visits. The great majority of the time, reassurance, dietary changes, and laxatives are effective treatment for both the patient and the family. Often the possibility of Hirschsprung's disease causes concern, but extensive diagnostic studies are usually not needed; a good history and physical examination will suffice.

Although constipation in the newborn is usually easy to treat, it can be quite distressing for the family. Infants are noted to strain excessively and clearly have difficulty passing stools, although the stool consistency and frequency are normal. Physical findings are also normal, including anal tone. The difficulty in passing stool is thought to represent a delay in maturation of intestinal motility and is self-resolving; glycerin suppositories may be helpful.[73] As the child gets older, constipation can be due to anal fissure, diet, behavior problems, or, rarely, an ectopic anus. Constipation in children may present as watery diarrhea and incontinence due to overflow around impacted stool. Constipation is often seen after surgery for imperforate anus and Hirschsprung's disease. Initial therapy consists of disimpaction, dietary counseling, and stool softeners. Mineral oil, starting at 2ml per kg will be taken by many children. The dose can be doubled, if needed. Once the child has leakage of mineral oil, no benefit is gained with increasing the dose. Other agents such as lactulose and Colace can also be useful.

Bulking agents are also helpful, but many children will not voluntarily take the available products. Increasing the crude fiber in the diet and sprinkling raw bran on the food is useful in providing bulk. The author usually avoids stimulant agents as they are rarely necessary, although they may be helpful in establishing a bowel training regimen in patients after operation for imperforate anus.

If a treatment regimen of bulking agents or laxatives is not curative, further diagnostic studies and evaluation as outlined in Chapter 6 may be warranted. All children with soiling may benefit from a bowel training regimen. Daily enemas effectively assure evacuation. Although not commonly needed, long-term use of enemas may occasionally be beneficial in certain patients.[74] Rectal myomectomy for the patient with recalcitrant constipation has been described but is not widely practiced.[26] Abdominal colectomy is rarely indicated in children and the author has no experience with this procedure for constipation.

Anterior ectopic anus as a cause of constipation is controversial. The true anteriorly displaced anus is common, and many patients will be asymptomatic. Two large series were published in the late 1970s; little additional information has appeared until recently.[75,76] Unfortunately, there has been inadequate long-term follow-up following operation. It is important to distinguish an anterior anus, which is surrounded by sphincter muscles, from a very low imperforate anus with a fistula to the perineum. The latter is clearly best managed by an anoplasty. In the rare patient with an anterior anus and refractory constipation, a cutback may be reasonable.[77]

Rectal Prolapse

Rectal prolapse can be caused by several factors including constipation, increased intraabdominal pressure, protracted diarrhea, cystic fibrosis, anatomic causes, or infections. Alternatively, it can be idiopathic.[78,79] Prolapse must be distinguished from intussusception with a transanal mucosal prolapse. This condition can be distinguished by history and physical examination. A probe or cotton-tipped applicator can be inserted alongside the intussusceptum, whereas in rectal prolapse it cannot be inserted past the dentate line. Rectal prolapse may be the initial presentation of cystic fibrosis, as over 10 percent of patients with prolapse have cystic fibrosis. Conversely, however, most patients with cystic fibrosis do not have prolapse.[78] All children who present with rectal prolapse should be tested for cystic fibrosis.

A search for the underlying cause should be made so that a reasonable treatment plan can be formulated. Rectal prolapse in childhood will usually resolve with resolution of the underlying cause. Stool softeners and bulking agents are the initial treatment. Should this fail, injection of a sclerosing agent such as hypertonic saline or 5% phenol circumferentially injected around the anus is successful in up to 90 percent of cases.[80] Surgical treatment should be undertaken cautiously since the problem is usually self-limited. Numerous operations are recommended for rectal prolapse and include a posterior sagittal approach, transanal mucosal sleeve resec-

tion, posterior repair and suspension, and a modification of the Thiersch technique (Chapter 7).[81-84] The author prefers the transanal sleeve resection, a modified Delorme procedure, as it is relatively simple with low risk.[82]

Fistula In Ano

Perianal abscess and fistula can be seen at any age but is much more common in children under 1 year of age than in older children. Infants may have low grade fever or irritability. Examination reveals an obvious abscess in the perianal area. Perirectal abscess with systemic sepsis is uncommon in children with the exception of immunosuppressed patients or patients with cancer, in whom *Pseudomonas* can cause significant perianal/perineal infection. This can usually be treated with antibiotics alone.[85] Drainage for routine perianal abscess is performed in the clinic and other than routine cleansing, little else is required. Those infants who present with recurrent infection, or in whom a chronic tract is established, should be treated by operative fistulotomy. This is curative and recurrence is rare. Crohn's disease should be considered in older children and adolescents with recurrent fistulae and abscess.

Other Anorectal Problems

Anal fissure can occur in young children and is the most common cause of rectal bleeding in children less than 1 year of age. The child will often complain of pain, but in the young infant, the presenting symptom is usually blood in the stool. Anal fissure should be searched for in the patient with constipation. Pain from defecation can lead to a fear of having bowel movements and consequently to stool retention. This fear may persist even after the fissure has healed. The fissure is usually visible on inspection of the perianal area. If a fissure is present, rectal examination should be avoided as it will alienate the patient and provide little useful information. Treatment includes stool softeners and bulking agents. For the patient with persistent pain or bleeding, a lateral sphincterotomy is indicated.

Unfortunately, perianal condyloma can also be seen at almost any age. The etiology is papilloma virus in most cases. The mode of transmission has been questioned, but most authorities believe that the large majority of cases result from sexual transmission.[86,87] The question of abuse should be raised in every child with perianal condyloma. Social services should be included in the child's care. In the occasional patient with minimal disease, topical therapy can be attempted. This approach, however, can be quite traumatic to the young child, and patients requiring repetitive treatments should be managed in the operating room. A careful examination under anesthesia for vaginal and intrarectal spread should be performed. Fulguration with electrocautery or laser therapy is usually successfully (Chapter 21). Recurrence after fulguration is uncommon.

Some of the other more common adult diseases such as pilonidal disease, hemorrhoids, and inflammatory bowel disease are uncommon in the preadolescent. In the older child, management is the same as in the adult.

Familial polyposis can be present in the young child under surveillance. Timing for colectomy is judgmental, as is the decision to perform an abdominal versus total colectomy.

In general, a conservative approach to most acquired diseases in children is warranted. Many will resolve with time and in those requiring surgery, the rate of success is high and morbidity low for experienced surgeons.

References

1. Hamilton WJ, Mossman HW. *Human Embryology.* Baltimore: Williams & Wilkins; 1976:351–363.
2. Gray SW, Skandalakis JE. *Embryology for Surgeons.* Philadelphia: WB Saunders; 1972:187–216.
3. Smith EI, Gross RE. The external sphincter in cases of imperforate anus: a pathologic study. *Surgery.* 1961;49:807–812.
4. Okamoto E, Ueda T. Embryogenesis of intramural ganglia of the gut and its relation to Hirschsprung's disease. *J Pediatr Surg.* 1967;2:437–443.
5. Hirschsprung H. Stuhltragheit Neugeborener in Folge von Dilatation und Hypertrophie des Colons. *Jahrb Kinderheillkol.* 1887;27:1–7.
6. Roed-Peterson K, Erichsen G. The Danish pediatrician Harald Hirschsprung. *Surg Gynecol Obstet.* 1988;166:181–185.
7. Ladd WE, Gross RE. *Abdominal Surgery of Infancy and Childhood.* Philadelphia: WB Saunders; 1941:141–154.
8. Swenson O, Bill AH. Resection of rectum and rectosigmoid with preservation of the spincter for benign spastic lesions producing megacolon: an experimental study. *Surgery.* 1948;24:212–220.
9. Swenson O. My early experience with Hirschsprung's disease. *J Pediatr Surg.* 1989;24:839–845.
10. Badner JA, Seiber WK, Garver KL, Chakravarti A. A genetic study of Hirschsprung disease. *Am J Hum Genet.* 1990;46:568–580.
11. Carter CO, Evans K, Hickman V. Children of those treated surgically for Hirschsprung's disease. *J Med Genet.* 1981;18:87–90.
12. Polley TZ, Coran AG. Hirschsprung's disease in the newborn. *Pediatr Surg Int.* 1986;1:80–83.
13. Kaplan P, de Chaderevian J-P. Piebaldism-Waardenburg syndrome: histopathologic evidence for a neural crest syndrome. *Am J Med Genet.* 1988;31:679–688.
14. Gauderer MWL, Rothstein FC, Izant RJ Jr. Ileal atresia with long-segment Hirschsprung's disease in a neonate. *J Pediatr Surg.* 1984;19:15–17.
15. Lally KP, Chwals WJ, Weitzman JJ, Black T, Singh S. Hirschsprung's disease: a possible cause of anastomotic failure following repair of intestinal atresia. *J Pediatr Surg.* In press.
16. Swenson O, Sherman JO, Fisher JH. Diagnosis of congenital megacolon: an analysis of 501 patients. *J Pediatr Surg.* 1973;8:587–594.
17. Teitelbaum DH, Qualman SJ, Caniano DA. Hirschsprung's disease. Identification of risk factors for enterocolitis. *Ann Surg.* 1988;207:240–244.
18. Brearly S, Armstrong GR, Nairn R, et al. Pseudomembranous colitis: a lethal complication of Hirschsprung's disease unrelated to antibiotic usage. *J Pediatr Surg.* 1987;22:257–259.
19. Wilson-Storey D, Scobie WG, McGenity KG. Microbiological studies of the enterocolitis of Hirschsprung's disease. *Arch Dis Child.* 1990;65:1338–1339.
20. Luukkonen P, Heikkinen M, Huikuri K, Jarvinen H. Adult Hirschsprung's disease. Clinical features and functional outcome after surgery. *Dis Colon Rectum.* 1990;33:65–69.
21. Wheatley MJ, Wesley JR, Coran AG, Polley TZ Jr. Hirschsprung's disease in adolescents and adults. *Dis Colon Rectum.* 1990;33:622–629.
22. Rosenfield NS, Ablow RC, Markowitz RI, et al. Hirschsprung disease: accuracy of the barium enema examination. *Radiology.* 1984;150:393–400.
23. Berdon WE, Baker DH. The roentgenographic diagnosis of Hirschsprung's disease in infancy. *Am J Radiol.* 1965;93:432–446.
24. Ikawa H, Kim SH, Hendren WH, Donahoe PK. Acetylcholinesterase and manometry in the diagnosis of the constipated child. *Arch Surg.* 1986;121:435–438.
25. Loening-Baucke VA. Anorectal manometry: experience with strain gauge pressure transducers for the diagnosis of Hirschsprung's disease. *J Pediatr Surg.* 1983;18:595–600.
26. Mishalany HG. Seven years' experience with idiopathic unremitting chronic constipation. *J Pediatr Surg.* 1989;24:360–362.

27. Andrassy RJ, Isaacs H, Weitzman JJ. Rectal suction biopsy for the diagnosis of Hirschsprung's disease. *Ann Surg.* 1981;193:419–424.

28. Schofield DE, Devine W, Yunis EJ. Acetylcholinesterase stained suction rectal biopsies in the diagnosis of Hirschsprung's disease. *J Pediatr Gastroenterol Nutr.* 1990;11:221–228.

29. Challa VR, Moran JR, Turner CS, Lyerly AD. Histologic diagnosis of Hirschsprung's disease. The value of concurrent hematoxylin and eosin and cholinesterase staining of rectal biopsies. *Am J Clin Pathol.* 1987;88:324–328.

30. Carcassonne M, Guys JM, Morisson-Lacombe G, Kreitmann B. Management of Hirschsprung's disease: curative surgery before 3 months of age. *J Pediatr Surg.* 1989;24:1032–1034.

31. Foster P, Cowan G, Wrenn EL Jr. Twenty-five year's experience with Hirschsprung's disease. *J Pediatr Surg.* 1990;25:531–534.

32. Sieber WK. Hirschsprung's disease. In: Welch KJ, Randolph JG, Ravitch MM, O'Neil JA Jr, Rowe MI, eds. *Pediatric Surgery.* Chicago: Yearbook Medical Publishers; 1986:995–1016.

33. Soave F. A new surgical technique for treatment of Hirschsprung's disease. *Surgery.* 1964;56:1007–1014.

34. Duhamel B. Retrorectal and transanal pull-through procedure for the treatment of Hirschsprung's disease. *Dis Colon Rectum.* 1964;7:455–460.

35. Boley SJ. New modification of the surgical treatment of Hirschsprung's disease. *Surgery.* 1964;56:1015–1017.

36. Martin LW, Caudill DR. A method for elimination of the blind rectal pouch in the Duhamel operation for Hirschsprung's disease. *Surgery.* 1967;62:951–953.

37. Weitzman JJ. Management of Hirschsprung's disease with the Swenson procedure with emphasis on long-term follow-up. *Pediatr Surg Int.* 1986;1:100–104.

38. Sherman JO, Snyder ME, Weitzman JJ, et al. A 40-year multinational study of 880 Swenson procedures. *J Pediatr Surg.* 1989;24:833–838.

39. Polley TZ, Coran AG, Wesley JR. A ten-year experience with ninety-two cases of Hirschsprung's disease. Including sixty-seven consecutive endorectal pull-through procedures. *Ann Surg.* 1985;202:349–355.

40. Canty TG. Modified Duhamel procedure for treatment of Hirschsprung's disease in infancy and childhood: review of 41 consecutive cases. *J Pediatr Surg.* 1982;17:773–778.

41. Caniano DA, Teitelbaum DH, Qualman SJ. Management of Hirschsprung's disease in children with Trisomy 21. *Am J Surg.* 1990;159:402–404.

42. Ikeda K, Goto S. Diagnosis and treatment of Hirschsprung's disease in Japan. An analysis of 1628 patients. *Ann Surg.* 1984;199:400–405.

43. Kimura KM, Nishijima E, Muraji T, Tsugawa C, Matsutmo Y. Extensive aganglionosis: further experience with the colonic patch graft procedure and long-term results. *J Pediatr Surg.* 1988;23:52–56.

44. Kottmeier FK. Jongco B, Velceck FT, Friedman A, Klotz DH. Absorptive function of the aganglionic ileum. *J Pediatr Surg.* 1981;16:275–278.

45. Martin LW. Surgical management of total colonic aganglionosis. *Ann Surg.* 1972;176:343–346.

46. Matas R. The surgical treatment of congenital anorectal imperforation considered in the light of modern operative procedures. *Trans Am Surg Assoc.* 1897;15:453–553.

47. Stephens FD, Smith ED. Classification, identification and assessment of surgical treatment of anorectal anomalies. *Pediatr Surg Int.* 1986;1:200–205.

48. McLorie GA, Sheldon CA, Fleisher M, Churchill BM. The genitourinary system in patients with imperforate anus. *J Pediatr Surg.* 1987;22:1100–1104.

49. Hoekstra WJ, Scholtmeijer RJ, Molenaar JC, Schreeve RH, Schroeder FH. Urogenital tract abnormalities associated with congenital anorectal anomalies. *J Urol.* 1983;130:962–963.

50. Parrott TS. Urologic implications of anorectal malformations. *Urol Clin North Am.* 1985;12:13–21.

51. Tunell WP, Austin JC, Barnes PD, Reynolds A. Neuroradiologic evaluation of sacral abnormalities in imperforate anus complex. *J Pediatr Surg.* 1987;22:58–61.

52. Wangensteen OH, Rice CO. Imperforate anus. *Ann Surg.* 1930;92:77–85.

53. Donaldson JS, Black CT, Reynolds M, Sherman JO, Shkolnik A. Ultrasound of the distal pouch in infants with imperforate anus. *J Pediatr Surg.* 1989;24:465–468.

54. Mezzacappa PM, Price AP, Haller JO, Kassner EG, Hansbrough F. MR and CT demonstration of levator sling in congenital colorectal anomalies. *J Comput Assist Tomogr.* 1987;11:273–275.

55. Pringle KC, Sato Y, Soper RT. Magnetic resonance imaging as an adjunct to planning an anorectal pull-through. *J Pediatr Surg.* 1987;22:571–574.

56. Stevenson RJ, Sheldon C, Ildstad ST. Percutaneous transperineal pouch localization in low imperforate anus: a new approach. *J Pediatr Surg.* 1990;25:273–275.

57. Moore TC. Advantages of performing the sagittal anoplasty operation for imperforate anus at birth. *J Pediatr Surg.* 1990;25:276–277.

58. Shepard R, Kiesewetter WB. Hyperchloremic acidosis as a complication of imperforate anus with recto-urinary fistula. *J Pediatr Surg.* 1966;1:62–69.

59. Stephens FD. Malformation of the anus. *Aust N Z J Surg*. 1953;23:9–24.

60. Kiesewetter WB, Turner CR. Continence after surgery for imperforate anus: a critical analysis and preliminary experience with the sacro-perineal pull-through. *Ann Surg*. 1963;158:498–512.

61. DeVries P, Pena A. Posterior sagittal anorectoplasty. *J Pediatr Surg*. 1982;17:638–643.

62. Pena A. Results in the management of 322 cases of anorectal malformations. *Pediatr Surg Int*. 1988;3: 94–104.

63. Ditesheim JA, Templeton JM Jr. Short-term v. long-term quality of life in children following repair of high imperforate anus. *J Pediatr Surg*. 1987;22:581–587.

64. Ong N-T, Beasley SW. Long-term continence in patients with high and intermediate anorectal anomalies treated by sacroperineal (Stephens) rectoplasty. *J Pediatr Surg*. 1991;26:44–48.

65. Kiesewetter WB, Chang JHT. Imperforate anus: a five to thirty year follow-up perspective. *Prog Pediatr Surg*. 1977;10:111–120.

66. Swenson O, Donnellan WL. Preservation of the puborectalis sling in imperforate anus repair. *Surg Clin North Am*. 1967;47:173–193.

67. Vade A, Reyes H, Wilbur A, Gyi B, Spigos D. The anorectal sphincter after rectal pull-through surgery for anorectal anomalies: MRI evaluation. *Pediatr Radiol*. 1989;19:179–183.

68. Rangecroft L. Neonatal small left colon syndrome. *Arch Dis Child*. 1979;54:635–637.

69. Stewart DR, Nixon GW, Johnson DG, Condon VR. Neonatal small left colon syndrome. *Ann Surg*. 1977;186:741–746.

70. Bowers RFJ, Sieber WK, Kiesewetter WB. Alimentary tract duplications in children. *Ann Surg*. 1978; 188:669–674.

71. LaQuaglia MP, Feins N, Eraklis A, Hendren WH. Rectal duplications. *J Pediatr Surg*. 1990;25:980–984.

72. Matson DD, Jerva MJ. Recurrent meningitis associated with congenital lumbo-sacral dermal sinus tract. *J Neurosurg*. 1966;25:288–297.

73. Silverman A, Roy CC. *Pediatric Clinical Gastroenterology*. St Louis: CV Mosby; 1983:391–411.

74. Katz C, Drongowski RA, Coran AG. Long-term management of chronic constipation in children. *J Pediatr Surg*. 1987;22:976–978.

75. Leape LL, Ramenofsky ML. Anterior ectopic anus: a common cause of constipation in children. *J Pediatr Surg*. 1978;13:627–630.

76. Hendren WH. Constipation caused by anterior location of the anus and its surgical correction. *J Pediatr Surg*. 1978;13:505–512.

77. Tuggle DW, Perkins TA, Tunell WP, Smith EI. Operative treatment of anterior ectopic anus: the efficacy and influence of age on results. *J Pediatr Surg*. 1990;25:996–998.

78. Zempsky WI, Rosenstein BJ. The cause of rectal prolapse in children. *Am J Dis Child*. 1988;142: 338–339.

79. Corman ML. Rectal prolapse in children. *Dis Colon Rectum*. 1985;28:535–539.

80. Wyllie GG. The injection treatment of rectal prolapse. *J Pediatr Surg*. 1979;14:62–64.

81. Pearl RH, Ein SH, Churchill B. Posterior sagittal anorectoplasty for pediatric recurrent rectal prolapse. *J Pediatr Surg*. 1989;24:1100–1102.

82. Chwals WJ, Brennan LP, Weitzman JJ, Woolley MM. Transanal mucosal sleeve resection for the treatment of rectal prolapse in children. *J Pediatr Surg*. 1990;25:715–718.

83. Ashcraft KW, Garred JL, Holder TM, Amoury RA, Sharp RJ, Murphy JP. Rectal prolapse: 17-year experience with the posterior repair and suspension. *J Pediatr Surg*. 1990;25:992–995.

84. Groff DB, Nagaraj HS. Rectal prolapse in infants and children. *Am J Surg*. 1990;160:531–532.

85. Angel C, Patrick CC, Lobe T, Rao B, Pui C-H. Management of anorectal/perineal infections caused by *Pseudomonas aeruginosa* in children with malignant diseases. *J Pediatr Surg*. 1991;26:487–493.

86. Cohen BA, Honig P, Androphy E. Anogenital warts in children. Clinical and virologic evaluation for sexual abuse. *Arch Dermatol*. 1990;126: 1575–1580.

87. McCoy CR, Applebaum H, Besser AS. Condyloma acuminata: an unusual presentation of child abuse. *J Pediatr Surg*. 1982;17:505–507.

CHAPTER 4

PREOPERATIVE AND POSTOPERATIVE MANAGEMENT

Anthony M. Vernava III
and Phillip Dean

Introduction

The decision to perform an operative procedure is a fundamental aspect of surgical practice and the selection of an appropriate operation requires an accurate and current understanding of the disease. Operative results in patients with anorectal disease are, in part, determined by the adequacy of preoperative preparation and postoperative management. Advances in knowledge relating to preoperative and postoperative care have decreased the risk of perioperative complications and have facilitated the safe transition of many anorectal procedures from the inpatient to the outpatient setting.

The rapid and uncomplicated recovery of a patient following anorectal surgery depends as much on perioperative management as on intraoperative technique. Any serious medical problem, such as a nutritional deficiency, must be correctly identified and adequately treated prior to surgery. Decisions regarding perioperative antibiotics, anesthesia and analgesia, wound care, dietary manipulation, bowel and bladder function, and physical activity affect morbidity and mortality. As such all of these factors play a decisive role in ensuring a successful operative result and a satisfied patient.

Preoperative Preparation

Preoperative Evaluation

A thorough preoperative evaluation of patients undergoing anorectal procedures begins with an accurate and complete history and physical examination. A complete medical history as well as a thorough understanding of the patient's social situation can identify associated factors that could complicate a surgical procedure.

A cardiac evaluation is mandatory in all patients who undergo general or regional anesthesia. Patients with no prior clinical evidence of heart disease have a 0.15 percent risk of perioperative myocardial infarction,[1] so a routine cardiac history and physical examination are adequate for preoperative evaluation. Patients with a prior myocardial infarction, angina, congestive heart failure, or other cardiac risk factors may require more extensive cardiac evaluation.[1]

Interest in identifying patients at risk for postoperative pulmonary complications originates from the early surgical observation that these are the most frequent causes of postoperative morbidity and mortality.[2] Patients who undergo anorectal surgery are at relatively lower risk than those who undergo thoracic or abdominal surgery. Nonetheless, patients with concomitant lung disease are at risk for pulmonary complications and deserve special attention, particularly after a general anesthetic.

Other health risks and concerns include obesity, diabetes mellitus, liver disease, and renal failure; all represent an increased risk for complications following any surgical procedure. Medications should not be discontinued prior to surgery but new ones should be started only if strongly indicated. Advanced age may be a relative risk factor and warrants consideration of preoperative medical evaluation.

Classification of a patient's preoperative physical condition is of value in predicting the overall risk of operative mortality. The American Society of Anesthe-

Table 4-1 ASA Physical Status Classification

Class	Description
I	Healthy patient
II	Mild systemic disease—no functional limitations
III	Severe systemic disease—definite functional limitation
IV	Severe systemic disease that is a constant threat to life
V	Moribund patient not expected to survive 24 hours with or without operation

siologists' Physical Status Classification (Table 4-1) is useful in determining the relative operative and anesthetic risk and thereby helps in the selection of an appropriate form of treatment for the patient.[3]

Preoperative laboratory data required will vary according to the patient's physical status, the procedure to be performed, and the type of anesthesia. A complete blood count should generally be obtained, in women over age 12, in males over 60 years of age, and in any patient with a history of blood loss or whose surgery has the potential of significant blood loss. Coagulation studies are indicated in patients with hepatic disease, history of bleeding disorder, or use of anticoagulants.

Anemia should be investigated prior to operation. Urinalysis is often indicated in patients with anorectal complaints, and evidence of a urinary tract infection should elicit concern in patients with inflammatory or neoplastic disease. In these latter patient groups such an infection could represent a fistula. Liver function should be assessed in patients with neoplastic disease. Chest radiographs and an electrocardiogram should generally be obtained in patients over the age of 40 and in younger patients with suggestive cardiac or pulmonary histories. In otherwise healthy individuals routine preoperative screening examinations such as serum hematology and chemistry, urinalysis, chest radiographs, and arterial blood gas evaluation rarely provide information that will alter perioperative management.[4,5]

It is obvious but must be stated that a complete and accurate preoperative diagnosis of the patient's lesion and any synchronous lesions is essential to a safe and effective perioperative course. Rigid and flexible proctosigmoidoscopy, colonoscopy, endorectal ultrasound, and MRI or CT scanning are all currently employed diagnostic modalities that may be selected in addition to physical examination and anoscopy to help identify and plan effective therapy for anorectal pathology. These evaluations are discussed in Chapter 2.

Preparation of the Gastrointestinal Tract

It is no longer plausible to perform major elective anorectal surgery without preoperative cleansing of the bowel and prophylactic antibiotics.[6] There is clear evidence that prophylactic antibiotics significantly reduce the morbidity and mortality of operations upon the colon and rectum[7] and they should be a routine part of any major elective anorectal procedure, such as a sphincter repair, an anoplasty, or a transanal excision of a villous tumor or carcinoma. The advantages of mechanical bowel cleansing and prophylactic antibiotics in preparing the colon and rectum have been well documented.[7-12]

Mechanical preparation of the colon and rectum is essential prior to major anorectal surgical procedures to provide a clean operative field and to facilitate operative manipulation in the anorectal region. Methods for bowel preparation include cathartics such as magnesium sulfate and enemas, whole gut saline lavage, and oral lavage solutions containing polyethylene glycol (PEG). Unlike other preparation methods, PEG lavage results in no fluid or electrolyte abnormalities, explosive gas production, or increased wound infection rates.[8,9] PEG lavage also shortens preoperative hospitalization, uniformly results in an excellent bowel preparation, and is preferred by patients.[8-11] A recent survey of 352 clinically active board-certified colorectal surgeons in the United States and Canada revealed that 206 (58%) used PEG lavage.[13] An example of the bowel preparation employed by the authors is shown in Table 4-2. On the day prior to operation, the patient is placed on a clear liquid diet. That same day, the patient is given 4 liters of a PEG colonic lavage solution to ingest over several hours. On this schedule, with diarrhea persisting for only approximately 2 to 3 hours following ingestion of the solution, the patient is allowed a full night's rest prior to the operation. An intravenous infusion is started to prevent dehydration if the patient has a significant risk for cardiovascular disease.

The role of antibiotics in preparation for bowel surgery remains one of the more controversial issues in surgical care. Both oral and systemically administered antibiotics have demonstrated efficacy in reducing infection rates in patients who undergo operative procedures on the alimentary tract,[7] and a combination of both may be most effective. Adequate data are not available to fully evaluate the use of oral and/or systemic antibiotics in anorectal surgery, though in two recent surveys of colon and rectal surgeons 80 to 90 percent used both oral and systemic antibiotics routinely in their bowel preparation for elective colorectal surgery.[13,14]

Although available information on the synergy between oral and systemic antibiotic prophylaxis is inconclusive, there continues to be a theoretical advantage

Table 4-2   Example of a Bowel Preparation

1. Begin bowel preparation on the day prior to operation.

2. Low residue diet until 10:00 A.M.

3. NPO after midnight.

4. Patient to drink four liters of Go-lytely the afternoon prior to operation.
   Beginning at 10:00 A.M., the patient should drink an 8- to 10-ounce glass of the solution every 10 to 15 minutes until the entire amount of solution is ingested or the diarrhea is clear.

5. Phospho—soda enema the evening prior to operation and on the morning of operation.

6. Neomycin (1 g P.O.) at 1:00 P.M., 2:00 P.M., and 11:00 P.M. on the day prior to operation.

7. Metronidazole 500 mg P.O. (or erythromycin base 1 g P.O.) at 1:00 P.M., 2:00 P.M., and 11:00 P.M. on the day prior to operation.

8. Begin intravenous fluids: 5% dextrose in 0.45% normal saline with 20 mEq kCl/l at 75 to 125 ml/h on the evening prior to operation.

9. Cefoxitin 1 g intravenous piggyback (drip) *or* cefotetan 1 g intravenous piggyback (drip) on call to the operating room.

to the use of both methods of administration. The potential benefits, ease of administration and the extremely low incidence of associated complications, make the use of combined oral and parenterally administered antibiotics an attractive addition to mechanical colonic bowel preparation for major anorectal procedures. The authors' choice combines mechanical bowel cleansing with both oral and parenteral antibiotics. The prophylactic parenteral administration of a broad spectrum cephalosporin is maintained for no longer than 24 hours perioperatively and begins immediately prior to surgery (Table 4-2). A second-generation cephalosporin (cefoxitin, cefotaxime, cefotetan) provides adequate coverage of the obligate and facultative anaerobic as well as aerobic organisms which are responsible for infectious complications following anorectal surgery.

Routine minor anorectal procedures such as hemorrhoidectomy, fistulotomy, sphincterotomy, and incision and drainage of an abscess do not require either mechanical or antibiotic bowel preparation. Septic problems following these minor anorectal surgical procedures are rare and are limited to local wound infection. One or two phosphate enemas given the morning

of surgery should adequately prepare the rectum and anal canal for these brief procedures. Wound complications are more likely related to inadequate postoperative care than to the absence of prophylactic antibiotics.

Ostomy and Stomal Considerations

Many patients undergoing colorectal procedures have stomas or diseases whose management may require the formation of an ostomy. Preoperative education and preparation of the patient is essential for successful postoperative management. A critical component is the preoperative selection of a stomal site. Selecting the proper site is important so that the stoma can be brought through a scar-free part of the abdominal wall to allow a good seal of the faceplate of the ostomy equipment. The site should be chosen so that the appliance can be placed without abutting on bony prominences such as the iliac crest or the rib cage. Most people have a fat roll just below the umbilicus; in most patients, the optimum site for stoma placement is on the crest of that roll on the outer third of the rectus sheath (Fig. 4-1).

A template of the faceplate or the faceplate itself can be used to pick a site so that there is maximal contact between the faceplate and skin. This should be done in

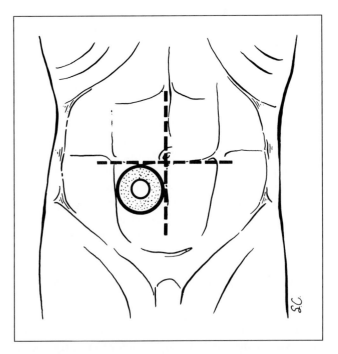

Figure 4-1.   Placement of a stoma site through the lower rectus abdominis muscle. Ileostomy is usually placed on the patient's right side and a colostomy is usually placed on the patient's left. (*From:* Beck DE, Harford FJ. In *Patient Care in Colorectal Surgery*. Boston: Little, Brown; 1991:96.)

all cases *before* the patient goes to the operating room. The site should be chosen with the patient in the supine, sitting, and standing position. Consideration should also be given to the type of clothing the patient wears. If the patient has had previous operations, several potential sites should also be selected. Once a site has been selected, it can be marked with either an indelible marker or a subcutaneous tattoo with methylene blue. If an indelible marker is used, the skin can be scratched after the patient is anesthetized so that the mark is not removed during the abdominal wall preparation. The assistance of an experienced enterostomal therapist can be helpful in difficult cases.

Patients with an existing stoma can undergo mechanical bowel preparation with minor modifications. A larger stomal pouch will accommodate the increased output associated with a lavage preparation. If a distal limb is present it may be cleansed with irrigations through a mucous fistula or with enemas.

Deep Venous Thrombosis Prophylaxis

Although deep venous thrombosis (DVT) is technically a complication of concern in the postoperative period, the concept of deep venous thrombosis prophylaxis must be addressed in the preoperative period. Deep venous thrombosis and subsequent pulmonary embolus (PE) are infrequent but constitute a major health risk to any patient undergoing general surgery. High risk factors include age over 40, obesity, malignancy, a history of DVT or PE, estrogen therapy, and a pelvic surgical procedure.[15] It is clear that prophylaxis against DVT should be considered in these patients.

Many methods for DVT prophylaxis have been advocated: intravenous and subcutaneous heparin (high and low doses), coumadin derivatives, dextran, and mechanical devices (graded compression and sequential compression stockings). Effective prophylactic treatment with either low dose subcutaneous heparin or sequential compression stockings can result in up to a 60 percent reduction in the incidence of DVT in these patients, with minimal associated morbidity.[15,16] Noncompression antithromboembolic stockings (TEDS) are of little value.[17]

Patients who undergo major anorectal procedures anticipated to last longer than 30 minutes, especially those in the lithotomy position and patients at otherwise high risk for DVT, should be considered for measures of DVT prevention. Minidose heparin (5000 U subcutaneously every 12 h) can be initiated 2 hours prior to operation and should be continued throughout the postoperative period until the patient is ambulatory. Alternatively, or in addition, intermittent sequential compression stockings are placed on both legs prior to operation and should remain functional until the patient is ambulatory. Patients who undergo minor anorectal procedures, such as hemorrhoidectomy, sphincterotomy, and fistulotomy require no such DVT prophylaxis unless specific risk factors are present.

Perioperative Management
Anesthesia and Analgesia

Anesthesia for anorectal procedures varies depending upon the operative requirements and patient compliance. Adequate anesthesia provides deep and prolonged analgesia of the anal canal and relaxation of the anal sphincters. Useful types of anesthesia include local infiltration with or without intravenous sedation, locoregional blocks, epidural and spinal anesthesia, and general anesthesia.

Local infiltration anesthesia and locoregional blocks are advantageous because they can be done rapidly and may be safely performed in an office setting. The authors prefer to use a mixture of 0.5% lidocaine and 0.25% bupivacaine in a 1:1 mixture, with the addition of epinephrine at a final concentration of 1:200,000. This mixture combines the rapid onset of lidocaine with the long duration of analgesia characteristic of bupivacaine. The addition of epinephrine not only prolongs the analgesic effect but also reduces capillary bleeding; caution should be exercised when using epinephrine in patients with coronary and cerebrovascular disease. Many surgeons elect to add hyaluronidase to the local anesthetic mixture at a concentration of 3 U/ml. The mucolytic properties of this enzyme allow the anesthetic solution to spread more rapidly throughout the tissues and results in less anatomic distortion of tissue at the injection site. However this property may also increase the toxicity of the local anesthetics used.[18]

Most minor anorectal procedures can be satisfactorily performed using local or locoregional anesthesia; intravenous sedation complements the local anesthetic. General, spinal, or epidural anesthesia may be indicated when maximum pelvic relaxation is required, when a prolonged surgical procedure is anticipated, and when local injection may be contraindicated. An example of the latter indication is the presence of extensive local sepsis. Local anesthetic may be used concomitantly when employing general or spinal anesthesia. This improves relaxation in the anal canal, improves local hemostasis, and allows a lighter level of general anesthesia. For all of these reasons, the authors feel that local anesthetic should be routinely employed. Anesthetic techniques are discussed in more detail in Chapter 5.

Postoperative Care

General Considerations

There is no easy postoperative routine for anorectal procedures. Many procedures can be performed on an outpatient basis and only patients with the most complicated conditions will spend more than a few days in the hospital. Analgesia must be provided as detailed above and the patient should be meticulously instructed on wound care techniques and diet. Discharge from the hospital usually depends on patient comfort.

The role of dietary restriction and bowel control is unclear. The authors advocate a period of complete dietary restriction followed by several days of a low residue diet for major anorectal procedures such as endoanal advancement flap for rectovaginal fistula and plication sphincter repair for incontinence. Routine anorectal procedures such as hemorrhoidectomy or sphincterotomy require no such precautions and the patient is allowed to resume a diet as tolerated following recovery from anesthesia, although fluids are restricted until the patient voids. The first bowel action usually occurs 24 to 48 hours after surgery, and if it does not occur a laxative is prescribed. A psyllium stool bulking agent should be given regularly to prevent constipation; stool softeners are of little value. The authors' routine postoperative instructions for anorectal surgical patients is given in Table 4–3.

Pain Management

One of the most important postoperative concerns for the surgeon is pain management, not only for patient comfort but also to ensure patient compliance, increase mobility, and prevent complications. Although pain is often the chief presenting symptom of many anorectal diseases it is also the single most important reason why patients avoid minor anorectal surgery. For many anorectal procedures postoperative pain is due to the incisional wounds and is exacerbated by the first several bowel movements. Adequate analgesia must be provided without constipating the patient; thus agents such as codeine should be employed with caution. Nonetheless, narcotic analgesia is appropriate for the first few postoperative days by intramuscular injection, oral routes, or patient-controlled analgesia (PCA pump).

Local measures of pain relief play an important role in the management of postoperative pain. Frequent sitz baths provide an excellent means of wound cleansing and provide substantial relief from pain and muscle spasm. Topical anesthetic ointments can be employed but are often of limited use and may induce an allergic reaction. Open wounds generally produce greater sub-

Table 4–3   Postoperative Instructions for Anorectal Surgical Patients

1. The following medicines or prescriptions will be sent home with you:
   - Psyllium seed preparation: 2 doses daily in full glass of water.
   - A prescription for pain reliever with instructions will be given to you.
   - Analgesic ointment: Apply externally with cotton dressing after each bath and bowel movement.

2. Postoperative office visits are essential to ensure proper healing of your rectal wounds. Please call the office to make your first appointment as instructed.

3. Sitz baths, comfortably warm, should be taken three times a day, especially after bowel movements. Have the water as hot as can be tolerated. Bath should last no longer than 20 minutes.

4. Some bloody discharge, especially after bowel movements, can be expected after rectal surgery. If there is prolonged or *profuse* bleeding, call us at once.

5. Bowel movements after rectal surgery are usually associated with some discomfort. This will diminish as the healing progresses. You should have a bowel movement at least every other day. If 2 days pass without a bowel movement, take an ounce of milk of magnesia and repeat in 6 hours if no results.

6. The use of dry toilet tissue should be avoided. After bowel movements use facial tissue, cotton, or Tucks pads to clean yourself, or if possible take a sitz bath.

7. A general diet is recommended, including plenty of fruit and vegetables. Try to drink six to eight glasses of water a day.

8. No strenuous exercise or heavy lifting should be attempted until healing is well underway. Climbing stairs, walking, and car riding and driving may be done in moderation.

9. If you have any questions about your postoperative care, feel free to call the physician anytime at home or the office.

jective pain complaints than closed wounds and may require a longer duration of analgesic administration.

Extensive anorectal procedures such as a plication sphincter repair, a complex anoplasty, and a rectovaginal fistula repair involve longer periods of hospitalization and lend themselves more readily to newer methods of pain control. Epidural administration of local anesthetic agents or opioids provides analgesia that is superior to that from systemically administered narcotics and is associated with a lower incidence of side effects.[19-22] Our anecdotal experience with this technique suggests that patients ambulate earlier and have improved wound care. The invasive nature of this technique limits its use to selected patients in whom conventional pain control is expected to fail. Patient-controlled analgesia also provides improved pain relief over conventional methods[19,23] but, like epidural analgesia, is only occasionally required for patients after anorectal surgery.

Wound Healing and Wound Care

Anorectal procedures are carried out in a field where numerous and varied bacterial organisms are present. Contrary to what one would logically expect in such a medium, postoperative suppurative complications are rare whether the wound is closed or left open. Wounds in the anorectum generally heal to completion without complication. Primary closure of noninfected anorectal wounds is preferred, although fistulotomy and abscess wounds should be left open to heal secondarily and packing or drains should rarely be used.

Healing of a large open wound is achieved by contraction of the granulation tissue and epithelial cells from the wound edge. Large open wounds such as this require a prolonged time to heal; moreover, the resulting scarring can result in a painful stricture. In the absence of wound sepsis these wounds can be safely closed by a variety of techniques. Skin grafting can be safely performed in the perianal region if primary wound closure is impossible. Skin flaps may also be used to provide wound coverage and sensation. Many different flaps have been described and flap closure should be tailored to the particular needs of the wound. These approaches are discussed in Chapters 12 and 14.

Wound care consists primarily of keeping the wound as clean as possible. A sitz bath, with or without a mild antiseptic solution, is recommended three times daily and after each bowel movement to ensure cleanliness. The wound should be inspected daily while patients are hospitalized. It is unnecessary, unwise, and uncomfortable for the patient to undergo a digital rectal exam in the early postoperative period.

Complications of Anorectal Procedures

Numerous complications can occur following anorectal operative procedures, although most are quite rare.[24] Suppuration can occur but is unusual. Constipation or impaction can occur owing to postoperative pain and the fear of pain. The patient must be assured that stool bulking agents and/or laxatives should be used as they will make bowel action much more comfortable. Temporary incontinence of mucus and flatus commonly occurs following many anorectal procedures and usually improves with time. Permanent incontinence to solid stool following an anorectal procedure should be avoidable by proper operative techniques. Hemorrhage is a well-known complication following hemorrhoidectomy and transanal tumor excision, and may require reoperation.

Most properly constructed anorectal wounds heal to completion without significant stricture formation and do not require dilation. The passage of stool through the anal canal is usually all that is required. Postoperative anal dilation is painful, usually unnecessary and should be avoided. Indication for anal dilation exists, however, when a well-lubricated index finger cannot be gently inserted into the anal canal. Gentle anal dilation can usually be performed in the office using an anoscope, although an anesthetic may be required in the operating room for more severe strictures. Such stenosis may require a formal corrective procedure such as anoplasty.

Acute urinary retention is the most common complication of surgery for benign anorectal disease (10%).[25] The precise causes are unknown, but proposed etiologies include inadequate pain control, excessive rectal packing, and the administration of excessive perioperative fluids. Urinary retention is more common in patients given a large fluid volume in the perioperative period and is also more common in patients who receive a long-acting local anesthetic or spinal anesthesia.[26] Fluid restriction in the early postoperative period is advocated in most patients to decrease the risk of this complication. In addition, some surgeons advocate the use of bethanecol[27] although its efficacy is unclear. An occasional patient may require bladder catheterization. Urinary retention invariably resolves within 2 to 3 days postoperatively.

References

1. Freeman WK, Gibbons RJ, Shub C. Preoperative assessment of cardiac patients undergoing noncardiac surgical procedures. *Mayo Clin Proc.* 1989;64:1105–1117.

2. Zibrak JD, O'Donnell CR, Marton K. Indications for pulmonary function testing. *Ann Intern Med.* 1990;112:763–771.

3. Ross AF, Tinker JH. Anesthesia risk. In: Miller

RD, ed. *Anesthesia*. 3rd ed. New York: Churchill Livingstone; 1990:715–742.

4. Turnbull JM, Back C. The value of preoperative screening investigations in otherwise healthy individuals. *Arch Intern Med*. 1987;147:1101–1105.

5. Macpherson DS, Snow R, Lofgren RP. Pre-operative screening: value of previous tests. *Ann Intern Med*. 1990;113:969–973.

6. Condon RE. Bowel preparation for colorectal operations. *Arch Surg*. 1982;117:265. Editorial.

7. Conte JE Jr, Jacob LS, Polk HC Jr. *Antibiotic Prophylaxis in Surgery. A Comprehensive Review*. Philadelphia: JB Lippincott; 1984.

8. Beck DE, Harford FJ, DiPalma JA. Comparison of cleansing methods in preparation for colonic surgery. *Dis Colon Rectum*. 1985;28:491–495.

9. Beck DE, Fazio VW, Jagelman DG. Comparison of lavage methods for preoperative colonic cleansing. *Dis Colon Rectum*. 1986;29:699–703.

10. Wolff BG, Beart RW Jr, Dozois RJ, et al. A new bowel preparation for elective colon and rectal surgery: prospective and randomized clinical trial. *Arch. Surg*. 1988;123:895–900.

11. Dueholms S, Rubinstein E, Reipurth G. Preparation for elective colorectal surgery: a randomized blinded comparison between oral colonic lavage and whole gut irrigation. *Dis Colon Rectum*. 1987;30:360–364.

12. Johnston D. Bowel preparation for colorectal surgery. *Br J Surg*. 1987;74:553–554.

13. Solla JA, Rothenberger DA. Preoperative bowel preparation. A survey of colon and rectal surgeons. *Dis Colon Rectum*. 1990;33:154–159.

14. Beck DE, Fazio VW. Current pre-operative bowel cleansing methods: a survey of American Society of Colon and Rectal Surgeons members. *Dis Colon Rectum*. 1990;33:12–15.

15. NIH Consensus Development Conference. Prevention of venous thrombosis and pulmonary embolism. *JAMA*. 1986;256:744–749.

16. Hyers TM, Hull RD, Weg JG. Antithrombotic therapy for venous thromboembolic disease. *Chest*. 1987;95:375–515.

17. Browse NL, Jackson BT, Mayo ME, Negus D. The value of mechanical methods of preventing postoperative calf vein thrombosis. *Br J Surg*. 1974;61:219–223.

18. Clery AP. Local anaesthesia containing hyaluronidase and adrenaline for anorectal surgery: experience with 576 operations. *Proc R Soc Med*. 1973;66:680–681.

19. Lutz LJ, Lamer TJ. Management of postoperative pain: review of current techniques and methods. *Mayo Clin Proc*. 1990;65:584–596.

20. Cousins MJ, Mather LE. Intrathecal and epidural administration of opioids. *Anesthesiology*. 1984;61:276–310.

21. Bromage PR, Comparesi E, Chestnut D. Epidural narcotics for postoperative analgesia. *Anesth Analg*. 1980;59:473–480.

22. Rawal N, Sjostrand VH, Dahlstrom B. Postoperative pain relief by epidural morphine. *Anesth Analg*. 1981;60:726–731.

23. Bennett RL, Batenhorst RL, Bivins BA, et al. Patient-controlled analgesia: a new concept of postoperative pain relief. *Ann Surg*. 1982;195:700–705.

24. Ferrari BJ, Ray JE, Gathright JB, eds. *Complications of Colon and Rectal Surgery: Prevention and Management*. Philadelphia: WB Saunders; 1985.

25. Prasad ML, Abcarian H. Urinary retention following operations for benign anorectal disease. *Dis Colon Rectum*. 1978;21:490–492.

26. Petros JG, Bradley TM. Factors influencing postoperative urinary retention in patients undergoing surgery for benign anorectal disease. *Am J Surg*. 1990;159:374–376.

27. Gottesman L, Milsom JW, Mazier WP. The use of anxiolytic and parasympathomimetic agents in the treatment of postoperative urinary retention following anorectal surgery. *Dis Colon Rectum*. 1989;32:867–870.

CHAPTER 5

OPERATIVE AND ANESTHETIC TECHNIQUES

*Alan G. Thorson and
Garnet J. Blatchford*

Operative Techniques

Anorectal surgery encompasses a large variety of procedures and techniques. A number of different procedures may be described for the management of a particular disease process. Similarly, a variety of different techniques may be used to accomplish a particular procedure. For example, a lateral internal sphincterotomy may be accomplished by any of several techniques. Although this situation is sometimes an indication that no single alternative has been proved to give a consistently good result, at other times it may simply signify that all of the alternatives are equally effective. Selection of such alternatives may be largely based on the personal preference of the surgeon.

At least a portion of operative technique is due to an individual surgeon's personal style and can be taught effectively only on a one-to-one basis. Other techniques cannot be passed on but remain as an individual surgeon's signature on all of his or her work. At the other end of the spectrum are techniques that can be commonly applied to all anorectal operations. These latter techniques serve as basic fundamentals for successful anorectal surgery.

In general, three factors are critical to a successful anorectal operation: proper positioning of the patient, adequate lighting, and proper instrumentation. The application of these factors to anorectal surgery is unique because of the confining anatomy of the anus and rectum.

Patient Position

Proper positioning of the patient is essential to allow optimum exposure for definition of both the anatomy and the pathology. Ideally, the patient should be positioned in such a way as to allow an assistant easy access to the operating field. A well-trained assistant can shorten operating time by providing good exposure and assisting with some of the more complicated maneuvers required when operating in a small deep space. These factors can result in a safer and more accurately reproducible procedure.

Four basic patient positions are used in anorectal surgery; lithotomy, left lateral, prone, and Sims' or modified Sims' left anterolateral position. Each has certain advantages and disadvantages for specific situations. Familiarity with all of these positions will allow the surgeon the flexibility needed to deal effectively with the problems seen in the anorectal region. It is a mistake to believe that any one position is always the best. Such recalcitrance will only lead to times of exasperation as the pathology slides out of the view of the operating surgeon.

The lithotomy position was popularized by Milligan, Morgan, and colleagues when they described a technique of ligation and excision of hemorrhoids.[1] This position keeps the upper body supine as the lower extremities are flexed at the hips and the knees in some type of stirrup arrangement (Fig. 5-1). This position is favored by many anesthesiologists because it provides easy access to the airway. The disadvantage is to the surgeon doing the procedure. For many anorectal procedures, exposure is limited and the option for an actively participating assistant is virtually eliminated.

The lithotomy position is, however, frequently an excellent choice during transanal excision of low posterior lesions. Unless one likes to operate standing on one's head, it is a poor choice for an anterior and most lateral lesions. An exaggerated lithotomy position with

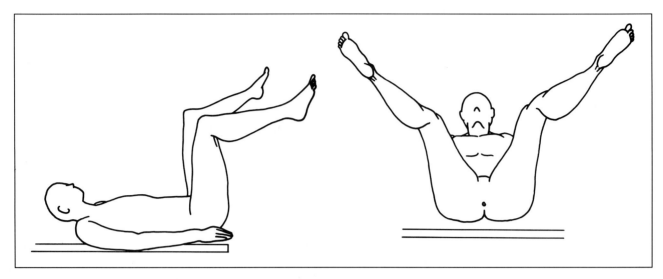

Figure 5-1. A slightly modified lithotomy position using mild flexion of the knees.

the lower extremities doubly flexed to bring them cephalad to the buttocks, which are themselves placed beyond the edge of the operating table, is another alternative. This position can provide excellent exposure during Altmeier type perineal rectosigmoidectomy for rectal prolapse (Fig. 5-2). With the attachment of a small instrument tray to the end of the table, the table can be raised to the proper level to allow the operating surgeon to stand. With the lower extremities out of the way, an assistant can actively participate in this procedure, which is done entirely outside of or caudal to the anal canal.

The left lateral position has been championed by the Ferguson Clinic in their descriptions of hemorrhoidec-

tomy technique (Fig. 5-3).[2] This position does allow an assistant easy access, but the assistant does not have the same view of the operative field that the surgeon has. In some instances, this may render the assistant unable to be of full benefit to the surgeon and may actually increase the overall operative time. Moreover, the upper buttock, in a natural response to gravity, coapts with the lower buttock, further compromising visibility.

The left lateral position can be particularly useful in the office for examinations. Although the prone–jackknife position is probably the most popular position in the United States for rigid proctosigmoidoscopy, this examination can also be performed with the patient in the left lateral position. The patient is maintained in the

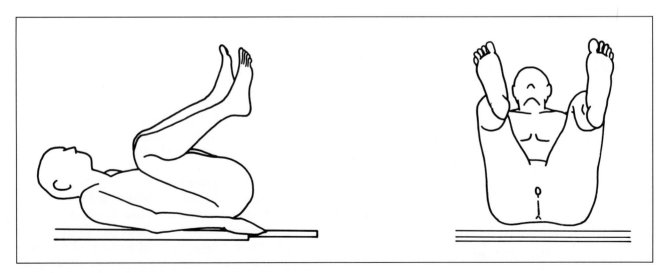

Figure 5-2.   An exaggerated lithotomy position with the buttocks extending over the edge of the table. The addition of an instrument tray to the table makes this position ideal for perineal rectosigmoidectomy.

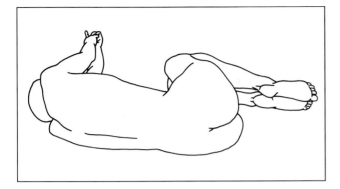

Figure 5-3.   Full left lateral position with both knees and hips flexed and both arms extended.

full lateral position with the left side down. The left thigh and leg are extended straight to the bottom of the table and the right thigh and leg flexed into a near knee-chest position. The buttocks are brought far to the edge of the table and even allowed to extend over the edge just enough so that the patient need not fear falling. As shown in Fig. 5-4, the back is slightly flexed. This position is particularly suited to the female patient well advanced in pregnancy, to some amputees, and to patients with spinal cord or other neurologic injuries.

A prone position has been described for use in Buie[3] and Fansler[4] type hemorrhoidectomies. A soft but firm roll is placed under the hips of the prone patient. Placement is critical since positioning of the roll too far caudally will lead to poor exposure by not elevating the buttocks high enough to separate them. A low roll will also cause discomfort in the thighs during a local anesthetic and postoperatively from a general or regional anesthetic. A roll placed too far cephalad may restrict venous return through the inferior vena cava. The result may be transient hypotension and the possibility of increased intraoperative bleeding. Excessive compression of the abdomen can also impair ventilation. An additional roll is placed beneath each ankle to keep the toes off of the surface of the operating table. All pressure

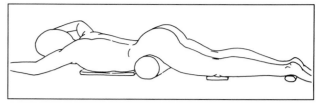

Figure 5-5.   The prone position. The hip roll must be carefully positioned directly under the hips. The knees, elbows, and toes must be padded. Chest rolls ease respiratory expansion.

points including knees and elbows need to be carefully monitored and adequately padded (Fig. 5-5).

The prone position has much to offer for most anorectal surgery. The entire operating team including surgeon, assistant surgeon, and scrub nurse have a full and unobstructed view of the operative field. Thus, the assistant and nurse can always see the maneuvers of the surgeon and be there to offer the best chance for improved efficiency. Lighting of any type is enhanced. Anorectal anatomy is clearly delineated and any bleeding drains automatically away from the operative field.[5] Disadvantages include the anesthesiologist's concern about the airway and patient complaints of pain over the pubis and low backache during a local anesthetic.[6]

The left anterolateral, or modified Sims', position[6] starts with the patient prone, both arms crossed in front of the head or under the forehead. A slight lateral positioning is then obtained by placing a blanket or small roll under the right chest. The left thigh and leg are maintained in an extended position and the right thigh and leg mildly flexed on a pillow (Fig. 5-6). For local anesthetics, this position appears to eliminate complaints of pubic pain and low backache. It may limit visualization of the right posterior quadrant[6] but appears a good alternative for sphincterotomies, fistulotomies, and pilonidal cysts being treated under local anesthetic.

Lighting

Proper lighting is critical to all anorectal surgery. Improper lighting can result in blind dissections leading to

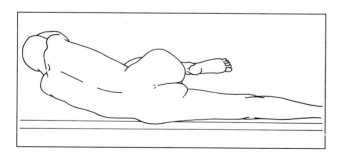

Figure 5-4.   A modified left lateral position for use in the office for patients with special needs such as pregnancy, amputations, or spinal cord injuries.

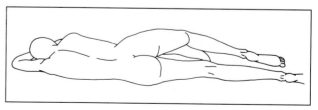

Figure 5-6.   The left anterolateral (modified Sims') position for use with local anesthetics when doing sphincterotomies, simple fistulotomies, and pilonidal disease.

compromise in patient care and operative outcome. Most anorectal operations are performed in a deep dark tunnel which is not easily illuminated to satisfactory levels. The standard overhead lighting found in most operating rooms is generally inadequate for anorectal surgery. When overhead lighting is properly positioned to allow visualization of the anal canal, it is most frequently eclipsed by the head or hands of the operating surgeon. For this reason the use of a headlight is extremely effective in maintaining adequate illumination. The Luxtec® (Luxtec Corporation, Technology Park, Sturbridge, Massachusetts) fiberoptic light is one of several good commercially available headlights.

A properly adjusted headlight will focus the light in the surgeon's line of sight. The surgeon's hand maneuvers will always allow a line of sight to the operative field and it is through this line of sight that the beam of light is now descending to that field. Shadowing from the surgeon's head is no longer a concern.

The use of a headlight should not be limited to the operating room. The typical office examining room has far less adequate lighting than do most operating rooms. The use of a headlight in the examining room is a quick and thorough solution to this problem. We have found the Welch Allyn (Welch Allyn, Inc., Skaneateles Falls, New York) physician headlight to be an excellent and inexpensive light source for anorectal examination in the office setting (Fig. 5-7). It allows light to be focused directly into the anal canal. Failure to provide adequate illumination at this point in the patient's evaluation may lead to incomplete or even inaccurate diagnosis.

Instrumentation

Proper instrumentation makes the difference between smooth, efficient, low-effort anorectal surgery and its nemesis: the awkward, frustrating, and frequently dangerous manipulation of one of the body's most sensitive, specialized, and socially indispensable organs. Instrument selection is based on the setting (office vs. operating room) and the pathologic condition. The basic considerations consist of anoscopes, speculums, retractors, and supporting materiel including needle holders, needles, suture, forceps, and electrocautery.

Anoscopes

One must be careful to distinguish between the instruments that are used in the office and those used in the operating room. Office instruments are generally smaller in caliber than are operative instruments to ensure patient comfort. They are adequate for diagnostic work but really do not offer enough exposure for most operative maneuvers. We have found the Vernon–David anoscope modified with the handle of the Hirshman anoscope to be the ideal office anoscope. The Vernon–David scope itself is well tolerated by patients, and the longer handle borrowed from the Hirshman scope provides better control over the instrument while keeping one's hand out of the visual pathway (Fig. 5-8).

The Hinkel–James anoscope is ideal for rubber-band ligation. It is longer and provides a larger diameter orifice through which to manipulate the ligating instrument. It is open on one side, allowing easy identification of the hemorrhoid as it falls into the lumen. Despite its length, it is tapered to allow for excellent tolerance by the patient (Fig. 5-9).

Speculums

Speculums are generally used only for operation (Fig. 5-10). They may be bi-valved or tri-valved. Speculums

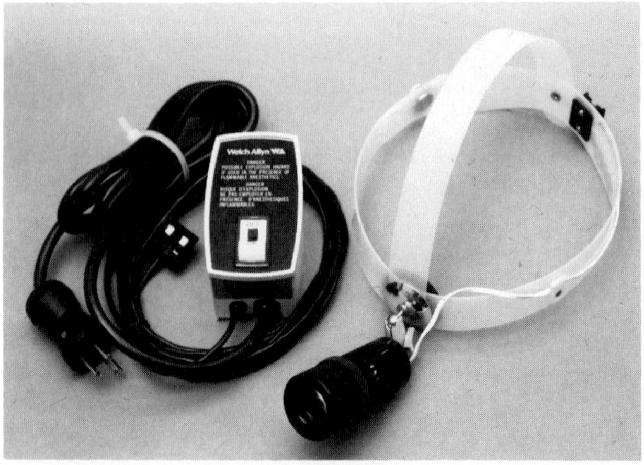

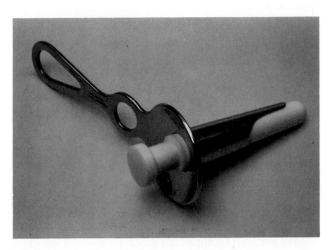

Figure 5-7. The Welch-Allyn physician headlight is an ideal office light source for anorectal examination (Welch Allyn, Inc., Skaneateles Falls, New York).

Figure 5-8. Vernon–David anoscope with Hirshman handle.

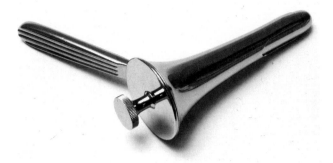

Figure 5-9. Hinkel–James anoscope. Well-suited for rubber-band ligation.

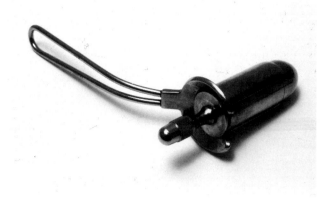

Figure 5-11. The Fansler operative anoscope.

have a tendency to pinch mucosa and thus are poorly tolerated in the unanesthetized patient. This is particularly true of fenestrated speculums. We find such fenestrated instruments very difficult to work with and would not recommend them. However, the nonfenestrated bi-valve type instrument, such as the Pratt, is very useful in evaluating the anesthetized anal canal. With gentle dilation, it can be slowly opened to allow a wide operative field. Opening it to a mild degree of tension allows the accurate and rapid identification of the caudal edge of the internal sphincter. This will be palpable as a firm cord. This technique is very useful while performing internal sphincterotomies and during rectal mucosectomies. Nasal speculums can be useful in instances of severe stenosis where a speculum the size of a Pratt instrument cannot be placed in the anal canal.

The Fansler operative anoscope is our preferred instrument for operative hemorrhoidectomy (Fig. 5-11).

It provides an ample operating field to one side of the anal canal while all other quadrants are tucked neatly behind the lumen of the remainder of the instrument. This instrument is too large to be used in the unanesthetized canal.

Retractors

The Sawyer, Hill–Ferguson, Ferguson–Moon, and other similar retractors are all alike in providing an anal "spoon" or "cup" which will expose about 40 to 50 percent of the circumference of the anal canal (Fig. 5-12). The small size of these retractors leads to minimal dilation and distortion of the hemorrhoidal cushions, but also provides limited room for maneuvering of instruments. We have been blinded to bleeding vessels hidden by the tamponade of the larger Fansler scope. In this situation, the judicial use of a Ferguson–Moon type retractor will often allow the identification of such a

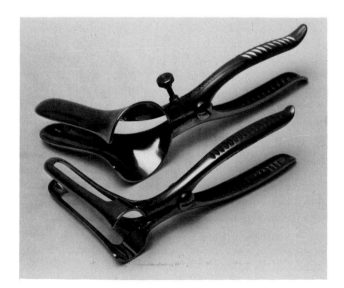

Figure 5-10. (*Upper*) Pratt speculum. (*Lower*) Fenestrated speculum.

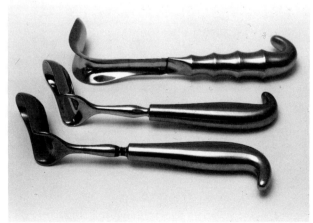

Figure 5-12. (Top to bottom) Sawyer, Ferguson–Moon, and Hill–Ferguson anal retractors.

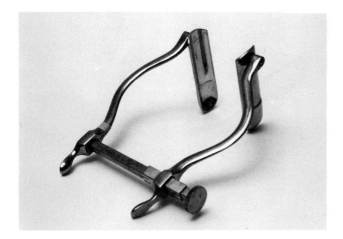

Figure 5-13. Buie–Smith self-retaining anal retractor.

vessel since the anal canal is not subjected to the same stretch and compression.

A number of self-retaining anal retractors, such as the Buie–Smith and Parks', are sometimes used in transanal excisions and mucosectomies (Figs. 5-13 and 5-14). We generally find that the frames of such retractors interfere with the instrumentation necessary to accomplish the desired task and prefer anal eversion in these situations (especially with mucosectomies). Eversion may be accomplished by using four-quadrant heavy sutures from the dentate line to well out on the buttocks or with the Lone Star retractor (Fig. 5-15) (Lone Star Medical Products, Houston, Texas).[7]

Supporting Materiel

Other considerations include selection of proper needle holders, suture material, needles, forceps, clamps, and cautery equipment.

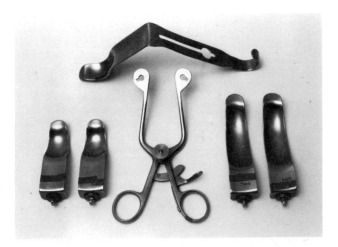

Figure 5-14. Parks' self-retaining anal retractor. The lateral blades are of two sizes and attach to the superior limbs. The central blade attaches to the joint to provide a tripod retraction system.

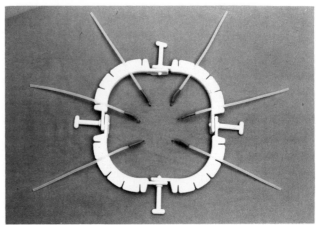

Figure 5-15. The Lone Star retractor. The plastic frame anchors the elastic stay hooks which are used to retract against the dentate line and evert the anus (Lone Star Medical Products, Houston, Texas).

The **needle holder** must be personally selected to the preference of the surgeon. In general, however, it must have adequate length to reach beyond the depth of the retractor being used while allowing the operator's hand to remain completely external to the anal canal. This usually means a nine-inch instrument of medium weight.

Absorbable **suture material** of chromic cat gut or polyglycolic acid is preferred. No suture removal is required and absorption is at a rate that will allow wounds to open in the face of infection rather than serving as a site for abscess formation. We prefer 3-0 chromic catgut suture for most hemorrhoidal and anal canal work. The slower absorbing suture material is more frequently used for low rectal work including transanal excisions and anal anastomoses.

When suturing is confined to the perianal skin, a cutting **needle** is preferred. When suturing in the rectal mucosa, a taper needle is preferred. For hemorrhoidal surgery, when the incision to be closed extends across both columnar and squamous epithelium, we prefer a taper-cut needle. It is less likely to tear the rectal mucosa than is a cutting needle and will still allow penetration of the perianal skin.

Our choice for tissue handling is a Debakey **forceps.** Some type of toothed forceps should be readily available in instances of complicated and edematous hemorrhoids and when operating for fistulae. An Allis or Babcock clamp is indispensable when operating in a scarred field or with fibrotic tissue and when elevating tissue, whether a hemorrhoidal cushion or a mucosal advancement flap.

To complete the basic anorectal surgery tray, an assortment of **probes** for use in identification and treatment of fistulas is necessary. We find it helpful to have a

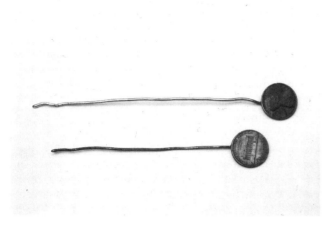

Figure 5-16.   A malleable probe to define fistula pathways.

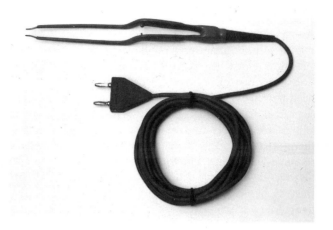

Figure 5-18.   Monopolar hand-activated bayonet-type electrocautery for use in hemorrhoidectomy.

malleable probe available in the operating room for investigating and documenting the pathway of a fistula. A "penny probe" has been the mainstay of our office for this purpose since shortly after its founding in 1919 (Fig. 5-16). A fine malleable probe with an eye at one end is helpful when placing a seton. Lockhart–Mummery grooved retractors are ideal for laying open a fistula once its course has been confirmed (Fig. 5-17).

The appropriate application of **electrosurgery** to operations on the anal canal provides rapid, effective hemostasis. We have found the use of a monopolar hand-activated bayonet-type cautery unit to be particularly helpful when performing hemorrhoidectomy (Fig. 5-18). Its use is ideal in allowing the simultaneous control and cauterization of bleeding vessels. A blade-type unit is much more effective when cautery is used for tissue cutting such as when elevating flaps or unroofing chronically inflamed fistula tracks. A needle tip cautery is helpful when coring out fistula tracks as described by Parks.[8]

Finally, a word about gauze **sponges.** We make liberal use of sponges in association with the cautery to control hemostasis. Rarely is it necessary to have suction at the operating table. However, the size of the sponge is critical to effective use in the anal canal. The 4 × 4 sponges are too large to pass through the operative scopes. The 2 × 2 sponges cannot absorb enough blood to be really helpful and they are easily lost in the rectum. It is the 3 × 3 that is the colorectal surgeon's friend when operating on the anal canal. There should always be a liberal supply at hand.

Anesthetic Techniques

The small area in which most anorectal operations are performed allows a number of anesthetic options to be easily considered. The importance of this selection should not be underestimated. Techniques of regional and local anesthesia can provide excellent relaxation and comfort to the patient in most instances. Unfortunately, not all patients are able to tolerate the thought of less than a general anesthetic for any operation involving their anorectal region. For these patients, general anesthesia becomes the anesthetic of choice. This is unfortunate because in most instances the benefits of regional and local anesthesia far outweigh their disadvantages and have much to offer in the way of safety over a general anesthetic.

All parties involved in an operation must be comfortable with the type of anesthetic selected. One must be familiar with the options as well as their advantages, disadvantages, and complications to be able to make the best choice. The following discussion centers on these issues rather than specifics of techniques which are well described in basic anesthesiology textbooks.[9,10]

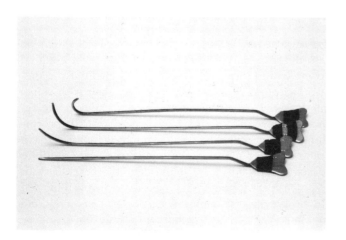

Figure 5-17.   Lockhart–Mummery grooved retractors.

Mode of Administration

As stated above, the choice of anesthetic must always be a joint effort on the part of the surgeon, patient, and anesthesiologist. If a patient has a real fear of an operation and a fear of regional or local anesthesia, it makes no difference how successful the anesthetic is. The patient will still be miserable and will have a miserable experience. As a result, the surgeon will also have a less than satisfactory experience. For this reason, it is good to have a working knowledge of the advantages and disadvantages of each type of anesthetic available so that this can be discussed openly and honestly with the patient. Many patients' fears of regional or local anesthesia can then be overcome and a good experience can result. Failure in this important part of the preparation of the patient for anorectal surgery can lead to unhappiness for all participants.

General Anesthesia

A patient's preference for general anesthesia may be based on a fear of the operation itself or a fear of the operating room. Some people's modesty makes it uncomfortable for them to be awake while they are exposed for an operation. Others worry that a local or regional anesthetic will wear off in the middle of the procedure, leaving them vulnerable to severe pain. Some patients worry about repeated needle punctures. Still others simply do not want to know what goes on in an operating room and believe that anything short of a general anesthetic will make them too aware of the course of events. If these fears can be identified, they can frequently be addressed and overcome by careful consultation among all parties involved.

There are real disadvantages to a general anesthetic. For all those procedures performed in the prone position, endotracheal intubation is required. There is a significant incidence of nausea and vomiting following general anesthesia. Patients with significant cardiac or pulmonary insufficiency may be at increased risk.

A distinct advantage of general anesthesia is total relaxation of the pelvic floor. This can be important when operating on complicated and high fistulas or when approaching the rectum for transanal excisions. Local anesthesia is frequently inadequate in these instances. If regional anesthesia is contraindicated by a neurologic condition, a back injury, anticoagulation, or for other reasons, general anesthesia may be the anesthetic of choice.

Regional Anesthesia

Regional anesthetics applicable to anorectal surgery consist of spinal and epidural blocks. Both provide for excellent relaxation of the anal canal and pelvic floor and are good options for anorectal surgery. Both are contraindicated in the presence of anticoagulation or if infection is present at the proposed site of injection such as might occur with pilonidal disease. Each has special considerations.

Spinal Anesthesia. The injection of a local anesthetic into the subarachnoid space leads to spinal anesthesia. The onset of action is predictable and within a few minutes. Autonomic function is lost first, followed by superficial pain sensation, temperature sensation, vibratory sensation, and then motor power and finally touch. The resultant sympathetic blockade places the patient at risk for hypotension and increases the demand for intravenous fluids. This and the direct effect of the block on the parasympathetics of the bladder may increase the incidence of urinary retention postoperatively.[11] The duration of the block depends on the local anesthetic agent selected for use. Procaine will provide anesthesia for approximately 60 minutes whereas bupivacaine may persist for 2.5 hours or longer.

A major disadvantage of spinal anesthesia is the risk of spinal headache. The incidence ranges from 3 to 16 percent. It is more common in younger patients with the peak incidence in the third decade. Risk is diminished with decreasing size of the needle used for puncture.[12] Spinal headache seems to occur when CSF leaks at the site of the puncture at a rate greater than CSF production with consequent traction on pain-sensitive intracranial structures. Treatment of spinal headache consists of bedrest, hydration, and analgesics. In severe cases, an autologous "blood patch" is effective about 90 percent of the time.[12]

There is a persistent fear that spinal anesthesia can lead to long-term neurologic injury including paraplegia. In fact, recent studies indicate that the risk of serious neurologic sequelae is exceedingly low when current methods of asepsis and management have been employed.[13]

Epidural Anesthesia. An injection of local anesthetic into the space surrounding the dura mater (the epidural space) within the spinal canal induces epidural anesthesia. The onset of anesthesia is slower than with spinal anesthesia. Larger volumes of local anesthetics are required. This and the increased vascularity of the epidural space compared to the subarachnoid space leads to some increased risk of systemic absorption and resulting toxicity. Although there is the same theoretical risk of hypotension with epidural blocks as with spinal blocks, the slower onset of action means less risk of a rapid fall in blood pressure, allowing more time for compensatory mechanisms to come into play. The result is less risk of clinically significant hypotension with epidural blocks.

The duration of action is partially dependent on the type of local anesthetic chosen as is true with spinal blocks. However, other factors such as volume and concentration of the local anesthetic are also important with epidural blocks. The vascularity of the epidural space leads to rapid absorption. This absorption can be slowed by administration of epinephrine. In fact, epinephrine is frequently used with epidural anesthesia for the purpose of decreasing absorption, thereby extending the duration of action and decreasing the risk of systemic toxicity.

A major advantage of epidural anesthesia is the capacity to place a catheter into the epidural space. This can be left in place and used for repeat injections in cases where prolonged anesthesia is needed. Since there is no dural puncture, spinal headache does not occur. On the other hand, if there is accidental dural puncture when placing an epidural injection, a spinal headache is a frequent occurrence owing to the large bore needle used.

Disadvantages include the fact that epidural anesthesia requires greater expertise to administer. Accidental vascular injection is more common because of the vascularity of the epidural space. As noted earlier, this increases the risk of systemic toxicity. An accidental injection into the subarachnoid space with the large volumes of anesthetic usually used in an epidural can result in a high spinal anesthesia with respiratory paralysis.

Caudal Anesthesia. Caudal anesthesia is really an epidural anesthetic placed through the sacral hiatus into the sacral or caudal canal. A caudal block requires a relatively large volume (15–20 ml) of local anesthetic. Onset of anesthesia is slow, being apparent in 5 minutes but requiring 15 minutes for complete block.

Caudal anesthesia is particularly suited to anorectal surgery. It provides a dense sacral block suitable for work on the anal canal. Its main advantage over lumbar epidural anesthesia is the lesser risk of accidental dural puncture, but if the injection is improperly placed above the S-2 level (the termination of the dural sac), spinal headache is nearly a certainty. Also, since a caudal block is routinely placed with the patient in the prone position, there is no need to reposition the patient after the block if the prone position is going to be used for operation.

Disadvantages of caudal block include a highly variable level of anesthesia related to variations in the capacity of the caudal canal and highly variable rates of drug diffusion. Variable anatomic abnormalities result in a failure rate of caudal anesthesia as high as 10 percent.[14] Since injection is made approximately 5 cm above the tip of the coccyx, this type of regional anesthesia is the most likely to be limited by perianal suppuration. Caudal blocks have the greatest systemic absorption of the techniques discussed here and thus the greatest risk of toxicity.

Local Anesthesia. Many anorectal procedures can be safely performed using local anesthesia (Table 5-1). Those procedures limited to the anal canal such as hemorrhoidectomy, sphincterotomy, and low, simple fistulas are particularly suited to local block. Procedures that require relaxation of the puborectalis or the pelvic floor are best performed under a regional block or a general anesthetic. These include most transanal excisions and complex fistulas.

The use of local anesthetic has many distinct advantages over other forms of anesthesia. It is well tolerated by even the poorest risk patients with little risk of postoperative problems. The need for intravenous fluid to compensate for peripheral vasodilation is minimal. The complication rate from the anesthetic itself is very low.

Although there are at least ten local anesthetic agents, we limit our use to two. This allows complete familiarity with the agents being used. Lidocaine 1% and bupivacaine 0.25% are our agents of choice for local infiltration in anorectal surgery. Both are used with epinephrine 1:200,000 for the purpose of vasoconstriction. The vasoconstrictive property aids in intra-

Table 5-1   Local Anesthetic Agents

| Agent | Usual Duration | Maximum Single Dose | | Dose/kg |
		With Epinephrine	Without Epinephrine	
Lidocaine (Xylocaine)	1–2 h	500 mg	300 mg	5–7 mg
Bupivacaine (Marcaine)	2–4 h	225 mg	175 mg	2–4 mg

Adapted from: Cousins MJ, Bridenbaugh PO. *Neural Blockade in Clinical Anesthesia and Management of Pain.* Philadelphia: JB Lippincott, 1990:112.

operative hemostasis and decreases the absorption rate, leading to a decreased risk of systemic toxicity and a prolonged effect. Limiting the number of agents used makes it easier to remember maximum dosage which is 500 mg for lidocaine and 225 mg for bupivacaine. *These maximums should not be exceeded.*

Injection of local anesthetic for anorectal surgery can be terribly uncomfortable for the patient if not done in a controlled manner. It is preferable to have the patient heavily sedated for the actual injection. This can be a concern if the patient is in the prone position. However, if the patient is maintained in the left lateral position during injection, sedation to the point of brief loss of consciousness may be used so long as airway control is maintained by the anesthesiologist.[15] When the patient is again fully awake with protective airway reflexes, full prone position may be obtained.

In the absence of such heavy sedation, mild sedation with slow, steady injection is the key to maintaining a comfortable patient. We prefer to mix equal parts of the lidocaine and the bupivacaine to take advantage of the rapid onset of the former and the long duration (2 to 4 h) of the latter. Initial injection is made bilaterally with a 1.2-cm 30-gauge needle. After the perianal skin has been infiltrated circumferentially in this manner, a 3.75-cm 25-gauge needle is used to make a submucosal injection circumferentially in the anal canal. We have not found it necessary to inject deeper than this needle will allow. Emphasis is placed on injecting in the posterolateral position bilaterally because this is where the heaviest concentration of nerves is found. The process is one of true infiltration with the needle being kept in constant motion. This decreases the risk of a significant vascular injection and resultant toxicity. Generally, an adequate block can be achieved with a total of 20 ml (100 mg lidocaine and 25 mg bupivacaine) of solution, although occasionally 30 ml (150 mg lidocaine and 37.5 mg bupivacaine) is required (Fig. 5-19).

It is possible to perform a bilateral pudendal nerve block during the infiltration of local anesthesia. This is done by inserting the nondominant index finger in the anal canal and palpating the ischial tuberosity. A 22-gauge spinal needle is then used to inject around the nerve. Generally, 5 to 10 ml of solution on each side provides a satisfactory block (Fig. 5-20).

The use of local infiltration can also benefit the patient undergoing general anesthesia. Once the block is in place, the general anesthetic agent need only maintain a level of anesthesia sufficient for tolerance of an endotracheal tube if the prone position is being used. If the patient is not intubated, even lighter anesthesia may be adequate. When epinephrine is used as a part of the local agent, the same hemostatic advantage described above can be realized. Finally, the local block will provide

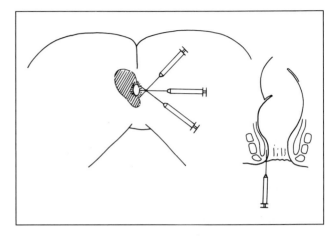

Figure 5-19.   Technique of local infiltration to block the anal canal. The shaded area represents the proportionate distribution of local anesthetic around the anal canal.

complete pain control during the initial postoperative period.

The user of local anesthetics must be familiar with the potential adverse effects and their management. True allergic reactions are rare. Most systemic reactions are due to excessive plasma levels caused by accidental intravascular injection. Infrequently, excessive dosage results in toxic plasma levels due to absorption from tissue.[16]

Signs of toxicity from local anesthetics are manifested in the central nervous and cardiovascular systems. Early signs of toxicity in the central nervous system are excitatory with restlessness, vertigo, tinnitus, and slurred speech. Progression can lead to seizures and ultimately to CNS depression. Toxicity to the cardiovascular system results in peripheral vasodilatation and myocardial depression. This is manifested

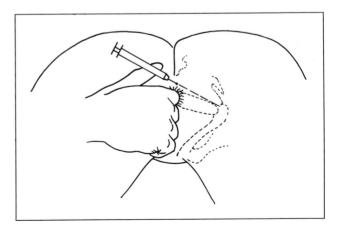

Figure 5-20.   Transanal placement of pudendal nerve block.

clinically by hypotension, prolonged P-R interval and widened QRS complex on ECG, decreased cardiac output, and ultimately AV block.[17]

Treatment of toxicity is symptomatic. Seizures are treated with diazepam in repeated 5-mg doses. Oxygen should be administered immediately. The airway must be cleared and protected and aspiration prevented. Intubation may be necessary. Hypotension should be treated with intravenous fluids and vasopressors.[18]

References

1. Milligan ET, Morgan CN, Jones LE, Officer R. Surgical anatomy of the anal canal, and the operative treatment of haemorrhoids. *Lancet.* 1937;2: 1119–1124.

2. Ferguson JA, Mazier WP, Ganchrow MI, Friend WG. The closed technique of hemorrhoidectomy. *Surgery.* 1971;70:480–484.

3. Atkinson KG, Baird RM. Modified Buie amputation for extensive hemorrhoidal disease. *Am J Surg.* 1978;135:862–864.

4. Fansler WA, Anderson JK. A plastic operation for certain types of hemorrhoids. *JAMA.* 1933;101: 1064–1066.

5. Goldberg SM, Gordon PH, Nivatvongs S. *Essentials of Anorectal Surgery.* Philadelphia: JB Lippincott; 1980:80.

6. Nivatvongs S. Alternative positioning of patients for hemorrhoidectomy. *Dis Colon Rectum.* 1980;23: 308–309.

7. Roberts PL, Schoetz DJ Jr, Murray JJ, Coller JA, Veidenheimer MC. Use of new retractor to facilitate mucosal proctectomy. *Dis Colon Rectum.* 1990;33:1063–1064.

8. Parks AG. Pathogenesis and treatment of fistula-in-ano. *Br Med J.* 1961;1:463–467.

9. Stoelting RK, Miller RD. *Basics of Anesthesia.* 2nd ed. New York: Churchill Livingstone; 1989: 89–90,173–188.

10. Dripps RD, Eckenhoff JE, Vandam LD, eds. *Introduction to Anesthesia: The Principles of Safe Practice.* 7th ed. Philadelphia: WB Saunders; 1988:211–258.

11. Greene NM. *Physiology of Spinal Anesthesia.* 2nd ed. Huntington, NY: Robert E Krieger; 1976:171–172.

12. Dripps RD, Eckenhoff JE, Vandam LD, eds. *Introduction to Anesthesia: The Principles of Safe Practice.* 7th ed. Philadelphia: WB Saunders; 1988:233.

13. Phillips OC, Ebner H, Nelson AT, Black MH. Neurologic complications following spinal anesthesia with lidocaine: a prospective review of 10,440 cases. *Anesthesiology.* 1969;30:284.

14. Stoelting RK, Miller RD. *Basics of Anesthesia.* 2nd ed. New York: Churchill Livingstone; 1989:186.

15. Poulard J-B, Cooperman A, Holtzman R, Margolis IB. Anorectal infiltration anesthesia in the prone position. *Dis Colon Rectum.* 1986;29:676–677.

16. Stoelting RK, Miller RD. *Basics of Anesthesia.* 2nd ed. New York: Churchill Livingstone; 1989:86.

17. Goodman LS, Gilman A, eds. *The Pharmacological Basis of Therapeutics.* 5th ed. New York: Macmillan Publishing Co; 1975:385, 396.

18. Dripps RD, Eckenhoff JE, Vandam LD, eds. *Introduction to Anesthesia: The Principles of Safe Practice.* 7th ed. Philadelphia: WB Saunders; 1988:221.

CHAPTER 6

FUNCTIONAL ANORECTAL DISORDERS AND PHYSIOLOGICAL EVALUATION

Ridzuan Farouk, Graeme Scott Duthie, and David Charles Craig Bartolo

The continence mechanism is a complex one involving local and spinal reflex arcs with a cerebral input acquired by learning. Somatic and visceral muscle function is integrated with a sensory input to attain continence. Interaction between these variables creates the complex physiological mechanism that converts the pelvic floor into a functioning sphincter, thereby maintaining continence.

Parameters and Techniques

Anal Canal Pressure

Method

Anal canal pressures may be measured in a number of ways. Each method is subject to its own disadvantages. Methods available include water-filled perfusion catheters,[1] water- or air-filled balloons,[2] sleeve catheters,[3] and pressure transducers.[4] Perfusion systems rely on the compliance of the system and the rate of perfusion. Furthermore, the pressure generated may induce contractions. Similar alterations in anorectal contractility may arise when using balloon systems. The sleeve catheters cannot distinguish between internal and external sphincter activities. Microtransducers avoid many of these problems by minimizing distention of the anus.

Figure 6-1 shows a water-perfused catheter and Figure 6-2 a microtransducer catheter.

Interpretation

The resting pressure undergoes regular fluctuations with an amplitude of 5 to 25 cm H_2O and a frequency of 10 to 20 per minute.[5] These fluctuations are termed *slow waves* and are thought to be generated by the internal sphincter[6] (Fig. 6-3). The frequency of the slow wave is higher in the lower anal canal, providing for a mechanism that propels small amounts of anal canal contents cephalad into the rectum[5] (Fig. 6-4). A gender difference does exist with males generally having higher pressures. No age relationship has been convincingly demonstrated.[7] Studies to date which do suggest lower pressures in the elderly have been performed in the chronically ill or on those taking several medications.[8] Other studies are flawed by a lack of information about their normal subjects.[9,10]

A zone of high pressure does exist approximately 2 cm from the anal verge,[11] which is caudal to the puborectalis sling. Zones of low pressure have also been identified within the anal canal.[11] Pressures are relatively low in the anterior aspect of the upper third of the anal canal, which corresponds to the area not closely attached to the puborectalis sling, and in the posterior aspect of the lower third of the anal canal.

The relative contributions of the several sphincters have been identified by pudendal nerve block.[12] We have shown a direct relationship between internal sphincter EMG frequency and resting anal canal pressures.[13] We know that division of the internal sphincter

Acknowledgments: Ridzuan Farouk is supported by a grant from the Medical Research Council. Graeme Scott Duthie is supported by a grant from the Wellcome Trust.

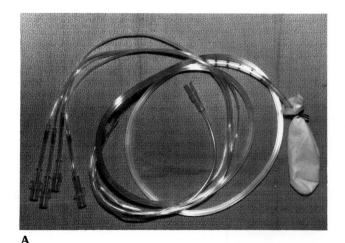

A

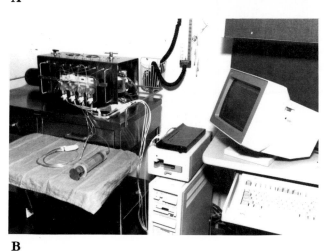

B

Figure 6-1. (A) Waterperfused catheter (Arndorfer Inc, Greenvale, Wisconsin) and perfussion hydralic pump attached to (B) IBM personal computer. Data are interpreted with a PC-Polygram Lower GI Package and hardware interface (Synetics, Inc, Irving, TX).

results in decreased resting pressures, and that the internal sphincter contributes approximately 85% of resting anal pressure.[14] The hemorrhoidal plexuses make a minor contribution to resting pressures,[14] although their influence is greater in subjects with hemorrhoids. These individuals generally have high resting anal pressures and exhibit ultra-slow anal pressure waves. Anal

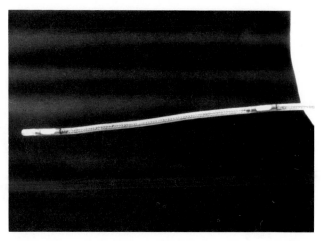

Figure 6-2. Pressure probe with microtransducers mounted at 2 and 6 cm from the catheter tip (Gaeltec Ltd., Isle of Skye, Scotland).

dilation abolished ultra-slow wave activity in 39% of one cohort of patients with hemorrhoids, in whom resting anal pressures fell. Patients with anal fissures[15] and some patients with idiopathic chronic constipation[16] also had ultra-slow wave activity.

When subjects voluntarily contract their anal sphincters, the anal canal pressures rise by between 175 and 270 percent (Fig. 6-5). The distribution of the contraction is generally symmetrical except at about 3 cm, where it is significantly lower anteriorly than posteriorly.[11]

The length of the anal canal can be assessed by manometric measurements.[17] Pressure rises sharply when the probe enters the anal canal. The probe is allowed to rest for 30 seconds to allow the pressure to stabilize and is then slowly withdrawn. This is termed the *pullthrough* technique. When measured by this method, the anal canal is 2.5 to 5 cm long.

Rectal Pressure

Basal pressures within the rectum range between 5 and 25 cm H_2O. The inflation of an intrarectal balloon is associated with an initial rise in pressure, often followed by a secondary increase in pressure due to rectal contrac-

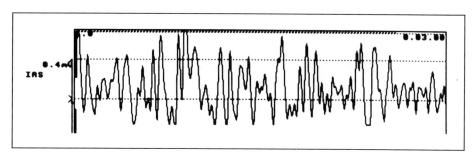

Figure 6-3. Normal internal sphincter EMG appearance.

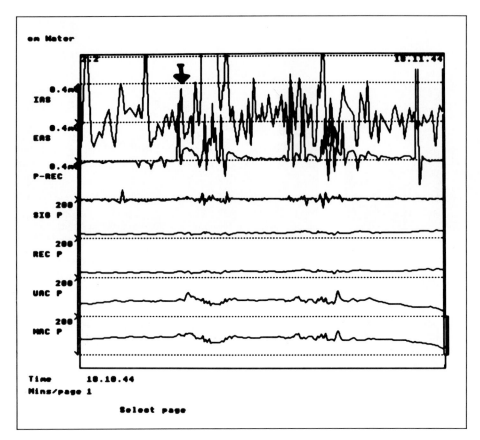

Figure 6-4. Anorectal sampling in a normal subject.

IAS = internal sphincter EMG.
EAS = external sphincter EMG.
P-REC = puborectalis EMGG.
SIG = sigmoid pressure.
REC = rectal pressure.
UAC = upper anal canal pressure.
MAC = Mid-anal canal pressure.

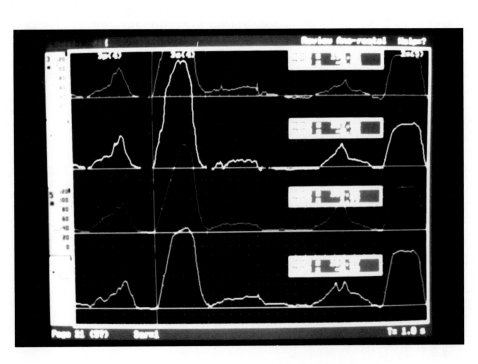

Figure 6-5. Squeeze pressure. Note the elevation over baseline of generally between 175% and 270%.

tion. A degree of accommodation then occurs and the rectal pressure gradually falls to a baseline value. Increasing the distending volume eventually leads to a failure to further accommodate and a large increase in rectal pressure, which may be associated with pain.[18] The contractile response of the rectum to distention is decreased or absent in patients with spinal cord lesions, suggesting a spinal input to this reflex.[19]

Normal Values

The range of normal values for anal canal pressures is somewhat dependent on the method of manometry. In our laboratory the normal range for resting pressure is between 70 and 110 cm H_2O.

The Rectoanal Inhibitory Reflex

Distention of the rectum with a small volume of air causes transient internal sphincter relaxation accompanied by a transient but significant fall in resting anal pressures.[19] Increasing the amount of air or water instilled causes prolonged inhibition of the internal sphincter accompanied by a similar fall in anal pressures. This reflex is termed the *rectoanal inhibitory reflex*.[19] It is conceivable that such laboratory investigations simulate defecation and anorectal sampling.[20] Figure 6-6 shows a balloon catheter that can be used to elicit reflexes. Figure 6-7 shows the reflex itself.

This reflex is absent after circumferential rectal myotomy and in patients with Hirschprung's disease,[21] suggesting that intrinsic myenteric nerve plexuses play a major role in it. Rectal distention leads to descending inhibition of the muscle fibers, possibly mediated by vasoactive intestinal peptide.[22] The role of the extrinsic autonomic system in this reflex is less clear.

Distention of the rectum with consequent relaxation of the internal sphincter causes the anal canal to assume a funnel shape to allow rectal contents access to the specialized sensory epithelium. This allows for sampling and conscious or subconscious perception of rectal contents. Increasing rectal distention leads to complete internal sphincter inhibition. During these episodes, the external sphincter contracts to maintain continence, but since the internal sphincter contributes most of the resting pressure, there is a net fall in anal pressures. If the rectal pressure wave persists, then the sphincter will be overcome as the external sphincter fatigues after 45 to 60 seconds. With the onset of rectal relaxation, the lower rectal contents are returned cephalad by contraction of the pelvic floor muscles, which allows the internal sphincter to recover its resting tone. Interestingly, internal sphincter relaxation will also occur following propulsive activity in the lower sigmoid colon in the presence of an empty rectum.[20] Some of the falls in anal pressures noted during ambulatory recordings may be related to such episodes of sigmoid contractions in the absence of sampling.[20]

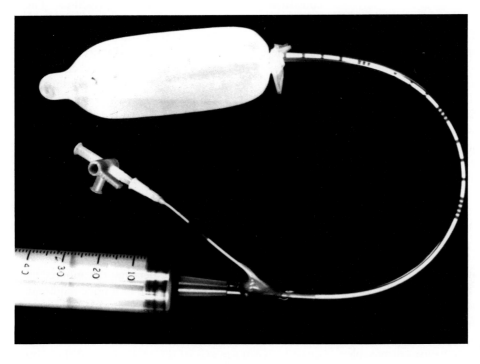

Figure 6-6. Balloon catheter for the assessment of the rectoanal inhibition reflex.

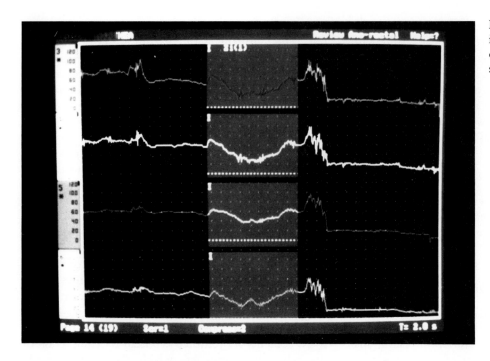

Figure 6-7. Rectoanal inhibitory reflex. Note the transient decrease in internal anal sphincter pressure.

Cinedefecography

An attempt to investigate defecation and its disorders in a physiological manner was described by Burhenne in 1964.[23] This method, which attempts to overcome the problems associated with static proctography, is known as cinedefecography.

Method

Fifty milligrams of a semisolid barium sulphate and potato starch mixture simulating stool may be instilled directly into the rectum. A liquid mixture would be evacuated in 2 seconds, whereas a semisolid mixture is evacuated by the rectum over 10 to 15 seconds, allowing better radiologic visualization. Fluoroscopic techniques are generally used with cineradiographic or video recording to reduce radiation dosage in defecography. The technique can be combined with synchronous anorectal manometry and striated muscle electromyography to allow integrated assessment. A dilute solution of barium sulphate is infused into the rectum until the subject reports a desire to defecate. The patient is seated on a specially designed radiolucent commode (Fig. 6-8). The anorectum is visualized by means of a 100-mm camera (Sircam 106, Siemens) at 0.6 mm focus from an x-ray source generating 125 kV at 1000 mA. In addition to being displayed on the image intensifier the image is stored for further study on a Sony U-matic™ videotape recorder. Commercially manufactured barium paste mixtures are available. These generally contain 200 ml (500 g) of barium paste in a ready-to-use, disposable caulking tube (Fig. 6-8).

Interpretation

We have studied the continence mechanism in the liquid-filled rectum using imaging techniques combined with anorectal manometry and EMG.[24] No contact between the anterior rectal wall and the top of the anal canal was observed during the Valsalva maneuver. Continence was associated with recruitment of the external sphincter and puborectalis EMG, with rectal pressures consistently being lower than anal pressures. These findings have been subsequently confirmed by other investigators.[25] A further study of sphincter repair for incontinence revealed that resting and squeeze anal pressures rose significantly in patients with a successful outcome, whereas the anorectal angle did not significantly alter.[26]

The anorectal angle is often assessed by proponents of the "flap valve theory"[27] and for the assessment of patients with other problems related to defecation such as the perineal descent syndrome, suspected rectal prolapse, rectocele, and the solitary ulcer syndrome. Interpretation is notoriously plagued by the large overlap of results between normal and symptomatic subjects.[28] It is frequently difficult to know what significance to ascribe to the radiologic abnormalities that are documented.

In addition, techniques for defining the anorectal angle lack consistency. Variations in technique require that normal values to be individually generated. Some investigators have measured the angle at the posterior rectal border. We believe the anorectal angle should be measured between the axis of the anal canal and the central axis of the rectum.

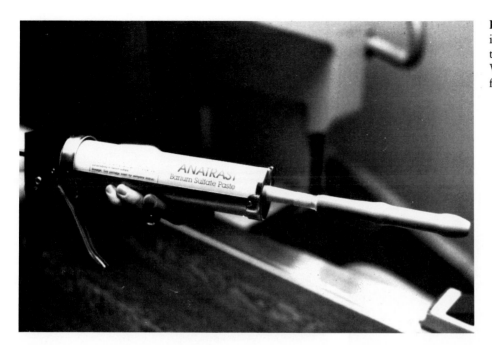

Figure 6-8. Anatrast caulking gun (Lafayette Pharmaceutical Corporation Inc., Fort Worth, TX) and the cinedefecogram.

Normal Values

Using the central anorectal angle, the average angle at rest is around 80°, with hip flexion increasing this angle to over 90° (Fig. 6-9). During defecation this angle opens to about 115° (Fig. 6-10). Squeezing of the anus and the Valsalva maneuver decrease the anorectal angle to between 85° and 100°, with the angle being more acute in anal squeezing (Fig. 6-11). Changing position from lateral decubitus to sitting straightens the resting angle, with no change from sitting to standing.[28,29]

The position of the anorectal junction is another parameter which may be assessed by defecography or scintigraphy in the measurement of perineal descent. Similar problems as for the anorectal angle exist for the assessment of the perineal plane because of different

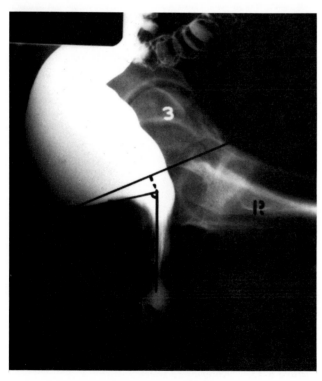

Figure 6-9.   Anorectal angle at rest.

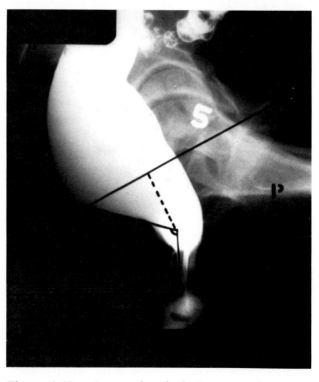

Figure 6-10.   Anorectal angle during evacuation.

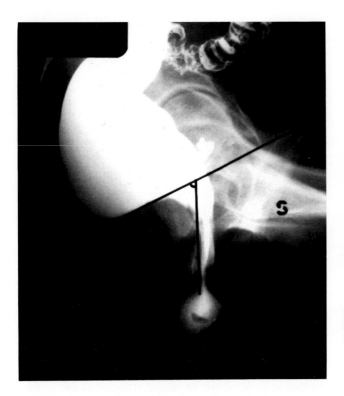

Figure 6-11.   Anorectal angle during squeezing.

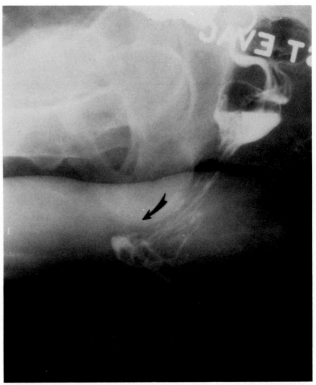

Figure 6-12.   Rectoanal intussusception (at arrow).

interpretations of which anatomic landmarks should be used. The anorectal angle at rest lies closest to a line joining the tip of the coccyx to the most anterior part of the symphysis pubis. This is the line of the perineal plane used by the authors. Radiologic assessment of descent is superior to use of a perineometer.[30] Perineal descent of between 1 and 3 cm occurs on straining in all patients. Descent in excess of this range is defined as a clinical entity: the descending perineal syndrome.[31]

Abnormal Findings

Perineal descent in excess of 3 cm; an increase in the anorectal angle during squeezing and, conversely, no change or a decrease in the anorectal angle during straining; and the presence of a rectal intussusception, rectocele, or enterocele are all considered abnormal. However, such findings are often present in normal subjects.[28,29,32]

Defecography is the only method for assessing anorectal function that provides anatomic detail of mucosal prolapse, intussusception (Fig. 6-12), rectocele (Fig. 6-13), and enterocele (Fig. 6-14). One study illustrated that half of both male and female groups of volunteers showed radiologic evidence of mucosal prolapse and intussusception. Of the 21 women studied, 17 also had a rectocele, which must therefore be considered the norm in women.[33] Because of this overlap, these

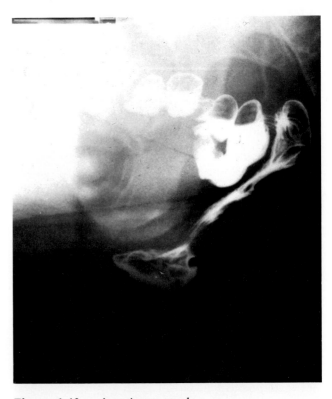

Figure 6-13.   Anterior rectocele.

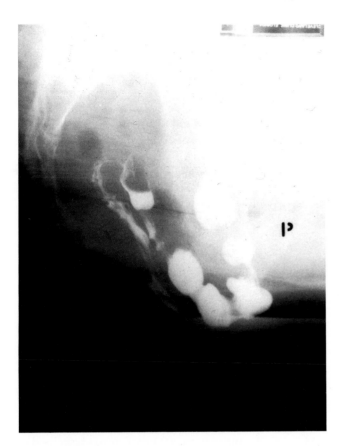

Figure 6-14.   Enterocele.

studies must be interpreted along with the clinical history before the treatment plan can be formulated.

Electromyography

Method

Electromyography (EMG) is one of the main techniques used to investigate the internal and external sphincters and the pelvic floor muscles. Individual muscle fibers derived from a motor unit summate to form the motor unit action potential. This potential can be recorded at a greater distance than that which is required to record individual muscle fiber activity.

Concentric Needle Electrodes.   Concentric needle electrodes are commonly used. They consist of bare-tipped steel wire 0.1 mm in diameter with an insulating resin (Fig. 6-15). The area of uptake of the electrode is small, and any electrical activity recorded can be assumed to originate where the electrode is inserted. However, individual muscle fiber action potentials cannot be identified reliably using concentric needle electrodes.

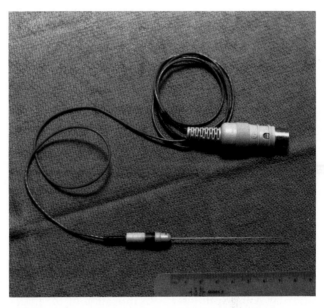

Figure 6-15.   Concentric EMG needle electrode.

Single-Fiber Electrodes.   A single-fiber EMG electrode that has an uptake radius of 270 microns can record the activity of individual muscle fibers within a motor unit. The electrode consists of a needle slightly narrower than 0.1 mm filled with resin (Fig. 6-16). A central wire opens at the midshaft of the electrode through a 25-μg leading off surface. The cannula of the electrode represents the reference electrode and a separate ground electrode is also required. An amplifier with a 500-Hz low frequency filter setting and a trigger delay line are required with the amplifier set at 2 to 5 ms per division. The mean duration of motor unit potentials consisting of more than one component recorded by this method is less than 8 ms.[34]

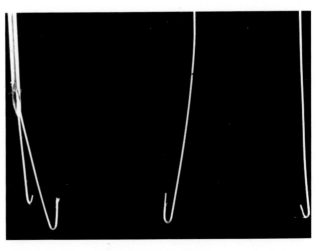

Figure 6-16.   Fine wires, 0.13 mm in diameter, bared and barbed, used for electromyography.

Ambulatory Electromyography. We have developed an ambulatory method of assessing individual patients using fine wire electrodes to measure the EMG activity of the internal sphincter, external sphincter, and puborectalis.[20] Two Teflon-coated steel wires, each 0.13 mm in diameter with the tips bared 1 mm and barbed, are introduced through a 21-gauge sterile hypodermic needle into these muscles. The small diameter of the wires and prior introduction of a local anesthetic to the area ensures that the procedure is comfortable and that the patient remains unaware of the presence of these electrodes once inserted. Electrical detection is related to a ground electrode placed low on the patient's back. All the wires are attached to an ambulatory recorder (Fig. 6-17).

Abnormal Findings

Internal Anal Sphincter. Examination of the internal sphincter in normal controls reveals electrical slow wave activity which is sinusoidal in nature at a frequency of 15 to 35 cycles per minute.[35] Several groups of pacemaker cells are present within the lower sphincteric portion, each group generating a slightly different frequency. This slow wave activity is not disrupted by general anesthesia or by pudendal nerve blockade.[12] The frequency of the internal sphincter slow wave has a linear relationship with resting anal canal pressures and is reduced in patients with neurogenic fecal incontinence[13] and full-thickness rectal prolapse (unpublished observations). No such correlation was found between the amplitude of slow waves and resting anal pressures.[13]

The internal sphincter is continuously active.[5] In vitro examination of isolated strips of sphincter muscle reveals it to be in a continuously tonic state[36] (see Fig. 6-3). This indicates that a pure myogenic origin is partially responsible for basal tone. Activity of the internal sphincter slow wave is not constant, and recruitment occurs following events that challenge the continence mechanism such as coughing. There is diminished activity during sleep, which is accompanied by a fall in resting anal canal pressures. Abolition of internal sphincter electrical activity occurs during rectal distention.[19] Should the rectal distention be sufficient, this abolition of activity becomes prolonged. Passage of flatus, fecal impaction within the rectum, and a rectal prolapse conceivably cause sufficient rectal distention to induce internal sphincter relaxation. In the case of the latter two conditions, fecal incontinence may result.

External Anal Sphincter. The external sphincter is continuously active even in subjects who are asleep, but the amount of activity is dependent on posture and activity.[37] It is a fatigable muscle, however, and voluntary contraction to maintain maximal squeeze and therefore continence lasts for less than a minute.

Distention of the rectum with 50 ml of air causes the recruitment of external sphincter activity, which precedes internal sphincter inhibition.[38] Continued distention of the rectum causes sustained external sphincter EMG activity until 150 to 200 ml of air has been used to inflate the rectal balloon. Complete inhibition of external sphincter activity then occurs (constant relaxation is achieved). Such activity of the external and sphincter can be inhibited by pudendal nerve block.[12] Patients with spinal transection above the third lumbar segment have normal resting external sphincter EMG activity with good recruitment while the patient is coughing.[39,40] Conversely, patients who have sustained sphincter injury may show either electrical silence (Fig. 6-18) or more commonly, polyphasia and patterns of denervation.

Digital traction on the anal canal leads to recruitment of the external sphincter and puborectalis EMG activity.[40] In normal subjects this EMG activity is sustained and followed by a sharp burst of EMG activity (the *closing reflex*)[40] when traction is released. Such evidence supports a cortical input to this reflex which is abolished by spinal injury. The "normal" response to defecation involves pelvic muscle relaxation in most subjects and it is unlikely that there is sustained recruitment of the external sphincter during defecation. The closing reflex is commonly seen at the end of defecation and appears to be a physiologic entity.

The puborectalis muscle forms a part of the pelvic floor musculature and exhibits almost identical electrophysiological characteristics with the external anal sphincter during coughing and straining. Indeed, the two muscles appear to function as a single unit during

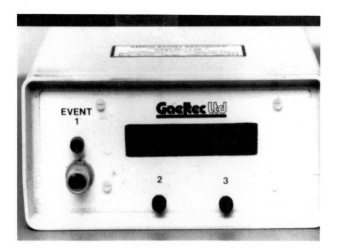

Figure 6-17. Ambulatory recorder used for integrated recordings of anorectal EMGs and pressures (Gaeltec Ltd., Isle of Skye, Scotland).

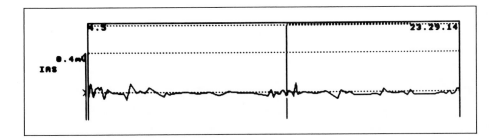

Figure 6-18. Sphincter electrical silence in idiopathic fecal incontinence.

such activity. Pudendal nerve blockade does not abolish pelvic floor contraction.[12] It has been traditionally assumed that the puborectalis and the external anal sphincter function as a single unit, but this assumption was challenged by the finding of differing responses of these muscles to rectal distention in the cat.[41] Ambulatory monitoring in humans, however, to a large extent confirms that these muscles often act in concert.

The degree of correlation between straining in the laboratory setting and normal defecation remains uncertain. Ihre studied pressure and EMG changes during evacuation of a rectal balloon in 11 patients.[42] External sphincter and puborectalis activity was inhibited in 8 subjects while the remainder exhibited continued sphincter activity during straining. We have studied 12 patients who, while straining, displayed inappropriate pelvic muscle contraction which exceeded 50 percent of basal activity. Ambulatory monitoring in 9 of these patients failed to confirm such inappropriate contraction on defecation.[43] Such observations should dictate caution in the interpretation of laboratory-based findings, particularly in the diagnosis of anismus.

Of Kerremans' subjects, 80 percent showed a temporary sustained increase in external sphincter EMG activity during straining.[5] Other observers have described initial external sphincter recruitment followed by complete inhibition while straining.[39] Paraplegic patients who are able to raise their intraabdominal pressures voluntarily also exhibit initial recruitment of pelvic floor activity followed by inhibition.[44]

Pudendal Nerve Assessment

Technique

Transanal pudendal nerve stimulation provides a method of assessing pelvic floor neuropathy.[45] A glove-mounted electrode (St. Mark's Pudendal Electrode 13L40, Dantec Electronics, Bristol, U.K.) is connected to a pulsed stimulus generator (Medelec Mystro) and the pudendal nerve is transanally stimulated as it passes over the ischial spines. The latent period between pudendal nerve stimulation and electromechanical response of the muscle is measured with an oscilloscope (Medelec Mystro). The electrode is shown in Figure 6-19. Generally each of the two nerves is stimulated three times and the average latency is accepted.

Interpretation

Prolonged pudendal nerve terminal motor latency is seen in the majority of patients with idiopathic fecal incontinence,[45] patients with a rectal prolapse,[46] and those with double anorectal and urinary incontinence.[47] Damage to the pudendal nerves is thought to occur in 60 percent of women who have sustained injury to the external sphincter.[48] Furthermore, 20 percent of women who undergo vaginal delivery without apparent injury to the external sphincter have prolonged pudendal nerve terminal motor latencies. Subsequent recovery occurs in 15 percent of these patients.[48] Normal pudendal nerve terminal motor latency is 1.6 to 1.9 ms for those below 55 years of age and 1.9 to 2.2 ms for those 55 years and over.

Determination of pudendal nerve conduction velocity is often complemented by the estimation of single muscle fiber density.[49] Fiber density is calculated using single-fiber EMG electrodes to estimate the mean number of single-fiber action potentials recorded within an uptake area in 20 different positions within the muscle. This is done by inserting four separate electrodes into the muscle and adjusting the position of the electrode within these individual insertions. Following injury to the motor unit, reinnervation will cause an increase in fiber density because more fibers within the uptake area will be innervated by a single axon. In normal subjects the fiber density of most muscles is less than two, although this increases slightly with age.[50] Normal fiber density, therefore, varies with age but is generally about 1.8 in a normal healthy adult external sphincter.

Perineometry

Up to 98 percent of normal subjects have been shown to exhibit a degree of pelvic floor descent on straining. One method of measuring the amount of descent is by defecography.[29,32,33] The perineometer is a custom-

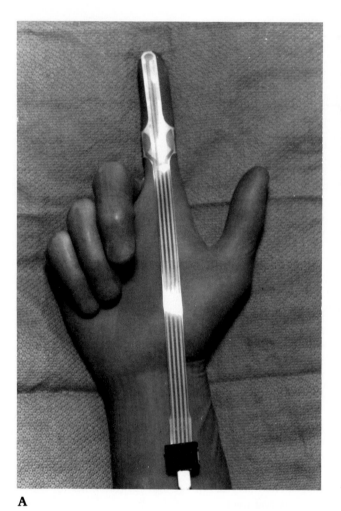

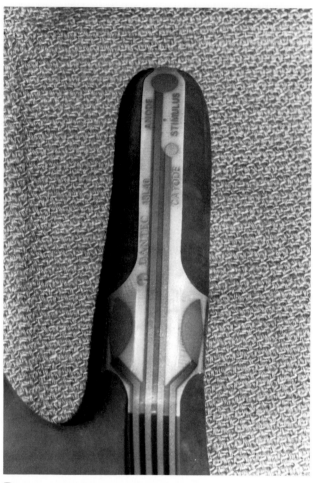

A

B

Figure 6-19.   (A) The Snash-Henry disposable pudendal nerve stimulatory electrode (Dantec Electronics, Skovlunde, Denmark). (B) Close-up view.

designed instrument used to measure such pelvic floor descent (Fig. 6-20). One purported advantage of this device is that it does not require exposure to radiation. In addition this instrument provides economy, safety, portability, reproducibility, and ease of operation.[51] Despite these advantages, it is not so accurate as radiographic assessment in the estimation of pelvic floor descent.[30]

Method

The perineometer consists of a central latex cylinder graduated in centimeters which is free to move in a vertical direction. This cylinder is flanked by two vertical steel limbs which can be adjusted along a horizontal plane. The patient is placed in a left lateral decubitus position. The latex cylinder is placed at the anal verge while the two steel limbs rest on the patient's ischial tuberosities. A note is taken of the perineal plane at rest using the graduated scale on the latex cylinder and the

patient is then asked to strain. A second recording of the new position of the perineal plane is then taken; the difference between the first and second readings is the amount of perineal descent.

Interpretation

In normal subjects the perineal plane at rest lies between 1.9 and 3.1 cm above the ischial tuberosities.[51] On straining the perineal plane descends by a mean of 1.6 cm to a position between 0 and 2.1 cm above the ischial tuberosities. There is no significant gender difference for these values. In patients with the descending perineal syndrome the perineal plane at rest is between 1 and 3 cm above the ischial tuberosities and descends by a mean of 1.2 cm below this plane on straining.

The perineometer has been shown to be a relatively insensitive instrument when compared with defecography in estimation of the amount of perineal descent. A significant number of patients with the descending per-

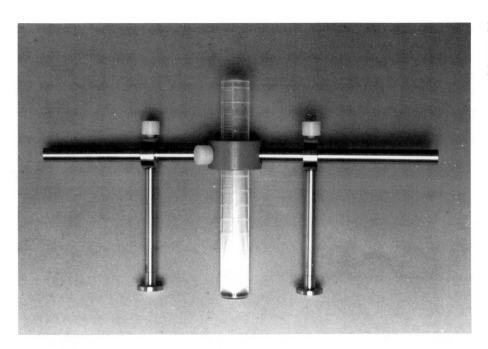

Figure 6-20. Perineometer. (Photo courtesy of Michael V. Kamm, M.D., London, England.)

ineal syndrome may not be diagnosed if the perineometer alone is used.[30]

Rectal Compliance

Rectal capacity determines the frequency and degree of urgency for defecation. Appreciation of rectal filling occurs with volumes as small as 10 ml, but its capacity often approaches 300 ml before there is an urgent desire to defecate. This can be assessed physiologically by instilling air or water at a steady rate into a rectal balloon. The change in volume is then compared with the rate of change of rectal pressure. Initially the proctometrogram shows small increases in rectal pressure per unit volume instilled, but the rise in pressure becomes progressively steeper as the maximum tolerated volume is approached. Thus values can be recorded of volumes causing the initial sensation of distention, the desire to defecate, urgency, and the maximum tolerated volume. These values provide an estimate of rectal compliance which is calculated by plotting volume versus pressure and calculating the gradient. Low compliance is seen in patients with a rectal prolapse,[52] radiation proctitis,[53] colitis (unpublished observations), and rectal neoplasms. Normal compliance can be restored by excision of the noncompliant rectum and construction of a neorectum.[54] This is possible by forming a pouch from a suitable length of colon following anterior resection or using terminal ileum in restorative proctocolectomy.

Patients with rectal prolapse are known to experience sustained internal sphincter inhibition with only minimal rectal distention.[52] This may occur because the rectum is full by virtue of being occupied by the prolapse or because the sphincter is disrupted. Repairing the prolapse by implanting foreign material may not improve the situation because such materials make the rectum rigid and therefore noncompliant. Our early experience with simple suture rectopexy with resection of redundant colon for full-thickness rectal prolapse reveals evidence of internal sphincter recovery based on EMG and anal resting pressure measurements (unpublished observations). This method of treatment has the additional advantage of not leaving the patient with an iatrogenic noncompliant rectum.

Sensitivity

Rectal filling is perceived as a fullness felt in the pelvis. Ability to appreciate this filling is thought to be related to stretch receptors within the rectal wall and pelvic floor. Such sensation therefore persists after rectal excision.[55] Balloon distention up to approximately 15 cm from the anal orifice leads to a rectal sensation of fullness whereas distention above this level elicits a colicky discomfort in the left iliac fossa.[56] Rectal sensation is thought to be related to rectal contractile activity. Cerebral evoked potentials have been elicited from electrical stimulation of the rectosigmoid.[57]

The anal canal mucosa is richly innervated from the anal canal margin to the dentate line.[58] A sensory input is received from the pudendal nerve.[12] Pudendal nerve block brings about a loss of sensation of the perianal and genital area with no impairment of rectal sensation. Maximal anal perception is thought to occur at the midanal canal which is composed of transitional epithelium.[58] Discrimination of sensation by the anal epithelium is less precise than that of adjacent perianal skin, however.

The role of anal sensation in the maintenance of continence has been questioned. Read and Read applied topical lignocaine into the anal canal of normal subjects without causing fecal incontinence.[59] There was, however, a significant reduction in the ability to maintain external sphincter contraction. Sensation may therefore prove crucial to patients with impaired sphincteric mechanisms in providing sufficient warning of impending incontinence. The relevance of this study is somewhat questionable because saline cannot be judged to be a physiologic simulator of feces.

Electrical Sensitivity

We assess anal mucosal sensitivity by estimating electrosensitivity.[60] A 14-gauge Nelaton catheter is used for this purpose by attaching two copper electrodes spaced 1 cm apart at the tip. Copper wires are connected to the electrodes and a constant current generator (Department of Medical Physics, Bristol Royal Infirmary, Bristol, U.K.) is used to apply a stimulus at 5 pulses per second (Fig. 6-21). Impaired anal sensitivity has been documented in all patients with anorectal disorders except those with anal fissures. Sensation improves following surgery for sphincter repair[26,61] and after rectopexy for prolapse[52] (Fig. 6-22). We attribute this improvement in anal sensation following surgery to the restoration of the prolapsed anal transition zone to anatomic normality.

Thermal Sensitivity

Rectal temperature is lower than that in the anal canal. The anal canal mucosa is highly sensitive to temperature changes between 32 to 42° C.[62] The temperature gradient between the rectum and anal canal is, however, only 0.2° C.[63] There is a regional thermal gradient between the rectum and lower, mid, and upper anal canal of 0.4, 0.2, and 0.1 degrees respectively. There is some debate regarding the importance of thermal sensitivity in health.[64] although in patients with neurogenic fecal incontinence the lower rectum has been shown to be significantly less sensitive to temperature changes.

Anorectal Sampling

The transitional zone within the anal canal is lined with a specialized sensory epithelium that can discriminate with a high index of accuracy variables such as temperature, pain, and light touch.[62] This epithelium in normal subjects is exposed to rectal contents on average seven times per hour (see Fig. 6-4).[20] Rectal contents distend mechanoreceptors within the rectal wall leading, by means of intrinsic nerve pathways, to inhibition

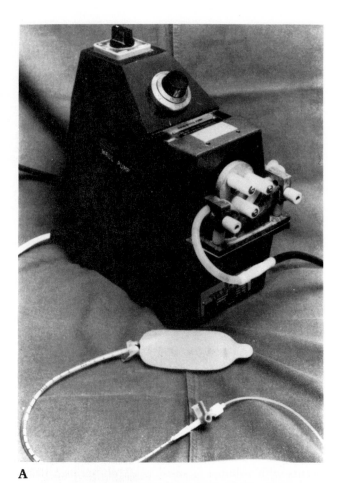

A

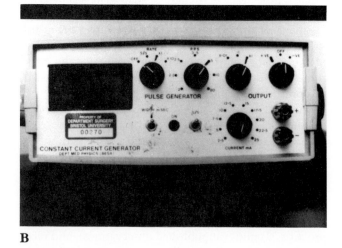

B

Figure 6-21.   (A) A constant infusion pump, as meter and balloon for measuring rectal compliance. (B) Current generator used to assess mucosal electrosensitivity.

of the internal sphincter. The cephalad anal canal opens and rectal contents are exposed to the anal transition zone. Such events are "covered" and continence is maintained by the external sphincter. Each episode lasts for less than 10 s, and therefore recruitment of the

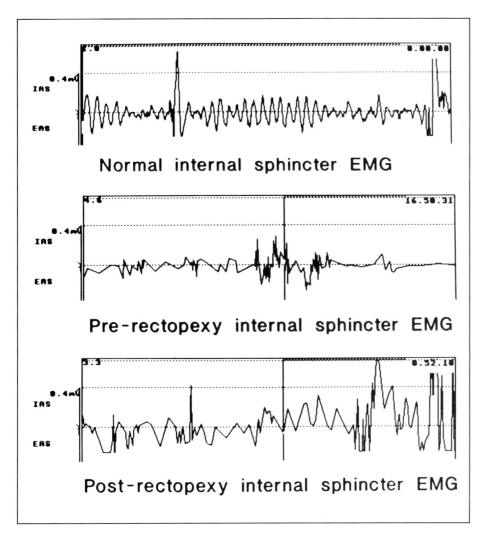

Figure 6-22.   Internal sphincter EMG recovery is associated with recovery of continence following rectopexy for rectal prolapse. (A) Normal EMG. (B) Pre-rectopexy. (C) Postrectopexy.

fatigable external sphincter is easily achieved. This process, termed *sampling,* and allows for differential appreciation of rectal contents. Fewer sampling episodes occur during sleep and prolonged fasting.[64,65] Figure 6-23 shows the sampling in a patient with neurogenic fecal incontinence. Figure 6-24 shows internal and sphincter EMG recovery after rectopexy for prolapse.

Integrated Anorectal Physiologic Assessment

Most current attempts to assess healthy and diseased subjects are nonphysiologic. As a result, increasingly sophisticated attempts are being made to assess these patients in a physiologic setting. Baseline measurements such as anal canal sensation and rectal compliance can still be a reliable indicator of anorectal disease. This can be supplemented by neurophysiologic investigations such as estimation of pudendal nerve terminal latencies and estimation of single fiber density of individual nerve motor units. A relatively recent and apparently useful

technique of assessing sphincter injuries in the laboratory setting is the use of endoanal ultrasound.[66,67]

We have developed a seven-channel ambulatory recording system that allows monitoring of patients within the more physiologic environment of their homes over a period of 12 to 24 hours.[20] Three EMG channels and four pressure channels are used in this system (Fig. 6-24). The recording is digitalized by the recorder and can be viewed in real-time mode or subsequently transferred for viewing and storage on disk facilities. This allows for an integrated assessment of EMG and pressure recordings in an ambulatory setting. This recording lasts for between 12 and 24 hours and allows for assessment of sphincter and pressure changes during sampling, passage of flatus, defecation, and micturition as well as other events that are not reproducible in a laboratory setting. These results are reproducible and have identifiable variables for patient groups. Progress in understanding the physiology and pathology of the continence mechanism may come from such integrated assessment.

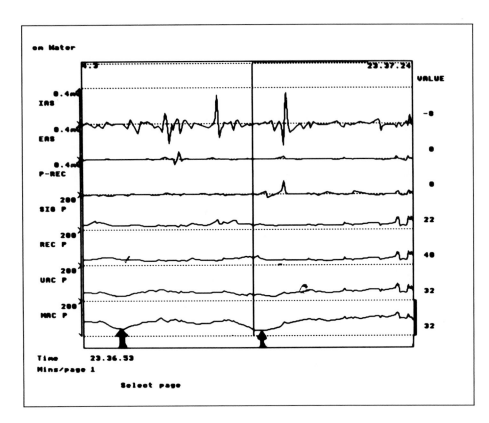

Figure 6-23. Anorectal sampling in a patient with neurogenic fecal incontinence.

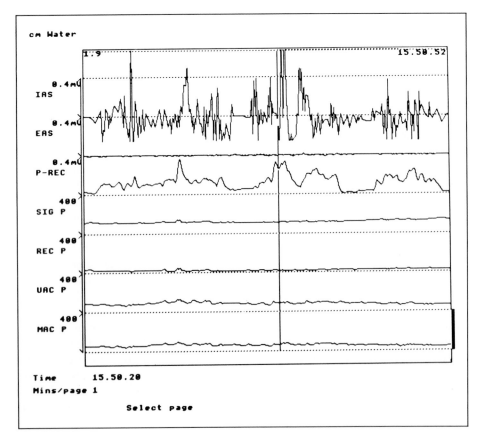

Figure 6-24. Example of EMG and pressure recordings using the integrated ambulatory monitoring system.

IAS = internal sphincter EMG.

EAS = external sphincter EMG.

P-REC = puborectalis EMGG.

SIG = sigmoid pressure.

REC = rectal pressure.

UAC = upper anal canal pressure.

MAC = Mid-anal canal pressure.

Applications of Physiology

Anismus

Diagnosis

Inappropriate contraction of the pelvic floor results in a pelvic outlet obstruction which causes difficulty in evacuation of rectal contents. Such inappropriate contraction of the pelvic floor muscles is termed *anismus*. Synonyms include nonrelaxing puborectalis syndrome and paradoxical puborectalis contraction. Anismus is attributed to the failure of the somatic component of the anal sphincter apparatus to relax to allow spontaneous defecation. The pathophysiology is unclear, however, with similar findings having been reported for the solitary ulcer syndrome, perineal pain, and in normal controls.[68,69] It is precisely because of this that the diagnosis of anismus has been questioned as a nonsignificant finding.[68]

The patient is often a young woman whose main problem is constipation. These patients are usually aware of the need to defecate but are unable to complete the act satisfactorily. Anismus is also associated with a number of neurologic disorders such as spina bifida and Parkinson's disease. The diagnosis is usually made by a combination of electromyography, manometry, and defecography.

As with many other anorectal conditions, these tests are usually performed in an unphysiologic environment. The presence of an investigator peering at one's perineum during attempted defecation can induce anismus in normal subjects, as attested by the finding that asymptomatic normal controls frequently exhibit anismus on defecography.[70] Our own experience is that more than 80 percent of these patients when monitored using ambulatory equipment within the home environment have no such inappropriate contraction of the pelvic floor during defecation.[43]

About half of our patients who have undergone subtotal colectomy and ileorectal anastomosis for slow-transit constipation have anismus. Outcome following surgery for their constipation was not affected by the associated anismus in these cases (unpublished observations). Our patients were a highly selected group from among tertiary referrals. Other groups have achieved a success rate of over 90 percent after thorough evaluation and selection of less than 10 percent of all clinically constipated patients.[71] Moreover success rates of 50 percent or less have resulted when colectomy was undertaken for colonic inertia coexistent with anismus.[72]

Treatment

Surgery as yet has no role in the treatment of anismus. Lateral or posterior division of the puborectalis has failed in the long term to provide any benefit.[73,74] Long anorectal myectomy and the injection of *Botulinum* toxin into the muscle greatly lowers anal pressure with either temporary or permanent fecal incontinence of up to 55 percent.[75] The long-term results of both methods are poor.[76]

In biofeedback training, the patient is shown a viewing screen of his or her own electromyographic tracings and manometric recordings. This allows an opportunity for the subject to exercise and discover which pelvic floor movements allow relaxation.[77,78] The equipment can be computerized and can be portable for home practice sessions.[79] The most favorable results have traditionally been obtained in children.[78] It remains speculative whether patients who improve using this technique would have improved spontaneously. One recent study reviewed 18 patients who underwent outpatient treatment of anismus with intraanal sensor biofeedback.[80] A mean of 10 hour-long sessions resulted in an increase in frequency of unassisted bowel movements from 0 to 7 per week in 89 percent of patients. Figure 6-25 shows a typical intraanal sensor along with the biofeedback computer.

Rectocele

Diagnosis

A large rectocele can cause a pelvic outlet obstruction with resulting constipation and an unsatisfactory feeling of incomplete rectal evacuation. The patient with symptoms arising from a rectocele is usually a middle-aged female, often with a history of a hysterectomy or anal surgery. A history of constipation is common and often there is concurrent rectal bleeding or pain. The patient may report that vaginal digitalization is required to overcome the stool pocketing that occurs. Visual and digital assessment of the anorectum combined with proctoscopy and vaginal speculum examination often confirms the diagnosis. An associated cystocele or enterocele may also be detected by such examination. Many such patients have other anorectal conditions such as hemorrhoids, anal fissure, anal stenosis, rectovaginal fistula, or fistula-in-ano.[81]

Electromyography and manometry have no direct contribution to the diagnosis and management of this condition. Defecography is frequently used to confirm the diagnosis of rectocele. Interpretation is fraught with difficulty as many asymptomatic women have rectoceles measuring up to 1.5 cm as seen on defecography.[33] The finding of a pelvic outlet obstruction in combination with a large rectocele on defecography combined with the history and physical findings is used to determine whether corrective surgery is required. In one retrospective study of outcome following surgery

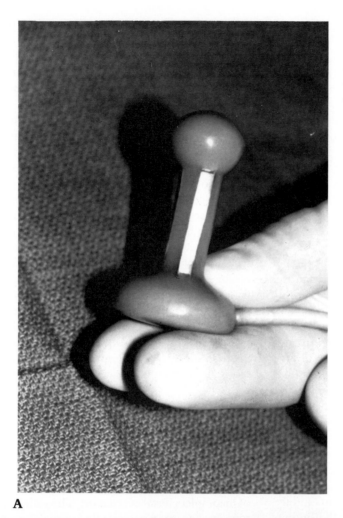

A

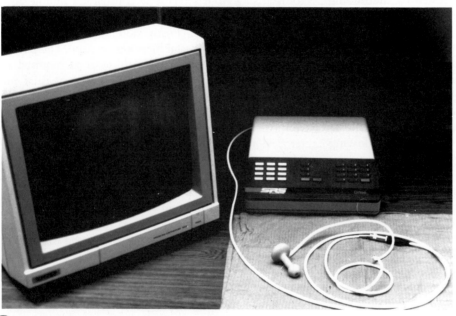

B

Figure 6-25. (A) Perry intraanal EMG-based sensor (PerryMeter™ anal EMG sensor EPS-21, Perry Meter Systems, Strafford, PA) which is attached to (B) Orion™ (Self Regulation Systems, Redmond, WA) biofeedback computer.

for rectocele, the indications for surgery were constipation (75%), rectal bleeding (34%), rectal pain (23%), vaginal digitalization (20%), stool pocketing (19%), large rectocele with associated cystocele or enterocele (11%), and recurrent rectocele (8%).[82]

Treatment

We have little experience of this condition and have not yet seen a patient with obstructed defecation in whom rectocele repair was considered appropriate. Transvaginal[83] or transanal[84] repair are used by other centers for this condition. While accepting that a few patients are symptomatic from stool pocketing, the majority appear to have a rectocele as an incidental finding and are symptomatic from other anorectal disorders such as fissures or hemorrhoids. The decision to perform "corrective" surgery is therefore deferred until the coexisting pathologic condition has been treated.

This approach appears to have been justified by a recent retrospective study. This study reported that concurrent surgery was performed in excess of 80 percent of patients who underwent rectocele surgery.[82] The most common concurrent procedures were for hemorrhoids (64%) and anal fissure (32%). The morbidity reported from this series was relatively high (34%); the most common complication was urinary retention (12.5%). Long-term review of outcome suggests that although there was general patient satisfaction of outcome in about 80 percent of cases, constipation, pain, and bleeding still occurred in a substantial number of patients. More alarming were the rates of incontinence and sexual dysfunction, each complication having been reported in just over a third of patients. The investigators correctly concluded that patient selection for rectocele surgery is difficult and that the concurrent presence of constipation and a rectocele does not imply an association. Patient selection can be improved by anorectal physiologic examination. However, this is certainly not a definitive means of decision making because of the considerable overlap of findings in normal controls and symptomatic patients.[28,29,32]

Descending Perineum Syndrome

Diagnosis

Clinical assessment is based on the presenting history and physical examination findings. The latter include inspection and digital assessment of the anorectum, proctoscopy, sigmoidoscopy, and a limited neurologic assessment of the lumbosacral plexus. Many of these patients do not suffer from fecal incontinence but instead report symptoms of obstructed defecation.[85] Those who are incontinent are graded in a manner

similar to that described by Browning and Parks:[86] grade A, continent to solid, liquid, and flatus; grade B, continent to solid and liquid but incontinent of flatus; grade C, continent to solid but incontinent of liquid and flatus; and grade D, completely incontinent.

Anorectal manometry, electromyography, mucosal electrosensitivity tests, and pudendal nerve latency evaluations are performed as previously outlined in this chapter.

The anorectal angle is measured radiologically. Patients are placed in the left lateral position on the x-ray table with the hips flexed 90° to the trunk. A 50-ml semisolid mixture of barium sulphate and potato starch is injected into the rectum through a small catheter. A plastic ball, 2 cm in diameter and attached to a beaded metal chain, is then inserted into the anal canal. The axis of the rectum is thus outlined with barium while the anal canal is outlined by the metal chain. The anorectal angle is defined as the angle between the central axis of the rectum and the anal canal as shown by the beads. The degree of perineal descent is determined by drawing a line between the tip of the coccyx to the most anterior part of the pubic symphysis, the pubococcygeal line. A perpendicular is then dropped from this line to the apex of the angle formed by the axis of the rectum and the axis of the anus. The distance of the pubococcygeal line to the anorectal angle is then recorded. If the anorectal angle lies above the pubococcygeal line, a positive measurement is recorded, whereas if the angle lies below the line, a negative value is recorded. Lateral radiographs are taken in the positions of rest, maximum sphincter contraction (squeeze), and when bearing down as if to stool (strain).

The findings from radiologic and neurophysiologic studies in continent and incontinent patients with the descending perineal syndrome are similar. This suggests that this syndrome may represent a stage in the development of idiopathic fecal incontinence. Alternatively, patients with perineal descent may develop incontinence secondary to a visceral neuropathy affecting the internal anal sphincter.[81]

Treatment

The treatment of patients with the descending perineal syndrome is often directed at the common presenting complaint of constipation. The treatment of such patients by lateral internal sphincterotomy or anal stretch may result in incontinence due to damage to an already neuropathic internal anal sphincter. The finding of abnormal perineal descent alone is not considered by our group to be an indication for surgical intervention. The development of idiopathic fecal incontinence may indicate the need for surgical intervention such as a postanal repair or anterior sphincteroplasty.

References

1. Harris LD, Winnans CS, Pope CE. Determination of yield pressures: a method for measuring anal sphincter competence. *Gastroenterology*. 1964;50: 754–760.

2. Duthie HL, Watts JM. Contribution of the external sphincter to the pressure zone in the anal canal. *Gut*. 1965;6:64–68.

3. Dent JA. A new technique for continuous sphincter pressure measurement. *Gastroenterology*. 1976;71: 263–267.

4. Mathias JR, Sninsky CA, Millar HD, Clench MH, Davis RH. Development of an improved multi-pressure sensor probe for recording muscle contraction in the human intestine. *Dig Dis Sci* 1985;30: 119–123.

5. Kerremans R. Morphological and physiological aspects of anal continence and defecation. Brussels: Editions Arscia; 1969.

6. Bouvier M, Gonella J. Nervous control of the internal anal sphincter of the cat. *J Physiol*. 1981;310: 457–469.

7. Loening-Buck V, Anuras S. Anorectal manometry in healthy elderly subjects. *J Am Geriatr Soc*. 1984; 32:636–639.

8. Bannister JJ, Abouzecky L, Read NW. Effect of aging on anorectal function. *Gut*. 1987;28:353–357.

9. Matheson DM, Keighly MRB. Manometric evaluation of rectal prolapse and fecal incontinence. *Gut*. 1981;22:126–129.

10. Hamel-Roy J, Devroede G, Arhan P, Tretault JB, Lemieux B, Scott H. Functional abnormalities of the anal sphincter in patients with myotonic dystrophy. *Gastroenterology*. 1984;86:1469–1474.

11. Taylor BM, Beart RW, Phillips SF. Longitudinal and radial variations of pressure in the human anal canal. *Gastroenterology*. 1984;86:693–697.

12. Freckner B, von Euler C. Influence of pudendal block on the function of the internal sphincter. *Gut*. 1975;16:482–489.

13. Duthie GS, Miller R, Bartolo DCC. Internal sphincter electromyographic frequency is related to anal canal resting pressure. Both are reduced in idiopathic fecal incontinence. *Gut* 1990;31:A619.

14. Hancock BD, Smith K. The internal sphincter and Lord's procedure for haemorrhoids. *Br J Surg*. 1975;62:833–836.

15. Hancock BD, Smith K. The internal sphincter and anal fissure. *Br J Surg*. 1977;64:92–95.

16. Arhan P, Devroede G, Jehannin B, et al. Idiopathic disorders of fecal continence in children. *Pediatrics*. 1983;71:774–779.

17. Nivatongs S, Stern HS, Fryd DS. The length of the anal canal. *Dis Colon Rectum*. 1981;24:600–601.

18. Arhan P, Faverdin C, Persoz B, et al. Relationship between viscoelastic properties of the rectum and anal pressure in man. *J Appl Physiol*. 1976;41: 677–682.

19. Denny-Brown D, Robertson EG. An investigation of the nervous control of defecation. *Brain*. 1935; 58:256–310.

20. Miller R, Lewis GT, Bartolo DCC, Cervero F, Mortensen NJMcC. Sensory discrimination and dynamic activity in the anorectum: evidence using a new ambulatory technique. *Br J Surg*. 1988;75: 1003–1007.

21. Lubowski DZ, Nicholls RJ, Swash M, Jordan MJ. Neural control of the internal anal sphincter function. *Br J Surg*. 1987;74:668–670.

22. Burleigh DE. Non-cholinergic, non-adrenergic inhibitory neurons in the human internal sphincter muscle. *J Pharm Pharmacol*. 1983;35:258–260.

23. Burhenne HJ. Intestinal evacuation study: a new roentgenologic technique. *Radiol Clin*. 1964; 33:79–84.

24. Bartolo DCC, Roe AM, Locke-Edmunds JC, et al. Flap valve theory of anorectal incontinence. *Br J Surg*. 1986;73:1012–1014.

25. Bannister JJ, Gibbons C, Read NW. Preservation of fecal continence during rises in intra-abdominal pressure: is there a role for the flap-valve? *Gut*. 1987;28:1242–1245.

26. Miller R, Bartolo DCC, Locke-Edmunds JC, Mortensen NJMcC. A prospective study of conservative and operative treatment for fecal incontinence. *Br J Surg*. 1988;75:101–105.

27. Parks AG. Anorectal incontinence. *Proc R Soc Med*. 1975;68:681–689.

28. Mahieu P, Pringot J, Bodart P, Defecography, I: description of a new procedure and results in normal patients. *Gastrointest Radiol*. 1984;9:247–251.

29. Ekberg O, Nylander G, Fork FT. Defecography. *Radiology*. 1985;155:45–48.

30. Oettle GJ, Roe AM, Bartolo DCC, Mortensen NJMcC. What is the best way of measuring perineal descent? A comparison of radiographic and clinical methods. *Br J Surg*. 1985;72:999–1001.

31. Parks AG, Porter NH, Hardcastle JD. The syndrome of the descending perineum. *Proc R Soc Med*. 1966;59:477–482.

32. Shorvon PJ, McHugh S, Diamant NE, Somers S, Stevenson GW. Defecography in normal volunteers: results and implications. *Gut* 1989;30:1737–1749.

33. Urlaschh JT, Tobon F, Hambrecht T, Ban D, Schuster MM. Electrophysiological aspects of human sphincter function. *J Clin Invest*. 1970; 49:41–48.

34. Swash M, Schwartz MS. *Neuromuscular Disorders: A Practical Approach to the Diagnosis and Management*. Berlin: Springer-Verlag; 1981.

35. Pennickx F. Morphological and physiological aspects of anal function. Leuven: Acco n.v.; 1981.

36. Burleigh DE, D'Mello A, Parks AG. Responses of isolated human internal anal sphincter to drugs and electrical field stimulation. *Gastroenterology*. 1979; 77:484–490.

37. Floyd W, Walls E. Electromyography of the sphincter ani externus in man. *J Physiol*. 1953;16: 638–644.

38. Gaston EA. The physiology of fecal continence. *Surg Gynecol Obstet*. 1948;87:280–290.

39. Parks AG, Porter NH, Melzack J. Experimental study of the reflex mechanism controlling the muscles of the pelvic floor. *Dis Colon Rectum*. 1962;5: 407–414.

40. Porter NH. Physiological study of the pelvic floor in rectal prolapse. *Ann R Soc Med*. 1962;286: 379–404.

41. Dubrovsky B. Effects of anal distension on the sphincter ani externus and levator ani muscles in cats. *Am J Physiol*. 1988;254:G100–G106.

42. Ihre T. Studies in anal function in continent and incontinent patients. *Scand J Gastroenterol*. 1974;9 (suppl 25):5–64.

43. Duthie GS, Bartolo DCC, Miller R. Laboratory tests grossly over-estimate the incidence of anismus. Surgical Research Society; Winter meeting, 1991; London.

44. Melzack J, Porter NH. Studies on the reflex activity of the external sphincter ani in spinal man. *Paraplegia*. 1964;1:277–296.

45. Kiff ES, Swash M. Slowed conduction in the pudendal nerves in idiopathic (neurogenic) fecal incontinence. *Br J Surg*. 1984;71:614–616.

46. Parks AG, Swash M, Urich AB. Sphincter denervation in anorectal incontinence and rectal prolapse. *Gut*. 1977;18:656–665.

47. Snooks SJ, Barnes RPH, Swash M. Damage to the voluntary anal and urinary sphincter musculature in incontinence. *J Neurol Neurosurg Psychiatry*. 1984;47: 1269–1273.

48. Snooks SJ, Setchell M, Swash M, Henry MM. Injury to the innervation of the pelvic floor musculature in childbirth. *Lancet*. 1985;2:546–550.

49. Stalberg E, Thiele B. Motor unit fibre density in the extensor digitorum comunis muscle. *J Neurol Neurosurg Psychiatry*. 1975;38:874–88.

50. Neill ME, Swash M. Increased motor unit fiber density in external sphincter muscle in anorectal incontinence: a single fiber EMG study. *J Neurol Neurosurg Psychiatry*. 1980;43:343–347.

51. Henry MM, Parks AG, Swash M. The pelvic floor musculature in the descending perineum syndrome. *Br J Surg*. 1982;69:470–472.

52. Duthie GS, Bartolo DCC. Pathophysiology and management of rectal prolapse. In: *Recent Advances in Surgery*. Oxford, England: Butterworth-Heineman; 1991.

53. Varma JS, Smith AN, Busuttil A. Correlation of clinical and manometric abnormalities of rectal function following chronic radiation injury. *Br J Surg*. 1985;72:875–878.

54. Keighley MRB, Yoshioka K, Kniot W, Heyer F. Physiological parameters influencing function in restorative proctocolectomy and ileo-pouch-anal anastomosis. *Br J Surg*. 1988;75:997–1002.

55. Lane RH, Parks AG. Function of the anal sphincter following colo-anal anastomosis. *Br J Surg*. 1977; 64:596–599.

56. Goligher JC, Hughes ERS. The sensibility of the colon and rectum. *Lancet*. 1951;2:543–547.

57. Freiling T, Enck P, Weinbeck M. Cerebral responses evoked by electrical stimulation of rectosigmoid in normal subjects. *Dig Dis Sci*. 1989;34:202–205.

58. Duthie HL, Gairns FW. Sensory nerve endings and sensation in the anal region of man. *Br J Surg*. 1960;47:585–595.

59. Read MG, Read NW. Role of anorectal sensation in preserving continence. *Gut*. 1982;23:345–347.

60. Roe AM, Bartolo DCC, Mortensen NJMcC. New method for assessment of anal sensation in various anorectal disorders. *Br J Surg*. 1986;73:310–312.

61. Miller R, Orrom WJ, Cornes H, et al. Anterior sphincter plication and levatorplasty in the treatment of fecal incontinence. *Br J Surg*. 1989;76: 1058–1060.

62. Miller R, Bartolo DCC, Cervero F, Mortensen NJMcC. Anorectal temperature sensation: a comparison of normal and incontinent patients. *Br J Surg*. 1987;74:511–515.

63. Rogers J, Hayward MP, Henry MM, Misiewicz VJ. Temperature gradient between the rectum and anal canal: evidence against the role of temperature sensation as a sensory modality in the anal canal of normal subjects. *Am J Surg*. 1988;78:1083–1085.

64. Kumar D, Waldron D, Williams NS, Browning C, Hutton MRE, Wingate DL. Prolonged anorectal manometry and external anal sphincter electromyography in ambulant human subjects. *Dig Dis Sci*. 1990;35:641–648.

65. Keighley MRB, Winslet MC, Yoshioka K, Lightwood R. Discrimination is not impaired by excision of the anal transition zone after restorative proctocolectomy. *Br J Surg*. 1987;74:1118–1121.

66. Law PJ, Kamm MA, Bartram CI. Anal endo-

sonography in the investigation of faecal incontinence. *Br J Surg.* 1991;78:312–314.

67. Burnett SJD, Spence-Jones C, Speakman CTM, Kamm MA, Hudson C, Bartram CI. Unsuspected sphincter damage following childbirth revealed by anal endosonography. *Br J Radiol.* 1991;64:225–227.

68. Jones PN, Lubowski DZ, Swash M, Henry MM. Is paradoxical contraction of puborectalis of functional importance. *Dis Colon Rectum.* 1987;30:667–670.

69. Barnes PRH, Lennard-Jones JE. Function of the striated anal muscle during straining in control subjects and constipated patients with a radiologically normal rectum or idiopathic megacolon. *Int J Colorectal Dis.* 1988;3:207–209.

70. Womack NR, Williams NS, Holmfield JHM, Morrison JFB, Simpkins KC. New method for the dynamic assessment of anorectal function in constipation. *Br J Surg.* 1985;72:994–998.

71. Wexner SD, Daniel N, Jagelman DG. Colectomy for constipation: physiologic investigation is the key to success. *Dis Colon Rectum.* 1991;34(10):891–896.

72. Kamm MA, Hawley PR, Lennard-Jones JE. Outcome of colectomy for severe idiopathic constipation. *Br J Surg.* 1988;29:969–973.

73. Barnes PRH, Hawley PR, Preston DM, Lennard-Jones JE. Experience of posterior division of the puborectalis muscle in the management of chronic constipation. *Br J Surg.* 1985;72:475–477.

74. Kamm MA, Hawley PR, Lennard-Jones JE. Lateral division of the puborectalis muscle in the management of severe constipation. *Br J Surg.* 1988;75:661–663.

75. Pinho M, Yoshioka K, Keighley MRB. Long-term results of anorectal myectomy for chronic constipation. *Br J Surg.* 1989;76:1163–1164.

76. Hallan RI, Williams NS, Melling J, Waldron DJ, Womack NR, Morrison JFB. Treatment of anismus in intractable constipation with botulinum A toxin. *Lancet.* 1988;1:714–717.

77. Bleinberg G, Kuipers HC. Treatment of the spastic pelvic floor syndrome by biofeedback. *Dis Colon Rectum.* 1987;30:108–111.

78. Keren S, Wagner Y, Heldenberg D, Golan M. Studies of manometric abnormalities of the rectoanal region during defaecation in constipated and soiling children: modification through biofeedback therapy. *Am J Gastroenterol.* 1988;83:827–831.

79. Binnie NR, Kawimbe BM, Papachrystomou M, Smith AN. EMG biofeedback as a domiciliary treatment of anismus. *Gut.* 1989;30:A714.

80. Wexner SD, Cheape JD, Jorge JMN, Heyman S, Jagelman DG. A prospective assessment of biofeedback for the treatment of paradoxical puborectalis contraction. *Dis Colon Rectum.* (In press.)

81. Read NW, Haynes WG, Bartolo DCC, et al. Use of anorectal manometry during rectal infusion of saline to investigate sphincter function in incontinent patients. *Gastroenterology.* 1983;85:105–113.

82. Arnold MW, William RCS, Aguilar PS. Rectocoele repair: four years' experience. *Dis Colon Rectum.* 1990;33:684–687.

83. Ramon De Alvarez R. *Textbook of Gynaecology.* Philadelphia: Lea & Febiger; 1977;491–503.

84. Khubchandani IT, Sheets JA, Stasik JA, Hakki AR. Endorectal repair of rectocoele. *Dis Colon Rectum.* 1983;26:792–796.

85. Bartolo DCC, Read NW, Jarratt JA, Read MG, Donnelly TC, Johnson AG. Differences in anal sphincter function and clinical presentation in patients with pelvic floor descent. *Gastroenterology.* 1983;85(1):68–75.

86. Browning GG, Parks AG. Postanal repair for neurogenic faecal incontinence: correlation of clinical results and canal pressures. *Br J Surg.* 1983;70:101–104.

CHAPTER 7

RECTAL PROLAPSE
AND INTUSSUSCEPTION

Robert D. Madoff

Rectal prolapse, or procidentia, is full-thickness protrusion of the rectum through the anal sphincters. Internal or "hidden" prolapse occurs when the rectum intussuscepts but does not pass beyond the anal canal. Prolapse of the rectal mucosa alone is related to hemorrhoidal disease and is discussed in Chapter 14.

Pathophysiology

In 1912, observing that rectal prolapse patients had deep anterior cul de sacs, Moschowitz proposed that rectal prolapse was a sliding hernia of the anterior rectal wall through a defect in the pelvic fascia.[1] A half century later, Broden and Snellman used cine defecography to demonstrate that full-thickness rectal prolapse begins as an internal intussusception of the rectum with a lead point 6 to 8 cm proximal to the anal verge.[2] This view was confirmed by Theuerkauf and associates, who used radiopaque markers applied to the rectal mucosa to demonstrate the intussusception.[3] Although rectal intussusception is now generally agreed to be the mechanism of rectal prolapse, it is only fair to point out that anterior intussusception and a sliding hernia of the anterior rectal wall are anatomically indistinguishable.[4]

Several pelvic anatomic abnormalities are frequently seen in patients with rectal prolapse. These include a deep cul de sac, diastasis of the levatores ani, a redundant sigmoid colon, a patulous anal sphincter, loss of posterior rectal fixation, and loss of a horizontal distal rectal segment.[4] The temptation has always been present to attribute an etiologic role to one or more of these factors, and many prolapse operations have been devised with the goal of correcting these anatomic derangements. Moschowitz described purse-string obliteration of the cul de sac,[1] Graham and colleagues anterior levator repair,[5] and Pemberton and Stalker sigmoidopexy[6] to restore normal anatomy. The fact that these operations are of historical interest only suggests that these anatomic abnormalities are not responsible for the development of rectal prolapse. The common operating room observation of "lax" colonic attachments in rectal prolapse patients has led to speculation regarding a possible generalized connective tissue disorder. One study in which increased joint mobility was noted in rectal prolapse patients supports this point of view,[7] but additional mechanical and biochemical data are needed to clarify this issue.

Patients with mental illness, particularly institutionalized patients, seem to have an increased incidence of rectal prolapse.[8] In rare instances, neurologic disorders, such as multiple sclerosis, tabes dorsalis, and lesions of the cauda equina, are associated with rectal prolapse.[9] The role of parity in the development of rectal prolapse is unclear, but Corman believes that nulliparous woman have the highest risk.[10] In children, risk factors for rectal prolapse include cystic fibrosis, whooping cough, and developmental abnormalities such as meningomyelocele, spina bifida, and exstrophy of the bladder.[10] Malnutrition and diarrheal states secondary to parasitic infections can lead to childhood rectal prolapse.[11] These problems are more common in developing countries.

Over the past decade considerable investigation has been carried out to elucidate the pathophysiology of prolapse-associated incontinence. Using anal manometry, Matheson and Keighley, found normal anal pressures in continent prolapse patients while incontinent patients with and without prolapse had decreased basal and squeeze anal pressures.[12] Neill and associates found decreased resting pressure but preservation of maximal squeeze pressure in continent prolapse patients.[13] Electromyographic evidence of pelvic sphincter reinnervation (and thus of previous denervation) was found in all incontinent prolapse but only in one of eight continent prolapse patients.

Denervation is believed to be due to traction injury of the pudendal nerves caused by the rectal prolapse. This mechanism is identical to that proposed for "idiopathic" incontinence in which denervation is induced by perineal descent, vaginal childbirth, or excessive straining at stool. Continent prolapse patients do not show manometric or electromyographic signs of denervation, suggesting that this denervation is necessary only for the development of incontinence and not for the development for rectal prolapse itself. Keighley and Shouler studied colonic function in continent and incontinent prolapse patients, patients with idiopathic fecal incontinence, and normal controls. Incontinent patients had increased sigmoid motility and normal whole gut transit, whereas continent prolapse patients had normal sigmoid motility but delayed whole gut transit. These data, if reproducible in larger series, suggest that differences in gut motility may in part determine which individuals with prolapse will develop fecal incontinence with time.[14]

Prolapse-associated constipation is poorly understood. Its incidence, when reported at all, ranges between 25 and 50 percent of patients. In a recent retrospective review, we found constipation to be present in 20 of 47 patients (43%) prior to prolapse surgery.[15] No series to date has well characterized this problem or differentiated infrequent defecation from difficult evacuation in the definition of constipation. In a small uncontrolled series, Metcalf and Loening-Bauke found a paradoxical increase in external anal sphincter EMG activity in six of seven prolapse patients during attempted defecation (when external anal sphincter relaxation would be expected).[16] The seventh patient, who did not increase his external anal sphincter activity with straining, showed no sphincter relaxation, again an abnormal study. This inability to relax the pelvic floor for defecation—in fact, the active obstruction of defecation in most patients—causes excessive straining that can lead to pudendal nerve injury. Five of the seven prolapse patients in this study were incontinent. These intriguing data require confirmation in other laboratories.

Continence is often restored following prolapse surgery, but the mechanism for this improvement remains obscure. Keighley and colleagues found that 64 percent of incontinent prolapse patients had their continence restored following Marlex® mesh rectopexy.[17] Surprisingly, there was no overall difference in basal or squeeze anal pressures following surgery. Holmstrom and associates, in contrast, did find an increase in resting anal pressure following Ripstein rectopexy and suggested that internal anal sphincter function improved following surgery.[18] Yoshioka and associates attempted to identify factors that would predict the return of continence following prolapse repair with Marlex® mesh rectopexy.[19] In this small study, preoperative anal pressures were significantly lower in the prolapse patients than in the controls and preoperative anorectal angles were significantly more obtuse in the prolapse group. Neither of the abnormalities changed significantly after surgery. Only two physiological parameters were identified that changed after operation: the extent of perineal decent during attempted defecation and median rectal emptying both decreased significantly. Several factors were predictive of improved postoperative continence, including delayed leakage during saline infusion tests, a narrow anorectal angle during pelvic floor contraction, minimal pelvic floor descent with straining, and a long anal canal at rest and during pelvic floor contraction. However, these factors taken together seem to indicate only that patients with milder forms of incontinence were more likely to improve following surgery.

A recent prospective physiological study of 23 female rectal prolapse patients who underwent surgical repair at the University of Minnesota confirmed this general notion.[20] Preoperatively, both resting and maximal voluntary anal pressures were significantly lower in incontinent than in continent prolapse patients, though there was considerable overlap in the actual values. A significant rise in these pressures was seen for the entire group following surgery. No direct correlation could be drawn between the extent of manometric improvement and functional result. The anorectal angle did not change following prolapse repair. Patients who remained incontinent had significantly lower resting and maximal voluntary anal pressures preoperatively than did those whose continence improved, though again overlap was seen between these two groups. Our data thus also suggest that incontinent patients with severe sphincter dysfunction preoperatively are least likely to improve following prolapse repair, and that factors other than the restoration of normal anal pressures or anorectal angles are responsible for the functional improvement seen following surgery.

Clinical Features

Rectal prolapse is uncommon and its true incidence is unknown. Prolapse can occur at any age, though it tends to occur at the extremes of life. In children, most prolapse occurs within the first three years of life and with an equal sex distribution.[10] In adults, a great majority of patients are female. The most frequent presentation of full-thickness rectal prolapse is protrusion. This initially occurs during defecation but later can occur with any activity that increases intraabdominal pressures, such as coughing or straining. Chronic prolapse can lead to ulceration, bleeding, and mucous discharge; fecal incontinence can occasionally be the presenting complaint. Rarely, rectal prolapse can become incarcerated and even gangrenous. Symptoms of incomplete rectal prolapse include rectal pressure, tenesmus, and a sensation of incomplete rectal emptying (see below).

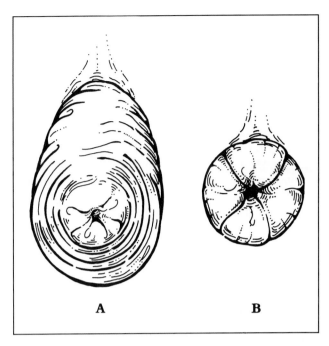

Figure 7-1. (A) Full-thickness rectal prolapse. Note concentric folds. (B) Rectal mucosal prolapse. Note radial folds. (*From:* Wassef R, Rothenberger DA, Goldberg SM. Rectal prolapse. *Curr Probl Surg.* 1986;23:402–451.)

Evaluation

Rectal prolapse may be obvious on initial examination or it may be necessary to have the patient strain in the sitting position to make the prolapse protrude. Corman correctly notes that the prone jackknife position commonly used for anorectal examination is the worst possible position for demonstration of rectal prolapse.[10] For children, Goligher recommends administration of a glycerin suppository to induce straining and to demonstrate the prolapse.[8]

Full-thickness rectal prolapse must be differentiated from rectal mucosal prolapse seen in association with advanced hemorrhoidal disease. This distinction is generally easy for the experienced examiner; most often by the typical concentric orientation of tissue folds of full-thickness prolapse or the radial folds of rectal mucosal prolapse (Fig. 7-1).[21] Several other features differentiate mucosal and full-thickness prolapse. In full-thickness rectal prolapse, a double rectal wall thickness can be palpated, the anus is in its normal position and a sulcus is present between the anus and the protruding rectum. Rectal mucosal prolapse rarely protrudes more than 5 cm, whereas full-thickness prolapse may protrude considerably farther. Chronically prolapsed tissue may have an inflamed, edematous, irregular surface. Biopsies may be necessary to differentiate these metaplastic changes from a prolapsing polypoid neoplasm.

With the prolapse reduced, digital rectal examination should be used to assess resting and squeeze anal pressures. Evidence of perianal skin maceration or excoriation should be noted. Endoscopic evaluation of the distal large bowel should be performed in all patients, preferably with the flexible sigmoidoscope. Biopsies should be taken from localized inflammation or ulceration to diagnose colitis cystica profunda or the solitary rectal ulcer syndrome and to exclude the presence of a colonic neoplasm. In adults, evaluation of the entire large bowel should be performed prior to any colonic surgery.

When internal intussusception is clinically suspected, or when colitis cystica profunda or solitary rectal ulcer syndrome is diagnosed, cine defecography should be obtained. This examination (described in Chapters 2 and 6) will diagnose or exclude the presence of internal rectal intussusception. Anal manometry provides an objective measure of anal sphincter function and may help predict the functional outcome of prolapse surgery but rarely alters the clinical approach to the patient. Colonic transit marker studies (Chapters 2 and 6) are indicated in severely constipated patients, as patients with slow transit constipation and normal pelvic outlet function deserve consideration of subtotal colectomy in association with their prolapse repair.[15] Electromyography can be used to evaluate the status of sphincter innervation but its role is generally limited to research.

Treatment

Management of rectal prolapse is surgical. Although well over one hundred procedures have been described for the treatment of rectal prolapse, a far smaller number remain in active use. Operations for prolapse can be classified into two groups on the basis of anatomic approach: transabdominal repairs and perineal repairs. Transabdominal repairs involve rectal fixation, large bowel resection, or a combination of resection and fixation. Results of these procedures are shown in Table 7-1. Perineal repairs include resection, rectal reefing and anal encirclement. The results of these three forms of perineal repair are presented in Tables 7-2 to 7-4.

Abdominal Procedures

Many techniques of transabdominal rectal fixation are highly effective in the repair of rectal prolapse (Table 7-1). Most surgeons use foreign material to fix the mobilized rectum to either the sacral hollow or promontory. Nylon, Teflon®, Marlex®, Ivalon®, Gore-Tex®, Vicryl®, and Dexon® have all been employed

with similar degrees of success. Other authors have enjoyed similar results through suture rectopexy of the lateral rectal attachments directly to the presacral fascia. No foreign material is used with this technique. Adequate rectal mobilization is believed essential for successful correction of rectal prolapse with the abdominal fixation technique. Most authors advocate complete posterior rectal mobilization to the level of the levators; our practice at the University of Minnesota also includes anterior rectal mobilization, to the level of the upper third of the vagina in women.

The most commonly performed operation in the United States for rectal prolapse is the anterior rec-

Table 7-1   Abdominal Suspension/Fixation Techniques

Author Year	Procedure	Material	No. patients Recurrence/Treated	Recurrence, %
Ripstein[22] 1952, 1972	Anterior sling	Teflon®/Marlex®	2/500	0
Morgan et al[23] 1980	Anterior sling	Teflon®	1/64	2
Holstrom et al[24] 1986	Anterior sling	Marlex®	4/97	4
Roberts et al[25] 1988	Anterior sling	Teflon®	13/130	10
Anderson et al[26] 1981	Posterior sling	Ivalon®	1/40	3
Atkinson and Taylor[27] 1984	Posterior sling	Ivalon®	4/40	10
Kuijpers and de Morree[28] 1988	Posterior sling	Teflon®	3/30	10
Arndt and Pircher[29] 1988	Posterior sling	Vicryl®/Dexon®	4/62	6
Yoshioka et al[19] 1989	Posterior sling	Marlex®	2/135	2
Goligher[30] 1980	Suture rectopexy	. . .	0/42	0
Carter[31] 1983	Suture rectopexy	. . .	1/32	3
Graham et al 1984	Suture rectopexy	. . .	0/23	0
Ejerblad and Kraus[32] 1988	Suture rectopexy	. . .	2/48	4
Blatchford et al[33] 1989	Suture rectopexy	. . .	1/42	2

Table 7-2   Perineal Rectosigmoidectomy: Selected References

Author Year	No. patients Recurrence/Treated	Recurrence, %
Hughes[34] 1949	65/108	60
Porter[35] 1962	55/110	50
Gabriel[36] 1963	16/131	12
Theuerkauf et al[3] 1970	3/13	39
Altemeier et al[37] 1971	3/106	3
Friedman et al[38] 1983	12/27	44
Gopal et al[39] 1984	1/18	6
Prasad et al[40] 1986	0/25	0
Ramanujam and Venkatesh[41] 1988	2/41	5
Williams et al[20] 1991	11/114	10

Table 7-3   Delorme Procedure

Author Year	No. patients Recurrence/Treated	Recurrence, %
Uhlig and Sullivan[42] 1979	3/44	7
Christensen and Kirkegaard[43] 1981	1/12	17
Gundersen et al[44] 1985	1/18	6
Monson et al[45] 1986	2/27	7
Houry et al[46] 1987	3/18	17

topexy or Ripstein procedure. Ripstein originally advocated anterior levator plication reinforced with a V-shaped fascia lata graft also affixed to the presacral facia.[22] Later, however, he modified his technique to what has become the classic Ripstein repair. The rectum is completely mobilized posteriorly and a loose sling is wrapped around the anterior wall of the rectum and sutured to the sacrum (Fig. 7-2). The rectum is pulled upward and its anterior wall is sutured to the sling. No pelvic floor repair is carried out. Morgan and associates[23] reported only two recurrences in Ripstein's series of 500 patients, though details of follow-up are completely lacking. Gordon and Hoexter polled members of the American Society of Colon and Rectal Surgeons and collected a series of 1111 rectal prolapse cases treated by the Ripstein procedure.[55] There was a 2.3 percent recurrence rate; 16.5 percent of patients experienced sling-related complications and 4 percent required reoperation. The Ripstein procedure has been criticized for causing obstructive complications due to the anterior

Table 7-4   Anal Encirclement Operations for Rectal Prolapse

Author Year	Material	No. patients	Success (%)	Failure (%)
Jackaman et al[47] 1980	Silicone® rod	52	44(85)	15(29)
Labow et al[48] 1980	Dacron®/Silastic®	9	9(100)	0
Hunt et al[49] 1985	Silastic® rod	41	22(54)	12(29)
Poole et al[50] 1985	Dacron® vascular graft	15	11(73)	6(40)
Vongsangnak et al[51] 1985	Wire (steel or silver)	25	15(60)	15(60)
Earnshaw and Hopkinson[52] 1987	Silicone® rod	21	16(76)	6(29)
Khanduja et al[53] 1988	Silicone® prosthesis	16	16(100)	4(25)

Modified from: Williams JG. Perineal approaches to repair of rectal prolapse. *Semin Colon Rectal Surg.* 1991;3(2): 198–204.[54]

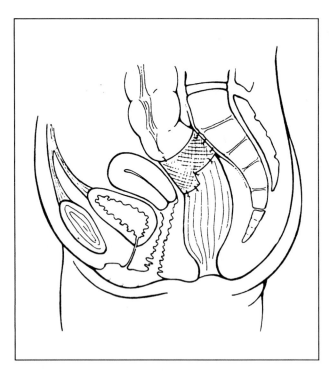

Figure 7-2. Anterior (Ripstein) rectopexy. (From: Wassef R, Rothenberger DA, Goldberg SM. Rectal prolapse. *Curr Probl Surg.* 1986;23:402–451.)

location of the sling that completely encircles the rectum. Sling stricture requiring reoperation has been reported in 1 to 3 percent of patients.[23] Other reports of constipation and fecal impaction complicating the Rip-

stein procedure must be interpreted with caution, as many patients who undergo prolapse surgery suffer preoperatively from evacuation difficulties.

Although U.S. surgeons have historically performed the Ripstein procedure for rectal prolapse, surgeons in the United Kingdom often prefer the posterior sling rectopexy described by Wells in 1959.[56] As initially described, the operation consisted of posterior rectal mobilization and fixation of a sheet of Ivalon to the sacral hollow. The Ivalon is wrapped around the lateral aspects of the mobilized rectum but the anterior rectal wall is left open (Fig. 7-3). This technique avoids complete rectal encirclement and is widely believed to obviate the obstructive complications of the Ripstein procedure. Indeed, Ripstein himself now uses a modified Wells procedure with placement of a posterior rather than anterior rectal sling.[57] Nonetheless, it is worth noting that Yoshioka and colleagues found an increase in constipation from 24 percent to 44 percent following posterior rectopexy for rectal prolapse.[19]

Results of the Wells procedure are depicted in Table 7-1. It is evident that the recurrence rates for anterior and posterior rectopexy are similar. Ivalon has fallen out of favor for many surgeons owing to its being extremely difficult to remove should an abdominal infection or a recurrent prolapse occur. Other surgeons shun its use because of experimental evidence of sarcoma induction in animal models although such carcinogenesis has not been observed in humans.

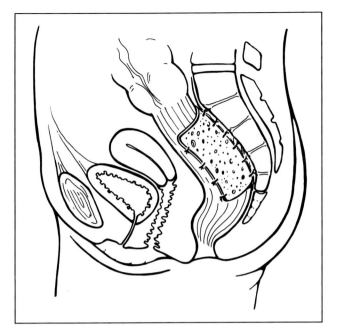

Figure 7-3. Posterior (Wells) rectopexy. (*From:* Wassef R, Rothenberger DA, Goldberg SM. Rectal prolapse. *Curr Probl Surg.* 1986;23:402–451.)

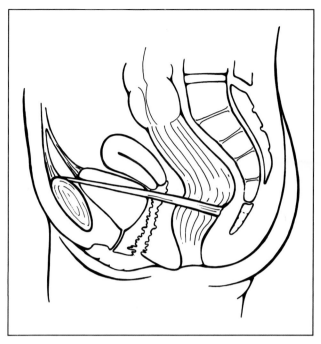

Figure 7-4. Puborectalis sling procedure (Nigro). (*From:* Wassef R, Rothenberger DA, Goldberg SM. Rectal prolapse. *Curr Probl Surg.* 1986;23:402–451.)

Two other sling-type rectal suspension procedures deserve mention. Loygue, modifying a procedure described by Orr in 1947, uses strips of nylon to suspend the lateral walls of the posteriorly mobilized rectum to the sacral promontory. A recurrence rate of 5.6 percent was reported in a series of 257 patients.[58] Nigro devised a unique suspension sling that loops behind the rectum and suspends it from the pubic tubercles bilaterally (Fig. 7-4). The goal of this procedure is to re-create the anorectal angle in a fashion anatomically similar to the puborectalis muscle. Nigro reported a series of 60 patients who underwent this procedure without any recurrences.

A number of surgeons have argued that the use of foreign material is not only unnecessary but also potentially dangerous in the event of intraabdominal infection. This latter issue is of particular importance when bowel resection is performed in association with rectopexy. In fact, very successful results have been reported in a number of series in which the lateral rectal attachments were sutured directly to the presacral fascia (Table 7-1). These collected results are similar to those reported with suspension procedures using foreign material.

Use of anterior resection for the treatment of rectal prolapse is based on the observation that the rectum becomes firmly adherent to the sacrum after anterior resection.[59] The largest series using this procedure was reported by Schlinkert and colleagues in 1985[60]: 113 patients underwent anterior resection for rectal prolapse, and prolapse recurred in 8 of the 92 patients (9 percent) who were available for follow-up. Morbidity was related to the level of anastomosis but the recurrence rate was not, and high anterior resection with anastomosis to peritonealized rectum was therefore recommended. One disadvantage of this approach is that 10 (22 percent) of the 46 patients whose continence was evaluated reported a deterioration in control, possibly related to loss of rectal reservoir function.

At the University of Minnesota, our approach has been to combine direct suture rectopexy with a convenient sigmoid resection. The rationale of the resection is severalfold: it prevents recurrence because the straightened left colon does not have adequate length to prolapse, it prevents volvulus of the elongated sigmoid colon following mobilization, and it may alleviate the symptoms of constipation that are frequently associated with rectal prolapse. For prolapse patients with documented slow-transit constipation and no pelvic outlet obstruction, subtotal colectomy with suture rectopexy has been performed with good results.[15]

Watts and associates reviewed the University of Minnesota experience of 138 patients undergoing rectopexy and sigmoid resection in 1985[61]: 102 patients were available for follow-up, and there were 2 recurrences (1.9 percent). Anastomotic complications occurred in 4 percent, and half of these required reoperation. In a more recent review of this series that also included patients who underwent more extensive bowel resection, full-thickness prolapse recurred in 6 percent of 47 patients.[15] An additional 9 percent of patients developed rectal mucosal prolapse. Husa and associates used a similar rectopexy and resection technique in 48 patients with a 9 percent recurrence rate.[62]

Perineal Procedures

Perineal prolapse repairs were initially described in the late 19th and early 20th centuries, prior to the modern era of safe abdominal surgery.[63-66] Because of the high recurrence rates in early series, these operations were largely supplanted by abdominal repairs when the later became safe for routine use. In general, perineal prolapse repairs have been reserved for patients for whom abdominal surgery is not advisable, although improved recent results with perineal rectosigmoidectomy have raised the question of whether this relatively simple and well-tolerated procedure should be offered to low risk patients as well.

At the University of Minnesota, our perineal procedure of choice is the rectosigmoidectomy (Fig. 7-5). Popularized in this country by Altemeier,[37] the operation was originally described by Mikulicz in 1889.[63] The operation can be carried out in the lithotomy or the prone jackknife position, under either general or re-gional anesthesia. The rectum is prolapsed and the outer cylinder of bowel is divided approximately 2 cm proximal to the dentate line. Stay sutures are placed in each quadrant. The inner cylinder of rectum and sigmoid is placed on traction and mesenteric vessels are sequentially ligated and divided. When the proximal bowel cannot be pulled down any farther, it is ready for division. At this point in the operation, levator repair can be carried out anteriorly, posteriorly, or in both positions. The specimen is then amputated, taking care to prevent retraction of the proximal colon into the abdomen. The anastomosis can be completed with either a sutured or stapled technique.[67]

Results of perineal rectosigmoidectomies have varied considerably between groups, but most recent studies have reported excellent anatomic results (Table 7-2). Many of the recent successful series have included levator repairs as part of the procedure. For example Gopal and associates included an anterior levator repair,[39] Ramanujam and Venkatesh a posterior levator repair,[41] and Prasad and colleagues a posterior levator repair with suture rectopexy.[40]

Williams recently reviewed the University of Minnesota experience with perineal rectosigmoidectomy[54]: 114 patients with a median age of 78 years underwent this operation between 1980 and 1990; 110 were available for follow-up. Preexistent medical disease was

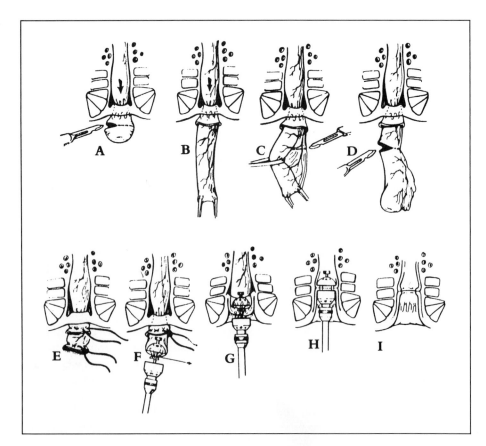

Figure 7-5.   Perineal rectosigmoidectomy. Stapled technique. (*From:* Wassef R, Rothenberger DA, Goldberg SM. Rectal prolapse. *Curr Probl Surg.* 1986;23: 402–451.)

present in 81 patients (71 percent). Median hospital stay was 4 days; 14 patients developed complications, mostly medical. There were three suture-line hemorrhages and no anastomotic leaks; there was no operative mortality. Of these patients 11 (10 percent) developed recurrent rectal prolapse 3 to 48 months following surgery; 6 of these patients underwent repeat rectosigmoidectomy.

The Delorme procedure involves stripping the mucosa from the redundant prolapsed rectum and reefing the denuded muscle wall to create a muscular pessary[65] (Fig. 7-6). Once rarely performed, this operation has enjoyed a resurgence of interest in the past decade. Like the perineal rectosigmoidectomy, the Delorme procedure can be performed in either the lithotomy or prone jackknife position using either regional or general anesthetic. The muscular stripping can be carried out with the prolapse either everted or reduced. Dilute epinephrine solution is injected submucosally to limit bleeding. The dissection begins at approximately 1 cm proximal to the detante line and is continued proximately until there is resistance to further dissection on the mucosal sleeve. The redundant mucosa is then excised and a mucosal anastomosis is completed with eight radially arrayed sutures that also take reefing bites of the exposed rectal wall.

The results of the Delorme procedure are depicted in Table 7-3. Although no single large experience is reported, several groups have now documented satisfactory results using this technique. Concurrent levator

repair can be performed in association with this procedure but requires a separate intersphincteric dissection to reach the levatores ani.

The simplest of all prolapse repairs is the anal encirclement procedure described by Thiersch in 1891.[66] The goal of this operation is to create a mechanical barrier that prevents the prolapse from protruding through the anal sphincter. No effort is made to correct the inciting internal intussusception. Anal encirclement procedures have two advantages over other prolapse repairs: simplicity of technique and the ability to perform the operation under local anesthesia. Two small incisions are made 180° apart with lateral incisions being preferred to allow burial of the knot in the ischiorectal fat. The encircling material is placed around the anal canal and secured. Too loose an encirclement is ineffectual; too tight an encirclement leads to difficult evacuation and local complications.

In the procedure's original description, silver wire was placed in the subcutaneous position. Difficulties with this technique including wire breakage, wire extrusion, infection, and skin sloughing have led to two types of modification. First, there is now a tendency to place the encircling material higher in the ischiorectal fossa than the subcutaneous tissue. Second, wire has been replaced with a variety of softer and more pliable materials to allow expansion of the anal canal with bowel movements. These newer materials have included Dacron-impregnated Silastic®,[48] knitted Dacron® vascular graft,[50] Silicon® rubber suture,[52] Silastic® rods,[49] and the Angelchik anti-reflex prosthesis.[68]

Results of anal encirclement operations are depicted in Table 7-4. Although several small series show good results, significant failure rates in the 25 to 40 percent range occur frequently. Furthermore, even though recent modifications may have improved results of anal encirclement for rectal prolapse, these modifications have also increased the magnitude of the procedure. Regional or general anesthesia is frequently necessary, and several authors advocate complete bowel preparation preoperatively. Once the simplicity of the Thiersch procedure is sacrificed, any advantage over perineal rectosigmoidectomy is lost.

Functional Results of Rectal Prolapse Surgery

Incontinence occurs in 35 to 100 percent of patients with prolapse (Tables 7-5 and 7-6) and is the most distressing complication of the disorder. Constipation is also frequently present though its incidence unknown. Studies of prolapse-associated "incontinence" and "constipation" uniformly suffer from inadequate definitions. Extent of incontinence is rarely if ever specified; few studies that mention constipation differentiate infrequent evacuation from difficult evacuation. "Success-

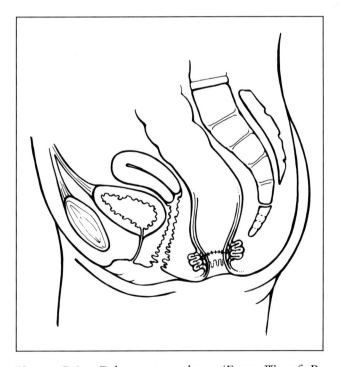

Figure 7-6. Delorme procedure. (*From:* Wassef R, Rothenberger DA, Goldberg SM. Rectal prolapse. *Curr Probl Surg.* 1986;23:402–451.)

Table 7-5 Restoration of Continence After Abdominal Prolapse Repair

Author Year	Procedure	No. patients	Incontinent (%)	Improved (%)
Graham et al[5] 1984	Suture rectopexy	23	9(39)	7(78)
Ejerblad and Kraus[32] 1988	Suture rectopexy	46	22(48)	15(68)
Blatchford et al[33] 1989	Suture reotopexy	42	27(64)	25(93)
Watts et al[61] 1985	Resection/rectopexy	61	25(40)	11(44)
Madoff et al[15] 1991	Resection/rectopexy	47	21(45)	8(38)
Husa et al[62] 1988	Resection/rectopexy	48	32(67)	30(94)
Roberts et al[25] 1988	Anterior sling	135	58(43)	45(78)
Holmstrom et al[24] 1986	Anterior sling	97	60(62)	34(57)
Boulos et al[69] 1984	Posterior sling	25	20(80)	16(75)
Yoshioka et al[70] 1989	Posterior sling	165	95(58)	74(78)

Table 7-6 Restoration of Continence After Perineal Prolapse Repair

Author Year	Procedure	No. patients	Incontinent (%)	Improved (%)
Ramanujam and Venkatesh[41] 1988	Rectosigmoidectomy/ levator repair	41	41(100)	32(78)
Friedman et al[38] 1983	Rectosigmoidectomy	27	11(41)	6(55)
Watts et al[61] 1985	Rectosigmoidectomy	18	4(23)	1(25)
Williams[54] 1991	Rectosigmoidectomy with levator repair without levator repair	11 93	11(100) 56(60)	10(91) 26(46)
Monson et al[45] 1986	Delorme	27	18(67)	15(83)
Houry et al[46] 1987	Delorme	18	9(50)	4(44)
Rogers and Jeffrey[71] 1987	Rectopexy/ levator repair	24	15(63)	15(100)
Prasad et al[40] 1986	Rectosigmoidectomy/ rectopexy/levator repair	25	25(100)	25(100)

Table 7-7   Effect of Prolapse Surgery on Constipation

Author Year	Procedure	Symptom/Results
Holmstrom et al[24] 1986	Anterior sling	Poor defecation Preoperative 27%, postoperative 43%
Husa et al[62] 1986	Sigmoidectomy/ rectopexy	Constipation Preoperative 39%, postoperative 10%
Broden et al[74] 1988	Anterior sling	Evacuation disturbance Preoperative 52%, postoperative 52%
Roberts et al[25] 1988	Anterior sling	Constipation 69% improved, 31% same or worse
Blatchford et al[33] 1989	Suture rectopexy	Constipation Preoperative 48%, postoperative 71%
Sayfan et al[72] 1990	Mesh rectopexy	3 of 3 persistent constipation 4 of 13 developed constipation
	Sigmoidectomy/ rectopexy	1 of 5 persistent constipation 0 of 8 developed constipation

ful" prolapse surgery requires not only restoration of normal anatomy but also restoration of normal bowel function.

The results of rectal prolapse surgery on incontinence are summarized in Tables 7-5 and 7-6. After fixation-type abdominal prolapse repair, improvement in continence can be expected in approximately two-thirds of cases. Results following anterior resection[60] and sigmoidectomy with rectopexy[15,61] are less impressive, raising the question whether bowel resection leads to more frequent or more liquid stool that may compromise continence. Unfortunately, trials comparing different operations for prolapse are rare, and those available involve very small numbers of patients.[72,73] Following perineal prolapse repair, the most successful results for restoration of continence are seen when associated levator repair is performed.

The effect of prolapse surgery on constipation is summarized in Table 7-7. The widely variable results obtained reflect not only the different operations used but also the differing definitions of constipation. This topic requires more careful prospective study before any conclusions can be drawn.

Internal Intussusception and Solitary Rectal Ulcer Syndrome

Solitary rectal ulcer syndrome (SRUS) is an uncommon nonmalignant condition characterized by rectal bleed-ing, copious mucous discharge, anal pain, and difficult evacuation. Despite its name SRUS can be associated with single or multiple rectal ulcers or none at all. When present, ulcers tend to occur on rectal valves and most commonly are found on the anterior rectal wall just above the anorectal ring.[75] Ulcers are characteristically shallow with a "punched out" gray-white base and a surrounding zone of hyperemia.[75] Colitis cystica profunda (CCP) is a related disorder whose symptoms are indistinguishable from those of SRUS. Instead of ulcerations, examination reveals firm nodules on the anterior rectal wall. Histologically, these are composed of normal colonic glands located submucosally and filled with pools of mucus.

SRUS has its peak incidence in the third to fourth decade, with the female predominance emerging after the age of 30.[75] The nature of the disordered defecation is highly characteristic: patients have a constant urge to defecate coupled with a sense of incomplete or unsuccessful evacuation.[76] These symptoms lead to numerous daily trips to the lavatory, many of which produce nothing more than frustration for the patient. Self-digitation to facilitate evacuation is not an uncommon practice among these patients.

The lesions of SRUS can be confused with benign and malignant neoplasms or with localized areas of inflammatory bowel disease, radiation proctitis, and pseudomembranous colitis. Biopsy is mandatory and establishes the diagnosis. Histologic findings include hypertrophy of the muscularis mucosa and fibromuscular obliteration of lamina propria.[77] CCP exists when dilated mucus-filled glands are displaced into the submucosa. This abnormal location can lead to a misdiagnosis of invasive carcinoma if note is not made of the histologically benign mucosa lining the glands.

Physiologic studies of patients with SRUS have sought to explain its etiology and prominent symptoms of disordered evacuation. Rutter and Riddell[78] demonstrated a paradoxical increase in external anal sphincter EMG activity with straining (when relaxation would be appropriate), but Jones and associates[79] found similar paradoxical puborectalis contraction in other unrelated anorectal conditions. Current thinking focuses on the relationship between SRUS and rectal intussusception and prolapse. Overt or internal rectal intussusception is present in up to 80 percent of patients with SRUS.[80-83] This relationship, from uncontrolled studies, must be interpreted in light of the high rate of internal intussusception found in normal volunteers undergoing defecography.[83] It should also be noted that internal intussusception is neither a necessary nor a sufficient condition for the development of SRUS, as patients can develop the syndrome without intussusception and not all patients with rectal intussusception develop SRUS. Despite these criticisms, it appears likely that in many cases a causal relationship between internal rectal intussusception and SRUS does exist. Supporting this notion is the fact that surgical approaches designed to correct rectal intussusception often are beneficial in the treatment of the rectal ulceration.

Treatment of SRUS is controversial. Once the diagnosis is established, virtually all patients should have a trial of medical therapy consisting of adequate fiber intake, defecation training with a strict prohibition against straining, and judicious use of laxatives and enemas to facilitate evacuation. Using a similar approach, Brandt-Gradel and colleagues reported a 71 percent healing rate for SRUS in 21 patients.[84] Keighley and Shouler, reviewing experience with 33 SRUS patients, found that 6 of 8 asymptomatic patients had spontaneous healing of their ulcers, and that an additional 9 of 13 patients could be treated successfully with medical management alone.[85]

A variety of surgical approaches to SRUS have been undertaken. Local excision of the rectal ulcer is not recommended, as this procedure does not address the responsible pathophysiology and the lesions tend to recur. Berman and associates performed the Delorme procedure on 31 patients in whom medical treatment of internal intussusception failed.[86] Fourteen patients were available for 6-month follow-up and all had relief of their preoperative symptoms. Keighley and Shouler reported 14 patients who underwent posterior Marlex rectopexy for SRUS.[86] Ulcers healed in 5 of 6 patients (83 percent) with full-thickness rectal prolapse, whereas only 2 of 8 patients (25 percent) without overt rectal prolapse healed. Nicholls and Simson devised an operation consisting of posterior Marlex rectopexy and anterior rectal wall Marlex stenting. In a series of 14 SRUS patients without overt rectal prolapse, rectal bleeding, mucous discharge, straining, and tenesmus were decreased in 100, 94, 79, and 86 percent respectively.[87] Defecation frequency and time spent attempting defecation markedly decreased postoperatively. These data taken together support conservative therapy for SRUS in the first instance. Should this approach fail, there is reasonable hope for improvement or cure following appropriate surgery aimed at correcting a demonstrable internal intussusception.

References

1. Moschowitz AV. The pathogenesis, anatomy and cure of prolapse of the rectum. *Surg Gynecol Obstet.* 1912;15:7–21.
2. Broden B, Snellman B. Procidentia of the rectum studied with cine radiography: a contribution to the discussion of causative mechanism. *Dis Colon Rectum.* 1968;11:330–347.
3. Theuerkauf FJ, Beahrs OH, Hill JR. Rectal prolapse: causation and surgical treatment. *Ann Surg.* 1970;171:819–835.
4. Goldberg SM, Gordon PH, Nivatvongs S. *Essentials of Anorectal Surgery.* Philadelphia: JB Lippincott; 1980.
5. Graham W, Clegg JF, Taylor V. Complete rectal prolapse: repair by a simple technique. *Ann R Coll Surg Engl.* 1984;66:87–89.
6. Pemberton J de J, Stalker LK. Surgical treatment of complete rectal prolapse. *Ann Surg.* 1939;109:799–808.
7. Marshaman D, Percy J, Fielding I, Delbridge L. Rectal prolapse: relationship with joint mobility. *Aust N Z J Surg.* 1987;57:827–829.
8. Goligher J. *Surgery of the Anus, Rectum, and Colon.* 5th ed. London: Bailliere Tindall; 1984.
9. Schoetz DJ, Veidenheimer MC. Rectal prolapse. Pathogenesis and clinical features. In: Henry MM, Swash M, (eds. *Coloproctology in the Pelvic Floor.* London: Butterworths; 1985.

10. Corman ML. *Colon and Rectal Surgery*. 2nd ed. Philadelphia: JB Lippincott; 1989.

11. Eriksen CA, Hadley GP. Rectal prolapse in childhood—the role of infections and infestations. *S Afr Med J* 1985;68:790–791.

12. Matheson DM, Keighley MRB. Manometric evaluation of rectal prolapse and fecal incontinence. *Gut.* 1981;22:126–129.

13. Neill ME, Parks AG, Swash M. Physiological studies of the anal sphincter musculature in faecal incontinence and rectal prolapse. *Br J Surg.* 1981;68: 531–536.

14. Keighley MRB, Shouler PJ. Abnormalities of colonic function in patients with rectal prolapse and rectal incontinence. *Br J Surg.* 1984;71:892–895.

15. Madoff RD, Williams JG, Wong WD, et al. Long term functional results of colon resection and rectopexy for overt rectal prolapse. *Am J Gastroent.* In press.

16. Metcalf AM, Loening-Baucke V. Anorectal function and defecation dynamics in patients with rectal prolapse. *Am J Surg.* 1988;155:206–210.

17. Keighley MRB, Fielding WL, Alexander-Williams JA. Results of Marlex mesh abdominal rectopexy for rectal prolapse in 100 consecutive patients. *Br J Surg.* 1983;70:229–232.

18. Holmstrom B, Broden G, Dolk A. Increased anal resting pressure following the Ripstein operation: a contribution to continence? *Dis Colon Rectum.* 1986;29:45–47.

19. Yoshioka K, Hyland G, Keighley MR. Anorectal function after abdominal rectopexy: parameters of predictive value in identifying return of continence. *Br J Surg.* 1989;76:64–68.

20. Williams JG, Wong WD, Jensen L, et al. Incontinence and rectal prolapse: a prospective manometric study. *Dis Colon Rectum.* 1991;34(3):209–216.

21. Carter HG. Treatment of procidentia of the rectum. *South Med J.* 1971;64:1238–1247.

22. Ripstein CB. Treatment of massive rectal prolapse. *Am J Surg.* 1952;83:68–71.

23. Morgan CN, Porter NH, Klugman DJ. Ivalon (polyvinyl alcohol) sponge in the repair of complete rectal prolapse. *Br J Surg.* 1972;59:841–846.

24. Holmstrom B, Broden G, Dolk A. Results of the Ripstein operation in the treatment of rectal prolapse and internal rectal procidentia. *Dis Colon Rectum.* 1986;29:845–848.

25. Roberts PL, Schoetz DJ Jr, Coller JA, Veidenheimer MC. Ripstein procedure. Lahey Clinic experience: 1963–1985. *Arch Surg.* 1988;123: 554–557.

26. Anderson JR, Kennenmonth AWG, Smith AN. Polyvinyl alcohol sponge rectopexy for complete rectal prolapse. *J R Coll Surg Edinb.* 1981;26: 292–294.

27. Atkinson KG, Taylor DC. Wells procedure for complete rectal prolapse. A ten year experience. *Dis Colon Rectum.* 1984;27:97–98.

28. Kuijpers JH, de Morree H. Toward a selection of the most appropriate procedure in the treatment of complete rectal prolapse. *Dis Colon Rectum.* 1988; 31:355–357.

29. Arndt M, Pircher W. Absorbable mesh in the treatment of rectal prolapse. *Int J Colorectal Dis.* 1988;3: 141–143.

30. Goligher JC. *Surgery of the Anus, Rectum, and Colon.* 4th ed. New York: Macmillan Publishing Co; 1980.

31. Carter AF. Rectosacral suture fixation for complete rectal prolapse in the elderly, the frail, and the demented. *Br J Surg.* 1983;70:522–523.

32. Ejerblad S, Kraus U. Repair of rectal prolapse by rectosacral suture fixation. *Acta Chir Scad.* 1988;154:103–105.

33. Blatchford GJ, Perry RE, Thorson AG, Christensen MA. Rectopexy without resection for rectal prolapse. *Am J Surg.* 1989;158:574–576.

34. Hughes ESR. In discussion on rectal prolapse. *Proc R Soc Assoc Med.* 1949;42:1007–1011.

35. Porter NH. Collective results of operations for rectal prolapse. *Proc R Soc Assoc Med.* 1962;55:1090.

36. Gabriel WB. Prolapse of the rectum. In: *Principles and Practice of Rectal Surgery.* 5th ed. Springfield, Ill: Charles C. Thomas; 1963:165–217.

37. Altemeier WA, Culbertson WR, Schowengerdt C, Hunt J. Nineteen years experience with the 1-stage perineal repair of rectal prolapse. *Am Surg.* 1971; 173:993–1001.

38. Friedman R, Muggia-Sulam J, Freund HR. Experience with the one-stage perineal repair of rectal prolapse. *Dis Colon Rectum.* 1983;26:789–791.

39. Gopal KA, Amshel AL, Shonberg IL, Eftaiha M. Rectal procidentia in elderly and debilitated patients. Experience with the Altmeier procedure. *Dis Colon Rectum.* 1984;27:376–381.

40. Prasad ML, Pearl RK, Abcarian H, Orsay CP, Nelson RL. Perineal proctectomy, posterior rectopexy, and postanal levator repair for the treatment of rectal prolapse. *Dis Colon Rectum.* 1986;29:547–552.

41. Ramanujam PS, Venkatesh KS. Perineal excision of rectal prolapse with posterior levator ani repair in elderly high-risk patients. *Dis Colon Rectum.* 1988; 31:704–706.

42. Uhlig BE, Sullivan ES. The modified Delorme operation: its place in surgical treatment for massive rectal prolapse. *Dis Colon Rectum.* 1979;22:513–521.

43. Christensen J, Kirkegaard P. Delorme's operation for complete rectal prolapse. *Br J Surg*. 1981;68: 537–538.

44. Gundersen AL, Cogbill TH, Landercasper J. Reappraisal of Delorme's procedure for rectal prolapse. *Dis Colon Rectum*. 1985;28:721–724.

45. Monson JR, Jones AN, Vowden P, Brennan TG. Delorme's operation: the first choice in complete rectal prolapse? *Ann R Coll Surg Engl*. 1986;68: 143–146.

46. Houry S, Lechaux JP, Huguier M, Moikhou JM. Treatment of rectal prolapse by Delorme's operation. *Int J Colorectal Dis*. 1987;2:149–152.

47. Jackaman FR, Francis JN, Hopkinson BR. Silicone rubber band treatment of rectal prolapse. *Ann R Coll Surg Engl*. 1980;62:386–387.

48. Labow S, Rubin R, Hoexter B, Salvati E. Perineal repair of procidentia with an elastic fabric sling. *Dis Colon Rectum*. 1980;23:467–469.

49. Hunt TM, Fraser IA, Maybury NK. Treatment of rectal prolapse by sphincteric support and using silastic rods. *Br J Surg*. 1985;72:491–492.

50. Poole GV Jr, Pennell TC, Myers RT, Hightower F. Modified Thiersch operation for rectal prolapse. Techniques and results. *Am Surg*. 1985;51: 226–229.

51. Vongsangnak V, Varma JS, Smith AN. Reappraisal of Thiersch's operation for complete rectal prolapse. *J Roy Coll Surg Edinb*. 1985;30:185–187.

52. Earnshaw JJ, Hopkinson BR. Late results of silicone rubber perianal suture for rectal prolapse. *Dis Colon Rectum*. 1987;30:86–88.

53. Khanduja KS, Hardy TG, Aguilar PS, et al. A new silicone prosthesis in the modified Thiersch operation. *Dis Colon Rectum*. 1988;31:380–383.

54. Williams JG. Perineal approaches to repair of rectal prolapse. *Semin Colon Rectal Surg*. 1991;2(3): 198–204.

55. Gordon PH, Hoexter B. Complications of the Ripstein procedure. *Dis Colon Rectum*. 1978;21: 277–280.

56. Wells C. New operation for rectal prolapse. *Proc R Soc Med*. 1959;52:602–603.

57. McMahan JD, Ripstein CB. Rectal prolapse. An update on the rectal sling procedure. *Am Surg*. 1987;53:37–40.

58. Orr TG. A suspension operation for prolapse of the rectum. *Ann Surg*. 1947;126:833–840.

59. Muir EG. Treatment of complete rectal prolapse in the adult. *Proc R Soc Med*. 1962;55:1086.

60. Schlinkert RT, Beart RW Jr, Wolff BG, Pemberton JH. Anterior resection for complete rectal prolapse. *Dis Colon Rectum*. 1985;28:409–412.

61. Watts JD, Rothenberger DA, Buls JG, et al. The management of procidentia. 30 years experience. *Dis Colon Rectum*. 1985;28:96–102.

62. Husa A, Salinio P, von Smitten K. Abdominal rectopexy and sigmoid resection (Frykman-Goldberg operation) for rectal prolapse. *Acta Chir Scand*. 1988;154:221–224.

63. Mikulicz J. Zur operativen Behandlung des Prolapsus Recti et Coli Invaginati. *Arch Klin Chir*. 1889; 38:74–97.

64. Miles WE. Rectosigmoidectomy as a method of treatment for procidentia recti. *Proc R Soc Assoc Med*. 1933;26:1445–1448.

65. Delorme E. On the treatment of total prolapse of the rectum by excision of the rectal mucus membranes or rect-colic. *Dis Colon Rectum*. 1985;28: 544–553.

66. Goldmann J. Concerning prolapse of the rectum with special emphasis on the operation by Thiersch. *Dis Colon Rectum*. 1988;31:154–155.

67. Vermeulen FD, Nivatvongs S, Fang DT, Balcos EG, Goldberg SM. A technique for perineal rectosigmoidoscopy using autosuture devices. *Surg Gynecol Obstet*. 1983;156:85–86.

68. Ladha A, Lee P, Berger P. Use of Angelchik antireflux prosthesis for repair of total rectal prolapse in elderly patients. *Dis Colon Rectum*. 1985;28:5–7.

69. Boulos PB, Stryker SJ, Nicholls RJ. The long term results of polyvinyl alcohol (Ivalon) sponge for rectal prolapse in young patients. *Br J Surg*. 1984; 71:213–214.

70. Yoshioka K, Helen F, Keighley MRB. Functional results after posterior abdominal rectopexy for rectal prolapse. *Dis Colon Rectum*. 1989;32:835–838.

71. Rogers J, Jeffery PJ. Intersphincteric repair and Ivalon sponge rectopexy for the treatment of rectal prolapse. *Br J Surg*. 1987;74:384–386.

72. Sayfan J, Pinho M, Alexander-Williams J, Keighley MRB. Sutured posterior abdominal rectopexy with sigmoidectomy compared with Marlex® rectopexy for rectal prolapse. *Br J Surg*. 1980;77:143–145.

73. Duthie GS, Bartolo DCC. A comparison between Marlex and resection rectopexy. *Neth J Surg*. 1989; 41:136–139.

74. Broden G, Dolk A, Holmstrom B. Evacuation difficulties and other characteristics of rectal function associated with procidentia and the Ripstein operation. *Dis Colon Rectum*. 1988;31:283–286.

75. Rutter KRP. Solitary rectal ulcer syndrome of the rectum: its relation to mucosal prolapse. In: Henry MM, Swash M, eds. *Coloproctology in the Pelvic Floor*. London: Butterworths; 1985:282–289.

76. Nicholls RJ. Internal intussusception—the solitary rectal ulcer syndrome. *Semin Colon Rectal Surg*. 1991;2(3):227–232.

77. Lowry AC, Goldberg SM. Internal and overt rectal procidentia. *Gastoenterol Clin North Am.* 1987;16 (1):47–70.

78. Rutter KRP, Riddell RH. Solitary ulcer syndrome of the rectum. *Clin Gastroenterol.* 1975;4:503–530.

79. Jones PN, Lubowski DZ, Swash M, et al. Is paradoxical contraction of puborectalis muscle of functional importance? *Dis Colon Rectum.* 1987; 30:667–670.

80. Mackle EJ, Manton Mills JO, Parks TG. The investigation of anorectal dysfunction in the solitary rectal ulcer syndrome. *Int J Colorectal Dis.* 1990;5: 21–24.

81. Mahieu PHG. Barium enema and defaecography in the diagnosis and evaluation of the solitary rectal ulcer syndrome. *Int J Colorectal Dis.* 1986;1:85–90.

82. Kuijpers HC, Schreve RH, Hoedemakers HC. Diagnosis of functional disorders of defecation causing the solitary rectal ulcer syndrome. *Dis Colon Rectum.* 1986;29:126–129.

83. Shorvon PJ, McHugh S, Diamant NE, Somers S, Stevenson GW. Defecography in normal volunteers: results and implications. *Gut.* 1989;30: 1737–1749.

84. Brandt-Gradel VVD, Huibregtse K, Tytgat GNJ. Treatment of solitary rectal ulcer syndrome with high-fiber diet and abstention of straining at defecation. *Dig Dis Sci.* 1984;29:1005–1008.

85. Keighley MRB, Shouler P. Clinical and manometric features of the solitary rectal ulcer syndrome. *Dis Colon Rectum.* 1984;27:507–512.

86. Berman IR, Manning DH, Dudley-Wright K. Anatomic specificity in the diagnosis and treatment of internal rectal prolapse. *Dis Colon Rectum.* 1985;28: 816–826.

87. Nicholls RJ, Simson JNL. Anteroposterior rectopexy in the treatment of solitary rectal ulcer syndrome without overt rectal prolapse. *Br J Surg.* 1986;73:222–224.

CHAPTER 8

ANAL INCONTINENCE

David Andrew Cherry and Marc Lehrer Greenwald

Anal continence is the ability to defer the call to stool to a socially acceptable time and place. Continence depends on a complex relationship between sphincter function, rectal and anal sensation, and "normal" pelvic anatomy. When stool or gas passes into the rectum, the rectum distends, initiating the relaxation of the internal sphincter via the rectoanal inhibitory reflex. The rectal contents then enter the anal canal where they are sampled by the sensitive anoderm. If passage of rectal contents is unwanted, afferent stimulation via the pudendal nerves augments the tonic activity in the puborectalis that decreases the anorectal angle and stimulates the external sphincter mechanism which tightens and lengthens the anal canal. Significant disruption of this process leads to incontinence.

Loss of control of solid feces is *complete anal incontinence,* whereas loss of control over flatus or liquid is *partial anal incontinence. Overflow incontinence* may be complete or incomplete and is more commonly associated with diarrheal syndromes and fecal impaction.[1] Anal incontinence is both psychologically traumatizing and incapacitating. Embarrassment, social ostracism, and poor physician acceptance often lead afflicted patients to minimize the degree of incontinence or to fail to report it altogether. For the same reasons the true incidence and prevalence of anal incontinence is unknown. A mail survey of 14,844 individuals ages 15 years or older in two London boroughs estimated the prevalence of anal incontinence to be 4.3 per 1000 population.[2] In contrast, higher prevalences—10.3 per 100—were found among patients residing in long-term care institutions for the elderly.[3]

A careful history is the first essential step toward understanding an individual's complaint of incontinence (Fig. 8-1). An adequate understanding of anorectal and pelvic floor anatomy and physiology will encourage a pointed investigation and subsequently a directed therapeutic approach to any individual's problem.[4]

Etiology

Pseudoincontinence

Pseudoincontinence (Table 8-1) caused by perineal soiling, frequency, and urgency must be distinguished from true anal incontinence. Soiling can be caused by prolapsing hemorrhoids, condylomata, poor hygiene, fistula-in-ano, or perianal dermatologic conditions. Similarly, frequency or urgency as a result of loss of the rectal reservoir, abnormal rectal compliance, or irritable bowel syndrome can imitate true anal incontinence.

Overflow Incontinence

Overflow incontinence is often associated with rectal fecal impaction. It has been shown that sphincter pressures in patients with fecal impaction are relatively normal, although anorectal sensation, compared to age-matched controls, is significantly decreased. Large rectal volumes are tolerated in recently disimpacted patients before fullness, pain, the desire to defecate, or reflex internal sphincter relaxation occurs. The decrease in rectal sensation, combined with a measurable decrease in anal and perianal sensation, plus a more obtuse anorectal angle found in these impacted patients, may be responsible for their overflow incontinence.[5,6] This disturbance of the continence mechanism permits soiling by interfering with the ability to contract the external sphincter consciously as liquid stool flows around the impacted fecal mass. Medications that alter mental status, stool consistency, or intestinal motility can be initiators of fecal impaction and incontinence. In addition, overflow incontinence may be associated with pelvic floor dysfunction, and appropriate investigation may be required.

Incontinence With Normal Pelvic Floor Function

Anal incontinence may occur in the presence of normal pelvic floor and sphincter function. In diarrheal states, an increased volume of liquid stool coupled with rapid colonic transit may overwhelm the normal mechanisms of continence. Shortened transit time and increased intraluminal quantities of liquid stool may be a consequence of intestinal resection, inflammatory bowel disease, laxative abuse, autonomic neuropathy, parasitic infestation, specific toxins, or other causes.

Incontinence With Abnormal Pelvic Floor Function

Disruption of the sphincter mechanism is one of the most common causes of anal incontinence. Previous surgical procedures and obstetric trauma represent the most common causes of sphincter mechanism injury.[7,8] The principal pathophysiologic conditions are complete or partial loss of the anal canal high pressure zone,[9] alterations in normal sampling mechanisms,[10] or both. When anorectal procedures that could jeopardize anal continence are being planned, patients should receive adequate information preoperatively about expected postoperative bowel function and the possibility of permanent incontinence.

Fistula Surgery

Fistula surgery is the most common operative procedure that results in anal incontinence. Complete anal incontinence is best avoided by preserving the anorectal ring. Nevertheless, partial incontinence may occur if even a small amount of the sphincter mechanism is divided. Clinical outcome correlates with the amount of sphincter cut as well as with a decrease in resting and voluntary contraction anal pressures.[11] Incontinence is best prevented by minimizing the amount of sphincter muscle cut and minimizing dilation of the anal canal. The use of a seton or "coring out" the fistulous tract may improve results by sparing the sphincter mechanism. Anal manometry may help identify preoperatively those patients with poor sphincter function who are at high risk of postoperative incontinence.

Obstetric Injury

Perineal tears and sphincter injuries as a result of vaginal deliveries are among the most common causes of surgically correctable incontinence seen in practice today. Primary repair of a third degree laceration is highly successful.[12,13] Episiotomies are incisions to facilitate delivery and shorten the second stage of labor. Nevertheless, it is unclear whether or not a routine episiotomy reduces the incidence of postdelivery sphincter injury and pelvic floor dysfunction. Although the incidence of third degree tears tends to be lower in mediolateral (0 to 9.0 percent) versus midline episiotomies (0.5 to 23.9 percent) the range of reported values is too broad to allow the inference that the mediolateral offers an advantage.[14] The incidence of incontinence associated with episiotomies has been difficult to assess.[12] However, in one study which included 106 women who had mediolateral episiotomies and 250 women who had median episiotomies, the incidences of complete anal incontinence were 1.9 and 1.2 percent, respectively.[15]

Despite primary repair, an infection, a localized hematoma, or breakdown of the wound may cause an immediately recognized rectovaginal fistula and/or sphincter dysfunction leading to incontinence. Unrecognized sphincter damage[16] and rectovaginal fistulas account for other causes of incontinence following vaginal delivery. Vaginal delivery can also cause pudendal nerve injury, and consequently sphincter weakness and incontinence.[17,18] One must always be cognizant of the "double pathology" involving both a nerve injury and a direct sphincter injury when investigating and treating obstetric trauma—induced anal incontinence. Surgical repair of the sphincter injury may not improve the patient's continence if the sphincter is also denervated.[19]

Internal Anal Sphincterotomy

Incision of the internal sphincter for the treatment of anal fissures, or for other reasons, may lead to a decrease in anal canal resting tone. Partial incontinence due to disruption of the internal sphincter may ensue. However, complete incontinence is rare unless the external sphincter or puborectalis is concomitantly damaged. The incontinence following isolated internal sphincterotomy may be temporary or permanent.

The *keyhole deformity* is a furrowed defect in the anal canal which follows an internal sphincterotomy, especially when performed in the posterior midline. Although classically it follows a midline posterior fissurectomy and sphincterotomy, it can occur after a variety of anal procedures. The defect results from excision of excessive anoderm and underlying muscle[20] and can lead to chronic leakage of mucus, an everted

ANAL INCONTINENCE HISTORY

Name _____

Age _____   Sex _____   Age at onset of incontinence _____

Stool consistency

☐ Liquid   ☐ Semiliquid   ☐ Formed/soft
☐ Formed/hard   ☐ Pellet

Status of incontinence

☐ Formed stool   ☐ Liquid stool   ☐ Flatus
☐ Day   ☐ Night   ☐ Day and night

Frequency (use of pad)

☐ Never   ☐ Sometimes   ☐ Always
☐ Day   ☐ Night   Duration of use _____

Sensation of call to stool   ☐ Normal   ☐ Variable   ☐ Absent

Sensation of at time of defecation   ☐ Normal   ☐ Variable   ☐ Absent

Ability to differentiate solid/liquid/gas   ☐ Normal   ☐ Variable   ☐ Absent

Urgency to evacuate   ☐ Yes   ☐ No

Excessive straining   ☐ Yes   ☐ No

Time required to evacuate _____

Painful evacuation   ☐ Yes   ☐ No

Sensation of incomplete evacuation   ☐ Yes   ☐ No

Number of bowel movements/24 hours _____

Frequent unsuccessful attempts to evacuate   ☐ Yes   ☐ No

Sensation of rectal prolapse   ☐ Yes   ☐ No

Rectal bleeding   ☐ Yes   ☐ No

Figure 8-1.   Anal incontinence history form.

anal canal, bothersome pruritus, and soiling of the undergarments. The keyhole deformity is best avoided by treating anal fissures with a lateral sphincterotomy rather than with either fissurectomy or posterior sphincterotomy. The desire to introduce a large anal retractor to facilitate rectal surgery in and of itself is not a good indication for a sphincterotomy.

Hemorrhoidectomy

Complete anal incontinence should be a rare and largely avoidable complication of hemorrhoidectomy. Yet, injury to the internal sphincter and subsequent incontinence can occur from blind clamping of hemorrhoidal tissue or from failure to create the proper plane of dissection. It has been suggested that partial incontinence may be a result of the removal of the "cushioning" hemorrhoid tissue itself, a tissue described as the corpus cavernosum of the anus.[21] Other investigators discount the importance of the anal vascular cushions for maintaining normal continence and contend that lower anal canal pressures account for posthemorrhoidal incontinence.[22] Rubber-band ligation is not associated with a reduction in anal canal pressures,[23] and this treatment may lead to fewer cases of incontinence following hemorrhoidal therapy.

Urinary incontinence   ☐ Yes   ☐ No

Alteration in social life
    ☐ Never   ☐ Sometimes   ☐ Always   ☐ Incapacitating

Medications _____

_____

Dietary inquiry _____

_____

Medical history

    Congenital anorectal disorders _____

    _____

    Therapeutic interventions—operative history, radiation _____

    _____

    Previous anorectal surgery/disease _____

    _____

    Anorectal trauma _____

    _____

    Obstetric history _____

    _____

    Systemic/neuromuscular disorders _____

    _____

    Gastrointestinal disorder, IBD, irritable bowel syndrome _____

    _____

    Psychiatric history _____

    _____

Figure 8-1. Anal incontinence history form. (*Continued*)

The Whitehead operation, when performed incorrectly, may lead to eversion of the rectal mucosa onto the anoderm. Incontinence results from destruction of normal sensory mechanisms, and soiling may occur as a direct outcome of an ectropion with leakage of mucus onto the perineum. Rarely, a hemorrhoidectomy will heal with a circumferential scar and result in partial incontinence from inadequate closure of the anal canal.

Submucosal hemorrhoidectomy has been shown to produce less alteration in the anal canal sensory mechanism than excisional hemorrhoidectomy. Nevertheless, this difference has not translated into improved function in the submucosal hemorrhoidectomy group.[24]

Stretching the Sphincters

Hemorrhoid or fissure therapy by intentional manual dilation as described in the Lord technique[25] can be followed by incontinence and sphincter damage, and therefore this technique should be avoided. Unintentional sphincter stretching during retraction for anal surgery may also adversely affect continence.[26,27] Use of adjustable bi-valve retractors[28] for anal procedures may decrease the incidence of unintentional anal dilation and postoperative incontinence, and intentional anal dilation to facilitate the introduction of large anal retractors should be avoided.

Table 8-1   Classification of Etiology of Anal Incontinence

PSEUDOINCONTINENCE

Perineal soiling	Urgency
rectal mucosal prolapse	noncompliant rectum
hemorrhoidal prolapse	irradiation
incomplete defecation	IBD
poor hygiene	absent rectal reservoir
fistula in ano	irritable bowel syndrome
dermatologic condition	
anorectal sexually transmitted disease	
anorectal neoplasms	

OVERFLOW INCONTINENCE

Impaction	Psychotropic drugs
Encopresis	Rectal neoplasms
Antimotility drugs	

INCONTINENCE WITH NORMAL PELVIC FLOOR

Diarrheal states	Systemic disease processes
IBD	CNS/spinal cord
short gut	neoplasm
laxative abuse	injury
infection	dementia/strokes
parasites	multiple sclerosis
bacteria	scleroderma
toxins	neuropathies (diabetic)
intermittent partial small bowel obstruction	

INCONTINENCE WITH ABNORMAL PELVIC FLOOR FUNCTION

Sphincter injury	
obstetric	imperforate anus
traumatic	myelomeningocele
iatrogenic	Pelvic floor denervation
neoplastic	pudendal nerve neuropathy
inflammatory	perineal descent syndrome
rectal prolapse	traumatic
Congenital abnormalities	aging
spina bifida	neoplastic infiltration

Modified from: Rothenberger DA. Anal incontinence. In: Cameron JL, ed. *Current Surgical Therapy*, 3rd ed. Philadelphia: BC Decker; 1989:186.

Sphincter Saving Operations

Low Anterior Resection. Low anterior resection performed in the mid third and distal third of the rectum can be associated with incontinence. Loss of the sigmoid–rectal reservoir, alterations in anal tone, and/or alterations in the anal rectal sensory mechanism are thought to be responsible.[29,30] These problems, usually seen in the early postoperative period, generally resolve within 6 months, although further improvement may continue for an additional year.[31-33] A small percentage of patients who undergo a low anterior resection suffer from partial incontinence, but incontinence to solid feces is exceedingly rare. The distal limit of an anastomosis that will not directly disturb the continence mechanism is the proximal anal canal. This point is just above the anorectal ring and is usually 4 cm from the anal verge. End-to-end anastomosis performed with staplers, particularly the development of the "double staple" technique, has permitted extremely low rectal anastomoses with acceptable function. However, if the anorectal ring is disturbed, partial or complete incontinence may occur.

Coloanal Anastomosis. The coloanal anastomosis is a method to preserve sphincter function in selected patients. By performing an end-to-end endoanal anastomosis, anal manipulation and alterations in sensory and anatomic relationships important in continence are minimized. Parks and Percy[34] reported functional results in 70 patients who underwent coloanal anastomosis following resection for carcinoma of the rectum. Of his patients, 39 had completely normal bowel function, while 30 others were continent with increased stool frequency. Only 1 of the 70 patients was incontinent. Other investigators who employ endoanal[35-37] and transsphincteric[38] coloanal anastomosis report similar favorable functional results. Continence appears to depend on the preservation of sphincter function and the avoidance of pelvic hematomas and ensuing sepsis which lead to pelvic fibrosis.[39]

Ileorectal Anastomosis. Ileorectal anastomosis is usually not associated with significant incontinence if adequate rectal length is preserved.[40] Nevertheless, caution in recommending this operation to the elderly is advised. Preexisting sphincter dysfunction due to aging and pelvic floor denervation may lead to incapacitating incontinence. This issue is discussed in more depth in the following pages.

Ileoanal Anastomosis. Ileoanal anastomosis following colectomy, mucosal proctectomy, and the formation of an ileal reservoir is associated with variable degrees of incontinence.[41-44] Contributing factors are thought to be loss of the rectal reservoir, disruption of sensory mechanisms and damage to the sphincter mechanism by coexisting perianal disease, or prolonged or excessive endoanal retraction.[26,45,46] Minimizing the duration of intraanal retraction or avoiding it with the use of Gelpi retractors[47] may improve postoperative continence. Some recent literature reports that avoidance of mucosectomy and performance of a double-stapled ileoanal anastomosis may result in better continence,[48,49,50a,50b] although one small prospective randomized trial did not show any difference in continence in patients with and without mucosectomy.[51]

Pelvic Floor Denervation

Any form of disruption of the normal sensory or motor innervation mechanisms of the pelvic floor can lead to incontinence. Pelvic floor denervation can be a result of pudendal nerve neuropathy, perineal descent syndrome, trauma, aging, neoplastic infiltration, or a combination of these problems[52,53] (see Table 8-1). What was once classified as "idiopathic incontinence" is now carefully evaluated by physiologic testing of the pelvic floor and categorized accordingly. Incontinence may result from occult pudendal nerve injury occurring during vaginal delivery, or from stretch injury associated with excessive perineal descent following chronic forceful straining during defecation.[54,55] It has been shown that the pudendal neuropathy associated with vaginal delivery may worsen over time, leading to neurogenic incontinence years after the initial insult.[18] Incontinent patients with measured pudendal neuropathy from presumed nerve stretch injury have also been shown to have dysfunctional internal sphincters when evaluated by electrophysiologic (EMG), manometric, and in vitro pharmacologic studies.[56] The presence of an abnormal internal anal sphincter in patients with neurogenic incontinence has also been demonstrated by anal endosonography. Law and associates[57] have reported a linear relationship between anal canal resting pressures and internal anal sphincter thickness in patients with "idiopathic" incontinence.

Progressive pelvic floor descent establishes a vicious cycle of repetitive neural stretch injury and continued denervation. A direct relationship has been reported between pelvic floor descent and pudendal nerve terminal motor latency in patients with idiopathic anal incontinence, thus correlating the degree of descent with the degree of neuropathy.[58]

Various studies have examined anorectal function in the elderly. Although the findings have been inconsistent regarding squeeze pressures, a significant decrease in anal resting pressures in older populations has been identified.[59,60] An age-related decrease in the number of spinal cord neurons has also been demonstrated,[61] and this, too, may be related to the incontinence associated with aging. Once denervation has occurred, muscular dysfunction is permanent.

Procidentia

Complete rectal prolapse, procidentia, is associated with incontinence in over 50 percent of cases reviewed.[62] In cases in which prolapse is associated with incontinence, electromyographic studies have documented evidence of denervation injury to the pelvic floor and sphincter muscles.[63,64] It is unclear whether denervation is caused by prolapse alone or is the result of nerve stretch injury from previous straining at defecation. Isolated prolapse without concomitant incontinence is rarely associated with electromyographic evidence of denervation injury.[64] Transabdominal repair of rectal prolapse has been associated with improvement of continence in 43 to 64 percent of patients, whereas perineal proctectomy has generally been associated with improvement in only 6 to 20 percent of patients.[65] Parks' postanal repair and sphincter plication techniques as secondary procedures have had varied success, although one report of perineal proctectomy combined with a posterior rectopexy and a postanal levator repair has shown a dramatic increase in postoperative continence.[66] Improved continence following abdominal and perineal proctopexy for prolapse may be a result of restoration of the anorectal angle or recovery from muscular dysfunction due to reversible muscular stretch injury.

Trauma

Blunt pelvic trauma or impalement injury may disrupt the sphincter mechanism. Also, severe pelvic fractures may cause direct nerve injury and neurogenic incontinence. If the source of incontinence is unclear, investigation is required to provide appropriate treatment. Anorectal trauma is discussed in more detail in Chapter 23.

Irradiation

Use of extracavitary or intracavitary radiation for the treatment of anal, rectal, cervical, prostatic, and uterine carcinomas can be associated with incontinence from damage to the sphincter mechanism and pelvic musculature. Radiation proctitis, loss of rectal compliance, and alteration of anorectal sensation are also contributing factors. Treatment of this problem can be difficult and generally begins with a high bulk diet and two to three daily cleansing enemas. If the incontinence is a result of radiation proctitis and altered rectal compliance in the presence of normal sphincter muscle function, resection and coloanal pullthrough may be beneficial. If the anal incontinence is due to sphincter muscle dysfunction, a permanent colostomy may be necessary. If anorectal symptoms continue after such diversion, a proctectomy may ultimately be required. The problems of radiation proctitis are further discussed in Chapter 25.

Imperforate Anus

Congenital anorectal malformations are classified according to the relationship of the termination of the bowel to the puborectalis sling. A high imperforate anus ends cephalad to the puborectalis, whereas a low imperforate anus ends below the puborectalis. Surgical repair is directed toward the establishment of a perineal opening with enough motor and sensory function to restore the normal mechanism of continence. Motor function is best reestablished by redirection of the bowel through the puborectalis sling and usually achieves gross continence of solids. Unfortunately, reestablishment of sensory function is unusual and its absence probably contributes to continued postoperative partial or complete incontinence. Treatment of imperforate anus is detailed in Chapter 3.

Miscellaneous

Rectal and anal neoplasms can invade the sphincter mechanism and cause anal incontinence. The presence of a tumor must always be excluded by a complete history and physical examination, and by appropriate evaluation. More proximal lesions can lead to overflow incontinence as a result of intermittent bowel obstruction and the rapid presentation of a large amount of liquid stool to a limited rectal reservoir. Chronic inflammatory conditions of the anorectum, such as amebic colitis, inflammatory bowel disease, and lymphogranuloma venereum, may lead to a disruption of sensory mechanisms and result in a loss of reservoir function and incontinence. On rare occasions, large villous adenomas produce large quantities of mucus which overwhelm the sphincter mechanism and present as incontinence.

Diagnosis

History

The most important factor in the successful treatment of anal incontinence is determination of the etiology. The history is the most reliable means of elucidating the etiology in the majority of patients (see Fig. 8-1). Many incontinent patients initially report symptoms other than true incontinence. The degree and duration of incontinence, together with any history of obstetric injury, anorectal surgery, or trauma should be documented (Table 8-2). A history of chronic straining, rectal prolapse, and urinary incontinence favors pelvic floor pathology as a cause of the anal incontinence. Assessment should include a neurologic review questioning the presence of pain in the perineum or lower back as well as sensory or motor changes in the lower extremities or buttocks. Symptoms of recent onset are of particular importance.

The degree of incontinence may be elucidated by questions regarding the use of protective pads, particularly the number of pads used per unit of time, and whether pads are required during both the day and the night. Often a patient will report not being able to leave the house unless he or she knows of an available bathroom at each destination. Dietary and medication history should be noted.

Physical Examination

Isolated sphincter dysfunction must be differentiated from general metabolic and neurologic disorders that may present as incontinence. In most patients with sphincter injuries, clinical evaluation by an experienced surgeon is all that is required for preoperative assessment and planning for proper repair (Table 8-3). Direct inspection of the perineum is essential. Spreading of the buttocks will reveal a patulous anus, loss of the perineal body, or muscular deficit in the anorectal ring. The

Table 8-2   Clinical Score for Anal Incontinence

Frequency	Incontinence of gas	Incontinence of liquid	Incontinence of solid	Significantly alters lifestyle
< 1/month	1	4	7	10
> 1/month < 1/week	2	5	8	11
> 1/week	3	6	9	12

The patient's incontinence score is determined by adding points from each column in the grid. Patients with scores above 12 are candidates for surgical repair.

Modified from: Miller R, Bartolo DCC, Locke-Edmunds NJM. Prospective study of conservative and experimental treatment for faecal incontinence. As cited by Rothenberger DA. Anal incontinence. In: Cameron JL, ed. *Current Surgical Therapy,* 3rd ed. Philadelphia: BC Decker; 1989:186.

Table 8-3   Physical Examination

INSPECTION
Perineal soiling
Scars
Mucosal ectropion
Prolapsing hemorrhoids
Rectal prolapse
Patulous anus
Loss of perineal body
Muscular deficit
Muscular contraction
Perineal descent with Valsalva
Fistula

PALPATION
Pinprick
  touch
  anal wink
Resting tone
Squeeze tone
Puborectalis motion
Puborectalis traction
Muscular defects
Anal canal length
Anorectal angle
Rectal content
Soft tissue scarring
Anal canal compliance

ENDOSCOPY
Neoplasm
Solitary rectal ulcer
Scarring
Mucosal lesions
Rectal intussusception

Adapted from: Rothenberger DA. Anal incontinence. In: Cameron JL, ed. *Current Surgical Therapy,* 3rd ed. Philadelphia: BC Decker; 1989:186.

presence of perineal soiling, scars from previous surgery or trauma, mucosal ectropion, prolapsing hemorrhoids, or complete rectal prolapse should be noted. Sensation is assessed by touch and gentle pinprick. Absence of the cutaneous anal wink reflex points to a neurologic origin of incontinence.[67,68] Direct palpation will reveal the tone of the sphincter musculature. Asking the patient to "squeeze" while the examining finger is in the anal canal and rectum will permit rapid assessment of the contractility of the sphincters. Sphincter defects and motion of the puborectalis can also be noted. Gentle traction by the examining finger on the puborectalis sling, followed by loss of sphincter tone, points to a neurologic etiology[69] of anal incontinence. The existence of inflammatory and neoplastic processes contributing to incontinence must be excluded by routine anoscopy and proctosigmoidoscopy. Endoscopic evaluation may reveal other diagnostic clues, such as a solitary rectal ulcer, which can be seen in incontinent patients with rectal prolapse. Finally, the ability of a patient to retain a 100-ml enema is a useful clinical guide in the assessment of incontinence. If a patient is able to retain the enema, careful consideration prior to extensive evaluation and eventual medical or surgical treatment is indicated.

Special Investigations

The traditional surgical treatment of anal incontinence has been based on clinical evaluation rather than on laboratory data. This approach is appropriate for most cases of uncomplicated sphincter injuries. However, in patients with sphincter dysfunction not attributable to direct muscular sphincter trauma, diagnosis and treatment can be more difficult. Pelvic floor morphology and the presence of complex reflex mechanisms have made isolated evaluation of the components of the continence mechanism very difficult. Yet, continued clinical research in the pelvic floor laboratory has allowed the development and refinement of several investigative tools which do permit some assessment of these components. These studies are discussed in more detail in Chapters 2 and 6.

Anal Manometry

The anal sphincters generate the basal resting and voluntary squeeze pressures. The aim of measuring anal canal pressures is to assess the resistance of the anal canal to the passage of gas, liquid, and solid material. There is a significant correlation between anal canal pressure and the force needed to expel a balloon from the rectum.[70] Despite this correlation, the manometric results of normal and incontinent patients overlap.[71,72] Manometry can assess the length of the sphincters in the anal canal, as well as resting and maximal voluntary contraction pressure, and the presence of the rectal anal inhibitory reflex. Such data may be helpful in planning the treatment of incontinence.

Direct traumatic sphincter injury is characterized by a low sphincter resting pressure, a low maximum voluntary contraction pressure, or both. In addition a shortened high pressure time and impaired anal canal sensation may be noted. Patients with isolated external sphincter injury will have near-normal resting tone and diminished maximum contraction pressure. Isolated division of the internal sphincter muscle will result in a drop in resting pressure[73] with maintenance of normal maximum voluntary contraction. Patients with idiopathic anal incontinence generally have low resting and maximum voluntary contraction pressures,[70,74,75] as well as a decrease in anal canal sensation.[10,76]

The correlation between external sphincter function and the degree of incontinence is a subject of debate. Early studies reported a significant relationship between manometric findings and incontinence,[77-79] whereas more recent work has demonstrated a lack of significant correlation between incontinence and anorectal function tests.[72] At present, precise indications for anal manometry in the study of anal incontinence are unclear. Data regarding the predictive value of preoperative manometric assessment for patients who undergo surgery for incontinence conflict.[80,81] It is desirable to identify the cause of a patient's incontinence, and anal manometry may augment the history and physical examination and help to distinguish those patients with incontinence from sphincter injury, neuropathic insult, or "double pathology."

Cine Defecography

Cine defecography is the radiographic visualization of the dynamics of defecation.[82,83] This simple technique involves filling the rectum with radiopaque contrast dye which has the consistency of stool. The patient is then positioned on a radiolucent commode and lateral fluoroscopic images are continuously recorded on videotape during defecation. Changes in the anorectal angle, perineal descent, configurational changes in the rectal wall, and the adequacy of evacuation can be observed. Causative or associated factors of incontinence that can be confirmed on cine defecography include occult rectal prolapse, increased perineal descent, increased anorectal angle, and shortened anal canal length.

Balloon Proctogram and Sphincterogram

To have incontinence of solid stool it is often necessary to have low sphincter pressures in combination with an obtuse anorectal angle. The balloon proctogram is one means of assessing the anorectal angle.[84] In this technique a flexible balloon filled with radiopaque dye is inserted into the anal canal and rectum. Lateral roentgenograms allow visualization of the anorectal angle during rest, maximum voluntary squeeze, and straining. Scintigraphic assessment of the anorectal angle[85] employs radioisotopes to obtain information about the anorectal angle.

To assess the anorectal angle and anal canal pressures simultaneously the balloon sphincterogram can be used.[86a] A contrast-filled balloon placed in the anal canal and rectum is used to assess the anorectal angle radiologically during sphincter contraction and rest, as is the case with balloon proctography. However, the balloon sphincterogram incorporates an open-ended system to record anal canal pressures simultaneously.

Balloon proctography and sphincterography can also be used to measure perineal descent and puborectalis motion, but these data may be more easily obtained with defecography. Since both manometry and defecography will provide the information obtained from balloon sphincterography, the technique is rarely used. The correlation between measurements of anorectal angle made with balloon proctography and those made with cine defecography is very poor.[86b]

Electromyography

Electromyographic investigation of the pelvic floor musculature allows important evaluation of the electrophysiological function of the external sphincter and the puborectalis muscle.[87] Electromyographic potentials that are multiphasic and of increased amplitude and duration are consistent with injury, denervation, and subsequent partial reinnervation of the puborectalis and external sphincter muscle fibers from adjacent intact neuromuscular units. If significant denervation has occurred, neurogenic pelvic floor dysfunction may result.

Electromyographic studies[53,63,64,88] in patients with idiopathic incontinence or incontinence associated with rectal prolapse suggest that neurogenic pelvic floor dysfunction may be responsible. Single-fiber electromyography allows the investigator to measure "muscle fiber density." An increased fiber density indicates a damaged neuromuscular unit that has undergone partial reinnervation.[53,87]

Once denervation injury has been documented by electromyography, the location of the neurologic lesion can be defined by evoked response electromyography techniques. The terminal external sphincter innervation can be assessed by stimulating the pudendal nerve transrectally, and more proximal innervation injuries can be localized by transcutaneous stimulation of the motor roots at the lumbar levels L-1 and L-4.[87] This technique can be used to assess pudendal, perineal, and spinal motor latencies. Injured segments of nerve axons have slower conduction velocities than normal segments. The slower conduction time in these damaged nerves is reflected in prolonged motor nerve latency times.[87,89] Measurement at different levels along the nerve axons allows localization of axon injury to the peripheral, root, or spinal level.

Rectal Compliance and Capacity

Alterations in rectal compliance can be responsible for incontinence. True rectal compliance is difficult to measure because the rectum is not a closed cavity. Despite these limitations, compliant water-filled balloons with internal pressure sensors can be employed to generate pressure/volume curves to derive estimates of rectal compliance. Some investigators have measured the rectal balloon volumes associated with patients' initial recognition of rectal fullness, the call to stool, acute urgency, pain, and maximum tolerable volume in continent and incontinent patients.[90–92] Significant differences between these two groups of patients have been found in one recent report,[91] but other reports contradict these findings.[90,92] It is hypothesized that surgical resection of the rectum, inflammation, radiation, or neoplastic infiltration may decrease rectal compliance and therefore allow for a more rapid rise in rectal pressure with rectal filling. When the rectal pressure becomes greater than the sphincter pressure, incontinence results. Moreover, a simple decrease in rectal capacity can contribute to incontinence. This may occur after a low colorectal or coloanal anastomosis.

Anal Endosonography

Anal endosonography was used by Law and associates[57] to examine 44 patients with anal incontinence; 11 patients had neurogenic incontinence, 14 patients had in- continence following obstetric trauma, and 19 patients had incontinence following surgical or other types of trauma. As mentioned earlier, Law found a linear relationship between anal canal resting pressure and internal sphincter thickness in patients with neurogenic incontinence and intact external sphincters. Also, patients with traumatic incontinence and combined internal and external sphincter defects had significantly lower anal canal resting pressures than patients with only external sphincter injuries. Of the 33 patients with traumatic incontinence, 25 had EMG mapping. External sphincter defects identified by anal endosonography correlated with defects identified by EMG in 19 of the 25 patients, and both endosonography and EMG evaluation failed to identify sphincter defects in the remaining 6 patients. In other words, Law found a 100% correlation between the results of endosonography and EMG evaluation in patients with traumatic incontinence. Anal endosonography will undoubtedly play an important role in the evaluation of the incontinent patient in the future.[93]

Treatment

Medical Therapy

Medical illness may cause changes in stool consistency or intestinal transit time which, even in the presence of normal pelvic floor function, may account for anal incontinence. Management in these patients should be directed at correction of identifiable underlying causes. A thorough investigation of diarrheal disorders should be conducted. Specific therapy in combination with constipating agents, dietary manipulation, or both will achieve satisfactory outcomes in many patients.

Prevention of excessive straining during defecation may prevent progressive perineal descent and denervation injury if prophylaxis is initiated early enough. Patient education, bowel training, and laxatives should be employed to minimize straining. Underlying pathologic conditions such as colonic neoplasms and functional pelvic outlet obstruction should be excluded.

Fecal impaction can account for anal incontinence in individuals with otherwise normal pelvic floor function. Overflow incontinence caused by fecal impaction should be excluded by physical examination in all incontinent patients. Therapies consisting of enemas, laxatives, and occasionally disimpaction in combination with a good bowel management program, patient education, and biofeedback in selected cases, are successful in the majority of individuals.[94]

The keyhole deformity can often cause significant soiling. Nonoperative therapy including instruction in personal hygiene with careful cleaning of the everted anus should be attempted. Bulk-forming or antimotility agents may help produce formed stool and minimize leakage for those patients with liquid or semisolid stool. A piece of cotton gauze placed between the buttocks and over the deformity may help prevent skin irritation. Operative correction is usually meddlesome, although some patients with severe deformities may require anoplasty.

Perianal strengthening exercises have been reported by patients to improve continence. Objective data that exercising actually improves sphincter function is lacking. Nevertheless, perineal exercises are simple to perform. Patients are instructed to contract the perineal muscle and hold the contraction for a count of 10 repeating the maneuver several times. The exercises are repeated at intervals throughout the day. Perianal electrical stimulation has also been reported to improve incontinence. One study using electrical stimulation of the dorsogenital nerve has shown a significant increase in resting and squeeze sphincter pressures in patients with pudendal nerve neuropathy.[95] Of 8 patients treated with this technique, 7 became continent by the end of the 2-month treatment period.

Biofeedback has become an accepted treatment alternative for anal incontinence.[96-101] The method involves the use of an anal probe connected to a transducer that monitors voluntary sphincter activity. The instrumentation can either be a balloon system which records pressure changes or an electromyographic plug which measures sphincter muscle activity. The patient is shown the normal response to voluntary contraction of the sphincter mechanism and then attempts to duplicate this response with the recording probe in place. A regimen is established with sphincter contraction repetition until the proper behavior is learned. It has been shown that patients who have had biofeedback training are able to sense rectal distention at much smaller volumes than could be detected in pretreatment examination. It has been postulated that this increase in rectal sensation is primarily responsible for the improvement in continence.[92,102] The "call to stool" is noticed by the patient because the distended rectum is appreciated at a point when the intraluminal rectal pressure is still lower than the anal sphincter pressure. This gives the patient time to reach the bathroom for a planned evacuation. MacLeod[99] used biofeedback to treat 113 patients with incontinence of several etiologies with 63 percent of patients having either complete recovery of incontinence or at least a 90 percent reduction in the frequency of incontinence. Of 31 patients with anal incontinence who were treated with biofeedback by Jensen and Lowry,[101] 28 also reported at least a 90 percent decrease in the frequency of incontinence. Intraanal EMG sensor–type biofeedback may be more valuable than manometric-based training or simple Kegel exercises.

Surgical Treatment

The importance of a sphincteric high pressure zone created by an intact and functional anorectal ring has been documented. An anatomically correct angle is also considered a component of the normal continence mechanism. Most current operative techniques attempt to restore the anorectal ring with its sphincter mechanism or the anorectal angle or both.

Acute trauma or obstetric injuries causing third- or fourth-degree lacerations of the perineum are best treated by immediate perineorrhaphy. If direct apposition of the severed muscle is performed at the time of injury without tension, results are satisfactory in the majority of patients (Fig. 8-2). Sepsis, hematoma formation, approximation under tension, faulty technique, or an unrecognized second sphincter injury can lead to unsatisfactory results requiring secondary repair. In the presence of excessive contamination or concomitant life-threatening injuries it is best to delay definitive sphincter repair. The addition of a diverting proximal colostomy is appropriate if the patient has multiple injuries, the perineal wound is large, or the patient has not been stabilized. Isolated obstetric injuries usually do not require a colostomy.

Delayed operative repair of the sphincter is the surgical treatment of choice for unrecognized anatomic disruption or failure of immediate repair. Secondary repair is performed only after all contaminated perineal wounds have healed, inflammation has subsided completely, and transient injury to the innervation of the external anal sphincter has subsided. This usually occurs in 3 to 6 months after the injury. During this waiting period, strong fibrous tissue forms at the injured muscle

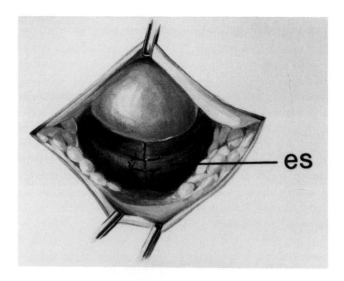

Figure 8-2.   Direct apposition: Immediate sphincter repair by direct apposition of external sphincter (es).

ends, which permits placement of secure sutures. Concomitant rectovaginal fistulas can be repaired at the same time as the sphincter muscle.

Candidates for surgical repair of the sphincter muscle must have at least one intact neuromuscular bundle with detectable voluntary anal sphincter contraction. As a general rule, at least 50 percent of the circumference of the sphincter must be present and actively contract.[103] Anal manometry and endosonographic[57,93] or electromyographic[104] sphincter mapping can be helpful in defining the anatomy of the sphincter injury if physical examination is inconclusive, although preoperative resting and squeeze pressures by themselves do not correlate with the success of the surgery.[105]

Overlapping Sphincteroplasty (Fig. 8-3)

Initial experience with delayed secondary repair of the severed sphincter muscle with end-to-end repair had a failure rate of 40 percent.[7] Failure was largely attributed to the suture material cutting through the muscle, which allowed retraction of the muscle ends.[106] To minimize the risk of disruption, overlapping sphincter repair is generally recommended.[106-110] This technique increases the contact surface area of severed muscle ends, thereby facilitating coaptation and adherence. Additionally, the overlapping technique calls for the placement of multiple mattress sutures which evenly distribute wound tension and prevent wound disruption. The overlap gives a margin of security that allows some retraction of the repaired muscle ends without complete disruption of the repair.

Preoperative management includes a full mechanical bowel preparation with the parenteral administration of antibiotics. A foley catheter is inserted in the operating room. The patient is placed in the prone jackknife position with the buttocks elevated over a 6-inch roll and taped apart. Shaving the patient is not necessary. Regional or general anesthesia may be used although a general anesthetic is preferred because the patient may become uncomfortable after a prolonged time in the jackknife position.

The operative site is infiltrated with a local anesthetic which contains a concentration of 1:200,000 epinephrine. This relaxes the muscles and facilitates hemostasis. A curvilinear incision is then made approximately 1.5 cm from the anal verge, parallel to the outer border of the superficial external sphincter, and the anoderm is mobilized from the underlying scar and sphincter mechanism. With extensive obstetric injuries (i.e., the traumatic cloaca) where the perineal body has been destroyed and the rectal mucosa is adjacent to the vaginal mucosa, the incision is created directly on the line separating the rectal and vaginal linings. The arc of the

incision for any overlapping sphincter repair should extend approximately 180 to 240 degrees, depending on the extent of the scar, to facilitate mobilization of the retracted underlying sphincter muscle. The incision should be extended laterally until unscarred ischiorectal fat is encountered. Initiating the flap dissection laterally in this unscarred area permits an easier entry into the proper plane, but care must be taken to preserve the neurovascular bundles, which enter the muscles posteriorly and laterally (Fig. 8-3A). The dissection continues medially and cephalad. Cephalad mobilization of the endorectal flap continues beyond the extent of the scar and may extend to the levator muscles if necessary. Defects in the mucosal tube, from rectovaginal fistulas or iatrogenic tears, should be repaired by simple suture during the mucosal dissection and before sphincter repair. The external sphincter is then dissected free from surrounding tissue for a distance of at least 2 cm (Fig. 8-3B). Although rarely necessary, stimulating electrodes may be used to identify the sphincter in difficult cases. Wide dissection permits approximation without tension.

After completion of the flap dissection, the sphincter is carefully examined. If there has been complete transection of the distal sphincter and only scar remains, an overlapping sphincteroplasty is performed. The scar tissue is first divided longitudinally in the midline; the severed scarred ends must be preserved (Fig. 8-3B). This divided scar tissue is used for placement of the sutures during the repair because it will hold the sutures more securely than the adjacent soft muscle. Once the midline scar tissue has been divided, the ends of the mobilized sphincter should be overlapped to re-create a tight anal canal without placing tension on the repair. Four to eight 2-0 synthetic absorbable mattress sutures are then carefully placed to maintain the overlapping snug position (Fig. 8-3C). The tendency for the sphincter ends to pull apart must be minimized by adequate mobilization and tension-free approximation. When all the sutures are in place they are tied snugly but not so tight as to cause muscular ischemia.

Most surgeons have not advocated separate dissection and plication of the internal and external sphincter muscles. However, separate imbrication of the internal sphincter with interrupted 2-0 absorbable sutures following a dissection of the intersphincteric plane has been described.[19] This technique results in statistically significant increases in both the squeeze and resting pressures as well as in the length of the high pressure tone. The use of anal endosonography to investigate patients with anal incontinence may support the preference for a separate repair of the external and internal sphincters.[57,93]

With less extensive injuries to the external sphincter,

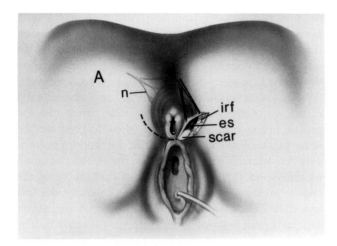

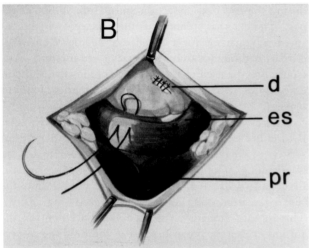

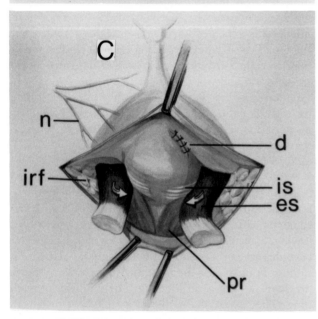

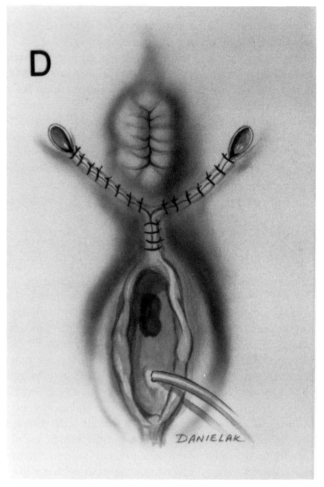

Figure 8–3.   (A) to (D) Overlapping sphincteroplasty: n = pudendal nerve. irf = ischiorectal fat. es = external sphincter. d = mucosal defect. is = internal sphincter. pr = puborectalis muscle.

mobilization of the sphincter mechanism may reveal intact but attenuated sphincter muscle. When presented with this unusual situation it may suffice to plicate the external sphincter with mattress sutures rather than to cut across intact sphincter muscle. An overlapping suture technique which can be used for this particular situation is illustrated in Figure 8-4.

For cases in which severe injuries exist and the entire sphincter mechanism has been disrupted, some surgeons have advocated an anterior plication of the exposed levators including the puborectalis.[111] The purpose of adding the levator plication is to lengthen the anal canal in hope of improving continence. The plication is carried out just prior to the overlapping sphincteroplasty. Four or five horizontal mattress sutures of 2-0 polypropylene are used to approximate the levators (Fig. 8-3C). A latticework of sutures may be used when the levators cannot be approximated without tension.

The wound is irrigated and hemostasis secured. The skin and the anoderm are then closed with fine interrupted absorbable sutures. Usually the wound is easily approximated in the shape of a T. This reconstitutes the normal separation between the rectum and vagina which is usually thinned with significant sphincter injuries. Reconstitution of the perineal body may be aided by reefing the transverse perineal or bulbocavernosus muscle but this is generally not necessary. The lateral ends or the center of the T is left partially open to facilitate drainage.[107,112] The final result is a reconstituted rectovaginal septum constructed of functional sphincter muscle encircling the anal canal (Fig. 8-3D). This repair concomitantly deals with rectovaginal fistula and cloacal type injuries where the mucosal defect can either be directly sutured or excised with creation of a sliding mucosal flap repair. These alternatives are discussed in Chapter 10.

Pain medication is used liberally, because the postoperative wound is generally quite uncomfortable. The patient is well hydrated and given a low residue diet for 3 or 4 days to minimize bowel movements and pain. Sitz baths are started on the first postoperative day. The foley catheter is removed when the pain has significantly decreased, usually on the third postoperative day. At this time the patient also starts a normal diet which includes daily psyllium seed for bulk. Laxatives or cautiously administered enemas may be used to prevent fecal impaction and stressing of the repair. If an enema is administered it should be given only by a physician or nurse and not self-administered by the patient. Discharge is possible on the fourth or fifth postoperative day. The patient is instructed to avoid strenuous activities, including sexual intercourse, and to continue daily sitz baths until the wounds are healed.

Results of late repair with overlapping sphincter plication are shown in Table 8-4. It is evident that good results can be obtained in the majority of patients. In a series from the University of Minnesota 93 patients with acquired anal incontinence were treated with overlapping sphincteroplasty between 1952 and 1982; the overall success rate was 82 percent.[107] Factors that adversely effect the outcome include advanced age (>65 years), a history of previous unsuccessful repair, and more than 10 years between the time of injury and repair. However, no patient should be denied a sphincteroplasty on the basis of age, previous failed repairs, or length of time following the injury.

Sphincter injury in more than one segment offers a challenge to the surgeon. Preoperative mapping by electromyography often allows identification of viable severed segments of sphincter muscle. Depending on the degree of injury sphincter overlap, direct end-to-end repair of mutiple segments and employment of a puborectalis muscular flap have been successful.[104]

Postanal Repair (Fig. 8-4)

Because of the theoretical importance of an adequate anorectal angle in the maintenance of continence, Parks devised an operation to restore the normal anorectal angle in selected incontinent patients with intact but

Table 8-4 Results Overlapping Sphincteroplasty

Surgeon	Period	No. patients	Cause of incontinence, %			Functional Result, %		
			Traumatic	Operative	Obstetric	Grade of Continence		
						1	2	3
Goldberg	1952–82	77	9	35	56	58	24	18
Parks	1961–82	97	27	60	13	78	13	9
Fazio	1975–84	50	5	10	85	70	10	15
Jagelman	1975–84	20	5	25	70	75	25	. . .
Belliveau	1981–84	13	. . .	8	92	92	8	. . .
Failes	1977–84	16	. . .	25	75	56	19	25
Polgase	1978–84	8	12	25	63	75	25	. . .
Goligher	1955–84	45	15	55	30	55	30	15
Alexander-Williams	1975–84	20	10	50	40	60	30	10
Keighley	1976–84	38	10	66	24	79	21	. . .
Abcarian[137]	1978–87	43	1	2	38	100	. . .	. . .
Wexner[10]	1988–91	. . .	0	6	94	76	19	5

Grade 1 = continent of solid and liquid.
Grade 2 = continent of solid stool only.
Grade 3 = incontinent or permanent colostomy.
Adapted from: Motson RW. Sphincter injuries: indications for, and results of sphincter repair. *Br J Surg.* 1985;72(suppl):S19–S21.

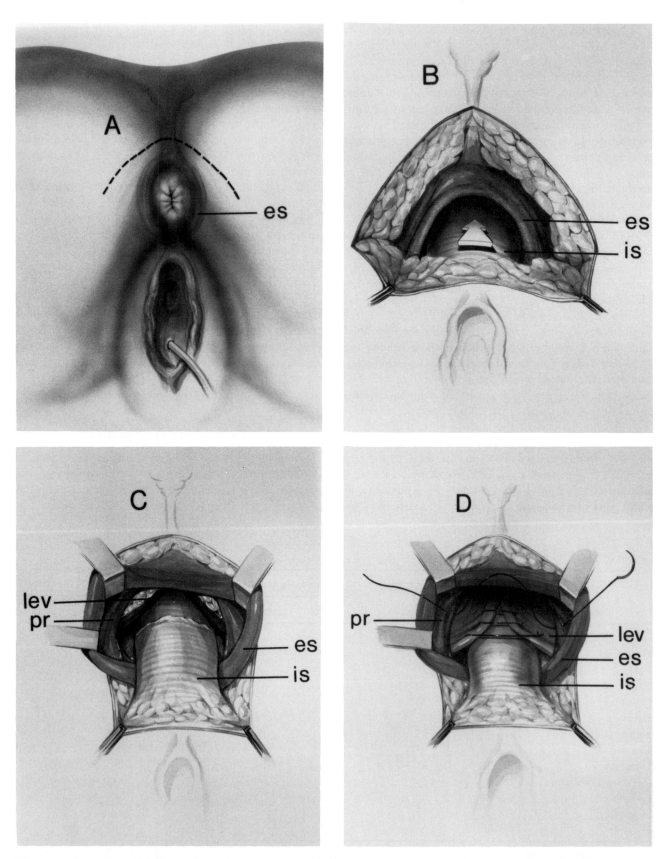

Figure 8-4.   (A) to (H) Postanal repair. es = external sphincter. is = internal sphincter. *Light arrow* indicates inter-sphincteric plane. lev = levator muscles. pr = puborectalis muscle. *Dark arrow* indicates postoperative anterior displacement of anorectal junction.

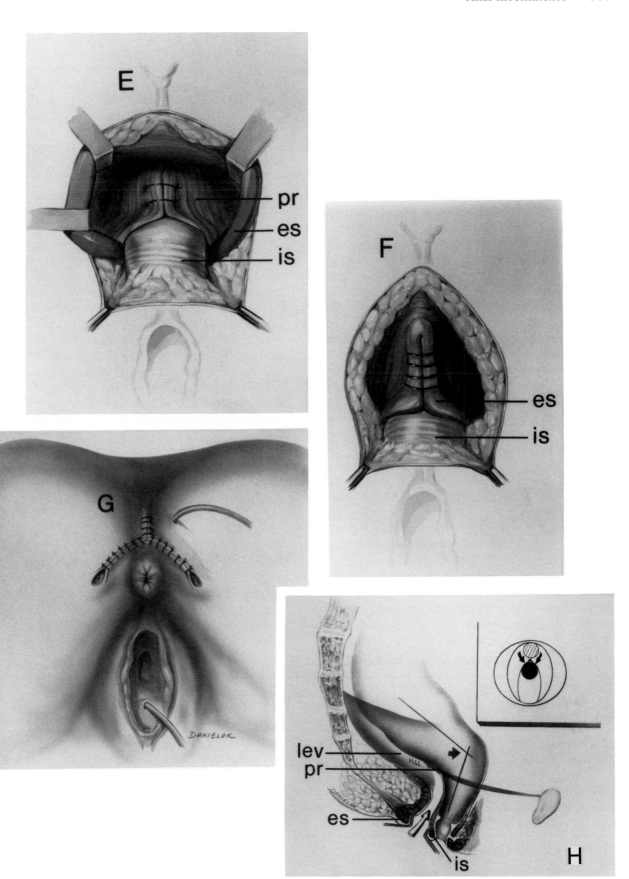

Figure 8-4. *(Continued)*

poorly functioning sphincters and a flat anorectal angle.[62] In this operation a posterior levatorplasty is thought to improve continence by making the anorectal angle more acute and lengthening the anal canal (see Fig. 8-4H). The postanal repair is particularly suited for idiopathic neurogenic incontinence and persistent incontinence following repair of rectal prolapse. Varied success rates with this procedure have been reported and are noted in Table 8-5.

Prior to surgery, the patient should undergo appropriate anorectal physiological evaluation to exclude sphincter injury or other causes for incontinence which might require alternative therapy. The preparation and positioning of patients for the postanal repair is the same as for patients undergoing an overlapping sphincteroplasty. Regardless of the use of regional or general anesthesia, the operative site is infiltrated with a local anesthetic which contains a concentration of 1:200,000 epinephrine to minimize bleeding during dissection. A curvilinear incision is made with its apex at the level of the coccyx, and a skin flap is developed (Fig. 8-4A). After careful identification of the intersphincteric groove, the dissection is carried cephalad in the intersphincteric plane by a combination of blunt and sharp dissection (Fig. 8-4B). Dissection is facilitated by staying in this avascular plane until the puborectalis muscle is reached. The rectosacral or Waldeyer's fascia is identified and divided by sharp dissection. The supralevator space is entered, the perirectal fat is pushed away, and the levator ani muscles are identified laterally (Fig. 8-4C). The repair is now performed by placing two or three 2-0 polypropylene sutures from one side of the pelvis to the other, incorporating the iliococcygeus muscle on either side. Since these muscles will not meet, the sutures are used to form a lattice to avoid tension and muscular necrosis (Fig. 8-4D). A second row of lattice sutures is then placed to approximate the pubococcygeus muscle without tension. The puborectalis

muscle limbs are also approximated to increase the efficiency of their pull and to further buttress the anorectal angle. These sutures should be tied without tension to avoid necrosis of the puborectalis muscle (Fig. 8-4E). Plicating sutures are also placed in the external sphincter muscle to increase its efficiency as well (Fig. 8-4F). Finally, the incision is closed over a closed suction drainage system. The postoperative care is similar to that for the patient who undergoes an overlapping sphincteroplasty.

Results for published series are presented in Table 8-5. Successful outcome has been thought to correlate with improved anal canal length, sensation, and anal canal pressures.[113,114] Other investigators have shown no correlation between improved continence and restoration of anal canal pressures or the anorectal angle and suggest improved continence may result from lengthening the anal canal and changes in tissue compliance following surgery.[115-117] The importance of an acute anorectal angle is further challenged by Orrom and associates,[114] who prospectively evaluated 16 patients who had anterior sphincteroplasties and levatorplasties and 17 patients who had postanal repairs for idiopathic anal incontinence. Ten patients in each group had satisfactory results; no significant change in the anorectal angle was demonstrated in the postanal repair group, whereas the angle was made significantly more obtuse in the anterior sphincteroplasty group. Failure of the postanal repair has been attributed to local sepsis and continuing neuropathic pelvic floor dysfunction.[113,118]

Perineorrhaphy

Plication of the perineal body in conjunction with a vaginal colporrhaphy is performed by some surgeons. Development of the rectovaginal septum by sharp dissection is followed by an excision of excess vaginal mucosa and then an approximation of the transverse

Table 8-5   Results of Postanal Repair for Anal Incontinence

Institution	Year	No. patients	A	B		C	D	Satisfactory, %	Unsatisfactory, %
General Hospital[138]	1982	114	37	—	67*	—	10	91.0*	9.0
St. Mark's Hospital[139]	1983	204	49	70		24	61	53.3	41.7
St. Elisabeth Hospital[116]	1984	16	11	—	1*	—	4	75.0*	25.0
London Hospital[115]	1988	16	6	8		0	2	87.5	12.5
Academic Hospital[117]	1989	39	6	—	11*	—	12	69.0*	31.0
Bristol Royal Infirmary[114]	1991	17	0	0		1	16	58.8	41.2

* Exact functional grade (B or C) not reported.
Grade A = continent to solid, liquid, and flatus.
Grade B = continent to solid and liquid only.
Grade C = continent to continent to solid only.
Grade D = Incontinent to solid, liquid and flatus.

perineal musculature by sutures to re-form the perineal body. Failure to recognize and repair concomitant injuries in the anal sphincter mechanism is usually accompanied by continued anal incontinence. Overlapping sphincteroplasty is clearly the operation of choice in incontinent patients with functional yet disrupted sphincter muscle.

Sphincter Plication

The perineal plication described in the foregoing section can be extended to include the external sphincter muscle, the puborectalis sling, or both.[119] After development of the rectovaginal septum, the external sphincter and the puborectalis is reefed in a cephalad direction. This is a technique used for transvaginal rectocele repairs. Some authorities believe that reefing procedures are more successful if they are combined with anoplasty.[8] Regardless, the series reported in the literature are too small to allow significant conclusions about this procedure.

The patient with intact nerve function and a thinned but intact external sphincter may benefit from a procedure that combines the reefing and overlap sphincteroplasty technique. With this technique the puborectalis is reefed anteriorly, and the dissected thinned external sphincter is fashioned into an S shape and sutured as if one were performing a classic anterior overlapping sphincteroplasty. The sphincter is not divided because there is no scar for the division line. This procedure will

provide bulk to both the sphincter mechanism and the perineal body (Fig. 8-5).

Sphincter Substitutes

Inadequate functional sphincter muscle mass due to destruction or disuse atrophy may preclude direct sphincter muscle repair. Insufficient muscle mass may be a result of a congenital defect, trauma, or neurogenic injury and may account for severe dysfunction despite an intact sphincter muscle. Encirclement procedures can be offered to these individuals with significantly disabling incontinence who refuse a colostomy. Reconstitution of a functional high pressure zone which substitutes for the sphincter mechanism requires bolstering of the weakened sphincter with some form of encirclement procedure using either muscle transfer techniques or circumferential synthetic prostheses.

Synthetic Encirclement Procedures (Fig. 8-6). Several investigators have attempted to bolster damaged nonfunctioning sphincter musculature by encirclement of the anus with synthetic material. These operations are all modifications of the Thiersch procedure originally described in 1891 for the treatment of prolapse and anal incontinence. Clearly, synthetic material cannot be expected to function as normal muscle, and to date the functional results have been less than optimal. Improvement in continence appears to rely on narrowing of the anal canal as a result of postoperative scarring. The best

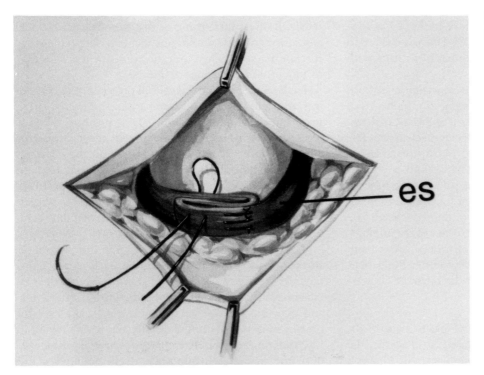

Figure 8-5. Sphincter plication. es = external sphincter.

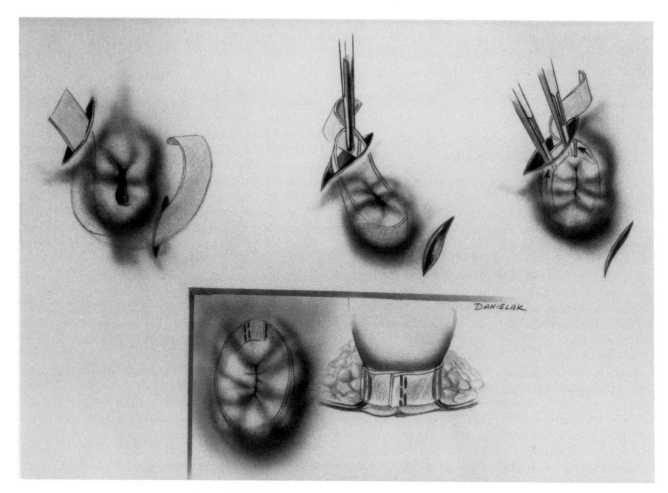

Figure 8-6.   Synthetic encirclement procedure.

material for this procedure appears to be a Dacron-impregnated Silastic sheet.[103,120-122] This has been used with limited success in a small number of patients with anal incontinence.

The operative procedure involves incision over both ischioanal fossae and the development of a tunnel deep enough to accommodate a 2-cm strip of Silastic material which is encircled around the sphincter mechanism. The Dacron sheet is tightened around the tip of an index finger and secured with staples. The wounds are closed in layers and the patient is discharged after the first in-hospital bowel movement. Data on functional results in patients with anal incontinence are limited. There is a high incidence of infection and extrusion of the implant. Functionally, the diameter of the anal canal is fixed and noncompliant. This repair has little to offer the patient and should be performed only in the rarest of circumstances.

Gracilis Muscle Transposition (Figs. 8-7 and 8-8). The gracilis muscle has been used to encircle the anus[123-125] and can be considered similar to the Thiersch

repair. It offers the advantage that the anal encirclement is performed with autologous viable tissue, rather than foreign material. Therefore the consequences of failure of this procedure are more limited.

Each patient should have a full preoperative mechanical and antibiotic bowel preparation. The patient is placed in the modified Lloyd–Davis position with the leg selected for harvesting the gracilis muscle prepared and draped free to allow repositioning during the operative procedure. The superficial medial location of the gracilis muscle in the thigh and the muscle's proximal blood supply allow division of the distal insertion site and proximal mobilization of the muscle without compromising viability.

The position of the muscle is first traced on the surface of the thigh from the pubic arch to the upper medial tubercle of the tibia. Incisions overlying the gracilis muscle in the upper and middle thirds of the thigh, and over the knee joint, are made. The tendon of the gracilis muscle is identified distally and severed from its insertion on the tibia. The muscle is carefully mobilized until the neurovascular bundle is encountered in the

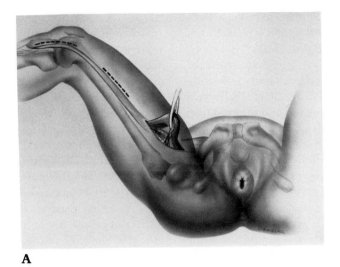

A

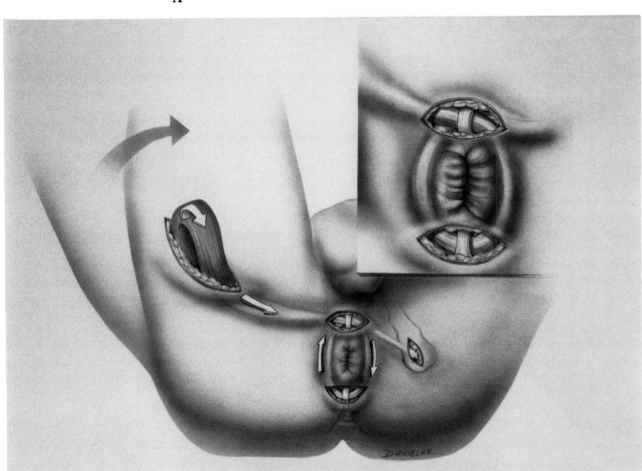

B

Figure 8-7.   Gracilis muscle transposition. (A) Harvesting of muscle. (B) Graft placement.

proximal third of the muscle. This neurovascular bundle is carefully preserved and defines the cephalad limit of the gracilis muscle dissection (Fig. 8-7).

Two incisions approximately 1.5 to 2 cm from the anal verge are made anteriorly and posteriorly, exposing but not cutting the midline raphe. A tunnel is fashioned between the anterior perineal incision and the proximal dissection of the gracilis muscle. The distal tendinous portion of the gracilis is then passed through this tunnel and under the anterior and posterior raphe to encircle the anus in the ischioanal space. The leg is then fully adducted to minimize tension on the gracilis and the tendinous end of the muscle is anchored to the contralateral tibial tuberosity with a strong nonabsorbable suture. When complete, the anal canal should allow one finger to pass snugly. Incisions are closed primarily without the use of drains (Fig. 8-8).

Immediate postoperative care consists of bed rest for 48 hours, followed by gradual ambulation. Although considered a "living Thiersch," the gracilis muscle can sometimes be relaxed purposefully at the time of defecation by assuming the squatting position and avoiding abduction of the thigh. Suppositories or enemas can be used to help establish a regular pattern of defecation and to promote complete evacuation of the rectum. Ultimately diphenoxylate or laxatives may be needed to optimize continence and effective evacuation.

Reports of the functional results of the gracilis muscle transposition have been limited by small series with little objective data concerning preoperative and postoperative pelvic floor physiology. Resting and voluntary pressures have not been shown to improve following the operation.[126] Table 8-6 summarizes the reported surgical data. Selected patients may benefit from gracilis muscle transposition when other means have failed or inadequate sphincter muscle is available for a classic sphincter repair. The repair has been more successful in patients who have suffered sphincter trauma, and less successful in patients with diarrhea or neurologic dysfunction.[127]

Gluteus Maximus Transposition.   Several cases have been reported in which the gluteus maximus muscle has been used in an encirclement procedure to reconstruct the anal sphincter mechanism.[128-130] First, the inferior 5 to 10 percent of each gluteal muscle is mobilized with preservation of its respective neurovascular supply. Each gluteal flap is then split in half to create posterior and anterior segments. These gluteal muscle segments are then wrapped around the anus and sutured together on the contralateral side. A small number of patients have undergone this procedure and successes have been reported. Pearl and associates[130] performed this operation on seven patients with incontinence related to a variety of causes. Six of the patients became continent of stool, while only two became continent to liquid and one became continent to gas. Subjectively, four of Pearl's patients reported "good" results and two reported "fair" results, while one patient's procedure failed. Three of the seven patients had significant wound infections requiring "prolonged hospitalization and intensive local wound care." Manometry testing pre- and postoperatively showed no change in resting pressures, although there was a marked increase in squeeze pressures. Another author[129] has reported one patient who had an increase in continence with gluteal reconstruction and who demonstrated tonic resting activity by EMG evaluation which was not present preoperatively. Further data will be required for a more complete evaluation.

Free Muscle Transplantation.   Free transplantation of the palmaris longus or a portion of the sartorius has been employed in cases of severe incontinence as a result of congenital absence of the puborectalis muscle or in cases in which the puborectalis has been severely damaged. Successful transplantation depends on reinnervation of the transplanted muscle following transplantation into the functional position of the puborectalis muscle. After reinnervation has taken place, the muscle becomes part of the reflex mechanism of the pelvic floor

Table 8-6   Results of Gracilis Muscle Transposition for Anal Incontinence

Study	No. patients	Postoperative Function			
		Excellent	Good	Fair	Poor
Corman[127] 1985*	14	7	. . .	4	3
Leguit[140] 1985	10	2	5	2	1

* 5 year follow-up.
Excellent = continent all the time.
Good = continent all the time; may require enemas or suppositories.
Fair = continent to formed feces not liquid stool; may use a pad or have trouble regulating bowels.
Poor = incontinent to formed stool; obstruction; required colostomy.

because it shares a common innervation with the surrounding pelvic musculature. The goal is to duplicate puborectalis function. Limited experience with this technique has proved successful in very selected patients.[131]

Ostomies

Patients who suffer from incapacitating anal incontinence in whom all options for controlling the problem have been exhausted will often benefit from a colostomy. Ideally, the most distal available colon should be used for the stoma. When adequate distal colon is not available, an ileostomy may be preferable to a proximal right colostomy.[132]

Future Considerations

Artificial and Electrically Stimulated Neoanal Sphincters

Several case reports have described the creation of an electrically stimulated neoanal sphincter using transposed gracilis muscle and a subcutaneously implanted stimulator. This was first described in a patient who had persistent incontinence following a previous gracilis muscle transposition.[133] The patient became continent as the "fast-twitch" gracilis muscle was retrained by the stimulator to act as a "slow-twitch," fatigue-resistant sphincter muscle. Williams and associates[134] recently reported success with gracilis transposition and immediate implantation of the electrical stimulator in five of six patients. This technique has also been described as a part of a staged reconstruction for a patient who had an abdominoperineal resection for rectal cancer.[135]

Implantation of an artificial anal sphincter is another therapeutic possibility for patients with neurogenic incontinence or incontinence due to the destruction of the anal sphincter mechanism. An inflatable artificial sphincter originally designed for treating urinary incontinence has recently been implanted in a few patients with neurogenic anal incontinence with good functional results.[136] Five of five patients regained continence of solid and semisolid stool, but they had difficulty with liquid stool. The artificial sphincter was removed from one patient because of infection. It is hoped that a modified device, created expressly for anal incontinence, will one day provide a realistic alternative to a colostomy in these very unfortunate patients.

References

1. Lane RH. Clinical application of anorectal physiology. *Proc R Soc Med.* 1975;68:28–30.
2. Thomas TM, Egan M, Walgrave A, Meade TW. The prevalence of faecal and double incontinence. *Community Med.* 1984;6:216–220.
3. Tobin GW, Brocklehurst JC. Faecal incontinence in residential homes for the elderly: prevalence, aetiology and management. *Age & Ageing.* 1986;15:41–46.
4. Cherry DA, Rothenberger DA. Pelvic floor physiology. *Surg Clin North Am.* 1988;68:1217–1230.
5. Read NW, Abouzekry L, Read MG, Howell P, Ottewell D, Donnelly TC. Anorectal function in elderly patients with fecal impaction. *Gastroenterology.* 1985;89:959–966.
6. Read NW, Abouzekry L. Why do patients with faecal impaction have faecal incontinence? *Gut.* 1986;27:283–287.
7. Blaisdell PC. Repair of the incontinent sphincter ani. *Surg Gynecol Obstet.* 1940;70:692–697.
8. Stricker JW, Schoetz DJ Jr, Coller JA, Veidenheimer MC. Surgical correction of anal incontinence. *Dis Colon Rectum.* 1988;31:533–540.
9. Bartolo DCC. Pelvic floor disorders: incontinence, constipation, and obstructed defecation. *Perspect Colon Rectal Surg.* 1988;1:1.
10. Miller R, Bartolo DCC, Cervero F, Mortensen NJ. Anorectal sampling: a comparison of normal and incontinent patients. *Br J Surg.* 1988;75:44–47.
11. Sainio P. A manometric study of anorectal function after surgery for anal fistula, with special reference to incontinence. *Acta Chir Scand.* 1985;151:695–700.
12. Legino LJ, Woods MP, Rayburn WF, McGoogan LS. Third and fourth degree perineal tears: experience at a university hospital. *J Reprod Med.* 1988;33:423–426.
13. Go PM, Dunselman GA. Anatomical and functional results of surgical repair after total perineal rupture at delivery. *Surg Gynecol Obstet.* 1988;166:121–124.
14. Thacker SB, Banta DH. Benefits and risks of episiotomy: an interpretative review of the English language literature, 1860–1980. *Obstet Gynecol Survey.* 1983;38:322–338.
15. Rageth JC, Buerklen A, Hirsch HA. Spatkomplikationen nach Episiotomie. *Z Geburtshilfe Perinatol.* 1989;193:233–237.

16. Mellerup-Sorensen S, Bondesen H, Istre O, Vilmann P. Perineal rupture following vaginal delivery. Longterm consequences. *Acta Obstet Gynecol Scand.* 1988;67:315–318.

17. Snooks SJ, Henry MM, Swash M. Faecal incontinence due to external anal sphincter division in childbirth is associated with damage to the innervation of the pelvic floor musculature: a double pathology. *Br J Obstet Gynecol.* 1985;92:824–828.

18. Snooks SJ, Swash M, Mathers SE, Henry MM. Effect of vaginal delivery on the pelvic floor: a 5-year follow-up. *Br J Surg.* 1990;77:1358–1360.

19. Wexner SD, Marchetti F, Jagelman DG. The role of sphincteroplasty for fecal incontinence reevaluated: a prospective physiologic and functional review. *Dis Colon Rectum.* 1991;34:22–30.

20. Mazier P. Keyhole deformity: fact or fiction. *Dis Colon Rectum.* 1985;28:8–10.

21. Stelzner F. The morphological principles of anorectal continence. *Prog Pediatr.* 1976;9:1.

22. Read MG, Read NW, Haynes WG, Donnelly TC, Johnson AG. A prospective study of the effect of haemorrhoidectomy on sphincter function and faecal continence. *Br J Surg.* 1982;69:396–398.

23. Arabia Y, Gatehouse D, Alexander-Williams J, et al. Rubber band ligation or lateral subcutaneous sphincterotomy for treatment of hemorrhoids. *Br J Surg.* 1977;64:737–740.

24. Roe AM, Bartolo DCC, Vellacott KD, Locke-Edmunds J, McMortensen C. Submucosal versus excisional haemorrhoidectomy: a comparison of anal sensation, anal sphincter manometry and postoperative pain and function. *Br J Surg.* 1987;74:948–951.

25. Lord PH. A new regime for the treatment of haemorrhoids. *Proc R Soc Med.* 1968;61:935.

26. Keighley MRB. Abdominal mucosectomy reduces the incidence of soiling and sphincter damage after restorative proctocolectomy and J-pouch. *Dis Colon Rectum.* 1987;30:386–390.

27. Goligher JC, Graham NG, Clark CG, de Dombal FT, Giles G. The value of stretching the sphincters in relief of post-hemorrhoidectomy pain. *Br J Surg.* 1969;64:609.

28. Rothenberger DA, Vermeulen FD, Christenson CE, et al. Restorative proctocolectomy with ileal reservoir and ileoanal anastomosis. *Am J Surg.* 1983;145:82–88.

29. Williams NS, Price R, Johnson D. The long term effects of sphincter preserving operations for rectal carcinoma on function of the anal sphincter in man. *Br J Surg.* 1980;67:203–208.

30. Suzuki H, Motsumoto K, Amuno J, Fujioka M, Honzumi M. Anorectal pressure and rectal compliance after low anterior resection. *Br J Surg.* 1980;67:655–657.

31. Bennett RC. The place of the pull through operation in the treatment of carcinoma of the rectum. *Dis Colon Rectum.* 1976;19:420–424.

32. Williams NS. The rationale for preservation of the anal sphincter in patients with low rectal cancer. *Br J Surg.* 1984;71:575–581.

33. Heald RJ. Towards fewer colostomies—the impact of circular stapling devices on the surgery of rectal cancer in a district hospital. *Br J Surg.* 1980;67:198–200.

34. Parks AG, Percy JP. Resection and sutured colo-anal anastomosis for rectal carcinoma. *Br J Surg.* 1982;69:301–304.

35. Enker W, Stearns M, Janov A. Peranal coloanal anastomosis following low anterior resection for rectal carcinoma. *Dis Colon Rectum.* 1985;28:576–581.

36. Rudd W. The transanal anastomosis: a sphincter-saving operation with improved continence. *Dis Colon Rectum.* 1979;22:102–105.

37. Vernava AM, Robbins PL, Brabbec GW. Restorative resection: colo-anal anastomosis for benign and malignant disease. *Dis Colon Rectum.* 1989;32:690–693.

38. Lazorthes F, Fages P, Chiotasso P, Buget R. Synchronous abdominal trans-sphincteric resection of low rectal cancer: new technique for direct colo-anal anastomosis. *Br J Surg.* 1986;73:573–575.

39. Lane R, Parks A. Function of the anal sphincters following colo-anal anastomosis. *Br J Surg.* 1977;64:596–599.

40. Goligher JC, Duthie HL, DeDombal FT, McK Watts J. The pull through abdominal anal excision for carcinoma of the middle third of the rectum: a comparison with low anterior resection. *Br J Surg.* 1965;52:323–335.

41. Taylor BM, Cranley B, Kelly KA, Philips SF, Beart RW, Dorois RR. A clinico-physiological comparison of ileal pouch-anal and straight ileoanal anastomosis. *Ann Surg.* 1983;198:462–468.

42. Nicholls J, Pescatori M, Motson RW, Pezim ME. Restorative proctocolectomy with a three-loop ileal reservoir for ulcerative colitis and familiar adenomatous polyposis: clinical in 66 patients followed for up to 6 years. *Ann Surg.* 1984;199:383–388.

43. Fonkalsrud EW. Endorectal ileoanal anastomosis with isoperistaltic ileal reservoir after colectomy and mucosal proctectomy. *Ann Surg.* 1984;199:151–157.

44. Dozois RR. Ileal 'J' pouch-anal anastomosis. *Br J Surg.* 1985;72(suppl):S80–S82.

45. Pescatori M, Parks AG. The sphincteric and sensory components of preserved continence after ileoanal reservoir. *Surg Gynecol Obstet*. 1984; 158:517–521.

46. Becker JM. Anal sphincter function after colectomy, mucosal proctectomy, and endorectal ileoanal pull-through. *Arch Surg*. 1984;119: 526–531.

47. Rothenberger DA, Wong WD, Buls JG, Goldberg SM. The S ileal pouch-anal anastomosis. In: Dozios RR, ed. *Alternatives to Conventional Ileostomy*. Chicago: Year Book Medical Publishers; 1985:345–366.

48. Johnston D, Holdsworth PJ, Nasmyth DG. Preservation of the entire anal canal in conservative proctocolectomy for ulcerative colitis: a pilot study comparing end to end ileo-anal anastomosis without mucosal resection with mucosal proctectomy and endoanal anastomosis. *Br J Surg*. 1987;74:940–944.

49. Keighley MRB, Yoshioka K, Kmiot W, Heyer W. Physiological parameters influencing function in restorative proctocolectomy and ileopouch anal anastomosis. *Br J Surg*. 1988;75:997–1002.

50a. Kmiot WA, Keighley MRB. Totally stapled abdominal restorative proctocolectomy. *Br J Surg*. 1989;76:961–964.

50b. Wexner SD, James K, Jagelman DG. The double-stapled ileal reservoir and ileoanal anastomosis. *Dis Colon Rectum*. 1991;34(b):487–494.

51. Seow-Cheon, Tsunoda A, Nicholls RJ. Prospective randomized trial comparing anal function after hand sewn ileoanal anastomosis with mucosectomy versus stapled ileoanal anastomosis without mucosectomy in restorative proctocolectomy. *Br J Surg*. 1991;78:430–434.

52. Percy JP, Neill ME, Kandiah TK, Swash M. A neurogenic factor in faecal incontinence in the elderly. *Age & Ageing*. 1982;11:175–179.

53. Neill MH, Swash M. Increased motor unit fiber density in the external anal sphincter muscle in anorectal incontinence: a single fiber EMG study. *J Neurol Neurosurg Psychiatry*. 1980;43:343–347.

54. Parks AG, Swash M, Ulrich H. Sphincter denervation in anorectal incontinence and rectal prolapse. *Gut*. 1977;18:656–665.

55. Womack NR, Morrison JFB, Williams NS. The role of pelvic floor denervation in the etiology of idiopathic fecal incontinence. *Br J Surg*. 1986; 73:404–407.

56. Lubowski DZ, Nicholls RJ, Burleigh DE, Swash M. Internal anal sphincter in neurogenic fecal incontinence. *Gastroenterology*. 1988;95:997–1002.

57. Law PJ, Kamm MA, Bartram CI. Anal endo-sonography in the investigation of faecal incontinence. *Br J Surg*. 1991;78:312–314.

58. Laurberg S, Swash M, Snooks SJ, Henry MM. Neurologic cause of idiopathic incontinence. *Arch Neurol*. 1988;45:1250–1253.

59. Wald A. Constipation and fecal incontinence in the elderly. *Gastroenterol Clin North Am*. 1990; 19:405–418.

60. Enck P, Kuhlbusch R, Lubke H, Frieling T, Erckenbrecht JF. Age and sex and anorectal manometry in incontinence. *Dis Colon Rectum*. 1989; 32:1026–1030.

61. Gardner E. Decrease in human neurons with age. *Anat Rec*. 1940;77:529–536.

62. Parks AG. Anorectal incontinence. *Proc R Soc Med*. 1975;68:681–690.

63. Snooks SJ, Henry MM, Swash M. Anorectal incontinence and rectal prolapse: differential assessment of the innervation of the puborectalis and external anal sphincter muscles. *Gut*. 1985; 26:470–476.

64. Neill ME, Parks AG, Swash M. Physiological studies of the anal sphincter in faecal incontinence and rectal prolapse. *Br J Surg*. 1981;68:531–536.

65. Goldberg SM. Rectal prolapse. *Curr Probl Surg*. 1986;23:402–451.

66. Prasad ML, Pearl RK, Abcarian H, Orsay CP, Nelson RL. Perineal proctectomy, posterior rectopexy, and postanal levator repair for the treatment of rectal prolapse. *Dis Colon Rectum*. 1986;29:547–552.

67. Henry MM, Parks AG, Swash M. The pelvic floor musculature in the descending perineum syndrome. *Br J Surg*. 1982;69:470–472.

68. Henry MM, Parks AG, Swash M. The anal reflex in idiopathic faecal incontinence: an electrophysiological study. *Br J Surg*. 1980;67: 781–783.

69. Hardcastle JD, Porter NH. Anal incontinence. In: Morson BC, ed. *Disease of the Colon, Rectum and Anus*. New York: Appleton Century Crofts; 1969: 251–260.

70. Read NW, Harford WV, Schmulen AC, Read MG, Santa Ann C, Fordtran JS. A clinical study of patients with faecal incontinence and diarrhea. *Gastroenterology*. 1979;76:747–756.

71. Kuypers JHC. Faecal incontinence. *Int J Colorectal Dis*. 1987;2:177.

72. Felt-Bersma RJF, Klinkenberg-Knol EC, Meuwissen SGM. Anorectal function investigations in incontinent and continent patients. *Dis Colon Rectum*. 1990;33:479–486.

73. Schuster MM. Motor action of the rectum and anal sphincters in continence and defecation. In:

Code CF, ed. *Handbook of Physiology*. Washington DC: American Physiology Society; 1968:4:2121–2139.

74. Read NW, Bartolo DCC, Read MG. Differences in anal function in patients with incontinence to solids and in patients with continence to liquids. *Br J Surg*. 1984;71:39–42.

75. Hiltunen KM. Anal manometric findings in patients with anal incontinence. *Dis Colon Rectum*. 1985;28:925–928.

76. Miller R, Bartolo DCC, Cervero F, Mortensen NJ. Anorectal temperature sensation: a comparison of normal and incontinent patients. *Br J Surg*. 1987;74:511–515.

77. Bartolo DCC, Read NW, Jaratt JA, Read MG, Donnelly TC, Johnson AG. Differences in anal sphincter function and clinical presentation in patients with pelvic floor descent. *Gastroenterology*. 1983;85:68–75.

78. Kuypers JHC. Anal manometry, its applications and indications. *Neth J Surg*. 1982;34:153–158.

79. Matheson DM, Keighley MRB. Manometric evaluation of rectal prolapse and faecal incontinence. *Gut*. 1981;22:126–129.

80. Keighley MRB, Fielding JWL. Management of faecal incontinence and results of surgical treatment. *Br J Surg*. 1983;70:463–468.

81. Scott ADN, Henry MM, Phillips RKS. Clinical assessment and anorectal manometry before postanal repair: failure to predict outcome. *Br J Surg*. 1990;77:629–630.

82. Mahieu P, Pringot J, Bodart P. Defecography, I: description of a new procedure and results in normal patients. *Gastrointest Radiol*. 1984;9:247–251.

83. Mahieu P, Pringot J, Bodart P. Defecography, II: contribution to the diagnosis of defecation disorders. *Gastrointest Radiol*. 1984;9:253–261.

84. Preston DM, Lennard-Jones JE, Thomas BM. The balloon proctogram. *Br J Surg*. 1984;71:29–32.

85. Barkel D, Pemberton JH, Philips SF, Kelly KA. Scintigraphic assessment of the anorectal angle. *Surg Forum*. 1986;37:183–186.

86a. Lahr CJ, Jensen L, Goldberg SM, Rothenberger DA. Balloon topography. *Dis Colon Rectum*. 1986;29:1–5.

86b. Jorge JMN, Wexner SD, Marchetti F, et al. How reliable are the currently available methods of anorectal angle measurement? *Dis Colon Rectum*. 1992;35(3). In Press.

87. Swash M. Anorectal incontinence: electrophysiological tests. *Br J Surg*. 1985;72(suppl):S14–S22.

88. Bartolo DCC, Jarratt JA, Read NW. The use of conventional EMG to assess external sphincter neuropathy in man. *J Neurol Neurosurg Psychiatry*. 1983;46:1115–1118.

89. Kiff ES, Swash M. Slowed conduction in pudendal nerves in idiopathic (neurogenic) faecal incontinence. *Br J Surg*. 1984;71:614–616.

90. Bielefeldt K, Enck P, Erckenbrecht JF. Sensory and motor function in the maintenance of anal continence. *Dis Colon Rectum*. 1990;33:674–678.

91. Rasmussen O, Christensen B, Sorensen M, Tetzschner T, Christiansen J. Rectal compliance in the assessment of patients with fecal incontinence. *Dis Colon Rectum*. 1990;33:650–653.

92. Ferguson GH, Redford J, Barrett JA, Kiff ES. The appreciation of rectal distention in fecal incontinence. *Dis Colon Rectum*. 1989;32:964–967.

93. Burnett SJD, Speakman CTM, Kamm MA, Bartram CI. Confirmation of endosonographic detection of external anal sphincter defects by simultaneous electromyographic mapping. *Br J Surg*. 1991;78:448–450.

94. Denis P, Colin R, Galmiche JP, Muller JM, et al. Traitement de l'incontinence fécale de l'adulte. Résultats en fonction des données cliniques et manométriques, d'inténêt de la rééducation par apprentissage instrumental. *Gastroenterol Clin Biol*. 1983;7:857–863.

95. Binnie NR, Kawimbe BM, Papachrysostomou M, Smith AN. Use of the pundendo-anal reflex in the treatment of neurogenic faecal incontinence. *Gut*. 1990;31:1051–1055.

96. Engel BT, Nikoomanesh P, Schuster MM. Operant conditioning of rectosphincteric responses in the treatment of fecal incontinence. *N Engl J Med*. 1974;290:640–649.

97. Cerulli MA, Nikoomanesh P, Schuster MM. Progress in biofeedback conditioning for fecal incontinence. *Gastroenterology*. 1979;76:742–746.

98. Wald A. Biofeedback for neurogenic fecal incontinence: rectal sensation as a determinant of outcome. *J Pediatr Gastroenterol Nutr*. 1983;2:202–206.

99. MacLeod JH. Management of anal incontinence by biofeedback. *Gastroenterology*. 1987;93:291–294.

100. Olness K, McParland FA, Piper J. Biofeedback: a new modality in the management of children with fecal soiling. *J Pediatr*. 1980;96:505–509.

101. Jensen LL, Lowry AC. Biofeedback: a viable option for anal incontinence. *Dis Colon Rectum*. 1991;34:P6. Abstract.

102. Riboli EB, Frascio M, Pitto G, Reboa G, Zanolla R. Biofeedback conditioning for fecal incontinence. *Arch Phys Med Rehabil* 1988;69:29–31.

103. Schoetz DJ. Operative therapy for anal incontinence. *Surg Clin North Am*. 1985;65:35–46.

104. Christiansen J, Pedersen IK. Traumatic anal incontinence: results of surgical repair. *Dis Colon Rectum*. 1987;50:189–191.

105. Jacobs PPM, Scheuer M, Kuypers JHC, Vingerhoets MH. Obstetric fecal incontinence. *Dis Colon Rectum*. 1990;33:494–497.

106. Parks AG, McPartlin JF. Late repair of injuries to the anal sphincter. *Proc R Soc Med*. 1971;64:1187.

107. Fang DT, Nivatvongs S, Vermeulen FD, Herman FN, Goldberg SM, Rothenberger DA. Overlapping sphincteroplasty for acquired anal incontinence. *Dis Colon Rectum*. 1984;27:720–722.

108. Corman ML. Anal sphincter reconstruction. *Surg Clin North Am*. 1980;60:457–463.

109. Hagihara PF, Griffin WO. Delayed correction of anorectal incontinence due to anal sphincteral injury. *Arch Surg*. 1976;111:63–66.

110. Motson RW. Sphincter injuries: indications for and results of repair. *Br J Surg*. 1985;72 (suppl):S19–S21.

111. Rothenberger DA. Anal incontinence. In: Cameron JL, 3rd ed. *Current Surgical Therapy-3*. Philadelphia: BC Decker; 1989:185–194.

112. Slade MS, Goldberg SM, Schottler JL, Balcos EG, Christenson CE. Sphincteroplasty for acquired anal incontinence. *Dis Colon Rectum*. 1977; 20:33–35.

113. Browning GG, Parks AG. Post anal repair for neuropathic faecal incontinence: correlation of clinical results and anal canal pressures. *Br J Surg*. 1983;70:101–104.

114. Orrom WJ, Miller R, Cornes H, Duthie G, Mortensen NJ, Bartolo DCC. Comparison of anterior sphincteroplasty and postanal repair in the treatment of idiopathic fecal incontinence. *Dis Colon Rectum*. 1991;34:305–310.

115. Womack NR, Morrison JFB, Williams NS. Prospective study of the effect of postanal repair in neurogenic faecal incontinence. *Br J Surg*. 1988; 75:48–52.

116. van Vroonhaven TJ, Schouten WR. Postanal repair in the treatment of anal incontinence. *Neth J Surg*. 1984;36:160–162.

117. Scheuer M, Kuijpers HC, Jacobs PP. Postanal repair restores anatomy rather than function. *Dis Colon Rectum*. 1989;32:960–963.

118. Snooks SJ, Swash M, Patil MRC, Henry M. Electrophysiological and manometric assessment of failed postanal repair for anorectal incontinence. *Dis Colon Rectum*. 1984;27:733–736.

119. Block IR, Rodriquez S, Olivares AL. The Warren operation for anal incontinence caused by the disruption of the anterior segment of the anal sphincter, perineal body and rectovaginal septum. *Dis Colon Rectum*. 1975;18:28–34.

120. Labow S, Hoexter MD, Moseson MD, Rubin RJ, Salvati EP, Eisenstat TE. Modification of silastic sling repair for rectal procidentia and anal incontinence. *Dis Colon Rectum*. 1985;28:684–685.

121. Horn HR, Schoetz DJ, Coller JA, Veidenheimer MC. Sphincter repair with a silastic sling for anal incontinence and rectal procidentia. *Dis Colon Rectum*. 1985;28:868–872.

122. Larach SW, Vazquez B. Modified Thiersch procedure with silastic mesh implant. *South Med J*. 1986;79:307–309.

123. Pickrell KL, Broadbent TR, Masters FW, Metzger JT. Construction of a rectal sphincter and restoration of anal continence by transplanting the gracilis muscle. *Ann Surg*. 1952;135:853–859.

124. Nieves PM, Valles TG, Aranguren G, Maldonado D. Gracilis muscle transplant for correction of traumatic anal incontinence. *Dis Colon Rectum*. 1975;18:349–354.

125. Corman ML. Gracilis muscle transposition. *Contemp Surg*. 1978;13:9–16.

126. Yoshioka K, Keighley MRB. Clinical and manometric assessment of gracilis muscle transposition for fecal incontinence. *Dis Colon Rectum*. 1988; 31:767–769.

127. Corman ML. Gracilis muscle transposition for anal incontinence: late results. *Br J Surg*. 1985; 72(suppl):S21–S22.

128. Onishi K, Maruyama Y, Shiba T. A wrap-around procedure using the gluteus maximus muscle for the functional reconstruction of the sphincter in a case of anal incontinence. *Acta Chir Plast*. 1989;31:56–62.

129. Iwai N, Kaneda H, Tsuto T, Yanagihara J, Takahashi T. Objective assessment of anorectal function after sphincter reconstruction using the gluteus maximus muscle. *Dis Colon Rectum*. 1985;28:973–977.

130. Pearl RK, Prasad ML, Nelson RL, Orsay CP, Abcarian H. Bilateral gluteus maximus transpositions for anal incontinence. Presented at the 89th Annual Convention of the American Society of Colon and Rectal Surgeons; 1990; St Louis, Missouri. *Dis Colon Rectum*. In Press.

131. Hakelius L. Free muscle transplantation. In: Henry MM, Swash M, eds. *Coloproctology and the Pelvic Floor: Pathophysiology and Management*. London: Butterworths; 1985:2611–2617.

132. Williams NS, Nasmyth DG, Jones D, Smith AH. De-functioning stomas: a prospective controlled trial comparing loop ileostomy with loop transverse colostomy. *Br J Surg*. 1986;73:566–570.

133. Baeten C, Spaans F, Fluks A. An implanted neuromuscular stimulator for fecal continence following previously implanted gracilis muscle: report of a case. *Dis Colon Rectum*. 1988;31:134–137.

134. Williams NS, Hallan RI, Koeze TH, Pilot MA, Watkins ES. Construction of a neoanal sphincter by transposition of the gracilis muscle and pro-

longed neuromuscular stimulation for the treatment of faecal incontinence. *Ann R Coll Surg Engl.* 1990;72:108–113.

135. Williams NS, Hallan RI, Koeze TH, Watkins ES. Restoration of gastrointestinal continuity and continence after abdominoperineal excision of the rectum using an electrically stimulated neoanal sphincter. *Dis Colon Rectum.* 1990;33:561–565.

136. Christiansen J, Lorentzen M. Implantation of an artificial sphincter for anal incontinence. *Dis Colon Rectum.* 1989;32:432–436.

137. Abcarian H, Orsay CP, Pearl RK, Nelson RL, Briley SC. Traumatic cloaca. *Dis Colon Rectum.* 1989;32:783–787.

138. Keighley MRB. How I do it: postanal repair. *Int J Colorectal Dis.* 1987;2:236–239.

139. Henry MM, Simon JNL. Results of postanal repair: a retrospective study. *Br J Surg.* 1985; 72(suppl):S17–S19.

140. Leguit P, van Bal JG, Brummelkamp WH. Gracilis muscle transposition in the treatment of fecal incontinence. *Dis Colon Rectum.* 1985;28:1–4.

CHAPTER 9

FISTULA IN ANO AND ABSCESS

Carol-Ann Vasilevsky

Fistula in ano and anorectal abscesses represent different stages along the continuum of a common pathogenic spectrum. Although the abscess represents the acute inflammatory event, the fistula is representative of the chronic process.

Abscess

Etiology

Approximately 90 percent of abscesses result from non-specific cryptoglandular infection while the remainder result from causes listed in Table 9-1. According to the cryptoglandular theory proposed by Parks,[1] abscesses result from obstruction of the anal glands and ducts which are located around the anal canal and enter at the base of a crypt. Anal glands have been found to arise in the mid anal canal at the level of the crypts and pass to the submucosa, with two thirds passing into the internal sphincter and one third to the intersphincteric plane.[2] Obstruction of a duct causes an abscess. Persistence of anal gland epithelium in part of the tract between the crypt and the blocked part of the duct leads to the formation of a fistula.

Classification

Depending on their location in the anatomic spaces, abscesses are classified as (1) perianal, (2) ischiorectal, (3) intersphincteric, or (4) supralevator (Fig. 9-1). Perianal abscesses constitute the most common type of abscesses, whereas supralevator are the rarest. Infection may also spread circumferentially through the intersphincteric, ischiorectal, and supralevator spaces resulting in a horseshoe abscess.

Diagnosis

History

Pain, swelling, and fever are the hallmarks associated with an abscess. The patient with a supralevator abscess may complain of gluteal pain.[3] Rectal bleeding has been reported; fever may or may not be present.

Physical Examination

Erythema, swelling, tenderness, and possible fluctulance may be seen with perianal or ischiorectal abscesses. The intersphincteric or supralevator types present without external manifestations despite the patient's complaint of excruciating pain.[4] With the supralevator abscess, a tender mass may be palpated on rectal or vaginal examination.[3]

Management

The treatment of acute anorectal abscesses consists of incision and drainage.

Antibiotics

There is little if any role for antibiotics in the primary management of anorectal abscesses except in patients with valvular heart disease or prosthetic heart valves, extensive soft tissue cellulitis, prosthetic devices, diabetes, or immunosuppression.

It is wise not to allow fluctulance to develop since this will allow the inflammatory process to spread along tissue planes resulting in possible damage to the anal sphincters.

132 Fundamentals of Anorectal Surgery

Table 9-1 Etiology of Anorectal Abscess

NONSPECIFIC
Cryptoglandular

SPECIFIC
Inflammatory bowel disease
  Crohn's disease
  Ulcerative colitis
Infection
  Tuberculosis
  Actinomycosis
  Lymphogranuloma venereum
Trauma
  Impalement
  Foreign body
  Surgery
    episiotomy
    hemorrhoidectomy
    prostatectomy
Malignancy
  Carcinoma
  Leukemia
  Lymphoma
Radiation

Surgical Technique

Incision and Drainage

Perianal abscesses can be effectively drained under local anesthesia.[3,5] After the most tender point has been determined, the area is infiltrated with 0.5% lidocaine with 1:200,000 epinephrine. A cruciate incision is made and the skin edges are excised to prevent coaptation since this can result in either poor drainage or recurrence (Fig. 9-2 A–D). Packing is generally unnecessary.

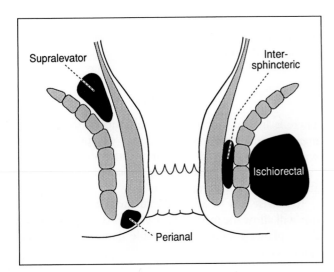

Figure 9-1. Classification of anorectal abscess

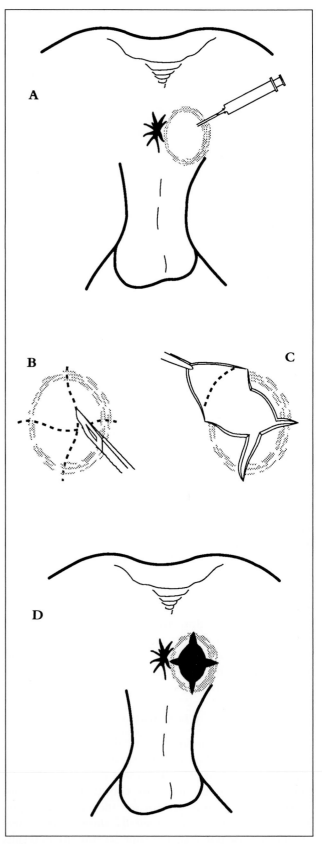

Figure 9-2. Drainage of abscess. (A) Injection of local anesthesia. (B) Cruciate incision. (C) Excision of skin edge. (D) Drainage cavity

Most ischiorectal abscesses can be incised and drained in a similar fashion unless they are large or of the horseshoe variety. In the case of the latter circumstance, drainage should be accomplished under general anesthesia. The source of infection of a horseshoe abscess is believed to be in the postanal space.[3] Under regional or general anesthesia, the patient is placed in the prone jackknife position and the primary opening is located in the posterior midline. The lower half of the internal sphincter is divided to drain the postanal space. Counter incisions are made over each ischiorectal fossa to allow drainage of the anterior extensions of the abscess[6] (Fig. 9-3). Again, there is no need for packing.

Since the diagnosis of intersphincteric abscess is entertained when the presenting symptom is pain out of proportion to the physical findings, an examination under anesthesia is mandatory to completely assess the cause of pain. Once the diagnosis is established, treatment consists of dividing the internal sphincter along the length of the abscess cavity. The wound is then marsupialized to allow adequate drainage and quicker healing time.

Catheter Drainage

An alternative method of treatment for selected patients is catheter drainage. To be suitable for this treatment, a patient should not be septic or in severe distress and should have stable vital signs and no history of a serious systemic illness.[7]

As for all anorectal surgery, the patient is placed in the prone jackknife position. The fluctulant point of the abscess is selected and the skin is prepared with a povidone-iodine solution. Local anesthesia consisting of 0.5% lidocaine is injected in a 1-cm area of skin and a stab incision is made to drain the pus. The lidocaine should be injected into the skin around rather than immediately over the point of maximal fluctulance because the acid environment may otherwise preclude adequate anesthesia (Fig. 9-4). A 10 to 16 French soft latex mushroom catheter is inserted over a probe into the abscess cavity. The shape of the catheter tip when released will hold the catheter in place, thus sutures are not required (Fig. 9-5). The external portion of the catheter is shortened to leave 2 to 3 cm outside the skin,

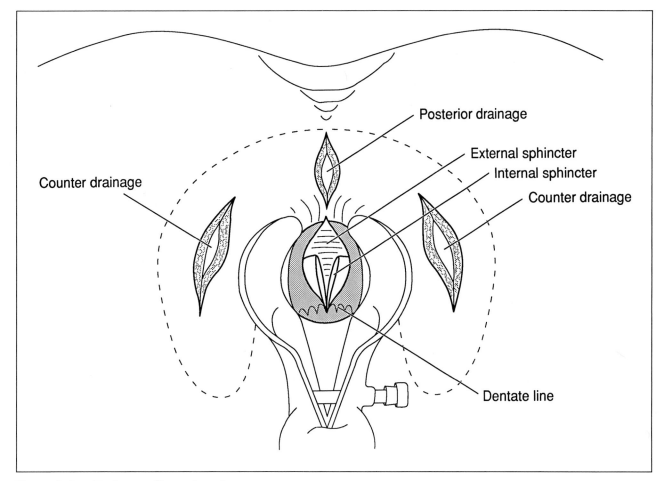

Figure 9-3. Drainage of horseshoe abscess.

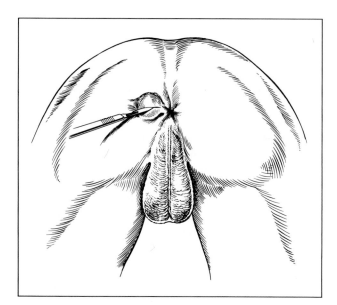

Figure 9-4.   Stab incision into edge of abscess cavity.

with the tip at the depth of the abscess cavity (Fig. 9-6). The chances of the catheter falling out or into the cavity are thereby reduced. A small bandage is placed over the catheter and the patient is discharged home. Antibiotics are not used and a mild non-codeine-containing analgesic is prescribed.

Patients are instructed to keep the area clean and to return for evaluation in 7 to 10 days. If the cavity has closed around the catheter and drainage has ceased, the catheter is removed. Proctoscopic and anoscopic examinations are performed to exclude an associated fistula. Patients with anal fistulas are scheduled for elective fistulotomy. If the abscess cavity has not healed, the catheter is left in place or replaced with a smaller one. Patients are observed until healing has occurred.

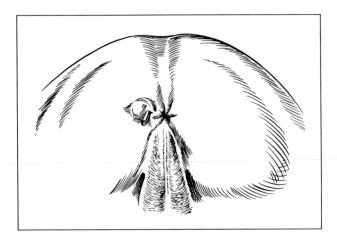

Figure 9-5.   Catheter in abscess cavity.

Several portions of the technique described above merit additional comment. First, the stab incision should be placed as close to the anus as possible, thereby minimizing the amount of tissue that must be opened if a fistula is found following resolution of inflammation (Fig. 9-4). Second, the size and length of the catheter should correspond to the size of the abscess cavity (Fig. 9-6). A catheter that is too small or too short may fall into the wound. If the patient waits too long for follow-up, the skin may seal and thus the patient may require a second incision to retrieve the catheter or to relieve an abscess that might have recurred. Third, the length of time that the catheter should be left in place requires clinical judgment. Factors involved in this decision include the size of the original abscess cavity, the amount of granulation tissue around the catheter, and the character and amount of drainage. If there is doubt, it is better to leave the catheter in place a longer period. Finally, follow-up care is very important. As with any outpatient procedure it is essential that the patient have easy and responsive access to the physician after the procedure in the event that problems arise. An adequate physical examination including proctoscopy after the inflammation has resolved is essential to exclude an associated fistula or other disease processes.

Catheter drainage of large ischiorectal abscesses has several advantages.[7] Patients are treated as outpatients, thus eliminating hospital and operating room costs, and many patients are spared larger procedures with associated morbidity and cost. The use of a soft catheter causes very little discomfort and packing and dressing changes are eliminated. Since there is little morbidity, patients can return to work more quickly.

Before treating a supralevator abscess, it is essential to determine its origin since it may arise from an upward extension of an intersphincteric abscess, an ischiorectal abscess, or downward extension of a pelvic abscess. The treatment in each case will be different. If the origin is an intersphincteric abscess, the abscess should be drained through the rectum and *not* through the ischiorectal fossa since a suprasphincteric fistula in ano will result. If it arises, however, from an ischiorectal abscess, the abscess should be drained as such and *not* through the rectum; otherwise an extrasphincteric fistula in ano will occur (Fig. 9-7). If the abscess is of pelvic origin, it may be drained through the rectum, the ischiorectal fossa, or the abdominal wall through percutaneous drainage depending on the direction to which it is pointing.

A point of controversy is whether a primary fistulotomy should be done at the time of initial abscess drainage. Those who support this procedure[6,8-11] feel that in the acute phase one can better trace the suppurative process because of the presence of pus. Primary

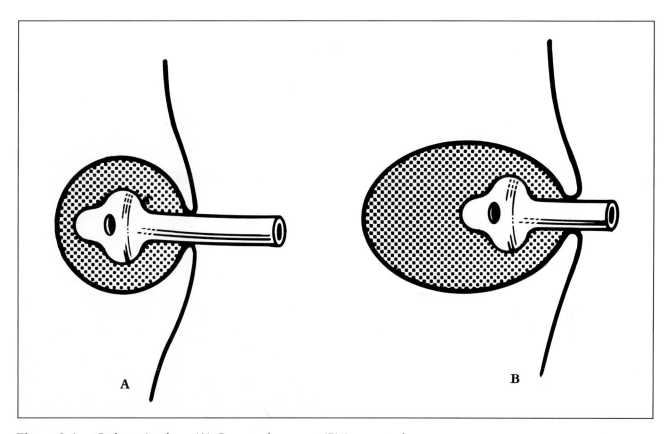

Figure 9-6.   Catheter in place. (A) Correct placement. (B) Incorrect placement

fistulotomy, of course, eliminates the source of infection and decreases the risk of recurrence. Fucini reported no recurrences in 51 out of 58 primary fistulotomies when internal openings could be identified.[11] No major

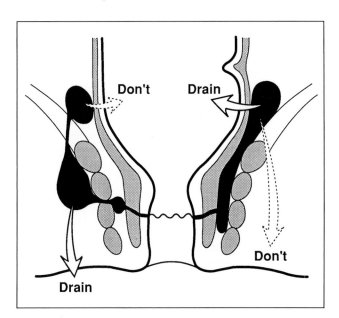

Figure 9-7.   Correct drainage routes for supralevator abscess.

incontinence was reported, but impaired control of flatus was seen in 17 percent. In 8 patients in whom incision and drainage was performed because of failure to identify an internal opening, recurrences were reported in 87 percent.[11]

Opponents,[5,12] however, are reluctant to perform primary fistulotomy in the presence of acute inflammation since this may create false passages and thereby lead to neglect of the main source of infection. Failure to report an internal opening has been reported to occur in as high as 66 percent of patients.[10] In addition, 34 to 50 percent of patients will undergo abscess drainage alone.[5,12] Of those patients whose abscesses that are drained, 11 percent may develop a fistula in ano while 37 percent may develop a recurrent abscess.[5] This is seen most often in conjunction with ischiorectal abscesses.[5] If the internal opening of a low transsphincteric fistula is readily apparent at the time of abscess drainage, primary fistulotomy is feasible with the following exceptions: (1) patients with Crohn's disease, (2) patients with AIDS, (3) elderly patients, (4) patients with high transsphincteric fistulas, (5) women with anterior fistulas and episiotomy scars.

Primary fistulotomy should be attempted only by a surgeon with a sound knowledge of the regional anatomy. Insistence upon finding a fistula may encourage creation of a false passage and unnecessary division of sphincter muscle.[11]

Postoperative Care

Patients are instructed to continue a regular diet and to take a bulk-forming agent and a non-codeine-containing analgesic. Sitz baths several times a day are routinely prescribed. Patients are seen in the office for follow-up in a month or, for intersphincteric or supralevator abscesses, 2 weeks postoperatively.

Necrotizing Anorectal Infection

Rarely, anorectal abscesses may result in necrotizing infection and death. Factors thought to be operative include delay in diagnosis and management, virulence of the organism involved, bactermia and metastatic infections, or underlying disorder such as diabetes, blood dyscrasia, heart disease, chronic renal failure, hemorrhoids, and previous abscess or fistula.[6]

Symptoms and Signs

Widespread cellulitis and crepitation may be present (Fig. 9-8). In addition, a black spot may appear early and indicates a widespread necrotizing infection.[13]

Treatment

Treatment consists of intravenous hydration, restoration of electrolyte balance, and insertion of a foley catheter. If fluid is present in the area of crepitation, a Gram stain test should be done to distinguish between clostridial and nonclostridial infections. Even if no fluid is present, the tissue should be aspirated with a needle and syringe to obtain material for the test. For gram-positive rods seen on Gram stain, antibiotics administered should include sodium penicillin G in doses of 24 to 30 million units per day and an aminoglycoside. For nonclostridial crepitant infections, therapy is influenced by the presence of tissue necrosis and predominance of staphylococci on Gram stain. Antibiotics should include a cephalosporin, an aminoglycoside, and anaerobic coverage.

Surgical treatment consists of wide radical debridement with a colostomy if indicated. Repeated debridement under anesthesia may be required. Fecal diversion may also be accomplished with a "medical colostomy" consisting of enteral or parenteral nutrition. Although it has been suggested that suprapublic catheters be used, this should be done only if the urinary tract is the source of infection.[14]

Although antibiotics and adequate surgical drainage are thought to be sufficient, the use of hyperbaric oxy-

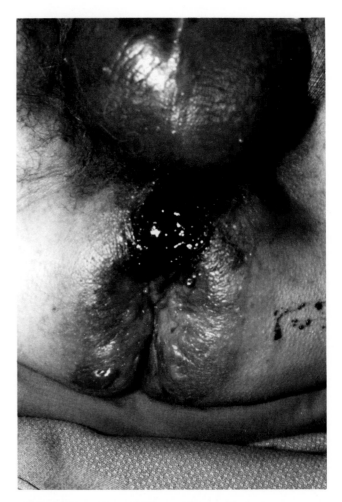

Figure 9-8.   Necrotising anorectal infection

gen (HBO) has been advocated as an adjunct to treatment, particularly in patients with diffuse spreading infections who do not have chronic obstructive pulmonary disease.[13] HBO is delivered as 100% oxygen through an orinasal mask or endotracheal tube at 3 ATM for one or two cycles each lasting 2 hours. Experiments in dogs have shown 95 percent survival with all three treatments compared to 55 percent with HBO and antibiotics and 70 percent with surgery and antibiotics alone.[15]

Anal Infection and Hematologic Diseases

Acute anorectal suppuration poses an interesting and often life-threatening problem in patients with acute hematologic diseases. In patients with acute leukemia, mortality rates of 45 to 78 percent have been reported. There is a definite relationship between the number of circulating granulocytes and the incidence of perianal infection in patients with hematologic diseases. In one study, patients with neutrophil counts below 500 per cubic millimeter had an incidence of anorectal infections of 11 percent whereas those with counts greater than 500 per cubic millimeter had an incidence of 0.4 percent.[16] Glenn and associates[17] reported that 63 percent of anorectal infectious episodes occurred when less then 500 neutrophils were present per cubic millimeter. The risk of developing anorectal infection in this patient population has been found to be related to the severity and duration of neutropenia.[18] Glenn's group found that the most important prognostic indicator was the number of days of neutropenia during the infectious episode.[17]

The most common presenting symptoms include fever, which precedes pain, and urinary retention. Point tenderness and poorly demarcated induration constitute the earliest signs,[18] while external swelling and fluctulance often appear late in the course of infection.[17]

Controversy surrounds the treatment of acute anorectal infections in patients with hematologic malignancies. Surgery has generally been avoided since what may seem to be a simple incision and drainage may produce scant or no pus and may instead cause hemorrhage, poor wound healing, or expanding soft tissue infection.[17]

Any patient with perianal pain is assumed to have a perianal complication and is started on precautionary measures which consist of no digital rectal examinations, suppositories, or enemas.[19] Sitz baths, stool softeners, and analgesia are advised. On aspiration of most abscesses in this group, the most common organisms have been found to be *E. coli* and group D streptococcus.[17] Consequently, infections are successfully controlled with a third-generation cephalosporin combined with anaerobic coverage or an extended spectrum penicillin in combination with an aminoglycoside and an antianaerobic antibiotic. This combination has been associated with an 88 percent success rate.[17]

Barnes and colleagues[18] recommend an aggressive surgical approach. Through this approach 13 of 15 patients who were severely neutropenic with neutrophil counts of less than 100 per cubic millimeter recovered with incision and drainage. It must be noted that these patients were found to have extensive soft tissue infection. Since appropriate antibiotic coverage has been found to control infection successfully, surgery has generally been recommended only if there is obvious fluctulance, progression of soft tissue infection, or persistent sepsis after a trial of antibiotic therapy.[17]

With severe neutropenia of less than 500 neutrophils per cubic millimeter, low dose radiation therapy of 300 to 400 rads for a period of 1 to 3 days has been suggested. Spontaneous drainage or subsidence of induration have been found to occur in 3 to 5 days.[19] A randomized controlled study, however, has failed to confirm the utility of this approach.[20]

Fistula in Ano

A *fistula* is defined as an abnormal communication between any two epithelium-lined surfaces. A *fistula in ano* is an abnormal tract or cavity communicating with the rectum or anal canal by an identifiable internal opening.

Classification

The most helpful yet complicated classification of fistula in ano is that described by Parks et al (Table 9-2).[21] It has been suggested that its use is particularly applicable to the treatment of recurrent fistulas.[11]

Intersphincteric Fistula in Ano

This fistula is caused by a perianal abscess. The tract passes within the intersphincteric plane (Fig. 9-9A). This is the most common type of fistula and accounts for approximately 70 percent of fistulas.[21] A high blind tract passing from the fistula tract to the rectal wall may occur; in addition, the tract may also pass into the lower rectum. The infectious process may pass into the intersphincteric plane and terminate as a blind tract. There is no downward extension to the anal margin, and thus no external opening is present. Infection may also spread in the intersphincteric plane to reach the pelvic cavity to lie above the levator ani muscles. Last, an intersphincteric fistula may originate in the pelvis as a pelvic abscess but manifest itself in the perianal area.

Table 9-2   Classification of Fistula In Ano

I. *Intersphincteric*
   A. Simple low tract
   B. High blind tract
   C. High tract with rectal opening
   D. Rectal opening without perineal opening
   E. Extrarectal extension
   F. Secondary to pelvic disease

II. *Transsphincteric*
   A. Uncomplicated
   B. High blind tract

III. *Suprasphincteric*
   A. Uncomplicated
   B. High blind tract

IV. *Extrasphincteric*
   A. Secondary to anal fistula
   B. Secondary to trauma
   C. Secondary to anorectal disease
   D. Secondary to pelvic inflammation

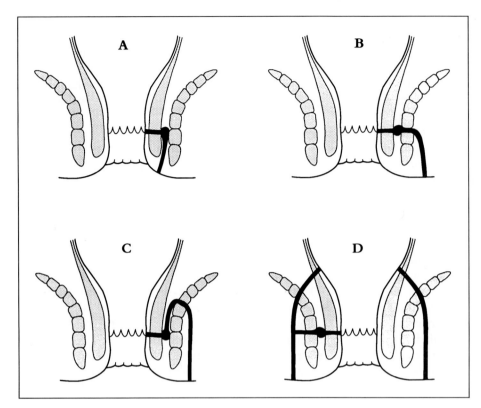

Figure 9-9. Classification of fistula in ano. (A) Intersphincteric. (B) Transsphincteric. (C) Suprasphincteric. (D) Extrasphincteric.

Transsphincteric Fistula in Ano

In its usual variety this lesion results from an ischiorectal abscess and constitutes approximately 23 percent of fistulas seen.[21] The tract passes from the internal opening through the internal and external sphincter to the ischiorectal fossa (Fig. 9-9B). A high blind tract may also occur in this situation in which the upper arm of the tract may pass into the levator ani muscles and thereby into the pelvis. One form of a transsphincteric fistula is the rectovaginal fistula. This is discussed further in Chapter 10.

Suprasphincteric Fistula in Ano

This lesion results from a supralevator abscess and accounts for approximately 5 percent of fistulas in some series.[21] The tract passes above the puborectalis after arising as an intersphincteric abscess. The tract curves downward lateral to the external sphincter in the ischiorectal space to the perianal skin (Fig. 9-9C). A high blind tract may also occur in this variety and result in a horseshoe extension.

Extrasphincteric Fistula in Ano

This constitutes the rarest type of fistula and accounts for 2 percent of fistulas seen.[21] The tract passes from the rectum above the levators and through the levators to the perineal skin via the ischiorectal space (Fig. 9-9D). This may result from foreign body penetration of the rectum with drainage through the levators, from penetrating injury of the perineum, or from Crohn's disease or carcinoma or its treatment. The extrasphincteric fistula may be iatrogenic secondary to vigorous probing during fistula surgery which is, in fact, the most common cause.[6]

Diagnosis

History

Patients with a fistula in ano will recount a history of an abscess that has been drained surgically or drained spontaneously. In addition, patients will complain of drainage, bleeding, pain with defecation, or decrease in pain with drainage.

Physical Examination

A secondary opening may be seen to be discharging pus. This may be elicited on digital rectal examination. In most cases, the primary internal opening is not apparent. The number of external openings and their location may be helpful in identifying the primary opening. According to Goodsall's rule (Fig. 9-10), an opening seen posterior to a line drawn transversely across the perineum will originate from an internal opening in the

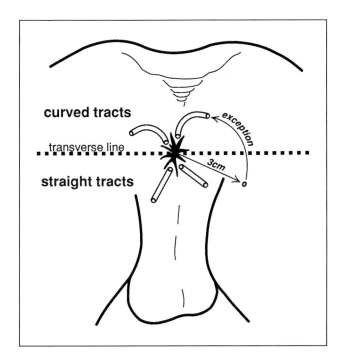

Figure 9-10.   Goodsall's rule.

posterior midline. An anterior external opening will originate in the nearest crypt. Generally, the greater the distance from the anal margin, the greater the probability of a complicated upward extension.

Digital rectal examination may reveal a cordlike structure. Sphincter tone should be adequately assessed preoperatively because of a possible risk of incontinence.

Anoscopy and sigmoidoscopy should always be done prior to operative management to attempt to identify the primary opening and to determine the presence underlying proctitis.

Investigations

Barium enema or colonoscopy and an upper gastrointestinal series with small bowel follow-up are indicated in those patients who have symptoms of inflammatory bowel disease and in patients with multiple or recurrent fistulas.

Although anal manometry is not generally required, it may be helpful in planning the operative approach in the elderly patient, the patient with Crohn's disease or AIDS, or in patients with a recurrent fistula.

Fistulography, which involves the injection of radiographic contrast through a small catheter placed into the secondary opening, may help delineate the tracts (Fig. 9-11). It is generally thought, however, to be unreliable and may provide false-positive results.[22] A recent retrospective review reported that information obtained from fistulography revealed unexpected pathology or altered planned surgical management in 48 percent of cases.[23] Its use may therefore be directed in the management of recurrent fistulas or in Crohn's disease where previous surgical exploration or disease may have altered anorectal anatomy.[23]

Anal endosonography is another evolving modality which is safe, accurate, and has a high degree of correlation with electromyography in the evaluation of external sphincter defects.[24] It is the only method avail-

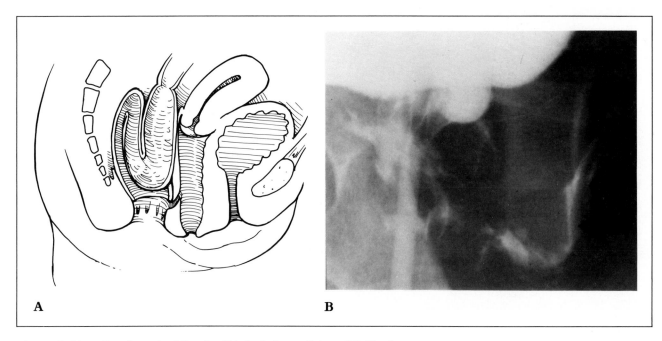

Figure 9-11.   Pouch vaginal fistula. (A) Artistic rendition. (B) Fistulogram.

able for direct assessment of the internal sphincter.[25] It may aid in the identification of complex fistulas[26] and may serve as an adjunct in the evaluation of complex suppuration to assess the adequacy of drainage[27] (Fig. 9-12). Ultrasonography cannot assess superficial, suprasphincteric, and extrasphincteric tracts or secondary supralevator and infralevator tracts.[28]

Management

The principles of fistula surgery are to eliminate the fistula, prevent recurrence, and preserve sphincter function. Success is usually determined by identification of the primary opening and dividing the least amount of muscle possible.

Several methods have been proposed to help identify the primary opening in the operating room:[3,29,30]

1. Passage of a probe or probes from the external to internal opening or vice versa
2. Injection of dye such as a dilute solution of methylene blue
3. Injection of milk or hydrogen peroxide
4. Following the granulation tissue present in the fistula tract

Surgical Techniques

Laying Open Technique

Although fistulectomy was once thought to be a satisfactory method of treatment, fistulotomy is preferred

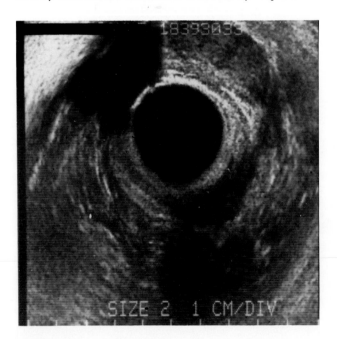

Figure 9-12.   Anal endosonogram

since a much smaller wound is created and injury to underlying sphincter is minimized. For the treatment of a simple intersphincteric fistula, the patient is placed in the prone jackknife position and local anesthesia consisting of 0.5% lidocaine with 1:200,000 epinephrine is injected along the fistula tract following insertion of an anal speculum. A probe is inserted from the external opening along the tract, and in a simple intersphincteric or low transphincteric fistula the tissue overlying the probe is incised. Granulation tissue is curetted and sent for pathologic evaluation. A probe is used gently to search for blind tracts or extensions. If none is found, the wound is marsupialized on either edge by sewing the edges of the incision to the tract with a running locked absorbable suture. There is no need to insert packing (Fig. 9-13 A–C).

When this "laying open" technique is used, it is safer to cut only a small portion of the muscle and insert a seton if a tract is seen to cross the sphincter at a high level (Fig. 9-14). The lower part of the internal sphincter is divided along with the skin to reach the secondary opening and a nonabsorbable suture or elastic is inserted through the fistulous tract. The ends of the suture or elastic are tied with several knots to create a handle for manipulation. The seton may stimulate fibrosis adjacent to the sphincter muscle to prevent gaping of the sphincter at a secondary stage repair. It allows delineation of the amount of remaining muscle and may act as a drain. Its use should be considered in high level fistulas, in anterior fistulas in women, patients with inflammatory bowel disease, in elderly patients with weakened sphincter muscles, in patients with previous fistula surgery, and in patients with concurrent fistulas.

A horseshoe fistula is caused by circumferential spread of infection leading to numerous secondary openings. The key to treatment lies in the identification of the internal opening, which is usually in the posterior midline. The lower part of the internal sphincter is divided, the external openings are enlarged, and the granulation tissue is curetted.

The treatment of an extrasphincteric fistula depends on its etiology. If the fistula arises secondary to an anal fistula, a secondary opening above the puborectalis is usually thought to be iatrogenic due to extensive probing of a transsphincteric fistula. The lower part of the sphincter is divided and the rectal opening is closed with a nonabsorbable suture. A temporary colostomy may be necessary, but a medical colostomy consisting of preoperative mechanical and antibiotic bowel preparation followed by enteral feeding may suffice. A foreign body may enter the rectum or be swallowed and forced through the rectal wall. Treatment consists of removing the foreign body, establishing drainage, closing the internal opening, and performing a colostomy to decrease

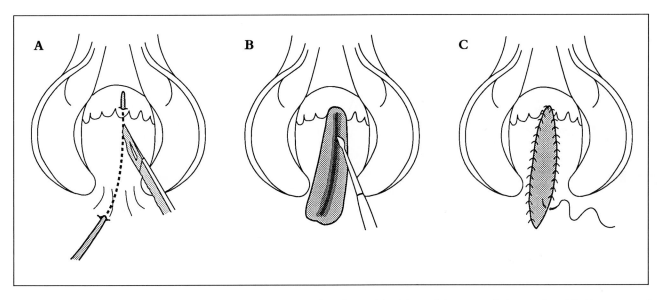

Figure 9-13.   Technique of laying open. (A) Insertion of probe and incision of tissue overlying probe. (B) Curettage of granulation tissue. (C) Marsupialization of wound edges.

rectal pressure. The fistula may also be a manifestation of Crohn's disease. This is discussed in detail in Chapter 25.

Finally, an extrasphincteric fistula may arise from downward tracking of a pelvic abscess. The abscess must be drained in order for the fistula to heal.

Anorectal Advancement Flap (Fig. 9-15 A–D)

The traditional laying open technique may be inappropriate for anterior fistulas in women and in patients with inflammatory bowel disease with high trans-

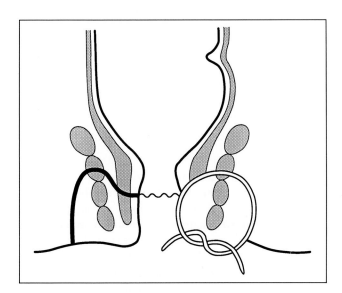

Figure 9-14.   Insertion of seton.

phincteric and suprasphincteric fistulas. Thus the use of an anorectal advancement flap has been proposed.[29,31] Following full mechanical and antibiotic bowel preparation, the fistulous tract is identified with a probe and the internal opening identified, excised, and closed with an absorbable suture. The external opening is made larger and the entire tract is either curetted or excised. A full-thickness flap of rectal mucosa and submucosa is dissected and advanced beyond the original internal opening and sutured to the anal canal distal to the internal opening. With associated inflammatory bowel disease, a diverting stoma may be useful. The main advantage of this technique over the traditional approach is that division of the sphincter muscle is not necessary, a factor which becomes important in patients with Crohn's disease. Because there is no perianal wound, less pain is experienced. In addition, more rapid resolution of fistulae has been reported.[31]

Anal Fistula in Crohn's Disease

The surgical treatment of fistula in ano with concomitant Crohn's disease has been relatively controversial. If anal Crohn's disease is present, a partial internal sphincterotomy may be done.[32] If no anal disease is present, the risks of nonhealing and anal incontinence are minimized.[33] This is discussed in more detail in Chapter 25.

Postoperative Care

Following the laying open technique, patients are placed on regular diets, bulk agents, and non-codeine-contain-

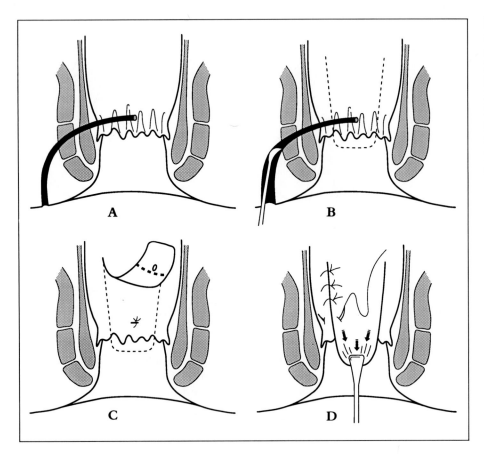

Figure 9-15. Anorectal advancement flap. (A) Transsphincteric fistula in ano. (B) Enlargement of external opening, curettage of tract, and outline of rectal flap. (C) Suture of internal opening, reflected rectal flap, and excision of flap apex. (D) Advancement of flap beyond internal opening and suturing to anal canal.

ing analgesia. The patient is instructed to take sitz baths several times a day to ensure good perianal hygiene. Patients are evaluated in the office at 2-week intervals to ensure that healing has occurred from the depths of the tract. Granulation tissue may be cauterized using silver nitrate sticks, and cotton-tipped swabs are often used to probe the depths of the incision to ensure that adequate healing is occurring.

Following the advancement flap technique patients are maintained on intravenous therapy and no oral nutrition is permitted 5 days to ensure adequate healing of the flap. Once this time has elapsed, the diet is progressed and routine management is instituted.

Complications

The most common complications reported immediately following fistula surgery include urinary retention, hemorrhage, fecal impaction, thrombosed external hemorrhoids; early complications were found to occur in less than 6 percent of cases.[34] Later complications including pain, bleeding, pruritus, tenderness, and poor wound healing have been reported to occur in 9 percent of cases.[33] With attention to detail these complications can be reduced to a minimum. In addition,

not performing primary fistulotomy at the time of acute suppuration will avert most complications.

Recurrent Fistulous Abscess

Recurrence rates following fistula surgery have ranged from 0 to 26.5 percent[3] (Table 9-3). The most common cause of recurrence is failure to identify the primary opening. Other reasons include an unrecognized lateral or upward extension of the fistulous tract, Crohn's disease, or missed diagnosis such as hidradenitis suppurativa.

Incontinence After Fistula Surgery

Incontinence rates range from 0 to 40 percent[35] (Table 9-3). Incontinence may follow fistula surgery for several reasons. Extensive division of the sphincter mechanism may have occurred. In an elderly patient or a patient with inflammatory bowel disease in whom the sphincter mechanism is already weakened, partial incontinence may result from division of an already weakened sphincter muscle. Prolonged packing following anorectal surgical procedures has also been thought to be contributory because packing leads to fibrosis of the sphincter and scar formation.

Table 9-3   Results of Fistula Surgery

Author	Year	No. Patients	Recurrence, %	Incontinence, %
Bennett[36]	1962	108	2.0	36
Hill[37]	1967	626	1.0	4
Lilius[38]	1968	150	5.5	13.5
Mazier[34]	1971	1000	3.9	0.001
Hamilton[39]	1975	57	7.0	. . .
Ani and Solanke[40]	1976	82	17.0	1.0
Hanley et al[41]	1976	31	0	0
Parks et al[21]	1976	158	0.0	17, 39*
Marks and Ritchie[42]	1977	793	. . .	3, 17, 25†
Ewerth et al[43]	1978	143	. . .	3.5
Adams and Kovalcik[44]	1981	133	3.8	0.8
Kuijpers[45]	1982	51	4.0	10.0
Vasilevsky and Gordon[35]	1985	160	6.3	0.7, 2.0, 3.3‡
Fucini[11]	1991	99	3.0	0, 0.2, 0.5§

* 17% without division of seton-contained muscle; 39% with division of seton-contained muscle.
† 3% solid stool, 17% liquid stool, 25% flatus
‡ 0.7% solid stool, 2.0% liquid stool, 3.3% flatus
§ 0 solid stool, 0.2% liquid stool, 0.5% flatus

References

1. Parks AG. Pathogenesis and treatment of fistula-in-ano. *Br Med J.* 1961;1:463–469.
2. Morson BC, Dawson IMP. *Gastrointestinal Pathology.* London: Blackwell Scientific; 1979: 715–718.
3. Goldberg SM, Gordon PH, Nivatvongs S. *Essentials of Anorectal Surgery.* Philadelphia: JB Lippincott; 1980:100–127.
4. Parks AG, Thomson JPS. Intersphincteric abscess. *Br Med J.* 1973;2:537–539.
5. Vasilevsky CA, Gordon PH. The incidence of recurrent abscesses or fistula-in-ano following anorectal suppuration. *Dis Colon Rectum.* 1984;27: 126–130.
6. Abcarian H. Surgical management of recurrent anorectal abscess. *Contemp Surg.* 1982;21:85–91.
7. Beck DE, Fazio VW, Lavery IC, Jagelman DG, Weakley FL. Catheter drainage of ischiorectal abscesses. *South Med J.* 1988;81:444–446.
8. Abcarian H. Acute suppurations in the anorectum. In: Nyhus LM, ed. *Surgery Annual,* vol 8. New York: Appleton Century Crofts; 1976:305–333.
9. Hanley PH. Anorectal abscess fistula. *Surg Clin North Am.* 1978;58:487–503.
10. Read DR, Abcarian H. A prospective survey of 474 patients with anorectal abscess. *Dis Colon Rectum.* 1979;22:566–569.
11. Fucini C. One stage treatment of anal abscesses and fistulas. A clinical appraisal on the basis of two different classifications. *Int J Colorectal Dis.* 1991;6: 12–16.
12. Scoma JA, Salvati EP, Rubin RJ. Incidence of fistulas subsequent to anal abscesses. *Dis Colon Rectum.* 1974;17:357–359.
13. Bubrick MP, Hitchcock CR. Necrotizing anorectal and perineal infections. *Surgery.* 1979;86:655–662.
14. Bode WE, Ramos R, Page CP. Invasive necrotizing infection secondary to anorectal abscess. *Dis Colon Rectum.* 1982;25:416–419.
15. Demello FJ, Haglin JJ, Hitchcock CR. Comparative study of experimental *Clostridium perfringens* infection in dogs treated with antibiotics, surgery and hyperbaric oxygen. *Surgery.* 1973;73:936–941.
16. Vanheuverzwyn R, Delannoy A, Michaux JL, Dive

C. Anal lesions in hematologic diseases. *Dis Colon Rectum* 1980;23:310–312.

17. Glenn J, Cotton D, Wesley R, Pizzo P. Anorectal infections in patients with malignant diseases. *Rev Infect Dis*. 1988;10:42–52.

18. Barnes SG, Sattler FR, Ballard JO. Perirectal infections in acute leukemia. Improved survival after incision and debridement. *Ann Intern Med*. 1984;100:515–516.

19. Sehdev MK, Daviing MD, Seal SH, Stearns MW. Perianal and anorectal complications in leukemia. *Cancer*. 1973;31:149–152.

20. Levi JA, Schempff SC, Slawson RC, Wiernik PH. Evaluation of radiotherapy for localized inflammatory skin and perianal lesion in adult leukemia: a prospectively randomized double-blind study. *Cancer Treat Rep*. 1977;61:1301–1305.

21. Parks AG, Gordon PH, Hardcastle JD. A classification of fistula-in-ano. *Br J Surg*. 1976;63:1–12.

22. Kuijpers HC, Schulpen T. Fistulography for fistula-in-ano: is it useful? *Dis Colon Rectum* 1985;28:103–104.

23. Weisman RI, Orsay CP, Pearl RK, Abcarian H. The role of fistulography in fistula-in-ano. Report of five cases. *Dis Colon Rectum*. 1991;34:181–184.

24. Law PJ, Kamm MA, Bartram CI. A comparison between electromyography and anal endosonography in mapping external anal sphincter defects. *Dis Colon Rectum*. 1990;33:370–373.

25. Law PJ, Kamm MA, Bartram CI. Anal endosonography in the investigation of fecal incontinence. *Br J Surg*. 1991;78:312–314.

26. Law PJ, Talbot RW, Bartram CI, Northover JMA. Anal endosonography in the evaluation of perianal sepsis and fistula-in-ano. *Br J Surg*. 1989;76:752–755.

27. Cataldo P, Senagore J, Luchtefeld MA, Mackeigan JM, Mazier WP. Intrarectal ultrasound in the evaluation of perirectal abscesses. Poster presentation at American Society Colon and Rectal Surgeons; May 1991; Boston.

28. Choen S, Burnett S, Bartram CI, Nicholls RJ. Comparison between anal endosonography and digital examination in the evaluation of anal fistulas. *Br J Surg*. 1991;78:445–447.

29. Fazio VW. Complex anal fistulae. *Gastroenterol Clin North Am*. 1987;16:93–114.

30. Gordon PH. Management of anorectal abscess and fistulous disease. In: Kodner IJ, Fry RD, Roe JP, eds. *Colon Rectal and Anal Surgery*. St Louis: CV Mosby; 1985:91–107.

31. Lewis P, Bartolo DCC. Treatment of transsphincteric fistulae by full thickness anorectal advancement flaps. *Br J Surg*. 1990;77:1187–1189.

32. Levien DH, Surreu J, Mazier WP. Surgical treatment of anorectal fistula in patients with Crohn's disease. *Surg Gynecol Obstet*. 1989;169:133–136.

33. Sohn N, Koreltz BI, Weinstein MA. Anorectal Crohn's disease: definitive surgery fistulas and recurrent abscesses. *Am J Surg*. 1984;139:394–397.

34. Mazier WP. The treatment and care of anal fistulas: a study of 1000 patients. *Dis Colon Rectum*. 1971;14:134–144.

35. Vasilevsky CA, Gordon PH. Results of treatment of fistula-in-ano. *Dis Colon Rectum* 1985;28:225–231.

36. Bennett RC. A review of orthodox treatment for anal fistula. *Proc R Soc Med*. 1962;55:756–757.

37. Hill JR. Fistulas and fistulous abscesses in the anorectal region: personal experience in management. *Dis Colon Rectum*. 1967;10:421–434.

38. Lilius HG. Fistula-in-ano, an investigation of human foetal anal ducts and intramuscular glands and a clinical study of 150 patients. *Acta Chir Scand*. 1968;383(suppl):1–88.

39. Hamilton CH. The deep postanal space: surgical significance in horseshoe fistula and abscess. *Dis Colon Rectum*. 1975;18:642–645.

40. Ani AN, Solanke TF. Anal fistula: a review of 82 cases. *Dis Colon Rectum*. 1976;19:51–55.

41. Hanley PH, Ray JE, Pennington EE, Grablowsky OM. A ten-year follow-up study of horseshoe-abscess fistual-in-ano. *Dis Colon Rectum*. 1976;19:507–515.

42. Marks CG, Ritchie JK. Anal fistulas at St. Mark's Hospital. *Br J Surg*. 1977;64:84–91.

43. Ewerth S, Ahlberg J, Collste G, Holmstrom B. Fistula-in-ano: a six year follow-up study of 143 operated patients. *Acta Chir Scand*. 1978;482(suppl):53–55.

44. Adams D, Kovalcik PJ. Fistula-in-ano. *Surg Gynecol Obstet*. 1981;153:731–733.

45. Kuijpers JH. Diagnosis and treatment of fistula-in-ano. *Neth J Surg*. 1982;34:147–152.

CHAPTER 10

RECTOVAGINAL FISTULAS

Ann C. Lowry

Rectovaginal fistulas are epithelium-lined communications between the rectum and the vagina. They are fortunately uncommon. One investigator found that the rectovaginal fistulas represent less than 5 percent of all anorectal fistulas.[1] When they occur, however, these fistulas are usually quite troublesome for the patient and for the surgeon. As recently as 1980, they were described in the following manner: "Fistula involving the vagina is an ancient scourge with its evil reputation as a surgical problem well-earned—a common tale being one of repeated failure."[2]

Etiology

Both congenital and acquired disorders may cause rectovaginal fistulas (Table 10-1). Congenital fistulas are usually associated with other anomalies. Their evaluation and treatment is complex and well described in pediatric surgical texts.

In unselected series, the incidence of a given etiology varies. In the Mayo Clinic series of 252 patients, 24 percent of cases were secondary to inflammatory bowel disease, 12 percent to congenital anomalies, and 11 percent to childbirth injuries.[3] Bandy and associates from Duke University found that 30 percent were related to radiation injury, 20 percent to obstetric trauma, 16 percent to neoplasm, and 11 percent to inflammatory bowel disease.[4] The difference in findings presumably reflects institutional referral patterns. When only low rectovaginal fistulas are reviewed, obstetric trauma and perianal infection are the dominant causes. Hibbard reported that 92 percent of his 24 cases were due to obstetric injury.[5] Of the 32 fistulas in Russell and Gallagher's series,[6] infection caused 18 and childbirth injury 15. In two other series, obstetric trauma was the major

cause, resulting in 62 percent and 74 percent of low rectovagnial fistulas respectively.[7,8]

Obstetric injury is the most common of the traumatic causes. Failure to recognize a fourth degree laceration, inadequate repair, or development of postoperative infection may result in a fistula. Prolonged labor with persistent pressure on the rectovaginal septum occasionally causes necrosis resulting in a fistula.[9] Fortunately, rectovaginal fistulas after vaginal deliveries are not common. Venkatesh and associates reviewed 22,050 vaginal deliveries: 25 of those patients (0.1 percent) developed rectovaginal fistulas.[10] Pepe and associates reported 1 rectovaginal fistula per 2635 deliveries.[11]

Rectal and vaginal operations may be complicated by low rectovaginal fistulas whereas pelvic operations may result in high rectovaginal fistulas. Hysterectomy, especially those performed for endometriosis with dense pelvis adhesions, is the operation most often resulting in high fistulas. Stapled low anterior anastomosis may result in a rectovaginal fistula if the stapler includes a portion of vaginal wall or if the anastomosis leaks.

Any infectious process contiguous with the rectovaginal septum can produce a rectovaginal fistula. Perianal or Bartholin gland infection may cause low rectovaginal fistulas. Diverticular disease is the most frequent infectious cause of high fistulas, although tuberculosis and lymphogranuloma venereum have been reported.[12]

Both ulcerative colitis and Crohn's disease can produce a rectovaginal fistula. Early studies reported a higher incidence of ulcerative colitis. Once the pathologic distinction between ulcerative colitis and Crohn's colitis had been made, Crohn's disease has been reported more frequently. Bandy and colleagues reported an 11 percent incident of Crohn's disease among their series of rectovaginal fistulas; none of the patients had ulcerative colitis.[4] Radcliffe and colleagues reviewed

145

Table 10-1   Etiology of Rectovaginal Fistula

CONGENITAL DISORDER

ACQUIRED DISORDERS
Trauma
  Operative
  Obstetric
  Violent
Infection
Inflammatory bowel disease
Radiation
Carcinoma

886 females with Crohn's disease and an intact colon[13]: 90 of them (9.8 percent) developed a rectovaginal or anovaginal fistula. DeDombal and associates found a rectovaginal fistula had developed in 10 of 275 women (3.6 percent) with ulcerative colitis.[14] They noted that the incidence increased with the severity of a flare: from 0.2 percent in years when patients had mild attacks to 2.1 percent in severe attack years. In Crohn's disease rectovaginal fistulas, like other forms of perianal disease, may precede intestinal symptoms.[15]

Irradiation used in the treatment of pelvic carcinomas, especially carcinoma of the cervix or endometrium, can cause a rectovaginal fistula. The incidence varies from 0.3 percent to 6 percent.[16-18] Proctitis is followed by ulceration of the anterior rectal wall 4 to 5 cm above the dentate line. One third to one half of such ulcers will progress to a rectovaginal fistula. Most fistulas develop between 6 months and 2 years after treatment. High dosages of radiation and previous hysterectomy increase the incidence of fistula formation.[19,20]

Primary, recurrent, or metastatic neoplasms can cause a rectovaginal fistula. Generally they result from colorectal, cervical, vaginal, or uterine carcinoma. Rarely, leukemias,[12] and giant condylomata[21] lead to these fistulas.

Symptoms

Whatever the cause, patients with rectovaginal fistulas are usually symptomatic. Their symptoms depend upon the size, location, and etiology of the fistula. Most frequently patients complain of the passage of flatus or liquid stool via the vagina. Malodorous vaginal discharge may accompany recurrent episodes of vaginitis. Intestinal symptoms of diarrhea, tenesmus, rectal bleeding, mucous discharge, and abdominal cramping sec-ondary to the underlying disorder may dominate the clinical picture. Alternatively, fecal incontinence secondary to associated sphincter injury or the underlying disease process may be the most troublesome symptom.

Evaluation

The goals of examination of the patient are to locate the fistula, determine the etiology, and assess the extent of any underlying disorder and associated injuries. The cause may be apparent from the history. If not, careful questioning about intestinal symptoms is important. Failure to recognize an underlying condition such as inflammatory bowel disease can lead to repeated failure of corrective procedures.

Most often, the fistula is palpable as a pit in the anterior midline on rectal examination and visualized easily on rectovaginal examination. If it is small, the opening of the fistula may appear only as depression or pitlike defect. On vaginal examination, the dark red mucosa in the fistula tract contrasts with the light vaginal mucosa. Stool or signs of vaginitis may be noted. The use of a probe is usually too painful for the patient.

Ancillary studies may occasionally be necessary to confirm the presence of a fistula. An elusive rectovaginal fistula can be identified after insertion of a vaginal tampon and by instilling an enema containing methylene blue into the rectum. After the enema is retained for 15 to 20 minutes, the tampon is removed. If no staining is seen, the diagnosis of a rectovaginal fistula is probably incorrect. Contrast studies should be done to exclude a colonic or enteric source.

For patients in whom the etiology is clearly perineal trauma or infection, proctoscopy completes the examination. If inflammatory bowel disease is suspected, appropriate endoscopic and contrast studies should be performed. Evaluation of a primary carcinoma is dictated by its location and stage. In patients with a history of radiation treatment thorough evaluation is necessary. It is critical that recurrent carcinomas be distinguished from irradiation change. A rectal ulcer with a gray, friable base with an elevated perimeter is suggestive of carcinoma. Examination under anesthesia with appropriate biopsies may be necessary before a therapeutic decision is made. Allen-Mersh and colleagues reported an equal incidence of radiation-induced and malignant fistulas.[18] In another series, 5 of 11 patients with fistulas arising after radiation had recurrent carcinoma.[22]

In all patients the status of the anal sphincter must be assessed. Fecal incontinence may be secondary to the fistula, the underlying disease, or anal sphincter dysfunction. The symptoms may be attributed to the fistula when there is actually significant sphincter impairment.

In patients with rectovaginal fistulas secondary to obstetric trauma, the incidence of significant sphincter injury and fecal incontinence may be as high as 25 percent.[8] Assessment should include physical examination and anal manometry. One should note the presence of perianal soiling and the size of the perineal body. Perianal sensation, sphincter tone, and extent of scarring anteriorly should be determined. Anal manometry and EMG provide objective measurement of sphincter and pudendal nerve function. These tests should be used in any patient in whom there is doubt about the adequacy of her sphincter muscle. Their investigations are discussed in more detail in Chapters 2 and 6.

Classification

There are many types of rectovaginal fistulas and at least as many techniques for repair. Classification of the fistula aids in selecting therapy. Size, location, and etiology are the criteria used to classify fistulas as simple and complex categories (Table 10-2). Simple rectovaginal fistulas include small, low fistulas caused by infection or trauma. Large, high fistulas and those caused by inflammatory bowel disease, irradiation, or carcinoma are classified as complex. Fistulas less than 2.5 cm in diameter are considered small; greater than that are deemed large. Location has been described in various ways in terms of the rectum, vagina, and rectovaginal septum.[23-26] Using the rectovaginal septum makes the location clear to both general surgeons and gynecologists. Essentially simple fistulas are ones with healthy, well-vascularized surrounding tissue which can be successfully repaired with local techniques. Fistulas that are complex because of location or diseased regional tissue often require more complicated repairs that involve resection or the introduction of healthy tissue. Multiply recurrent fistulas are also associated with decreased blood supply secondary to scarring and are therefore considered complex.

Table 10-2   Classification of Rectovaginal Fistulas

SIMPLE
Low or mid vaginal septum
<2.5 cm in diameter
Trauma or infection

COMPLEX
High vaginal septum
>2.5 cm in diameter
Inflammatory bowel disease, radiation, or neoplasm
Multiply failed repairs

Simple Rectovaginal Fistulas

For patients with simple fistulas, preoperative considerations, other than the choice of technique, are few. If the patient is sufficiently symptomatic to warrant repair, the repair need not be delayed until childbearing has been completed. However, waiting for resolution of inflammation or infection in the surrounding tissue is critical for successful repair. A waiting period of 3 to 6 months is often recommended but delay is unnecessary if the regional tissue is soft and pliable. A small but unknown percentage of fistulas close during the waiting period.

Simple fistulas may be approached through the vagina, perineum, or rectum (Table 10-3). Of note, none of the repairs for simple fistulas requires a diverting colostomy. Evaluation of the patient's continence and of her perineal body should play a major role in the choice of repair. In patients with a simple rectovaginal fistula, good continence, and intact anterior sphincter and perineal body, success has been reported with each of the approaches. If scar has replaced the anterior sphincter muscle, the lack of well-vascularized tissue between the rectum and vagina reduces the chance of success. In those patients a procedure directed at repair of the anal sphincter is most appropriate.

Sliding flap advancements are the most popular transanal approach. Although many modifications exist, the repairs all include closure of the rectal side of the fistula and coverage with a flap. The endorectal flap advancement promoted by Goldberg utilizes a flap of mucosa, submucosa, and circular muscle over reapproximated internal sphincter.[27] A standard mechanical and antibiotic bowel preparation is used as discussed in Chapter 4. The procedure may be performed under local anesthesia with sedation but either caudal block or general anesthesia is generally preferred. A urinary catheter is inserted and the patient positioned prone over

Table 10-3   Repairs for Simple Rectovaginal Fistulas

TRANSANAL PROCEDURES
Sliding flap advancement
Layered closure

VAGINAL PROCEDURES
Inversion of fistula
Layered closure

PERINEAL PROCEDURES
Fistulotomy
Conversion to complete perineal laceration/layered
   closure
Sphincteroplasty

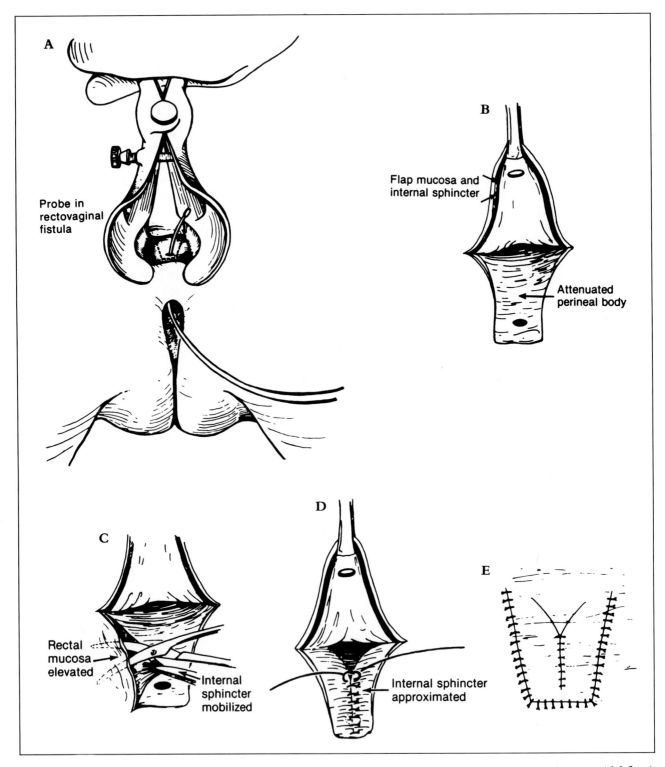

Figure 10-1. (A) With the patient in the prone position, an anoscope is introduced into the rectum. A trapezoidal flap is outlined. (B) A flap of mucosa, submucosa, and circular muscle is mobilized. (C) The internal sphincter is mobilized from the anoderm and rectal mucosa. (D) The internal sphincter is approximated over the fistula. (E) The flap is sutured in place resulting in a two-layer closure. (*From:* Goldberg SM, Nivatvongs S, eds. *Rectovaginal Fistulas in Essentials of Anorectal Surgery*. Philadelphia: JB Lippincott; 1980.)

a hip roll with her buttocks spread with tape. A perianal nerve block with local anesthetic containing epinephrine relaxes the sphincters and aids with hemostasis. A headlight and bivalve anoscope provide exposure. The tract is identified by palpation and careful probing.

A rectal flap is designed making the base at least twice the width of the apex to assure adequate vascular supply. The flap consists of mucosa, submucosa, and circular muscle (Fig. 10-1 A and B). Mobilization usually begins distally, but at times scar tissue makes the plane difficult to identify there. In those cases, it is helpful to identify the correct plane proximally and proceed distally. The flap should be mobilized a minimum of 4 cm cephalad—more if necessary to prevent tension on the suture line. Once the flap has been created, the internal sphincter is mobilized laterally on both sides. The tract is curetted free of granulation tissue. The muscle is then approximated either transversely or longitudinally to close the rectal opening. The flap is then sutured over the closure (Fig. 10-1 C, D, and E). The vaginal side is left open for drainage.

Patients are given perioperative antibiotic coverage. Regular diets with bulk agents to avoid constipation are prescribed. Intercourse and vaginal tampons are proscribed for 6 weeks.

Hoexter uses a technique that differs in several ways.[28] He makes an elliptical incision around the fistula and raises a 4-cm flap of mucosa and submucosa. He then excises the fistular tract. The attenuated sphincter fibers and scar are approximated. Circular muscle and internal sphincter are then closed. This closure is covered with the flap. Hilsabeck uses a flap of rectal mucosa and submucosa.[29] Mengert and Fish mobilize the entire anterior rectal wall as a flap.[30] It is not clear how important these technical variations are.

Success rates for endorectal flap procedures vary from 78 to 100 percent (Table 10-4).[6,29-35] Complications have been few and minor. Fever, urinary tract infection, and spinal headaches have been reported.[6,29-35] The hospital stay is brief and patient discomfort minimal.

Alternative techniques include perineal and vaginal procedures. The early perineal repair consisted of fistulotomy and drainage. It is mentioned only to be condemned because of frequent postoperative incontinence. Belt and Belt reported that all 8 patients who underwent a fistulotomy required a second operation for incontinence.[31]

Conversion of the fistula to a complete perineal laceration followed by a layered closure is a popular perineal technique.[36] Preoperatively a mechanical and antibiotic bowel preparation is performed. The patient is placed in lithotomy position. The bridge of skin and perineal body, often predominantly scar tissue, is divided (Fig. 10-2A). The fistulous tract is excised. The vaginal mucosa is mobilized for exposure. The rectal mucosa and submucosa are closed with absorbable suture (Fig. 10-2B). The levator ani and external sphincter muscles are carefully identified and approximated (Fig. 10-2 C and D). The perineal body is reconstructed, and the vaginal mucosa closed if possible (Fig. 10-2D. It is controversial whether a concomitant sphincterotomy is necessary.

Several small studies report success in 100 percent of patients (Table 10-5).[5,11,37,38] Reported complications include bleeding, wound hematoma, and urinary tract dysfunction. In most studies, postoperative continence is not mentioned. However, Tancer and coauthors state that all 9 patients were continent of flatus and stool after this type of repair.[38]

Two techniques, inversion and layered closure, are performed through the vagina. Both procedures are done with the patient in lithotomy position. For inversion, the fistula is exposed by anterior pressure on the rectal side.[36] The vaginal mucosa is incised circumferentially and dissected free from the fistula. A pursestring suture is inserted and the needle passed through to the rectal side. Tying the suture inverts the fistula into the rectum. The muscle layers and then vaginal mucosa are closed over the inversion. Given reported success in 8 of 11 fistulas repaired this way.[37]

In the more common layered closure, a longitudinal elliptical incision is made around the fistula.[36] If required for exposure, a mediolateral episiotomy is performed. The vaginal mucosa is circumferentially dissected for 2 to 3 cm. The fistular tract is then excised. All scar tissue should be removed but excessive excision can result in tension on the repair. The rectal mucosa is then closed, followed by the rectal muscle, rectovaginal septum, and finally the vaginal mucosa. This method of vaginal repair results in healing in 84 to 100 percent of fistulas (Table 10-6).[3,5,9,38] Complications are uncommon and include bleeding, vulvar hematomas, cellulitis,

Table 10-4 Outcome of Transanal Flap Advancements

Author	No. patients	Success, %
Mengert and Fish[30] (1955)	9	100
Belt and Belt[31] (1969)	8	100
Russell and Gallagher[6] (1977)	21	78
Hilsabeck[29] (1980)	9	100
Hoexter et al[32] (1985)	35	100
Jones et al[33] (1987)	12	75
Stern and Drezink[34] (1987)	8	87.5
Lowry and Goldberg[35] (1991)	85	78
Wise et al[7] (1991)	34	96

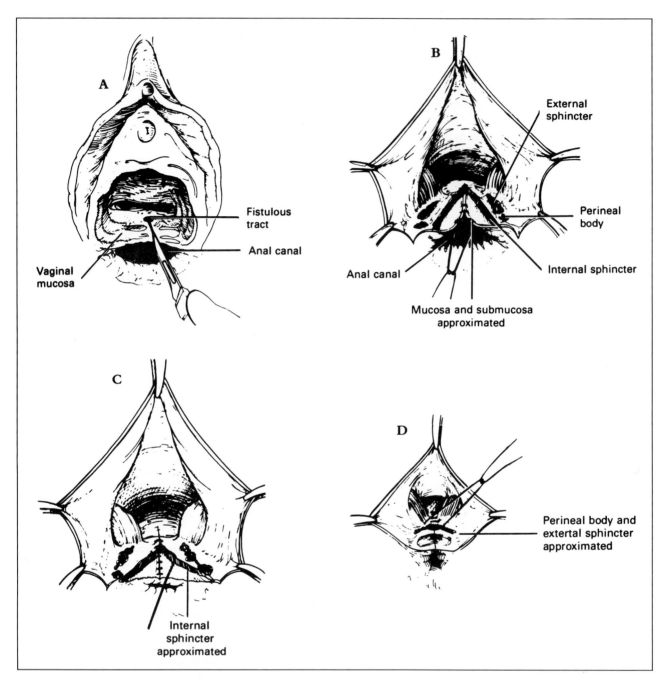

Figure 10-2. (A) With the patient in lithotomy position, the perineal body and remaining anterior sphincter are divided to the fistula. (B) The layered closure begins with rectal mucosa. (C) The internal sphincter is mobilized and approximated. (D) The external sphincter and levator ani muscles are reunited. The perineal body is reconstructed. (*From: Goldberg SM, Nivatvongs S, eds. Rectovaginal Fistulas in Essentials of Anorectal Surgery. Philadelphia: JB Lippincott; 1980.*)

and urinary retention.[5,38] A rectoperineal fistula at the site of the episiotomy has also been reported.[38]

The surgeon's preference usually determines the choice of repair for simple rectovaginal fistulas with an intact perineal body. The argument for an endorectal flap advancement is that the repair is directed at the high pressure side of the fistula. Its advocates believe that correction of the high pressure side of the fistula optimizes the chance of cure.[6,7,12] Both the transanal approach and the vaginal approach avoid iatrogenic injury to the sphincter and possible postoperative incontinence. There are no studies directly comparing the tech-

Table 10-5 Outcome of Conversion to Perineal Laceration Layered Closure

Author	No. patients	Success, %
Given[37] (1970)	10	100
Hibbard[5] (1978)	10	100
Pepe et al[11] (1987)	9	100
Tancer et al[38] (1990)	9	100

Table 10-7 Outcome of Sphincteroplasty

Author	No. patients	Success, %
Mengert and Fish[30] (1955)	23	96
Russell and Gallagher[6] (1977)	9	78
Lowry and Goldberg[35] (1991)	29	93
Wise et al[7] (1991)	15	100

nique and results. Overall, however, the data indicate that in knowledgeable hands, simple rectovaginal fistulas can be successfully repaired in one of several ways.

Failure of any of these repairs may be related to infection, bleeding, or inadequate healthy tissue in the perineum. The number of previous attempts at repair correlates with failure regardless of the method used. The experience at the University of Minnesota with endorectal flap advancement showed that the number of prior repairs was a significant factor in outcome.[8] In patients with no previous repairs 82 percent healed; with one prior attempt 86 percent healed. If there had been two prior repairs, only 55 percent of the procedures were successful. None of the attempts in patients with three previous repairs healed. Using vaginal repairs, both Hibbard[5] and Lescher and Pratt[3] found that successful repairs were less likely in patients with a history of two or more previous attempts. These data are useful in planning subsequent treatment. If the failed procedure is the first attempt and by history and examination the sphincter muscle is adequate, an endorectal flap advancement is recommended. If the anterior sphincter muscle is attenuated or the patient has fecal incontinence, a plication sphincteroplasty corrects both the fistula and the sphincter dysfunction. Inflammatory bowel disease must be excluded in women with repeated recurrences. If no evidence for that diagnosis exists, the fistula should be considered as complex and an appropriate technique chosen.

If fecal incontinence, anterior sphincter defect, or abnormal anal manometry accompanies an otherwise simple rectovaginal fistula, a perineal approach is preferred. In this way, the sphincter dysfunction and the

rectovaginal fistula are corrected concurrently. An overlapping sphincteroplasty is the preferred method. The technique is described in detail in Chapter 8. Briefly, a curvilinear incision is made through the anoderm about 2 cm from the anal verge. A flap of anoderm, rectal mucosa, and submucosa is raised off the internal sphincter. The external sphincter is mobilized from the ischiorectal fat and scar tissue. The retracted ends of sphincter muscle are identified and overlapped in the midline. The endorectal flap is sutured to the reconstructed muscle and the perianal skin. The vaginal wall is reefed and the perineal body reconstituted. The incision is closed loosely. Russell[39] and Corman[23] used similar techniques with some modifications to correct fistulas associated with sphincter injury. Successful closure of the fistulas was achieved in 78 to 100 percent of patients (Table 10-7).[6-8,30]

Complex Rectovaginal Fistulas

For complex fistulas local repairs and flap advancements are not appropriate. Because the surrounding tissue is abnormal, the fistula site must be excised until healthy tissue is reached. Alternatively, well-vascularized tissue can be interposed to correct the problem. To accomplish these goals, abdominal procedures or tissue interposition techniques are necessary (Table 10-8). Careful preoperative assessment is mandatory since the patients are often older with more medical problems. Assessment of the patient's ability and motivation to undergo a major procedure is an important part of the evalua-

Table 10-6 Outcome of Vaginal Repair

Author	No. patients	Success, %
Hibbard[5] (1978)	11	100
Lawson[9] (1972)	53	89
Lescher and Pratt[3] (1967)	49	84
Tancer et al[38] (1990)	10	100

Table 10-8 Repairs for Complex Rectovaginal Fistulas

TISSUE INTERPOSITION

ABDOMINAL PROCEDURES
Low anterior resection
Coloanal anastomosis
Onlay patch anastomosis
Abdominoperineal resection
Diversion

tion. The fistulas also require more evaluation. Biopsies should be done if there is any suspicion of carcinoma. Radiologic and endoscopic examinations help determine the extent of associated disease and involvement of other organs. The presence of incontinence and its etiology must be determined.

Low anterior resection is one option. The end-to-end stapling devices and the double-staple technique allow resection of the diseased bowel and preservation of intestinal continuity. Operation should be deferred until tissue inflammation has subsided.

Parks and associates promoted a sleeve anastomosis technique to treat postirradiation rectovaginal fistulas.[40] Most authors perform diverting transverse loop colostomy as the initial procedure. After a sufficient interval to allow reduction of tissue induration the colon is sufficiently mobilized to allow nonradiated bowel to reach the anal canal. The rectum is then mobilized down to the level of the rectovaginal fistula and divided at that point. The irradiated colon is resected. Then, from a perineal approach, a distal rectal mucosectomy is performed. Curettage of the mucosa may be necessary in technically difficult cases. The normal colon is threaded through the muscle sleeve, covering the fistula. A colo-anal anastomosis is then carried out.

Parks and associates reported correction of fistulas with good functional results in 5 patients.[40] Nowacki and colleagues had one postoperative death in 15 patients[41]; of the remaining 14 patients, 11 achieved cure of the fistulas with normal bowel habits. Two developed small relatively asymptomatic recurrences and one a significant recurrence. Cooke and Wellsted used this technique on 59 consecutive patients[42]; 42 had rectovaginal fistulas. Technical success was achieved in 55 patients (93 percent); there were no deaths.

Bricker and Johnston devised an onlay patch anastomosis as an alternative approach to complex rectovaginal fistulas.[43] The rectosigmoid is mobilized and the rectovaginal fistula exposed. The rectosigmoid is then divided and an end sigmoid colostomy established. The distal rectosigmoid is rotated down upon itself so the open end may be anastomosed over the debrided edges of the fistulous opening in the rectum (Fig. 10-3). A combined abdominal and perineal approach may be necessary to complete the anastomosis. When healing is confirmed radiologically, the proximal sigmoid is sutured end-to-side to the loop of rectosigmoid. Slight modification of this technique allows concurrent correction of an associated rectal stricture. Bricker reported excellent or satisfactory results in 19 of 20 patients.[43]

Many tissue interposition methods have been described for rectovaginal fistulas. Their purpose is to avoid direct apposition of two suture lines and to introduce well-vascularized tissue to the area. Grafts of

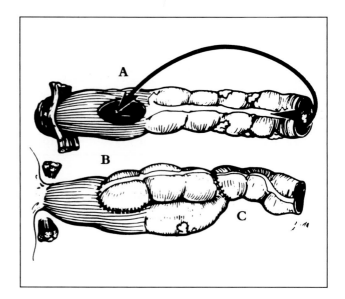

Figure 10-3. (A) After the rectum is freed from the vagina and the fistula debrided, the sigmoid colon is divided. (B) The sigmoid colon is rotated and the end anastomosed over the fistula. (C) After healing is complete, the proximal colon is anastomosed to the apex of the loop of sigmoid colon. (*From:* Goldberg SM, Nivatvongs S, eds. Philadelphia: JB Lippincott; 1980.)

omentum[24,44] and gracilis,[16] sartorius,[45] gluteus maximus[46] and rectus[16] muscles have all been successfully used. However, the bulbocavernosus muscle is the most commonly used. Preliminary diversion is established if the fistula is secondary to radiation injury. It is otherwise not necessary. With the patient in lithotomy position, a mediolateral episiotomy is made for exposure. Through the vagina, the margins of the fistula are mobilized and trimmed. The rectal defect is closed (Fig. 10-4). A vertical incision is made over one of the labia majora and skin flaps are raised. The fat pad and bulbocavernosus muscle are mobilized and passed through a subcutaneous tunnel to lie over the rectal closure (Fig. 10-5). The posterior pedicle is left intact to preserve the perineal branch of the pudendal artery. The vaginal mucosa is then closed over the flap. Both the labial and vaginal incisions are drained.

Zacharin cured 85 percent of patients with multiply recurrent fistulas using this techique.[47] Hibbard also recommends it for patients with two failed repairs.[5] White and associates reported success in 78 percent of radiation-induced fistulas.[48] Boronow succeeded with 84 percent.[49] Aartsen and Sindram achieved healing in all 14 radiation-induced fistulas.[50]

Abdominoperineal resection of pelvic exenteration may be indicated for extensive malignancy. Colpocleisis and permanent colostomy provide palliation in patients with poor general health.

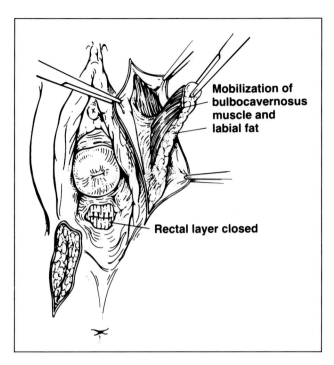

Figure 10-4. After the fistula has been excised and the edges have been debrided, the rectal muscles are closed. The bulbocavernosus muscle and labial fat pad are mobilized.

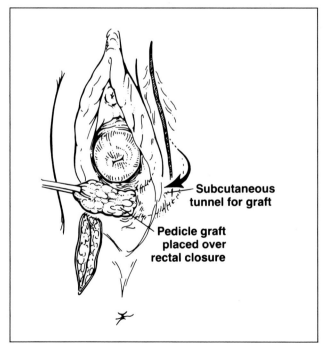

Figure 10-5. The graft of bulbocavernosus muscle and fat pad are passed through a subcutaneous tunnel to cover the rectal closure.

For complex fistulas, the etiology of the fistula is the primary determinant of therapy. Resection with anastomosis is the procedure of choice for high rectovaginal fistulas following hysterectomy, diverticular disease, or previous colon resections. Corman believes that for some fistulas secondary to hysterectomy, it suffices to separate the bowel from the vagina, close the opening, and interpose omentum, a peritoneal flap, or fascia.[23]

Overlapping sphincteroplasty and the Martius graft of bulbocavernosus muscle are appropriate for multiply recurrent low fistulas. The choice depends upon the patient's sphincter function.

If a carcinoma has produced a rectovaginal fistula, the fistula should be only a secondary consideration in choosing therapy for the neoplasm. In most cases, bowel resection—often abdominoperineal resection—will be necessary.

Irradiation-induced fistulas are particularly challenging because of the regional effect of the radiation. Traditionally, pessimism reigned and the only surgical procedure considered was a colostomy. Reasonably good results with a variety of repairs have led to cautious optimism. In symptomatic otherwise healthy patients without evidence of recurrent disease, attempt at repair is reasonable. In all such cases a temporary diversion is established and maintained for 6 to 12 months to allow the inflammatory reaction to subside.

Low anterior resection and coloanal procedures eliminate the diseased bowel, preventing a secondary carcinoma and future symptoms from radiation proctitis or stricture. The disadvantages are the technical difficulty and potential incontinence. Bricker[43] argues that his procedure is technically less difficult. The disadvantage is that the radiated bowel with its potential for bleeding, pain, and malignant degeneration is left in place.

Perineal tissue interposition methods avoid the risk of abdominal procedures and are therefore appropriate for high-risk patients. Again, the disadvantage is that the radiated bowel is not removed.

Rectovaginal fistulas in patients with inflammatory bowel disease have been treated with medical therapy, proximal diversion, proctectomy, and direct repair. There are reports of success with 6-mercaptopurine,[51] but most authors report no success with medical management.[52,53] Proximal diversion may relieve the patient's symptoms but rarely achieves permanent fistula closure. Proctectomy is indicated for markedly symptomatic fistulas when there is active proctitis unresponsive to medical therapy or sphincter destruction.

Many patients with rectovaginal fistulas secondary to Crohn's disease require proctectomy. In a review of 90 patients, 48 required proctectomy either as primary therapy or after failure of another form of treatment.[13] Most of the patients studied has severe proctocolitis;

symptoms from the fistula were the major indication for surgery in only 10 cases. Many surgeons have thought such an outcome inevitable.[23,54] In recent years, however, there has been growing interest in attempting local repair in patients without active proctitis. Several techniques have been reported. One group reported laying open low rectovaginal fistulas in patients with Crohn's disease.[55] All of the fistulas healed. Of the 9 patients, 6 maintained perfect continence while 3 were incontinent of liquid stool and flatus. Jones and coinvestigators performed endorectal flap advancements on 10 patients with rectovaginal fistulas and Crohn's disease.[35] The repair was successful in 6. Cohen recommends this technique.[56] In the study by Radcliffe and associates mentioned above,[13] the local repairs were done with endorectal flap advancement.[13] Others report success with conversion to a perineal laceration and layered closure. In Bandy's study,[4] 9 of 10 fistulas healed primarily; 2 recurred later during a flare of colitis. No mention is made of postoperative continence. Cohen

and associates used this method on 4 fistulas with success.[57] All patients were continent postoperatively, although intervals of almost 2 years were required to achieve control. Sher and coauthors performed vaginal repairs on 14 patients with Crohn's disease[15]: 13 (93 percent) of the repairs healed. The necessity for temporary diversion is quite controversial. Several authors support its use[15,52]; others believe it to be unnecessary.[4,8] The approach to rectovaginal fistulas in patients with Crohn's disease is evolving; there is a trend toward offering selected patients a local repair. Laying open the fistula should be avoided because of the risk of incontinence. The surgical management of rectovaginal fistulas in patients with Crohn's disease is discussed in detail in Chapter 25.

Rectovaginal fistulas test a surgeon's judgment and technical skill. With careful evaluation, consideration of the options, and meticulous technique, however, many patients can be cured of this "ancient scourge."

References

1. Laird DR. Procedures used in treatment of complicated fistulas. *Am J Surg.* 1948;76:701–708.
2. Zacharin KF. Grafting as a principle in the surgical management of vesicovaginal and rectovaginal fistulae. *Aust N Z J Obstet Gynecol.* 1980;20:10–17.
3. Lescher TC, Pratt JH. Vaginal repair of the simple rectovaginal fistula. *Surg Gynecol Obstet.* 1967; 124:1317–1321.
4. Bandy LC, Addison A, Parker RT. Surgical management of rectovaginal fistulas in Crohn's disease. *Am J Obstet Gynecol.* 1983;147:359–363.
5. Hibbard LT. Surgical management of rectovaginal fistulas and complete perineal tears. *Am J Obstet Gynecol.* 1978;130:139–141.
6. Russell TR, Gallagher DM. Low rectovaginal fistulas, approach and treatment. *Am J Surg.* 1977;134:13–18.
7. Wise WE, Aguelar PS, Padmanabtan A, et al. Surgical treatment of low rectovaginal fistulas. *Dis Colon Rectum.* 1991;34:271–274.
8. Lowry AC, Thorson AG, Rothenberger DA, Goldberg SM. Repair of simple rectovaginal fistulas—influence of previous repairs. *Dis Colon Rectum.* 1988;32(9):676–678.
9. Lawson J. Rectovaginal fistulas following difficult labour. *Proc R Soc Med.* 1972;65:283–286.
10. Venkatesh KS, Ramanyam PS, Larson DM, Haywood MA. Anorectal complications of vaginal delivery. *Dis Colon Rectum.* 1989;32:1039–1041.
11. Pepe F, Panella M, Arikan S, Panella P, Pepe G.

Low rectovaginal fistulas. *Aust N Z J Obstet Gynecol.* 1987;27:61–63.
12. Greenwald JC, Hoexter B. Repair of rectovaginal fistulas. *Surg Gynecol Obstet.* 1978;146:443–445.
13. Radcliffe AG, Ritchie JK, Hawley PR, Lennard-Jones JE, Northover JMA. Anovaginal and rectovaginal fistulas in Crohn's disease. *Dis Colon Rectum.* 1988;31:94–99.
14. DeDombal FT, Watts JM, Watkinson G, Goligher JC. Incidence and management of anorectal abscess, fistula and fissure in patients with ulcerative colitis. *Dis Colon Rectum.* 1966;9:201.
15. Sher ME, Bauer JJ, Gelernt I. Surgical repair of rectovaginal fistulas in patients with Crohn's disease: transvaginal approach. *Dis Colon Rectum.* 1991;34:641–648.
16. Graham JB. Vaginal fistulas following radiotherapy. *Surg Gynecol Obstet.* 1965;120:1019–1030.
17. Cooke SA, DeMoor NG. The surgical treatment of the radiation damaged rectum. *Br J Surg.* 1981;68: 488–492.
18. Allen-Mersh TG, Wilson ET, Hope-Stone HF, Mann CV. The management of late radiation-induced rectal injury after treatment of carcinoma of the uterus. *Surg Gynecol Obstet.* 1987;164: 521–524.
19. Perez CA, Breaux S, Bedevinek JM, et al. Radiation therapy alone in the treatment of carcinoma of the uterine cervix. *Cancer.* 1984;54:235–246.
20. Boronow RC. Repair of the radiation-induced vagi-

nal fistula utilizing the Martius technique. *World J Surg*. 1986;10:237–248.

21. Lock MR, Katz DR, Samoorian S, Parks AG. Giant condyloma of the rectum: report of a case. *Dis Colon Rectum*. 1977;20:154.

22. VanNagel JR, Parker JC, Maruyama Y, Utley J, Luckett P. Bladder or rectal injury following radiation therapy for cervical cancer. *Am J Obstet Gynecol*. 1974;119:727.

23. Corman M. Rectovaginal fistulas. In: *Colon and Rectal Surgery*. 2nd ed. Philadelphia: JB Lippincott Co.; 1989.

24. Bentley RJ. Abdominal repair of high rectovaginal fistula. *J Obstet Gynecol Br Commonw*. 173;30:364.

25. Daniels BT. *Rectovaginal Fistula: A Clinical and Pathological Study*. University of Minnesota Graduate School; 1949. Thesis.

26. Rosenheim NB, Genedry RK, Wodruff JD. An anatomic classification of rectovaginal septal defect. *Am J Obstet Gynecol*. 1980;134:439–446.

27. Stone JM, Goldberg SM. The endorectal advancement flap procedure. *Int J Colorectal Dis*. 1990;5: 232–235.

28. Hoexter B. Rectovaginal fistula. In: Fazio V, ed. *Current Therapy in Colon and Rectal Surgery*. Toronto: BC Decker; 1990:28–32.

29. Hilsabeck JR. Transanal advancement of the anterior rectal wall for vaginal fistulas involving the lower rectum. *Dis Colon Rectum*. 1980;23:236–241.

30. Mengert WF, Fish SA. Anterior rectal wall advancement: technic for repair of complete perineal laceration and rectovaginal fistula. *Obstet Gynecol*. 1955;5:262–267.

31. Belt RL, Belt RL Jr. Repair of anorectal vaginal fistula utilizing segmental advancement of the internal sphincter muscle. *Dis Colon Rectum*. 1969;12: 99–104.

32. Hoexter B, Labow SB, Moseson MD. Transanal rectovaginal fistula repair. *Dis Colon Rectum*. 1985;28:572–575.

33. Jones IT, Fazio VW, Jagelman DG. The use of transanal rectal advancement flaps on management of fistulas involving the anorectum. *Dis Colon Rectum*. 1987;30:919–923.

34. Stern HS, Drezink Z. Rectovaginal fistula. *Adv Surg*. 1987;21:245–262.

35. Lowry AC, Goldberg SM. Management of simple rectovaginal fistula. In: Cameron JL, ed. *Current Surgical Therapy, 4*. In press.

36. Hudson CN. Rectovaginal and other fistulas between the intestine and genital tract. In: Smith R, Rob C, Dudley H, eds. *Operative Surgery, Colon, Rectum and Anus*. 3rd ed. London: Butterworths; 1977.

37. Given FT. Rectovaginal fistula: a review of 20 years' experience in a community hospital. *Am J Obstet Gynecol*. 1970;108:41–46.

38. Tancer ML, Lasser D, Rosenblum N. Rectovaginal fistula or perineal and anal sphincter dysruption or both after vaginal delivery. *Surg Gynecol Obstet*. 1990;171:43–46.

39. Russell TR. Low rectovaginal fistulas. In: Cameron JL, ed. *Current Surgical Therapy, 3*. Toronto: BC Decker; 1989:194–198.

40. Parks AG, Allen CLO, Frank JD, McPartlin JF. A method of treating post-irradiation rectovaginal fistulas. *Br J Surg*. 1978;65:417–421.

41. Nowacki MP, Szawlowski AW, Borkowski A. Parks' coloanal sleeve anastomosis for treatment of postirradiation rectovaginal fistula. *Dis Colon Rectum*. 1986;29:817–820.

42. Cooke SA, Wellsted MD. The radiation-damaged rectum. Resection with coloanal anastomosis using the endoanal technique. *World J Surg*. 1986;10: 220–227.

43. Bricker EM, Johnston WD. Repair of postirradiation rectovaginal fistula and stricture. *Surg Gynecol Obstet*. 1979;148:499–506.

44. Goligher JC. Rectovaginal fistula and irradiation proctitis and enteritis. In: *Surgery of the Anus, Rectum and Colon*. 5th ed. London: Baillieer Tindall; 1984.

45. Byron RL, Ostergard DR. Sartorius muscle interposition for the treatment of the radiation-induced vaginal fistula. *Am J Obstet Gynecol*. 1969;104: 104–107.

46. Stirnemann H. Treatment of recurrent rectovaginal fistula. *Am J Proctology*. 1969;20:52–54.

47. Zacharin KF. Grafting as a principle in the surgical management of vesicovaginal and rectovaginal fistulae. *Aust N Z J Obstet Gynecol*. 1980;20:10–17.

48. White AJ, Buchsbaum HJ, Blythe JG, Lifshets S. Use of the bulbocavernosus muscle (Martius technique) for repair of radiation-induced rectovaginal fistulas. *Obstet Gynecol*. 1982;60:114–118.

49. Boronow RC. Repair of the radiation-induced vaginal fistula utilizing the Martius technique. *World J Surg*. 1986;10:237–248.

50. Aarten ET, Sindram IS. Repair of the radiation induced rectovaginal fistulas with or without interposition of the bulbocavernous muscle. *Eur J Surg Oncol*. 1988;14:171–177.

51. Present DH, Korelitz B, Wisch N. Treatment of Crohn's disease with 6-mercaptopurine: a long-term randomized double blind study. *N Engl J Med*. 1980;302:981–987.

52. Harper PA, Kettlewell MG, Lee EC. The effect of split ileostomy in perianal Crohn's disease. *Br J Surg*. 1982;69:608–610.

53. Grant DR, Cohen Z, McLeod RS. Loop ileostomy

for anorectal Crohn's disease. *Can J Surg*. 1986;29:
32–35.

54. Faulconer HT, Muldoon JP. Rectovaginal fistula in
patient with colitis: review and report of a case. *Dis
Colon Rectum*. 1975;18:413–415.

55. Francois Y, Descos L, Vignal J. Conservative treatment of low rectovaginal fistula in Crohn's disease.
Int J Colorectal Dis. 1990;5:12–14.

56. Cohen Z. Crohn's disease: perianal. In: Fazio V,
ed. *Current Therapy in Colon and Rectal Surgery*.
Toronto: BC Decker; 1990:199–202.

57. Cohen JL, Shicke JW, Schoetz DT, Coller JA,
Veidenheimer MC. Rectovaginal fistula in Crohn's
disease. *Dis Colon Rectum*. 1989;32:825–828.

CHAPTER 11

PRURITUS ANI: DIAGNOSIS AND TREATMENT

Terry C. Hicks and Frank G. Opelka

Pruritus, derived from the Latin work *prurire* (meaning "to itch"), refers to the unpleasant cutaneous sensation that leaves the patient with a nearly uncontrollable desire to scratch.[1] Pruritus ani is not a diagnosis but a symptom complex that has both medical and surgical implications. The plethora of protean manifestations challenges the skill of all physicians to make the correct diagnosis and to institute appropriate therapy. The key to therapeutic success requires a systematic approach to the problem coupled with appropriate follow-up care. This will ensure that nonresponders are reevaluated so their therapy can be adjusted appropriately, while providing a safeguard against missing a potentially life-threatening diagnosis.

Incidence

Pruritus ani occurs in approximately 1 to 5 percent of the population; men are affected more commonly than women by a ratio of 4:1.[1-3] This condition is most common in the fifth and sixth decades of life, but it is not infrequent for the clinician to encounter adolescents and elderly persons with pruritus. On those rare occasions in which pruritus ani affects children, it is usually related to an infectious etiology.

Clinical Presentation

Pruritus may begin insidiously, with the patient complaining of the sensation of uneasiness or itching in the perianal region. As the area of involvement spreads and the intensity of itching increases, the patient reflexively begins scratching and clawing at the skin. This leads to further skin damage, excoriation, and potentially a secondary skin infection. This unfortunately creates a vicious cycle of itching and scratching, which exacerbates the symptoms. Some patients have such severe pruritus that their lifestyle is utterly destroyed, leading them to suicidal tendencies.[4] Most patients are aware of the symptoms in the evenings and are more predisposed to exacerbations in the summer months.

Pathophysiology

The perianal skin is richly supplied with sensory nerve endings that mediate a variety of sensations.[5] These sensations may be elicited by local irritation from excoriations, alkaline secretions, and various chemical irritants. The receptor apparatus for both itch and pain is located at the dermoepidermal junction of the skin and consists of a plexus of free nerve endings. Damage to cells in close proximity to these nerve endings causes a release of diffusable mediators that may stimulate the receptors. Slow-conducting neurons transmit the itch sensation to the lateral spinothalamic tracts through synapses that connect with secondary fibers and send the sensation to the thalamus. There is a question whether tertiary neurons relay an itch to the cortex. Greaves[5] pointed out that pain and itch are served by the same receptors and neural pathways, thus explaining the effectiveness of pain in relieving itch.

Etiologies

The etiology of pruritus ani is routinely categorized under the headings of idiopathic and secondary types. The specific etiologic factors responsible for the diagnosis of secondary pruritus ani are nearly encyclopedic. Yet despite comprehensive evaluations, more than one half of patients with pruritus ani are categorized as having an idiopathic etiology (Fig. 11-1). The major contributors to secondary pruritus ani are listed in Table 11-1. This list may be summarized by the eight D's in the diagnosis of pruritus ani (Table 11-2).

Personal Hygiene

Clinicians have long been aware of the irritant effect of feces on the perianal area, especially in cases of prolonged contact. Caplan[6] reported that in a group of 27 subjects who were patch tested with autogenous fresh feces 44 percent developed pruritus. From this group of 12 symptomatic patients, only 4 had a previous history of anal pruritus. The authors concluded that the quickly

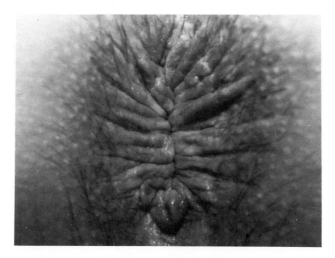

Figure 11-1.   Idiopathic pruritus ani.

developing symptoms were compatible with an irritant rather than an allergic effect. Marks[7] confirmed that, in pruritic patients, the stool pH paralleled the perianal skin pH. The authors attributed the excessive alkalinity

Table 11-1   Major Causes of Pruritus Ani

Personal hygiene	Poor cleansing habits resulting in chronic exposure to residual irritating feces; conversely, overmeticulous cleansing with excessive rubbing and soap use
Diet	Consumption of large volumes of liquids; coffee (caffeinated and decaffeinated, coffee-containing products), chocolate, citrus, spicy foods, tea, beer, and foods high in milk content; vitamin A and D deficiencies
Anatomic compromise	Obesity, deep anal clefts, excessive hair, tight-fitting clothing (tight clothing or clothing that impairs adequate ventilation), fistula, fissure, skin tags, prolapsing papilla, or mucosal prolapse
Systemic disease	Jaundice, diabetes mellitus, chronic renal failure, iron deficiency, thyrotoxicosis, myxedema, Hodgkin's lymphoma, polycythemia vera
Gynecologic conditions	Pruritus vulvae, vaginal discharge (endocervicitis, vaginitis)
Neoplasms	Bowen's disease, extramammary Paget's disease, squamous cell carcinoma, cloacogenic carcinoma, rectal or polypoid lesions
Diarrheal states	Irritable bowel syndrome, Crohn's disease, chronic ulcerative colitis
Radiation	Postirradiation changes
Psychogenic	Anxiety, neuroses, psychoses
Drugs	Quinidine; colchicine; antibiotics (tetracycline); IV hydrocortisone phosphate; ointments or creams that contain "caine" drugs; and nonprescription medications for personal hygiene such as perfumed soaps and ointments which may contain alcohol, witch hazel, or other astrigents
Dermatologic conditions	Psoriasis, seborrheic dermatitis, atropic dermatitis, lichen simplex, and lichen sclerosis.
Infections	Viruses: herpes simplex, cytomegalovirus, papillomavirus. Bacteria: *Staph. aureus,* erythrasma, mixed infections. Fungi: *dermatophytosis,* candidiasis. Parasites: pinworms, scabies, pediculosis. Spirochetes: syphilis.
Idiopathic	

Table 11-2   The Eight D's of Diagnosis of Pruritus Ani

1. Diseases of the anorectum

2. Diabetes and dyscrasias

3. Diseases of gynecologic origin

4. Diarrheal states

5. Drugs

6. Diet and deficiency of vitamins

7. Dermatoses

8. Disposition of patient

of the perianal skin in pruritus patients to lysozyme, a component of intestinal mucosecretions. In patients in whom continued fecal contamination can be identified as an etiologic factor, appropriate cleansing regimens often will alleviate symptoms. Another group of patients who may be plagued with pruritus secondary to their personal hygiene practices is known as the "overachiever group," noted to cleanse the perianal area meticulously. Their compulsive cleaning habits are usually associated with abrasive rubbing and the use of irritating alkaline soaps, which results in chronic pruritus. Physicians have categorized this as the "polishing the anus syndrome." These patients often obtain immediate resolution of symptoms once they adopt a perianal hygiene program that is less traumatic.

Anatomic Compromise

An estimated 25 percent of patients with pruritus ani have causative or contributory anorectal disorders.[3] These include anal fistula, fissure, skin tag, prolapsing anal papillae, or mucosal prolapse. These lesions may lead to seepage of fluid from the anal canal onto the perianal skin, which in turn can lead to inflammation, ulceration, and, if infected, suppuration. Surgical intervention to relieve pruritus is reported to be successful in fewer than 15 percent of all patients.[8] Thus, it becomes very important for the clinician to be highly selective in choosing surgical candidates, preferably only after an appropriate medical therapy has failed.

Patients who are obese may be predisposed to pruritus. Their anatomy can produce a persistently moist environment that may lead to difficulties in achieving appropriate personal hygiene. Patients with weak sphincter tone may have mucosal prolapse and fecal contamination of the perianal area, leading to pruritis. It also should be noted that patients wearing tight clothing (tight jeans, underwear, and girdles) or clothing that fails to allow proper ventilation are also predisposed to

this trapped moisture syndrome. Allan and associates[9] reported a physiologic study of 34 patients with pruritus. This study documented a marked increase in leakage through the anal sphincter in patients with pruritus ani compared with control subjects. The authors postulated that this increased leakage was caused by either the presence of coexisting anal disease or an exaggerated rectoanal inhibitory reflex.

Systemic Diseases

On occasion, systemic diseases may lead to generalized itching. Disease entities, including intrahepatic and extrahepatic biliary obstruction, may produce significant jaundice. Cholestatic jaundice has been associated with oral contraceptives, testosterone, and chlorpromazine. The itching associated with jaundice has long been attributed to elevated bile salt levels in the skin and blood, but this theory has not been substantiated. Administration of cholestyramine or colestipol hydrochloride is often helpful in reducing itching in this group of patients.[5]

Chronic renal failure is the most common systemic illness believed to elicit pruritus. Clinical manifestations are thought to be present in greater than 90 percent of patients on hemodialysis. The etiology of the itching is unclear. Ultraviolet B (UV-B) radiation is presently the most successful treatment.[5] Diabetes mellitus is often associated with vulvar and anogenital pruritus because of the disease's frequent presentation with candidiasis. Pruritus can also be associated with iron deficiency, with or without the presence of anemia, and it usually resolves with appropriate iron replacement. Patients with thyrotoxicosis or myxedema are also predisposed to generalized pruritus. Pruritus is a common complaint in patients with Hodgkin's disease. Symptoms often are exacerbated by alcohol. The pruritus of polycythemia vera is reported to be aggravated by bathing and showering with warm water. Researchers believe the symptoms are related to elevated blood histamine levels. These patients often respond to therapy with antihistamines or antiserotonin medications.[5]

Diet

Dietary factors represent the most significant cause of secondary pruritus ani. Diet may incite symptoms through three major pathways. First, it will help dictate the consistency of the stool, which in turn can lead to fecal soiling. Second, the components of the diet may lead to direct irritation secondary to their chemical make-up. Third, if an excessive volume of liquid is consumed, this could directly lead to more watery stools and pruritus strictly as a result of frequent contact irritation. Many food groups, such as coffee (caffeinated and decaffeinated), chocolate, citrus, spicy foods, tea, beer, and foods with a high milk content, have been implicated in initiating or promoting symptoms. Patients with vitamin A and vitamin D deficiencies are also believed to be predisposed to pruritus ani.[10]

The majority of patients with diet-induced pruritus ani can relate the onset of their symptoms to the ingestion of coffee or dairy products. Coffee is an irritant that can elicit pruritus when it is ingested in any form (fresh, instant, decaffeinated, or when used as a flavor additive to other foods, such as ice cream). An apparent threshold for coffee drinkers usually varies between 2 and 4 cups per day. A similar threshold, noted in milk-drinking patients, arises at ingestion of between 6 and 10 oz daily.[11] Pruritus caused by chocolate, tea, and cola is believed to be related to the xanthine content of these substances. Although beer has been implicated in eliciting pruritus ani, Smith and associates[12] found no correlation between alcohol ingestion and pruritus in their group of 75 patients. The appearance of diet-induced pruritus is often symmetric.[11]

Gynecologic Conditions

Pruritus ani often can be attributed specifically to diseases of gynecologic origin. Pruritus vulvae (Fig. 11-2) may extend posteriorly to involve the anal skin and can often be attributed to vaginal discharge or urinary incontinence. Irritation secondary to vaginal discharge may also lead to pruritus as the result of endocervicitis, trichomonal vaginitis, or candidal vaginitis. These disease processes cause a leukorrhea that irritates the perianal skin, and physicians should be prepared to perform pelvic examinations and to obtain appropriate cultures and stains in this subset of patients. Pruritus ani can frequently be reported in women during menopause independent of any identifiable local causes, probably secondary to estrogen deficiency.

Neoplasms

Neoplasms of the perianal region can be responsible for pruritus ani. The clinician must be cognizant of these potential etiologies and should exclude them by performing a careful physical examination and biopsy if necessary. Polypoid disease of the anorectum and villous lesions of the rectum may often lead to soiling. This may be secondary to changes in the normal anatomy or mucous secretions, as seen in the case of villous lesions. Bowen's disease is one unique form of squamous cell carcinoma in situ. This squamous carcinoma usually resides solely in the epidermal region but has invasive potential, estimated to be up to 5 percent of cases.[13,14] The disease can present as pruritus or may be found incidentally in an anorectal surgical specimen.

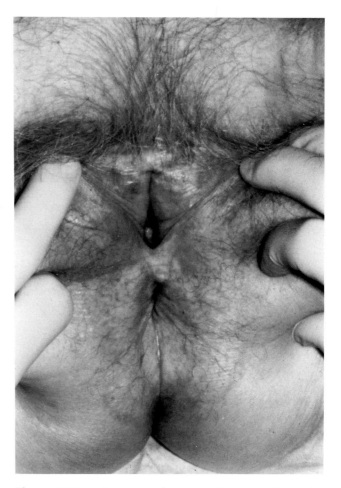

Figure 11-2.   Pruritus vulvae secondary to lichen sclerosis.

The lesion is characteristically an erythematous, hyperkeratotic plaque sharply demarcated from the surrounding skin. The size of the lesions ranges from a few millimeters to several centimeters. Because these lesions remain stable in size for long periods, they are often clinically overlooked or may be mistaken for psoriasis. If these lesions become pigmented, they can be confused with superficially spreading melanoma. The association of Bowen's disease with underlying systemic malignancies was reported by Graham and Helwig.[15] They discovered that as many as 33 percent of these patients developed an additional malignancy within 10 years of the diagnosis of Bowen's disease. However, recent reviews have not substantiated this association.[13,14,16] Small lesions may be treated successfully with topical 5-fluorouracil, but generous local excision with an adequate margin remains the preferred therapy.[16]

Extramammary Paget's disease is an intraepidermal neoplasm with a cellular composition similar to Paget's disease of the breast. Although the cell type of this lesion is still undefined, it is believed to be a pluripotential epithelial cell that borders on differentiation into sweat gland tissue. The lesions are usually red, indurated, scaling plaques often confused with eczema. Approximately 15 percent of such lesions are associated with an underlying cutaneous carcinoma or a breast or urogenital tumor.[17] The treatment for the noninvasive lesion is wide local excision. Invasive and recurrent lesions require special therapeutic considerations which are detailed in Chapter 16.[18]

Squamous cell carcinoma of the perianal region may also present as pruritus. The lesion is usually a nodular plaque with a warty appearance and is often confused with condyloma accuminata. It is usually treated with wide local excision. The clinician must be cognizant of this lesion's metastatic potential and should know its pattern of nodal spread. Basal cell carcinomas are rare tumors of the anorectal area. As described in Chapter 16, the characteristic appearance is similar to that found elsewhere on the body. This nodular growth, with its classic central depression, is usually treated by wide local excision. More radical surgery may be necessary for invasive or neglected tumors. Recent reports[19] indicate that in situ squamous carcinomas and cloacogenic carcinomas of the perianal region are being seen in increasing numbers in immunodeficient patients and in male homosexuals.[17,20] It is imperative that the clinician always biopsy any suspicious or nonresponding lesions of the perianal region.

Anorectal melanoma is a rare tumor of ectodermal origin. It is the most devastating perianal tumor. Regardless of the lesion's size, most melanomas have metastasized by the time of diagnosis. Unfortunately, these tumors usually do not respond to radiation or chemotherapy, and heroic efforts such as abdominal perineal resection yield only a 5 to 10 percent 5-year survival. Because of these dismal survival statistics palliative therapy is often the treatment plan.

Diarrheal States

Clinical and experimental data have shown that skin trauma secondary to moisture is one of the primary contributors to the production of pruritus ani. This can be seen not only in patients with colitis (Crohn's, ulcerative, or nonspecific), but also in patients who abuse laxatives or who ingest an excessively high-fiber diet. Patients with dumping or malabsorption syndromes, such as lactose intolerance, are also predisposed to pruritus. In the diarrheal patient, not only is the stool a direct skin irritant but the frequent hygiene it necessitates leads to abrasive trauma.

Radiation

Patients with rectal or anal canal cancers are often treated with a combination of chemotherapy and radiation. It is now generally understood that radiation therapy to the perineum can lead to pruritus. Radiation to the skin causes alterations in the normal cell cycle. Skin changes include erythema and edema (Fig. 11-3), which may progress to sclerosis and fibrosis. If the injury progresses, a full-thickness radiation burn will lead to ulcerations. Patients complain of pain, burning, and itching. Often radiation proctitis leads to diarrhea, which will further add to local anal skin irritation. Radiation proctitis can be managed with dietary measures

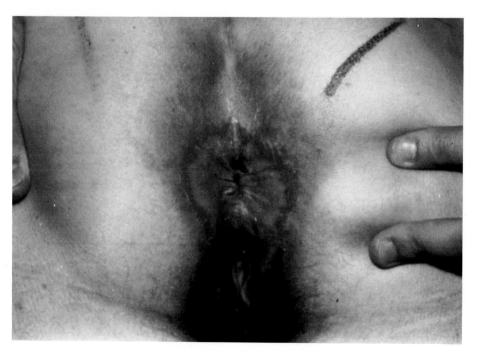

Figure 11-3. Perianal radiation dermatitis.

and bulking agents or a trial of hydrocortisone retention enemas. Radiodermatitis is difficult to treat. Initially, the physician should closely inspect the anoderm and biopsy all suspicious areas. Controlling pruritus is often difficult. Treatment should include cleansing the anoderm with a mild emollient soap substitute such as Balneol® and water. If this fails to control symptoms, a trial of topical hydrocortisone may be helpful.

Psychological Factors

The clinician should not underestimate the significance that psychological factors may play in the etiology of pruritus ani. Often, the patient suffering from pruritus can relate its onset to anxiety. The so-called "stress years" of midlife produce the largest patient population complaining of pruritus ani, perhaps suggesting more than a casual relationship with other etiologic factors. Smith and colleagues[12] evaluated the psychological profiles of 25 patients with pruritus ani by administering the Minnesota Multiphasic Personality Inventory. The authors found no statistically significant deviations from the clinical scales provided for non-pruritic patients, but it was noted that the pruritus patients demonstrated some possible tendencies toward "a relatively high degree of inhibition of aggression and denial of feeling of social and emotional alienation."[12]

Drugs

Several oral medications have been implicated in eliciting pruritus ani, by both contact irritation and increased leakage of fecal material from the anal opening. Quinidine and colchicine can initiate the acute onset of pruritus, although the patient may have been taking these medications in consistent dosages for years. Pruritus is usually controlled when the medication is stopped temporarily, which may be related to a threshold phenomenon. Mineral oil (taken orally) has also been detected as an offending agent; in this instance, pruritus is believed to be secondary to the pasty stool the patient develops and the associated perianal seepage. Ingestion of tetracycline also may cause pruritus by irritating the gut, which leads to a loose stool. In addition, tetracycline facilitates the occurrence of secondary perianal candidal infections. The intravenous administration of hydrocortisone phosphate has also been shown to produce pruritus ani. The application of certain topical ointments, creams, or cleansing agents may also elicit pruritus. Preparations containing the so-called "caines" notoriously produce intense inflammation in some susceptible patients. Many over-the-counter hygiene products, such as scented soaps, deodorants, toilet tissues, and laundry detergents, contain chemicals that may cause increased skin sensitivity and irritation. These chemicals include formaldehyde, alcohol, perfumes, and astringents. Many of these products elicit symptomatology by depriving the skin of its natural acidity. The increased use of anal wipes that are alcohol based or that contain witch hazel may lead to excoriation if used frequently or if left in contact with the skin for a prolonged period. Because of this, many of the new personal cleansing tissues are free of alcohol and witch hazel. Patients must be assisted in their selection of appropriate nonirritating, atraumatic perianal cleansing products.

Dermatologic Conditions

A large proportion of cases of pruritus ani may be attributable to nonmalignant dermatologic lesions. Perianal psoriasis (Fig. 11-4) may be a cause of refractory pruritus ani. The clinician should carefully inspect the patient for the presence of characteristic psoriatic patches elsewhere on the body, such as the scalp, knees, elbows, or other bony prominences. A perianal lesion

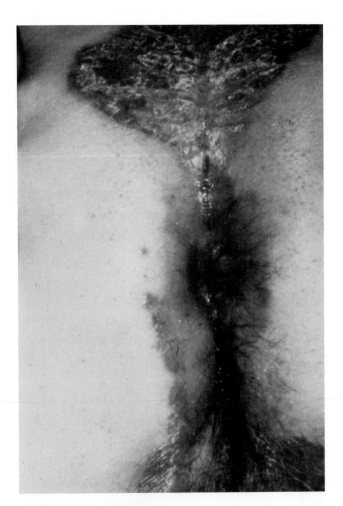

Figure 11-4.   Psoriasis.

may be the first or the only psoriatic lesion. Perianal psoriasis is usually found in the gluteal cleft spreading toward the sacrum. Although a perianal psoriatic lesion has a definitive border, it does not have the scaling of systemic psoriatic plaques. A multitude of treatment modalities exist for psoriasis. Initially, local lubrication to prevent fissuring and to maintain flexibility of the skin is important. Topical corticosteroids remain the most prescribed therapy, but coal tar applications remain beneficial despite their side effects of skin staining and odor.[21] For cases of psoriasis unresponsive to topical therapy, phototherapy often may be efficacious.[21]

When ultraviolet A light is used in conjunction with the photosensitizing properties of psoralen compounds, this treatment system is referred to as PUVA. Although PUVA is often effective in treating patients resistant to topical therapy, its long-term use is associated with an increase of cutaneous squamous cell cancers.[19] Methyltrexate and cyclosporin (when used in dosages lower than those required for transplant patients) have been shown to be effective systemic treatment agents, but only in highly selective resistant cases. Patients who receive these medications obviously must be informed of the risks and benefits of such dramatic therapy.[19]

Seborrheic dermatitis may also be a factor in perianal pruritus. Contact dermatitis may be allergic or irritant in nature. Allergic dermatitis is the result of a cell-mediated immune response to a specific exogenous allergen. This may be the chemical component of a plant or animal, a fabric, or a medicinal product. The most frequent offenders are poison ivy, poison oak, nickel, rubber compounds, procaine, neomycin, and the topical anesthetics of the "caine" family.[22] The lesions from contact dermatitis may vary from vesicles to eczemoid plaques with ill-defined borders. Dermatologic skin testing often can identify the offending agent. Treatment is aimed at prevention of allergen exposure supplemented by topical or systemic steroids if a reaction occurs. Nonallergenic contact dermatitis, or irritant dermatitis, is caused by exposure to such substances as acids, alkalis, the salts of metals, and hydrocarbons. The treatment is avoidance of exposure to these irritants and symptomatic measures on occasions when exposure leads to dermatitis. This may entail an inventory of all soaps, laundry detergents, and fabrics. There may be a temporal relation between the onset of pruritus and the acquisition of new clothing, soap, toilet tissue, or laundry detergent.

Lichen sclerosis et atrophicus is a rare condition most commonly referred to as lichen sclerosis (see Fig. 11-2). Its etiology is unknown, and it affects women in a ratio of 5:1 over men. In women, the disease often presents around the time of menopause and, in many cases, is associated with a previous episode of vaginitis. The lesions are elevated, ivory white, and macular. When several lesions coalesce, they form a "cigarette-paper crinkling" of the skin surface. There is no cure for the disease, and treatment is symptomatic, involving use of topical steroidal creams in conjunction with estrogen-containing creams.[16]

Atopic eczema is a chronic, relapsing pruritic dermatitis. It usually occurs in adults and is localized to the flexural surfaces of the face, neck, cubital or popliteal fossa, and hands. The dermatitis usually occurs in patients with a personal or family history of atopy or hay fever/asthma/urticaria. Lesions may present as papular, scaly, or chronic lichenified plaques. The etiology is unknown, it is believed to be IgE mediated.[16] Some researchers support food allergies and proteinaceous aeroallergens as possible etiologies. Patients with atopic dermatitis (Fig. 11-5) are likely to acquire bacterial and viral infections. Treatment is directed at skin hydration, corticosteroid administration, and antibiotics if secondary infections are present. Unfortunately, this is a chronic disease and relapses are common.

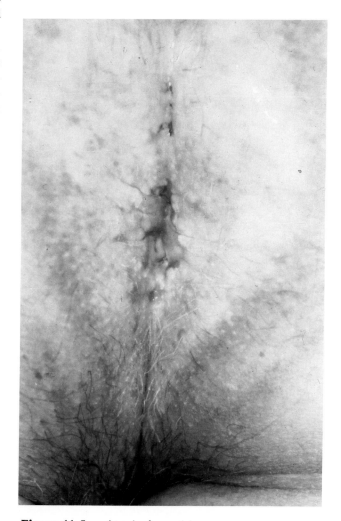

Figure 11-5. Atopic dermatitis.

Infections

Infectious agents must be considered in the differential diagnosis of secondary pruritus ani. The etiologic agents may be viral, bacterial, mycotic, parasitic, or of the spirochete family. Primary bacterial infections are an unusual occurrence, and when infectious agents can be documented they are usually superimposed on preexisting perianal skin trauma. Pruritus secondary to infectious agents often has an asymmetric appearance around the anus.[11]

Bacteria

Baral[22] successfully cultured *Staphylococcus aureus* from a small patient population with pruritus ani and reported that 100 percent of patients had resolution of symptoms after appropriate antibiotic therapy was instituted. Hidradenitis suppurativa (Fig. 11-6) as described in

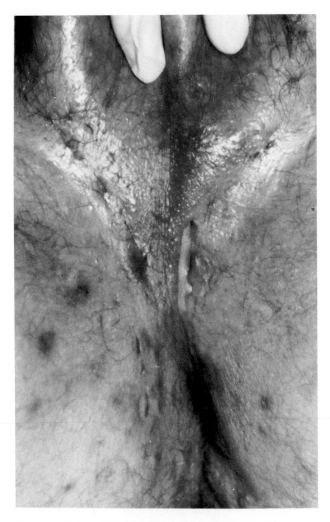

Figure 11-6. Hidradenitis suppurativa.

Chapter 13 may also cause pruritus. Erythrasma is an uncommon bacterial infection caused by *Corynebacterium minutissimum*.[23] These lesions initially present as a reddish scaly area that is well demarcated, but they eventually change to a tan color during the course of the disease. The diagnosis can be confirmed by using a Woods ultraviolet lamp, which allows the examiner to observe the characteristic red fluorescence of these lesions. Bowyer and McColl[23] diagnosed erythrasma in 15 of their 81 patients with pruritus ani but were only able to culture the organism in 3 patients. A 10-day course of erythromycin usually relieves the symptoms, but the condition sometimes recurs.

Viruses

Pruritis ani may be associated with the three major sexually transmitted viruses: herpes simplex virus (anogenital herpes), papillomavirus (condyloma accuminata), and cytomegalovirus (CMV). Patients with herpes simplex virus present with painful small vesicles surrounded by an erythematous areola. The vesicles usually rupture at approximately 48 hours, then progress over weeks to scaly eschars (see Fig. 21-6). The diagnosis can be confirmed by viral culture. Oral acyclovir is the current treatment of choice, and recent studies have indicated that the prophylactic use of this medication is successful in patients known to have frequent recurrences.[24] Condyloma accuminata are wart-like lesions found in the perianal region and the anal canal. The clinician should remember that the main reason for recurrence of this lesion is failure to eradicate anal canal lesions (see Fig. 21-10). Patients with immunodeficiency states are likely to develop CMV anal ulcerations or CMV colitis (see Fig. 22-1[25,26]). Biopsy of these lesions can confirm the diagnosis (see Fig. 22-2) but they are notoriously resistant to antiviral therapy.

Parasites

Parasitic infection should always be included in the differential diagnosis of patients with perianal pruritus. Pinworms (*Enterobius vermicularis*) are the most common cause of perianal itching in the pediatric age group. Jillson[27] challenged the common belief that pinworms elicit pruritus and proposed that symptoms actually are an uneasy crawling sensation and not itching. The diagnosis can be made by microscopically evaluating perianal skin samples collected on cellulose tape. It is imperative that other family members be evaluated so that they can be treated and recontamination does not occur. The symptoms usually occur in the evening, when these 6-mm long parasites migrate to the perianal skin. Scabies is a contagious skin infestation due to the mite *Sarcoptes scabiei* that can elicit severe pruritus. Although usually found on the finger webs or sides of the fingers, these lesions can often be identified in the perianal region. The diagnosis of scabies can be confirmed by demonstrating the mite or its products, such as ova or feces, from scrapings prepared on a slide with one drop of 10 percent potassium hydroxide.[28] Lesions appear initially as vesicles as the mite burrows its way into the stratum corneum. Treatment consists of the application of an appropriate scabeticide such as Kwell® lotion. The parasite *Pediculosis pubis* (crab or louse) can often be found grasping the base of a hair shaft and is noted to produce macular steel-gray spots, especially on the thighs and chest.[28] With careful examination under magnification this parasite strikingly resembles a crab. Management requires the treatment of all infected family members, appropriate delousing of all fomites such as clothes, bedding, and upholstery, and showering with an appropriate pediculocide such as Kwell®.

Mycotic organisms such as *Epidermophyton, Tricophyton,* or *Candida* can produce pruritus. Candidiasis of the perianal region as a primary source of pruritus is rare, identified in fewer than 1 percent of random skin scrapings.[16] These lesions are usually erythematous with classically well-defined borders. These infections are usually secondary to the overgrowth of bacteria after the use of antibiotics or topical corticosteroids or are associated with vaginal infections. Mycotic etiology can be confirmed by microscopic inspection or select cultures.

Spirochetes

Syphilitic lesions in their primary or secondary stages may have an associated exudate. Continued local irritation secondary to moisture may lead to maceration and pruritic complaints. During the primary stage of syphilis, a chancre may be identified approximately 18 to 20 days after infection with the spirochete. Usually this is a painless, noninflamed ulcer located at the anal verge. Though the lesion is not painful, the patient may often complain of tenesmus or uneasiness, and evaluation of the symptoms and the location and character of the lesion often lead it to be mistaken as a lateral fissure compatible with Crohn's disease. In the secondary stage of syphilis, a maculopapular rash is seen to convert to a red, indurated lesion that may or may not be pruritic. When syphilis is suspected, appropriate laboratory tests should be performed to confirm the diagnosis, and one should be especially suspicious of sexually transmitted diseases in patients practicing anal intercourse. The drug of choice for the treatment of syphilis remains penicillin, or tetracycline in penicillin-allergic patients.[13] The various treatment regimens are discussed in more detail in Chapter 21.

Approach to the Patient

For the physician whose patient has pruritus, formulating the correct diagnosis and instituting appropriate therapy can be challenging because of the multitude of pathologic etiologies of pruritus. The key to patient satisfaction is a systematic approach to the problem supported by appropriate follow-up care.

History

A carefully taken history can often aid in identifying the etiology of pruritus. The physician should first document the nature of the patient's complaints. This should include the onset of symptoms and their relationship to diet, medication, defecation, and anal hygiene practices. All medications should be identified, as most can contribute to pruritus. Special attention should be given to antibiotics, colchicine, quinidine, and topical medicines containing corticosteroids, estrogens, or "caines" drugs. Systemic illnesses, such as diabetes mellitus, chronic renal failure, or lymphoreticular diseases such as polycythemia vera or Hodgkin's disease should be identified. The history should also elicit any symptoms of inflammatory bowel disease or acolic stools. A history of anorectal surgery can be helpful in identifying patients with deformed anorectal anatomy, which in turn can lead to poor continence. The physician should also document whether the patient has allergies or any generalized dermatoses such as psoriasis or seborrheic dermatitis. A sexual history should include the patient's sexual orientation and specific practices, especially the practice of anal intercourse. The immune status of the patient is also important, not only in those with primary immunodeficient states or contracted states such as acquired immunodeficiency syndrome, but also in transplantation patients who are receiving immunosuppressive medications. A careful gynecologic history should be obtained from female patients and should include contraceptive practices and any history of inflammatory or ulcerative lesions. A brief psychological profile of the patient may be beneficial in identifying any association between symptoms and social or financial stresses with which the patient may be confronted.

Physical Examination

After completing a detailed medical history, the clinician should perform a meticulous physical examination. Initially, the general dermatologic evaluation may isolate conditions such as psoriasis, seborrheic dermatitis, or fungal or other infections. The patient should come to the examining suite without bowel preparation and with instructions not to have applied any creams or ointments to the perianal area. The examining room should be well stocked, with a bright light source and magnifying glass along with disposal enemas for bowel preparation and all clinical equipment necessary to obtain appropriate cultures, scrapings, or biopsies. The patient should then be assisted to the prone jackknife position (see Fig. 2-1) and a careful inspection of the perianal region should be performed, looking for signs of excessive moisture, soiling, excoriation, skin maceration (see Fig. 11-1), or any perianal dermatoses. After giving instructions to the patient to strain (Valsalva maneuver), the clinician can evaluate the perianal region for possible prolapsing hemorrhoidal tissue. An initial digital examination should be done without bowel preparation to evaluate the consistency of the stool and obtain a specimen for a stool Hemoccult test. The digital examination should include a 360° sweep of the anorectum, including an evaluation of the prostate gland in males. All abnormalities should be carefully documented, as should the resting and squeeze sphincter times.

Next, the clinician can complete any cultures, biopsies, or scrapings that are thought necessary to make an appropriate clinical diagnosis. Suspicious skin lesions can be biopsied using a punch biopsy technique. This technique involves subdermal infiltration of a few milliliters of 1 percent lidocaine with epinephrine (1:200,000) under the biopsy site. A punch biopsy tool is driven into the area with a circular motion. This is accomplished by swirling the punch between the thumb and index fingers. After the punch is 4 to 5 mm beneath the skin, it is gently raised and the resulting circular wedge of skin and subcutaneous tissue excised with a fine scissors. Bleeding should be minimal, and simple pressure should adequately effect hemostasis. A simple gauze dressing is all that is required. The punches are available in a number of sizes ranging in diameter from 1.0 mm to 1.0 cm. For convenience the authors use disposable punches. Two disposable enemas should then be administered to the patient, after which a careful sigmoidoscopy and anoscopy are performed. Patient evaluation for hemorrhoids, polyps, cancer, fistula, mucosal prolapse, stenosis, or evidence of previous surgery is documented. Sigmoidoscopy may be helpful in identifying patients who have proctitis, inflammatory bowel disease, rectal lesions, or active infections. The examiner should take special precautions in evaluating patients who engage in anal intercourse or who may be strong candidates for exposure to sexually transmitted diseases. The physician should decide on a case-by-case basis whether to perform pelvic examinations in female patients, but this may be helpful in difficult diagnoses.

Treatment

Once the clinician has acquired a comprehensive history, performed a thorough physical examination, and obtained appropriate cultures, scrapings, and biopsies, the primary cause for pruritus ani may be identified and appropriate therapy instituted. Treatment may include:

Conservative dietary changes to identify offending agents or their symptomatic thresholds

Initiation of appropriate medical therapy for infections, dermatoses, or systemic disorders

Surgical intervention for the few anatomic deformities which contribute to the pruritus

Unfortunately, the majority of patients with pruritus have no identifiable etiology and subsequently fall into the category of idiopathic pruritus ani.

To achieve success with this group of patients, the physician must provide a focused therapeutic approach which should include clear instructions tempered with realistic expectations for a response and a consistent follow-up pattern. Initially, it is important for the physician to maximize rapport with the patient. This can be accomplished first by displaying empathy for the patient's problems and second by providing reassurance of potential relief for the patient's symptoms. It is interesting to observe that once cancer has been excluded as an etiology most patients display a decreased level of anxiety about their condition. Anecdotally, the use of supplemental instruction sheets often leads to a higher degree of patient compliance (Fig. 11-7).

The patient should first be instructed about appropriate perianal hygiene. These initial efforts are directed toward keeping the perianal skin dry, clean, and slightly acidic. Any nonessential antibiotics should be discontinued, as should other irritants to the perianal area such as harsh toilet paper, soaps, and any personal hygiene products the patient may be applying to the area. The patient should also initially discontinue the use of any steroidal agents because of their harmful thinning of the perianal skin. Trauma incurred by scratching must be stopped, and for patients with severe symptoms, wearing white cotton gloves at bedtime may be necessary. An alternative to harsh toilet paper is small nonalcoholic towelettes, with appropriate drying of the perianal region with either a soft towel or a hair dryer. Substitute soap preparations such as Balneol® are useful and can be applied with the fingertips or moist cotton balls. During the day and at bedtime, the patient may find it helpful to apply a thin cotton pledget directly into the anal crease. The pledget should be small enough so that the patient

INSTRUCTIONS FOR PATIENTS

1. Our goal is to keep the skin of the anal area clean, dry, and slightly acidic.
2. During bath or shower, wash the outside of the anal area with water. Do not use soap in the anal area (it is alkaline and will increase your discomfort). If a cleansing agent is desired, apply Balneol with fingertips or wet cotton balls. When drying the anal area, avoid abrasive trauma or vigorous rubbing by patting the skin dry with a soft towel or using a hair dryer at low heat.
3. Following each bowel movement, make sure the anal area is clean of any residual stool or moisture. This may be accomplished with a nonalcoholic towelette. Be sure not to leave pads in contact with the skin for prolonged periods. Avoid the use of toilet paper on irritated skin. If persistent afterdrainage persists even after meticulous hygiene, rectal irrigation with a 4-oz syringe bulb and warm water may be useful.
4. In the morning and at bedtime, apply a thin cotton pledget directly in the anal crease. It should be small enough so that you are not conscious of its presence. You may dust the cotton with baby powder or cornstarch if needed. It is important to change the pledget often during the day if it becomes moist.
5. Soaking in a warm sitz bath for 20 minutes can provide relief. Do not add any soaps or skin softeners to the water, and be sure to dry the anal area thoroughly afterwards.
6. Maintain a soft, large, and nonirritating stool so that it can pass through the anal canal without causing mechanical or chemical trauma. This may be accomplished by the following:
   a. A bulking agent such as Konsyl, Metamucil, or Citrucil _____ tablespoons in _____ glasses of water of juice _____ times a day.
   b. Eat a high fiber diet that includes 8 to 10 glasses of water or juice a day, plenty of fruits and vegetables, and bran cereal every day.
   c. Avoid foods that cause bowel irritation, produce mucus, or aggravate drainage; these include dark colas, spicy foods, citrus foods and juices, coffee (regular or decaffeinated), beer, nuts, popcorn, milk, and foods known to produce gas or indigestion. 7-Up, ginger ale, and other light-colored soft drinks may be tolerated.
7. Wearing cotton gloves to bed can be of benefit if you scratch yourself while sleeping.
8. Recurrences are common and to be expected.
9. Don't become despondent over this, just be sure to reconsult your doctor so that appropriate corrections in therapy can be made.
10. You may apply a hydrocortisone cream, but only if it is directed by your physicians for use after a cleansing and drying routine.

Figure 11-7.   Patient care handout for pruritus ani.

is not conscious of its presence. Dusting the pledget with baby powder (nonperfumed) or cornstarch may improve moisture control.

The patient should also be counseled on dietary changes. As mentioned before, food products such as coffee, teas, cola, chocolate, beer, and tomatoes have been identified as offending agents, but there appears to be a threshold at which these products elicit pruritus.

For this reason, the patient should discontinue ingestion of these items and then slowly reinstate them into the diet in an attempt to isolate the offending agent. Once the offending agent, such as coffee, is identified, it may be possible to find the patient's threshold so that total abstinence from the product is unnecessary. Patients should discontinue any habit-forming cathartics and take a bulking agent instead so that the stool remains soft, large, and nonirritating. This will decrease trauma to the anal canal and help maintain better perianal hygiene.

In patients who continue to have uncontrolled leakage, rectal irrigation performed with a 4-oz bulb syringe and warm water is an acceptable adjunct. Daily sitz baths in warm water may also be helpful, but patients should not add any chemicals to the water. In the unfortunate patient who has intractable pruritus ani, many therapies have been tried: injection of alcohol- or oil-soluble anesthetics, injection of methylene blue, tattooing of the perianal skin with mercuric sulfide, surgical undercutting, and radiation therapy, all of which have had unacceptable results. These procedures have been associated with complications such as skin necrosis, lo-

cal sepsis, and sloughing of the perianal skin. The use of Berwick's solution followed by benzoin and talc at weekly intervals has been successful anecdotally in isolated cases. It should be noted that the use of sedation, tranquilizers, and biofeedback by well-trained practitioners may demonstrate some clinical benefit. Intermittent recurrences of the disease are common. The patient should be instructed not to become despondent but to reconsult the physician so that appropriate therapeutic corrections can be made. If symptoms continue despite aggressive therapy and appropriate changes in therapy fail to give the patient relief, a second opinion from a dermatologist, gynecologist, or internist should be considered.

References

1. Sullivan ES, Garnjobst WM. Pruritus ani: a practical approach. *Surg Clin North Am.* 1978;58:505–512.
2. Calnan CD, O'Neill D. Itching in tension states. *Br J Dermatol.* 1952;64:274–280.
3. Bowyer A, McColl I. A study of 200 patients with pruritus ani. *Proc R Soc Med.* 1970;63:96–98.
4. Goligher J. Pruritus ani. In: Goligher J, ed. *Surgery of the Anus, Rectum and Colon.* 5th ed. London: Balliere Tindall; 1984:237–245.
5. Greaves MW. The nature and management of pruritus ani. *Practitioner.* 1982;226:1223–1225.
6. Caplan RM. The irritant role of feces in the genesis of perianal itch. *Gastroenterology.* 1966;50:19–23.
7. Marks MM. The influence of the intestinal pH on anal pruritus. *South Med J.* 1968;61:1005–1006.
8. Daily TH. Pruritus ani. *Pract Gastroenterol.* 1980;4:1–4.
9. Allan A, Ambrose NS, Silverman S, Keighley MRB. Physiological study of pruritus ani. *Br J Surg.* 1987;74:576–579.
10. Friend WG. The cause and treatment of idiopathic pruritus ani. *Dis Colon Rectum.* 1977;20:40–42.
11. Friend WG. Pruritus ani. In: Fazio VW, ed. *Current Therapy in Colon and Rectal Surgery.* Toronto: BC Decker; 1990:42–45.
12. Smith LE, Henrichs D, McCullah RD. Prospective studies on the etiology and treatment of pruritus ani. *Dis Colon Rectum.* 1982;25:358–363.
13. Beck DE, Fazio VW, Jagelman DG, Lavery IC. Perianal Bowen's disease. *Dis Colon Rectum.* 1988;31:419–422.
14. Arbesman H, Ransohoff DF. Is Bowen's disease a predictor for the development of internal malig-

nancy? A methodological critique of the literature. *JAMA.* 1987;257:516–518.
15. Graham JH, Helwig EB. Bowen's disease and its relationship to systemic cancer. *Arch Dermatol.* 1959;80:133–159.
16. Arnold HL, Odom RB, James WD, eds. Syphilis. In: Yaws, Bejel, Pinta, *Andrews' Diseases of the Skin.* 8th ed. Philadelphia: WB Saunders; 1990:405–429.
17. Wexner SD, Smithy WB, Milsom JW, Dailey TH. The surgical management of anorectal disease in AIDS and pre-AIDS patients. *Dis Colon Rectum.* 1986;29:719–723.
18. Degefu S, O'Quinn AG, Dhurandhar HN. Paget's disease of the vulva and urogenital malignancies: a case report and review of the literature. *Gynecol Oncol.* 1986;25:347–354.
19. Stern RS, Lange R. Non-melanoma skin cancer occurring in patients treated with PUVA five to ten years after first treatment. *J Invest Dermatol.* 1988;91:120–124.
20. Wexner SD, Milsom J, Dailey TH. The demographics of anal cancers are changing: identification of a high-risk population. *Dis Colon Rectum.* 1987;30:942–946.
21. Martini MC, Marks JG. Contact dermatitis and contact urticaria. In: Sams WM, Lynch PJ, eds. *Principles and Practice of Dermatology.* New York: Churchill Livingstone; 1990:389–402.
22. Baral J. Pruritis ani and *Staphylococcus aureus.* *J Am Acad Dermatol.* 1983;9:962. Letter to Editor.
23. Bowyer A, McColl I. Erythrasma and pruritus ani. *Acta Derm Venereol (Stockh).* 1971;51:444–447.
24. Kaplowitz LG, Baker D, Gelb L, et al. Prolonged continuous acyclovir treatment of normal adults

with frequently recurring genital herpes simplex virus infection. *JAMA*. 1991;265:747–751.

25. Wexner SD. Cytomegalovirus ileocolitis and Kaposi's sarcoma in AIDS. In: Fazio VW, ed. *Current Therapy in Colon and Rectal Surgery*. Toronto:BC Decker; 1990:217–221.

26. Wexner SD, Smithy WS, Trillo C, et al. Emergency colectomy for cytomegalovirus ileocolitis in patients with acquired immune deficiency syndrome. *Dis Colon Rectum*. 1988;31:755–761.

27. Jillson OF. Pruritus ani: disputing the passage. *Cutis*. 1984;33:537, 541, 544, 548.

28. Morgan RT. Mite infestations in pediculosis. In: Sams WM, Lynch PJ, eds. *Principles and Practice of Dermatology*. New York:Churchill Livingstone; 1990:191–196.

CHAPTER 12

FISSURE IN ANO AND ANAL STENOSIS

James W. Fleshman

Fissure in Ano

History

Fissure in ano has been recognized as a common cause of anal pathology for many years. As early as 1829, Recamier recommended stretching the anal sphincter for the treatment of fissure in ano.[1] In 1833, Dupuytren recommended incising the fissure itself to relieve the patient of the pain.[2] In 1846, Demarquay reported performing subcutaneous sphincterotomy to treat fissure in ano.[3] Since that time, there has been a controversy over the treatment of fissure in ano. Martin in 1923 also recommended subcutaneous sphincterotomy.[4] Miles, however, recommended multiple "pectenotomy"[5] because he considered the cause of the fissure to be a band of scar tissue at the pectinate line which required release. Eisenhammer popularized lateral internal anal sphincterotomy for the treatment of fissure in ano in 1951 after originally recommending posterior midline sphincterotomy.[6] He is also credited with the concept that the internal anal sphincter fibers form the floor of the fissure. Dilation of the anal sphincter as proposed by Recamier is used extensively in some areas of the world. The lateral sphincterotomy is the most commonly used technique in the United States. Both techniques have their proponents and each technique has its complications.

Magnitude of the Problem

Fissure in ano is a common problem. It causes a significant morbidity and loss of working hours. In the last 5 years, 1214 office visits have been made by patients with fissure in ano to the Division of Colon and Rectal Surgery at Jewish Hospital. This represents 6.2 percent of total office visits. Nicholls reported that anal fissure comprised 15 percent of office referrals.[7] The majority

of these patients with fissure in ano have been successfully treated with conservative medical therapy. A total of 336 patients have been treated with lateral internal anal sphincterotomy. This represents 10 percent of all operative procedures performed by the division surgeons. Thus, it is apparent that this is a significant disease entity that requires attention by surgeons and physicians.

Symptoms

Patients who have a fissure in ano usually describe a tearing pain on defecation followed by blood on the stool or on the toilet paper. Rarely, blood will be noted in the toilet bowl water. The fissure is typified by a split in the skin during a solid constipated bowel movement followed by a tearing pain and then a dull ache or spasm in the anal canal. This ache eventually resolves over 1 to 3 hours. Patients may complain of continued pressure in the perineum. This symptom complex is usually reported as "hemorrhoids" when the patient arrives in the office. The patient has generally administered self-prescribed treatments such as ointments, local anesthethics, and steroid creams or suppositories and may complain of mucous discharge, itching, and occasionally soiling. The symptoms caused by fissure in ano may be acute in onset, intermittent, or chronic. The majority of patients seen in the office with this problem have had a previous episode which went untreated except by self-medication. However, the fear of cancer or other problems usually brings the patient to the office when the problem recurs.

Pathophysiology

The typical acute fissure is simply a split in the anoderm at the dentate line (Fig. 12-1). The fissure is usually noted in the anterior or posterior midline. The majority

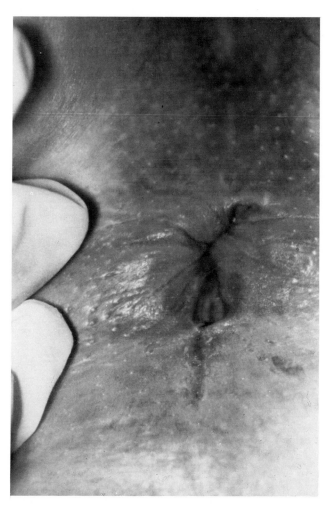

Figure 12-1. Chronic anal fissures in anterior and posterior midline.

(90 percent) of patients have a posterior midline fissure (Fig. 12-2A). An anterior midline fissure is seen in women more frequently than men. It has been reported in 10 to 20 percent of women and 1 to 10 percent of men with fissures.[8] A chronic fissure may eventually be associated with an external anal skin tag and a hypertrophied internal papilla at the mucosal edge of the fissure. The base of the acute fissure has a filmy white covering which is the connective tissue of the submucosa and longitudinal muscle fibers as they fan out from the intersphincteric groove to cover the underlying circular fibers of the internal sphincter. The base of the chronic fissure usually reveals fibers of the internal sphincter and the edges of the ulcer are slightly undermined and rolled.[7]

Differential Diagnosis

Idiopathic fissues, as described previously, are located anteriorly or posteriorly. Other types of fissures are located laterally (Fig. 12-2B).

Crohn's disease is the most common cause of anal fissure associated with other diseases. However, these fissures are usually not in the midline, are painless until much larger in size, and are associated with a thick edematous external skin tag. The base of the Crohn's fissure or ulcer will usually contain an exudate and granulation tissue. Eventual destruction of the underlying muscle and extension to the perirectal tissues may contribute to fistular disease. Fissures of Crohn's disease only become symptomatic when the skin tags are large, the ulcer burrows into the muscle deeply, the drainage affects the adjacent skin, or the external opening heals, resulting in pus under pressure. Biopsies of the skin tags and ulcers may occasionally reveal granulomata. Crohn's disease must be suspected in patients with fissures occuring in atypical positions around the anal canal since almost 10 percent of patients with Crohn's disease present with anal disease. Sphincterotomy may cause further sphincter damage and worsening the anal disease because of nonhealing. Conservative local or systemic therapy with metronidazole has been shown to be effective.

Anal tuberculosis may present as ulcerative, verrucous, lupoid, or miliary lesions in the anal canal.[9] A history of previous or concomitant pulmonary TB is found in 100 percent of patients with anal TB. Tuberculosis is spread to the anal canal by way of the lymphatic tissue, hematogenously, by direct extension or by the ingestion of contaminated food, milk, or swallowed saliva, especially after gastric acid–reducing procedures. A tuberculous ulcer should be suspected if the patient has no history of Crohn's disease and the ulcer is a nonhealing, nonmidline ulcer. Examination of a biopsy specimen by acid fast bacilli staining and culture will make the diagnosis. This problem is more common in patients immunocompromised during treatment for cancer or as a result of HIV infection. The treatment of anal tuberculosis is chemotherapy.

Foreign bodies such as fish bones, toothpicks, or metal pins may become lodged in the crypts of the dentate line and cause an anal ulcer. These are usually associated with an abscess locally.

Anal cancer (squamous, cloacogenic, and adenocarcinoma) occasionally causes pain, but anal cancer is usually a painless, nonmidline lesion with an atypical firm texture. The possibility of anal cancer existing in an anal ulcer has been used as a reason for excising a fissure. Any nonhealing anal fissure should be biopsied.

An anal fistula is sometimes present after the ulcer has become chronic and the skin is undermined. However, a perianal abscess can mimic symptoms of fissure in ano. Cytomegalovirus has caused symptoms similar to a common anal fissure in patients with AIDS. Likewise the syphilitic ulcer has been shown to produce an anal ulcer.[7] These are painful ulcers and may mimic the

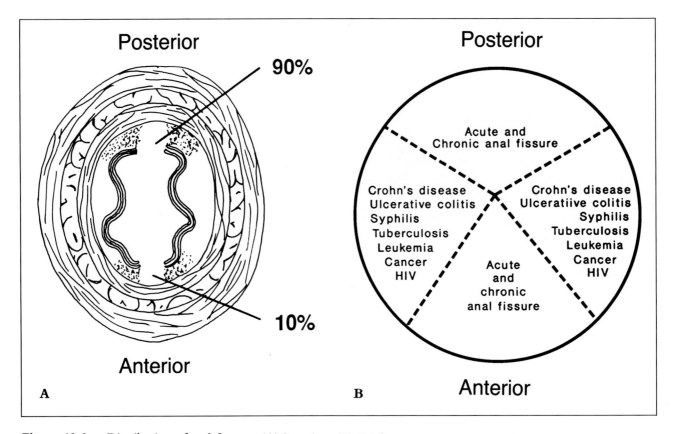

Figure 12-2.   Distribution of anal fissures. (A) Location. (B) Etiology.

symptom complex of the fissure in ano. A dark field examination will reveal the spirochetes. There is invariably a history of anal intercourse. Chlamydia, herpes simplex, and gonorrhea may also cause atypical or multiple anal fissures.

Diagnosis

The diagnosis of fissure in ano can usually be made by simply spreading the buttocks to inspect the anal canal. The fissure or the ulcer complex (skin tag, ulcer, and papilla) will be easily seen in the anal canal (see Fig. 12-1). Insertion of a cotton-tipped swab into the closed anal canal may also reveal the location of the fissure when a linear streak of blood is noted as the swab is withdrawn. Performance of digital rectal or proctoscopic examination during the initial visit when the patient is acutely symptomatic is painful and not well tolerated. Therefore, empiric medical therapy is generally indicated. A follow-up examination is much easier and should be performed at the subsequent visit when a patient is more comfortable.

Theory of Etiology

The fissure is generally reported after a hard bowel movement passes through the anal canal causing a stretching and tearing of the anal skin. The fissure is occasionally associated with profound severe diarrhea. This is sometimes the only reported change in bowel habits. Other patients will report diarrhea followed by a firm bowel movement with onset of the symptoms.

The fissure in ano is associated with several interesting findings. First, fissures are most commonly in the anterior or posterior midline. It has been suggested that the weak areas of the anal canal are in the anterior and posterior midline of the sphincter where decussating external sphincter fibers are found. During the passage of a firm stool, the mass is distributed anteriorly and posteriorly because of muscle mass laterally. A tear may occur in these areas because of the underlying weakness and lack of thick muscle.[10]

A second theory relies on the partial eversion of the anal canal during evacuation of stool from the rectal vault. This eversion is inhibited anteriorly and posteriorly because the skin is tethered to the sphincter mechanism in this area and encounters more tension or resistance to stretch.[7] As a result, there is more likely to be tearing in these areas.

Finally, the fissure may cause increased contraction in the internal anal sphincter, thereby increasing pressure in the anal canal. The increased pressure may cause ischemia owing to poor capillary filling in the area of the fissure.[11] The resting pressure can rise to levels higher than the venous pressure and capillary filling pressure of the muscle. Ischemia of the overlying skin is the result. The increased resting tone in the internal anal sphincter may be an intrinsic feature of the individual internal sphincter or the result of chronic spasm due to the patient's bowel habits. If the fissure causes recurring spasm in an anal canal with an already elevated resting tone, ischemia is perpetuated and the fissure becomes a chronic ulcer. As the ulcer is reactivated by passage of stool, more spasm occurs and the ulcer cannot heal.

Each of these theories has merit. In reviewing the onset of a fissure, the majority of patients describe passage of a firm bowel movement. However, patients also may describe diarrhea with intense efforts at control and resulting muscle spasm. Anal manometry has shown the resting pressure generated by the internal anal sphincter to be elevated in patients with anal fissure as compared with patients who do not have fissure in ano.[11,12] The external sphincter is normal. After treatment of the anal fissure with sphincterotomy or dilation and healing of the fissure, the anal pressures return to normal.[13,14] It is unknown whether the pressure is elevated prior to development of the fissure or whether the fissure causes an increase in the resting tone of the internal sphincter. Kuypers has shown that there is no muscle spasm in patients with anal fissure, simply increased pressure.[15]

Histologic studies have shown that an increased fibrosis of the internal sphincter in patients with fissure in ano.[16] Patients with Crohn's disease and ulcerative colitis who develop stenosis and spasm of the anal canal after chronic inflammation and ulceration also have increased fibrosis with an increased connective tissue: muscle ratio. There is also an increase in fibrosis in the internal sphincter of elderly patients.[17]

Even though the exact cause of anal fissure is not known we can suggest that constipation must play a role. A study by Jensen showed that withholding of dietary fiber and straining at constipated stools increased the incidence of fissure.[18]

Treatment

Medical Therapy

The majority of patients with fissure in ano will respond to medical therapy which consists of stool softeners, bulk agents, and topical anesthetic or corticosteroids. The initial episode of anal fissure has been shown to heal in 87 percent of patients treated with unprocessed bran twice a day.[19] Hydrocortisone ointment and local anesthetics have been shown to help 82 percent and 60 percent of these patients respectively.[19] Jensen also

showed that 15 g of unprocessed bran daily for 1 year reduced recurrence of the fissure to 16 percent in a study population.[18] An improvement in bowel movement regularity was also noticed in 82 percent of patients who reported irregular bowel movements before starting the bran. Since the daily recommended dietary fiber intake is 25 to 35 g and the calculated daily fiber intake for a western adult is approximately 10 to 14 grams per day, increasing the fiber intake by 15 g will usually place the patients in the recommended range. The addition of topical agents to fiber and hygiene did not appear to improve healing. Topical agents may be beneficial for relief of acute symptoms, however. Topical lidocaine or corticosteroid suppositories may bring immediate pain relief and some decrease in spasm. However, Jensen actually showed that 10 grams of unprocessed bran twice a day improved symptoms faster in patients than steroid ointments and local anesthetic alone.[19] He did not study bran and topical treatments in combination. It is possible that a combination of these may relieve local symptoms and allow healing to begin.

Anal dilation using dilators has not been helpful in treating anal fissures in adults,[20] even though it is usually successful in the treatment of fissures in children. McDonald and associates showed that the addition of an anal dilator was no more useful than stool softeners and topical anesthesia alone.[21]

The best recommendation for medical treatment seems to be an increase in dietary fiber by at least 15 g per day and a topical agent for symptom relief. These methods lead to healing of the fissure in the majority of patients with a first episode of fissure in ano and almost half of patients with chronic fissure.

Surgical Therapy

Surgical treatment for anal fissures should be reserved for chronic anal fissures or anal ulcers. The chronicity of the problem can be detected by the appearance of the anal fissure or ulcer. Nicholls suggested that the presence of a skin tag and papilla, undermined edges of the ulcer, and visible internal sphincter at the base of the ulcer indicated chronicity and the need for surgery.[8] A study in 1983 by Gough and Lewis showed that 40 percent of chronic fissures healed with conservative therapy using bran and topical anesthetics.[20] There is, therefore, some evidence to suggest that even chronic fissures should be treated initially with bran and topical agents. However, once conservative therapy has failed, one must proceed with surgical therapy. The surgical treatment of fissure in ano remains controversial. The possibilities include manual sphincter stretch, excision of the fissure, and internal anal sphincterotomy. Sphincterotomy may be performed in different areas of the anal canal and in different ways.

Sphincter Stretch

In 1965, Watts, Bennett, and Goligher described stretching of the anal sphincter to treat anal fissure.[22] Since then, numerous studies have compared four-finger anal stretching with sphincterotomy. The majority have shown that sphincter stretch or maximal anal dilation results in good healing of the anal fissure (Table 12-1). Weaver and associates described a technique of anal dilatation using four fingers for 4 minutes with 92 percent success.[23] Fissures recurred in only 5 percent of patients after initial healing. O'Connor reported 30 patients with fissure who underwent six-finger anal dilation and an increase in dietary fiber intake with 100 percent success and no recurrence.[24] The majority of authors agree that anal stretch is an uncontrolled fracturing of the internal anal sphincter. This also results in varying degrees of sphincter injury leading to incontinence of flatus and soilage. Nearly one third of patients who underwent dilation in Jensen's series had recurrence, and complications were higher in the dilated group.[25] The procedures were performed under local anesthesia which may account for the poor results. Weaver and associates found no difference between sphincterotomy and anal dilation when both were performed under general anesthesia.[23]

Excision of Fissure

There is no good evidence that the fissure should be excised to promote healing. The rationale for adding this to the procedure includes removal of the edges of the chronic ulcer to promote healing and to identify a possible anal cancer. Gingold reported on 86 patients who underwent sphincterotomy and fissurectomy with good success and no complications.[26] He did not report on long-term follow-up. All the patients that he treated returned to work in 3 days. Khubchandani and Reed concluded that excision of the fissure is not necessary. Time to healing and success in healing a fissure were not influenced by excision of the fissure.[27]

Sphincterotomy

A sphincterotomy can be performed in several different ways. Posterior midline sphincterotomy was initially recommended by Eisenhammer. He changed his technique to a lateral sphincterotomy to avoid the keyhole deformity and the soiling that resulted. Multiple sphincterotomies have been performed around the circumference of the anal canal.[5,28] Bilateral partial sphincterotomy has also been recommended.[27] The majority of U.S. surgeons perform a lateral internal anal sphincterotomy, using either an opened or a closed technique. Regional anesthesia, local anesthesia supplemented by sedation, or general anesthesia can be used. The open technique (Fig. 12-3) for the lateral internal sphincterotomy requires insertion of a Hill-Ferguson or other similar retractor into the anal canal. The intersphincteric groove and hypertrophied internal anal sphincter are identified and a radial incision is made over the intersphincteric groove. A curved hemostat is then used to enter the intersphincteric plane. The hypertrophied distal third of the internal anal sphincter is then delivered through the wound with the tip of the curved hemostat and divided using electrocautery. The wound can be left opened to drain any blood or closed with simple sutures of absorbable material.

A closed sphincterotomy (Fig. 12-4) is performed by placing a number 11 blade or a cataract blade into the intersphincteric groove through the skin in the mid lateral position with a Hill-Ferguson or similar retractor in place. The intersphincteric groove is thus readily identified. The edge of the knife blade is then turned toward the anal canal and with steady pressure the internal sphincter fibers are divided as the blade is withdrawn. A finger is placed in the anal canal as a guide to prevent a mucosal incision. The knife blade is removed and the remaining fibers are fractured with outward pressure from the finger within the anal canal. Bleeding is controlled with firm pressure from the finger within the anal canal for several minutes. The wound may be closed with a single suture of absorbable material.

Table 12-1 Outcome of Sphincter Stretch

Series	No. Patients	Success,* %	Recurrence, %	Incontinence†, %
Watts et al[22] (1965)	99	95	16	3.2
O'Connor[24] (1980)	30	100	0	0
Jensen et al[25] (1984)	28	96.5	28.6	Increased
Weaver et al[22] (1987)	59	92	5.1	51

* Healing of fissure.
† Includes soiling and incontinence of flatus.

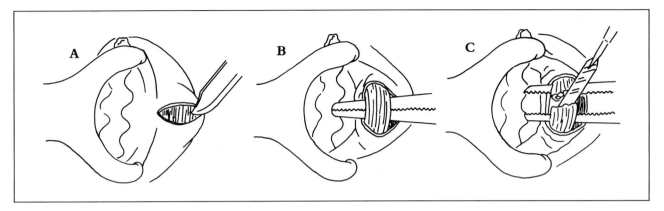

Figure 12-3.   Open lateral internal anal sphincterotomy. (A) Lateral midline over intersphincteric groove incised. (B) Hypertrophied internal sphincter delivered. (C) Internal sphincter divided.

There may be variations in the details of these techniques which can be tailored to individual patients or the surgeon's personal preference. For example, the closed technique can also be performed by placing the knife blade in the submucosal layer and moving the knife laterally. This may be the preferred technique in patients in whom the risk of HIV infection or AIDS is high. Some surgeons may also prefer not to deliver the internal sphincter over a curved hemostat, and to divide the

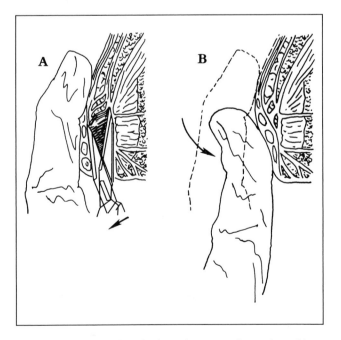

Figure 12-4.   Closed lateral internal anal sphincterotomy. (A) Straight knifeblade inserted into intersphincteric groove in lateral midline and drawn toward mucosa and outward to cut muscle. (B) Finger in anal canal pushed into muscle incision to fracture uncut fibers and stop bleeding.

muscle with scissors or scalpel in situ. Good surgical technique and complete hemostasis are necessary regardless of the technique applied.

The rate of recurrence of fissure in ano has been reported as high as 25 percent. A comparison of closed and open sphincterotomy from Walker, Rothenberger, and Goldberg in 1985 revealed a major complication requiring reoperation in 3 percent of patients.[29] These included bleeding, infection, or incomplete sphincterotomy. Early incontinence occurred in 86 percent of patients. The complication rate was 20 percent for closed and 55 percent for open sphincterotomy. The authors were able to follow a group of 100 successfully treated patients. Persistent minor incontinence was reported by 15 percent of patients. This is consistent with the incontinence rates reported in other series (Table 12-2). More recently, Lewis and associates found no difference between open and closed sphincterotomy.[30]

Lateral internal anal sphincterotomy can be performed in either the outpatient surgery setting or in the office. Local anesthesia may be acceptable. Some authors have suggested that local anesthesia is inadequate for performing lateral sphincterotomy because of a high recurrence rate and recommend that the procedure be performed only under general anesthesia.[31] However, these studies did not use sedation to supplement local anesthesia in the outpatient operating room to obtain an adequate operation.

The sphincterotomy originally described for fissure in ano was performed in the posterior midline. However, the use of the posterior midline sphincterotomy has been shown to be associated with a slightly higher incidence of incontinence to flatus and soilage (Table 12-3). The recurrence rate is no different from that of patients treated with lateral sphincterotomies. The procedure is sometimes performed in conjunction with fissurectomy.[28] However, it has been noted that this

Table 12-2 Outcome of Lateral Sphincterotomy

Series	No. Patients	Success,* %	Recurrence, %	Incontinence†, %
Abcarian[32] (1980)	150	100	1.3	30
Keighley et al[31] (1981)	71	100	25	2
Ravikumar et al[33] (1982)	60	97	0	5
Hsu and MacKeigan[28] (1984)	89	100	5.6	0
Jensen[25] (1984)	30	100	3	0
Walker et al[29] (1985)	100	100	0	15
Gingold[26] (1987)	86	96	3.5	0
Weaver et al[23] (1987)	39	93	5.1	2.5
Lewis et al[30] (1988)	50	94	6	6
Zinkin[34] (1988)	151	95	0	. . .
Khubchandani and Reed[27] (1989)	420	97	0	35

* Healing of fissure.
† Includes soiling and incontinence of flatus.

produces fragile scars.[32] It is generally accepted that if there is a small fistula associated with the anal ulcer, a posterior midline sphincterotomy should be performed to heal the ulcer and the fistula. However, there is a risk for keyhole deformity with soiling and leakage of flatus with this procedure.

Several series of patients have been reported after treatment with bilateral and multiple sphincterotomies. The multiple and bilateral sphincterotomies require superficial, partial sphincterotomy; a moderate amount of judgment is required in determining an adequate depth of the incision. There seem to be no differences among lateral, bilateral, and multiple sphincterotomy in terms of incontinence of flatus and soiling or recurrence of the anal fissure.[27,28]

In summary, 90 percent of conservatively treated fissures should be expected to heal. Surgical treatment of chronic fissures should result in a healing rate of 90 to 95 percent. The differences among the surgical techniques are the incidence of incontinence, soiling, and recurrence. Lateral internal anal sphincterotomy seems to be associated with the lowest incidence of incontinence and recurrence.

Anal Manometry

Anal manometry has been used to evaluate patients before and after lateral internal sphincterotomy. Manometric findings before treatment reveal high resting pressures with ultra-slow waves and a normally functioning external sphincter (Fig. 12-5). There is no evidence of spasm or abnormal resting anal inhibitory reflex.[11,12,15] The sphincter profile after lateral sphincterotomy reveals return of the resting pressure to normal levels and normal functions.[13] The external sphincter continues to function normally. These changes have been shown to be permanent.[37] There may be a change in the distal sphincter profile which reflects the division of the internal anal sphincter in the distal third of the fibers (Fig. 12-6). Anal manometry is useful in the evaluation of patients who report soiling and in patients with recurrent fissures after sphincterotomy. It has not been necessary to use anal manometry to diagnose primary anal fissure. In the rare case of a patient with a high resting pressure and an anal ulcer but inadequate squeeze one might wish to avoid any surgical procedure which would divide the internal

Table 12-3 Outcome of Midline Sphincterotomy

Series	No. Patients	Success,* %	Recurrence, %	Incontinence†, %
Bennett and Goligher[35] (1962)	127	100	7	43
Abcarian[2] (1980)	150	100	1.3	40
Bode et al[36] (1984)	121	100	4	25
Hsu and MacKeigan[28] (1984)	344	100	13	0.3
Khubchandani and Reed[27] (1989)	75	100	0	24

* Healing of fissure.
† Includes soiling and incontinence of flatus.

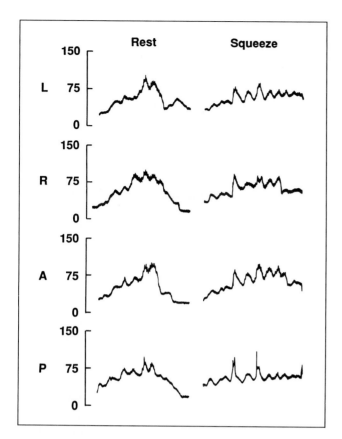

Figure 12-5. Anal manometry tracing in patient with fissure in ano. Rest profile with elevated rest pressure and ultraslow waves. Normal stationary squeeze pressures. L = left quadrant. R = right quadrant. A = anterior quadrant. P = posterior quadrant. Pressure in mm Hg.

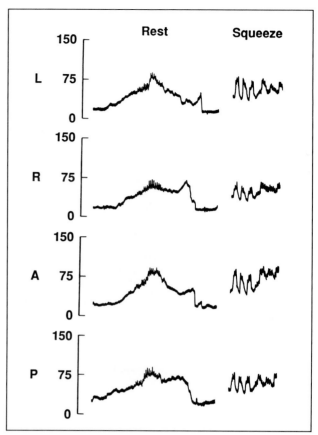

Figure 12-6. Anal manometry after left lateral anal sphincterotomy. Normal rest pressures, reduced rest pressure profile in distal third of left quadrant and normal squeeze. L = left. R = right. A = anterior. P = posterior. Pressure in mm Hg.

sphincter; complete incontinence might otherwise ensue. Anal manometry can be of help in diagnosing this rare situation.

Recurrent Fissure

Recurrent fissure has been treated by contralateral anal sphincterotomy.[7] Occasionally a band of scar tissue or an uncut band of hypertrophied sphincter will be detected in the area of the previous sphincterotomy, which may then be reincised. However, recurrence may be associated with anal stenosis and require other methods for dilating the anal canal.

Crohn's Disease and AIDS

Anal fissures in Crohn's disease and in patients with AIDS are generally caused by the disease, not by skin tearing from hard stools. In patients with Crohn's disease, the fissures are usually atypically placed around the anal canal and do not have the characteristic midline

position (Fig. 12-7). The ulcers are usually associated with large edematous skin tags with granulation tissue at the base. Frequently these ulcers or fissures are associated with adjacent fistulas. It is important to recognize the ulcers as being secondary to Crohn's disease, because a sphincterotomy performed on the patient with Crohn's disease of the anal canal can result in nonhealing of the wound and worsening of the condition. These fissures are best treated conservatively with local medical therapy including corticosteroid suppositories, 5 aminosalicylic acid suppositories, and Flagyl® orally or with local gel application. Occasionally anal Crohn's disease will also respond to 6-mercaptopurine.

Patients with AIDS anal disease can have anal fissures due to local invasion of cytomegalovirus, Kaposi's sarcoma, syphilis, or opportunistic pathogens present in the stool. The fissures occur in atypical positions but have many features of the usual anal fissure (Fig. 12-8). These fissures are usually difficult to heal, and symptomatic control is therefore the goal. Operative management is very rarely successful and may produce worsening anal sepsis. Special attention is needed to

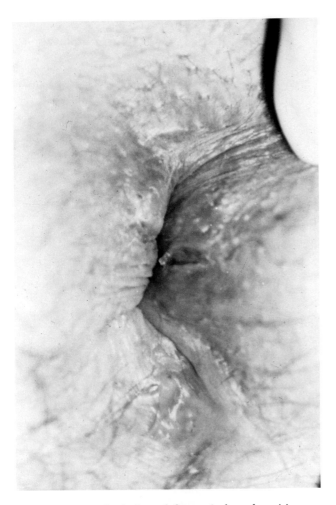

Figure 12-7.   Crohn's anal fissure in lateral position.

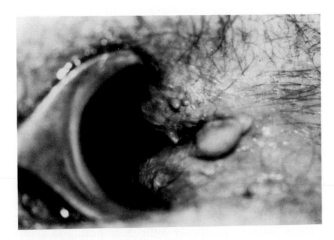

Figure 12-8.   Deep lateral anal fissure in patient with AIDS.

identify local crypt abscess disease since uncontrolled anaerobic gangrene is rapidly fatal. Only rarely will patients require lateral anal sphincterotomy. Close observation is needed to prevent perineal sepsis in these cases. The management of anal fissures in AIDS patients is discussed further in Chapter 22.

Anal Stenosis

Anal stenosis is an uncommon finding in the patient population seen by the colorectal surgeon. It has become more uncommon as the use of circumferential hemorrhoidectomy has been abandoned. Usually, anal stenosis is secondary to excisional hemorrhoidectomy with excision of the anoderm.[38] The resultant scar and stenosis also produce an ectropion, causing the Whitehead deformity. Other causes of anal stenosis include recurring anal fissure, chronic diarrhea, recurrent abscess and fistula requiring surgical treatment, anal Crohn's disease, radiation, and excision of perianal skin lesions as in Paget's or Bowen's disease. The majority of patients with stenosis have had anal surgery prior to presentation. Approximately 87 percent will have had a hemorrhoidectomy.[39] Anal stenosis occurs with approximately 1.2 percent of hemorrhoidectomies. Only 3 percent of patients with stenosis have had procedures for anal Crohn's disease. The remainder are divided among the other causes.

The treatment of anal stenosis depends on its position in the anal canal and the severity of the stenosis. High anal strictures that are covered entirely by mucosa are more difficult to treat than the low anal strictures at the level of the anoderm. Mild anal stenosis responds to more conservative therapy,[38] whereas severe anal stenosis may require more extensive surgical procedures.

Treatment

Medical Therapy

Medical therapy for anal stenosis combines bulking of the stool with dilation in the office using the finger or calibrated rubber dilators and topical anesthetic. The patient can perform this routinely at home. This is an ideal treatment for Crohn's disease or high-risk patients with otherwise weakened external sphincters.[40] The combination of repeated dilation and steroid suppositories may prevent early recurrence of the stenosis, but no well-controlled trials have been done to prove this. The presence of anal stenosis has been shown to cause megarectum in elderly patients.[41] These patients are usually nursing home residents who require daily enemas for constipation and daily routine care.

Surgical Therapy

The surgical treatment of anal stenosis includes lateral internal sphincterotomy, numerous advancement flaps, and occasionally a colostomy for diversion. Anal strictures may be associated with an ectropion, which is the protusion of a flap of mucosa out onto the anoderm as the scarring tissue retracts toward the perineum. The lateral internal sphincterotomy has been suggested as a means of treating anal stenosis that is mild and low in the anal canal. The results have been adequate, but this does not treat the ectropion. The sphincterotomy occasionally needs to be repeated.

There are several varieties of flaps to manage anal stenosis. Some also address the problem of the ectropion. The flaps are either mucosal or skin. Some are rotational or advancement flaps. Others are island flaps.

Mucosal Advancement Flap.   The mucosal advancement flap (Martin anoplasty) advances a pedicle of mucosa into the anal canal by way of an incision made through the stenotic area.[38] This results in a posterior mucosal ectropion that prevents repeat stricturing. Khubchandani revised the procedure to be used in a lateral sphincterotomy position.[42] This technique is simple and safe but causes mucous discharge and creates an ectropion. It is rarely used in our institution.

V-Y Advancement Flap.   Rosen described the use of the V-Y advancement flap to treat anal stenosis and ectropion.[43] The V-Y advancement flap advances a V-shaped portion of skin into the anal canal. The V is drawn with the wide base at the dentate line and incised through the skin (Fig. 12-9). The subcutaneous attachments in the lateral edges of the V are released to allow mobilization of the skin into the anal canal. The blood supply to the flap relies on perforating vessels in the subcutaneous fat. The skin is then closed behind the V at the external portion of the perineum to push the V into the anal canal and widen the stenotic area. This method may be used for the treatment of ectropion. Milsom and Mazier suggested that severe low stenosis should be treated with a V-Y advancement flap.[39] They showed a 96 percent success in treatment of these strictures using this method. This is a very simple method and follows basic principles of plastic surgery. However, the flap does not advance a wide portion of skin into the scar. The benefit is derived from soft pliable tissue inserted into the nonpliable scar. If more tissue is needed to allow the canal to dilate, this technique may be repeated on the opposite side of the anal canal.

Y-V Advancement Flap.   The Y-V advancement flap is a slightly different principle. Gingold recently re-

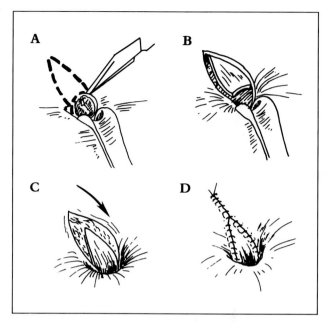

Figure 12-9.   V-Y advancement flap. (A) Lateral inverted V inscribed over ectropion. (B) Flap mobilized to preserve vasculature and stenosis divided or ectropion excised. (C) Flap advanced into anal canal. (D) Flap sutured in place with Y closure.

ported on 14 patients who were improved after Y-V advancement; these patients had strictures secondary to hemorrhoidectomy, chronic fissure, Paget's disease, and other causes.[44] The vertical limb of the Y is inscribed on the anal canal at the level of the stenosis, and the V of the Y drawn on the lateral perianal skin (Fig. 12-10). The skin is incised and the V-shaped flap of skin is freed laterally. Once again the blood supply of the flap is based on vessels in the underlying subcutaneous tissue. The V is then introduced into the stenoic anal canal to close the wound as a V-shaped incision. This can be used unilaterally or bilaterally with good results. The V is still attached to the buttock skin. If tension is too great the flap will not remain within the anal canal and stenosis can recur.

Island Flaps: Diamond and U.   Island flaps for the treatment of anal stenosis were first described by Caplin and Kodner to construct a diamond- or a U-shaped advancement flap.[45] The stenotic scar is first incised laterally at the dentate line (Fig. 12-11). A diamond-shaped island of skin from the lateral perineum is inscribed to match the defect in the anal canal made by this incision. The flap is then mobilized from its lateral subcutaneous attachments and advanced into the incision made in the stenotic anal canal. This flap of skin will open the stenosis widely when the lateral corners of

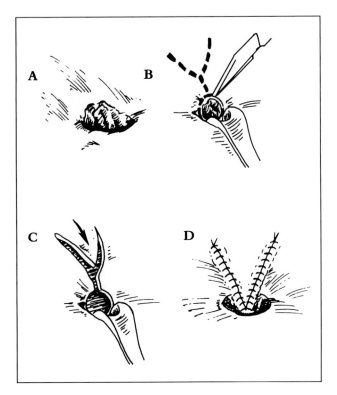

Figure 12-10.   Y-V advancement flap. (A) Ectropion and stenosis. (B) Y flap inscribed outside ectropion. (C) Ectropion excised, Y flap incised. (D) Flap sutured with V closure.

the diamond are sutured at the level of the stenosis. This flap allows advancement of maximal skin to the point of stenosis with minimal tension. A U-shaped flap as described by Pearl and associates is especially useful for patients with Whitehead deformity and ectropion.[46] The U is a broader-based version of the V-Y advancement flap but allows the ectropion to be excised across a

wide base and the inverted U advanced into the anal canal to fill the defect.

S-Plasty.   The S-plasty is best used for the treatment of Bowen's disease or Paget's disease where a large amount of skin has to be excised and new skin rotated into the area.[38] The S-plasty does not open a stricture as well as the advancement flaps. It is used to provide a wide area of skin to cover a perineum that is entirely excised for disease. The base of the S is drawn on to the lateral buttock and the necessary tissue excised (Fig. 12-12). The skin and subcutaneous tissue in the S are rotated down to the mucosal incision and sutured in place. The opposite curve of the S is treated similarly on the other side of the anal canal. This provides for adequate blood supply and avoids cross tension.

Each of these advancement flap procedures requires mechanical bowel preparation. Regional or local anesthesia is possible. Pearl and associates reported only 2 failures in 20 patients treated with island flap anoplasty for stricture.[46]

Each flap mentioned can be used easily and safely with good results, and each flap has an advantage in a particular setting. The surgeon should be experienced in all of them to best treat the patient. The advancement flap techniques require more mobilization of tissue, more suture lines, and a complete bowel preparation. Therefore, the anoplasty techniques should be reserved for the most severe problems after conservative measures have failed.

The complications of anoplasty include infection, failure of the anoplasty to correct the stenosis, and slough of the island flap. These can usually be avoided with adequate preparation and adherence to good technique.

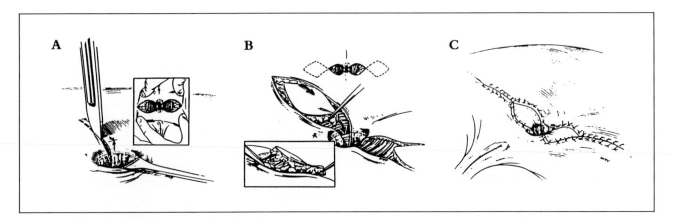

Figure 12-11.   Diamond island flap. (A) Stenosis incised in lateral midline and diamonds inscribed laterally to match defects. (B) Diamond flaps incised and advanced into anal canal. (C) Flaps secured with wide point at stenosis line.

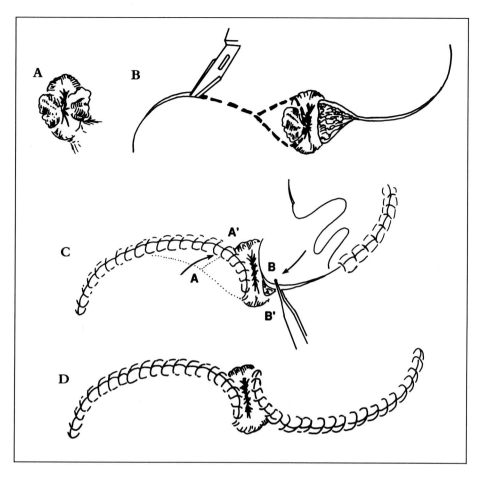

Figure 12-12. S-plasty: (A) Perianal skin lesions requiring removal of large skin area. (B) Area of perianal skin excised, lateral curves incised onto buttocks. (C) Curves of skin advanced into perianal defect and secured laterally. (D) S-shaped closure of rotated flaps.

Patients with strictures secondary to Crohn's disease, lymphogranuloma venereum, or syphilis usually respond best to repeated dilation.[39,40] Only rarely has anal stenosis secondary to inflammatory bowel disease been treated with anoplasty. The patients may require anoderm release incisions with repeated dilation. It is difficult to use anoplasty in these patients since the underlying disease process is continuous and may affect the healing.

References

1. Recamier JCA (1829). Quoted by OH Goodsall and WE Miles, *Diseases of the Anus and Rectum*, Part I. Longmans, London; 1900.

2. Dupuytren G. *Lecon Orales de Clinical Chirurgical*, 3. Paris: Germen-Bailliere; 1833:284.

3. Demarquay JW. Archives Generale Med (Paris). 1846;10:377.

4. Martin EG: Transcripts of the American Proctological Society. 1923:57.

5. Miles WE, Maingot R, eds. *Post Graduate Surgery*. London:Medical Publications Ltd; 1936.

6. Eisenhammer S. Surgical correction of chronic internal anal sphincter contracture. *South Afr Med J*. 1951;25:486.

7. Nicholls J. Fissure in ano and anorectal sepsis. *Verh Dtsch Ges Inn Med*. 1988;94:225–229.

8. Notaras MJ. Anal fissure and stenosis. *Surg Clin North Am*. 1988;68:1427–1440.

9. Whalen TV, Lieutenant MC, Kovalcik PJ, et al. Tuberculosis anal ulcer. *Dis Colon Rectum*. 1980;23:54–55.

10. Smith LE. Anal fissure. *Neth J Med*. 1990;37: S33–S36.

11. Gibbons CP, Read NW. Anal hypertonia in fissures: cause or effect? *Br J Surg*. 1986;73:443–445.

12. Lin JK. Anal manometric studies in hemorrhoids and anal fissures. *Dis Colon Rectum*. 1989;32: 839–842.

13. Cerdan FJ, Ruiz de Leon A, Azpiroz F, et al. Anal sphincteric pressure in fissure-in-ano before and after lateral internal sphincterotomy. *Dis Colon Rectum*. 1982;198:198–201.

14. Boulos PB, Araujo JG. Adequate internal sphincterotomy for chronic anal fissure: subcutaneous or open technique? *Br J Surg*. 1984; 71:360–362.

15. Kuypers HC. Is there really sphincter spasm in anal fissure? *Dis Colon Rectum*. 1983;26:493–494.

16. Brown AC, Sumfest JM, Rozwadowski JV. Histopathology of the internal anal sphincter in chronic anal fissure. *Dis Colon Rectum*. 1989;32:680–683.

17. Haas PA, Fox TA Jr. Age-related changes and scar formations of perianal connective tissue. *Dis Colon Rectum*. 1980;23:160–169.

18. Jensen SL. Maintenance therapy with unprocessed bran in the prevention of acute anal fissure recurrence. *J R Soc Med*. 1987;80:296–298.

19. Jensen SL. Treatment of first episodes of acute anal fissure: prospective randomized study of lignocaine ointment versus hydrocortisone ointment or warm sitz baths plus bran. *Br Med J*. 1986;292:1167–1169.

20. Gough MJ, Lewis A. The conservative treatment of fissure-in-ano. *Br J Surg*. 1983;70:175–176.

21. McDonald P, Driscoll AM, Nicholls RJ. The anal dilator in the conservative management of acute anal fissures. *Br J Surg*. 1983;70:25–26.

22. Watts JM, Bennett RC, Goligher JC. Stretching of anal sphincters in treatment of fissure-in-ano. *Br Med J*. 1964;342–343.

23. Weaver RM, Ambrose NS, Alexander-Williams J, et al. Manual dilatation of the anus vs. lateral subcutaneous sphincterotomy in the treatment of chronic fissure-in-ano. *Dis Colon Rectum*. 1987; 30:420–423.

24. O'Connor JJ. Lord procedure for treatment of postpartum hemorrhoids and fissures. *Obstet Gynecol*. 1980;55:747–748.

25. Jensen SL, Lund F, Nielsen OV, Tange G. Lateral subcutaneous sphincterotomy versus anal dilatation in the treatment of fissure in ano in outpatients: a prospective randomized study. *Br Med J*. 1984; 289:528–530.

26. Gingold BS. Simple in-office sphincterotomy with partial fissurectomy for chronic anal fissure. *Surg Gynecol Obstet*. 1987;165:46–48.

27. Khubchandani IT, Reed JF. Sequelae of internal sphincterotomy for chronic fissue in ano. *Br J Surg*. 1989;76:431–434.

28. Hsu TC, MacKeigan JM. Surgical treatment of anal fissure: a retrospective study of 1753 cases. *Dis Colon Rectum*. 1984;27:475–478.

29. Walker WA, Rothenberger DA, Goldberg SM. Morbidity of internal sphincterotomy for anal fis-sure and stenosis. *Dis Colon Rectum*. 1985;28: 832–835.

30. Lewis TH, Corman ML, Prager ED, et al. Long-term results of open and closed sphincterotomy for anal fissure. *Dis Colon Rectum*. 1988;31:368–371.

31. Keighley MR, Greca F, Nevah E, et al. Treatment of anal fissure by lateral subcutaneous sphincterotomy should be under general anesthesia. *Br J Surg*. 1981;68:400–401.

32. Abcarian HA. Surgical correction of chronic anal fissure: results of lateral internal sphincterotomy vs. fissurectomy-midline sphincterotomy. *Dis Colon Rectum*. 1980;23:31–36.

33. Ravikumar TS, Sridhar S, Rao RN. Subcutaneous lateral internal sphincterotomy for chronic fissure-in-ano. *Dis Colon Rectum*. 1982;25:798–801.

34. Zinkin LD. Left lateral internal sphincterotomy for anal fissure—as an office procedure. *N J Med*. 1988;85:43–45.

35. Bennett RC, Goligher JC. Results of internal sphincterotomy for anal fissure. *Br Med J*. 1962;1500–1503.

36. Bode WE, Culp CE, Spencer RJ, et al. Fissurectomy with superficial midline sphincterotomy: a viable alternative for the surgical correction of chronic fissure/ulcer-in-ano. *Dis Colon Rectum*. 1984;27:93–95.

37. Chowcat NL, Araujo JG, Boulos PB. Internal sphincterotomy for chronic anal fissure: long term effects on anal pressure. *Br J Surg*. 1986;73:915–916.

38. Rosen L. Anoplasty. *Surg Clin North Am*. 1988;68: 1441–1446.

39. Milsom JW, Mazier WP. Classification and management of postsurgical anal stenosis. *Surg Gynecol Obstet*. 1986;163:60–64.

40. Linares L, Moreira LF, Andrews H, Allan RN, et al. Natural history and treatment of anorectal strictures complicating Crohn's disease. *Br J Surg*. 1988;75:653–655.

41. Sandiford JA, Sabnis VM. Anal stenosis and megarectum in the elderly. *Am Surg*. 1980;46:307–309.

42. Khubchandani IT. Mucosal advancement anoplasty. *Dis Colon Rectum*. 1985;28:194–196.

43. Rosen L. V-Y advancement for anal ectropion. *Dis Colon Rectum*. 1986;29:596–598.

44. Gingold BS. Y-V anoplasty for treatment of anal stricture. *Surg Gynecol Obstet*. 1986;162:241–242.

45. Caplin DA, Kodner IJ. Repair of anal stricture and mucosal ectropion by simple flap procedure. *Dis Colon Rectum*. 1986;28:92–94.

46. Pearl RK, Hooks VH, Abcarian H, et al. Island flap anoplasty for the treatment of anal stricture and mucosal ectropion. *Dis Colon Rectum*. 1190;33: 581–583.

CHAPTER 13

HIDRADENITIS SUPPURATIVA
AND PILONIDAL DISEASE

Richard E. Karulf

Hidradenitis suppurativa and pilonidal disease are common treatment challenges for the surgeon. The origins of the colorectal referral pattern for these lesions stem from the proximity of these afflictions to the anus rather than the etiology of the diseases. High recurrence rates after initial therapy for both diseases highlight the difficulty in treating what appear to be simple cutaneous infections. A thorough understanding of these diseases and the several treatment options is required for successful therapy.

Pilonidal Disease

History

Most authors attribute the first report of this disease to Anderson in 1847[1] and the first series of patients to Warren.[2] The term *pilonidal* was first associated with this condition by Hodges in 1880.[3] It was derived from the Latin *pilus* meaning hair and *nidus* for nest. The intent of this term was to note the association of trapped hair in this unusual form of natal cleft skin infection.

Etiology

The etiology of pilonidal disease has been the source of debate for many years. The earliest authors who described pilonidal disease considered the lesions to be acquired. However, as human embryology received attention during the second half of the 19th century, the accepted treatment of pilonidal disease became based upon an assumption of an embryonic origin for suppuration.[4] Three main theories were put forth: (1) that it originated from remnants of the medullary canal, (2)

that it evolved from dermal inclusions due to faulty coalescence of the median raphe, and (3) that it represented a vestigial sex gland, homologous with the preen gland of birds.[5]

If the congenital theory is true, then removal of all epithelial tracts to the sacral fascia should be curative. However, a high recurrence rate even with removal of all tissues overlying the sacrum and coverage with rotation flaps derived away from the midline testifies for other factors as the cause for pilonidal disease.[6] These theories also could not account for the lack of intermediate stages between the congenital sinuses or tracts noted in childhood and the pilonidal disease seen in adults. Congenital tracts are usually located more superiorly, over the lumbar area rather than the sacrum, do not contain hair, frequently communicate with the spinal canal, and contain cuboidal epithelium rather than granulation tissue.[7,8]

The congenital theories for the origins of pilonidal disease remained unchallenged until 1946. At that time Patey and Scarff reopened the debate of congenital versus acquired disease by noting that the interdigital pilonidal sinuses of barbers were pathologically identical to postanal pilonidal sinuses.[9,10] Since then additional reports of hair causing pilonidal disease in the interdigital clefts[11] and periareolar skin[12] of barbers have appeared. In addition, pilonidal disease has been associated with loose hairs forming abscesses in the mammary ducts,[13] penis,[14] and umbilicus.[15] There are even reports of an identical inflammatory process associated with the fur of dogs,[16] the wool from sheep,[17] and feathers from bedding material.[18] These types of observations lend credibility to the theory that pilonidal disease is acquired.

Currently, the debate on the etiology of pilonidal disease centers on two main theories. One theory is that pilonidal disease is caused by a foreign body reaction to hairs embedded in the skin, commonly in the midline sacrococcygeal area. Patey and Scarff noted that although pilonidal tracts contain hair, they do not always contain hair follicles.[19] This would suggest that the hair and not the follicle is the source of the disease. The inflammation around the hair follows the path of least resistance and often travels in a cephalad and lateral direction, thus forming secondary tracts and openings.

An alternative theory, proposed by Bascom, is that the origin of pilonidal disease is in the hair follicles of the natal cleft.[20] Keratin occludes the follicle, which eventually becomes inflamed and ruptures into the surrounding fat, forming a pilonidal abscess. If the abscess drains, inflammation subsides and the mouth of the follicle reopens. The remnant of the follicle and abscess cavity, now a tube open at two ends, forms a draining pilonidal sinus. Vagrant hairs from the region gather in the glutel cleft and into the sinus. If the sinus cavity fails to heal promptly, epithelium migrates into the sinus from the edges of the follicle and forms an epithelium-lined tube.

Incidence

All forms of pilonidal disease are reported to be more common in men than in women with a relative frequency of 4 to 1.[21] It is known that the greatest incidence of pilonidal disease occurs between puberty and age 40.[22] Pilonidal disease was identified in 365 out of 31,497 men and 24 out of 21,367 women in a study of Minnesota college students.[23] The same study noted an association between pilonidal disease and obesity. Between 1950 and 1955, an average of 411 out of every 100,000 Navy personnel were treated at least once for pilonidal disease.[24] One author noted the association of pilonidal disease with hair on the glabella in Navy personnel.[25] During World War II, Buie referred to pilonidal disease as Jeep disease owing to its association with mechanized warfare.[26]

There are three common presentations for pilonidal disease. Nearly all patients have an episode of acute abscess formation. When this abscess resolves, either spontaneously or with medical assistance, many patients develop a pilonidal sinus. Although most sinus tracts resolve, a small minority of patients will go on to have chronic disease or recurrent disease after treatment. Treatment methods vary for each stage in pilonidal disease.

Abscess

Jensen and Harling used incision and drainage of first-episode acute pilonidal abscesses.[27] This simple treatment relieved symptoms in all patients and completely eradicated the lesions in 58 percent of patients within 10 weeks of the procedure. Between 20 and 40 percent of patients develop recurrent disease after this form of treatment. In attempts to lower the rate of recurrence, some authors have recommended adding excision of infected granulation tissue,[28] freezing,[29] and other techniques. None of these adjunctive measures has met with consistent success. Bascom reported a recurrence rate of only 15 percent after excision of only the epithelial pits.[30] This procedure is carried out with small (7-mm) incisions 5 days after initial incision and drainage.

Incision and drainage of acute abscesses is readily performed in an office setting using local anesthesia. The hair surrounding the natal cleft should be shaved to facilitate hygiene and healing. A 30-ml solution of 1% lidocaine with 1:100,000 epinephrine is injected with a 30 gauge needle as a field block around the area of inflammation. In cases of simple abscess with minimal cellulitis definitive treatment consists of incision, drainage, and curettage of the wall of the cavity. Cultures of the abscess contents may be taken but antibiotics are rarely required.

The wound is loosely packed open with plain gauze to prevent premature closure of the skin over the cavity and to absorb secretions. The wound is kept clean by irrigating the area twice daily with warm tap water using either a shower attachment, a sitz bath, or a dental Water-Pik®. It is important to dry the area painstakingly by blotting the skin dry or using a hair dryer to avoid maceration. The skin in the gluteal cleft is shaved during the weekly office visits. Also during these office visits, granulation tissue is cauterized and removed. Success is largely contingent upon diligent wound care by both the patient and the physician.

Sinus

Up to 40 percent of acute pilonidal abscesses treated by incision and drainage form a chronic sinus that requires additional treatment.[31] Although anaerobic organisms can usually be found in these chronic sinuses, antibiotic therapy is rarely required.[32] The majority of pilonidal sinuses resolve, regardless of treatment option, by age 40.[33] It is theorized that changes in body habitus (altered and increased fat deposition alters the gluteal cleft) and softening of body hair account for this change with age.

There is debate about the best method of treatment for the nonhealing pilonidal sinus. Many treatments have been reported and then abandoned, such as the use of thorium X.[34] One review of all articles published in the last 30 years on the treatment of pilonidal disease divided the procedures and analyzed them by broad category (Table 13-1).[35] Closed techniques (injection with phenol or coring out follicles and brushing the tracts) required shaving of the area but could be per-

Table 13-1   Comparison of Techniques by Mean Time to Healing and Mean Recurrence Rate Based on Minimum Follow-up in Several Review Articles.

Procedure	Mean Time to Healing, days	Recurrence, < 1-yr Follow-up, %	Recurrence > 1-yr Follow-up, %
Debride epithelial pit	42		
Debridement of pit and phenol injection	40	10	18
Lay open sinus	43	4	13
Lay open sinus and cauterize base	36		
Excision to fascia	73	14	13
Excision to fascia and marsupialization	27	6	4

Modified from: Allen-Mersh TG. *Br J Surg.* 1990;77:123–132.

formed on an outpatient basis. Mean healing time was about 40 days and recurrence rates were slightly higher than with other forms of treatment. Laying open the tracts (Fig. 13-1) with healing by granulation resulted in average healing time of 43 days and required frequent outpatient dressing changes. The incidence of recurrent sinus formation was generally less than 20 percent with this technique. Addition of cauterization of the cavity

decreased the average healing time to 36 days and reduced the reported recurrence rates. Wide and deep excision of the sinus alone (Fig. 13-2) resulted in an average healing time of 73 days. Recurrence rates were similar to those noted after simple laying open of the sinus. When partial closure of the wound (marsupialization) was added to wide and deep excision of the sinus (Fig. 13-3), healing time decreased to an average of 27

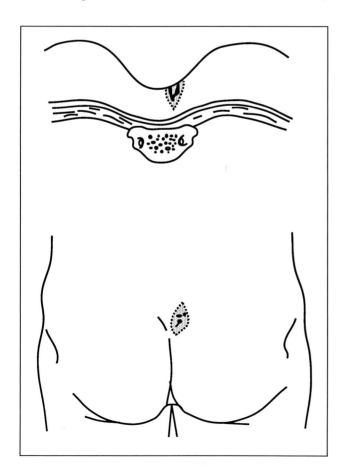

Figure 13-1.   Local excision of sinus.

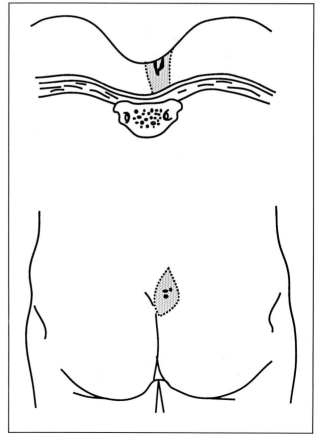

Figure 13-2.   Wide and deep excision of sinus to fascia.

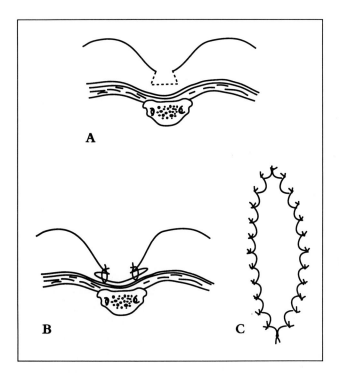

Figure 13-3. Laying-open technique. (A) Overlying tissue is excised. (B) Wound edges are sutured to base of wound. (C) Appearance of wound at completion of procedure.

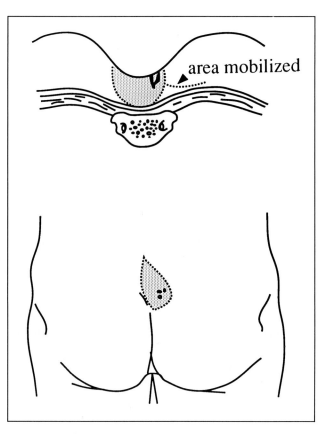

Figure 13-4. Asymmetric incision for recurrent pilonidal cyst. A flap of skin and subcutaneous fat is mobilized so that the incision is closed away from the midline.

days. Excision and primary closure resulted in wound healing within 2 weeks in successful cases. However, primary healing failed to occur in up to 30 percent of patients, and the average recurrence rate for these experienced surgeons was 15 percent. The same length of time for wound healing was reported for excision and primary closure whether oblique or asymmetric incisions were used (Fig. 13-4). The recurrence rate was less than 10 percent after primary closure.

Bascom reported less than 10 percent recurrence with excision of enlarged follicles.[36] This procedure involved an incision lateral to the midline to scrub the chronic cavity free of hair and granulation tissue (Fig. 13-5). Removal of the small midline pits was carried out with small (7-mm) incisions (Fig. 13-6). When epithelial tubes were present, they were removed through the lateral incision. The lateral wound was then left open but the midline incisions were closed with a removable 4-0 polypropylene subcuticular suture (Fig. 13-7).

Complex or Recurrent Disease

Even with proper treatment, a small subgroup of patients are left with persistent, nonhealing wounds. Repeated treatment of complex or recurrent disease with conventional measures rarely achieves satisfactory healing. A number of more aggressive treatments have

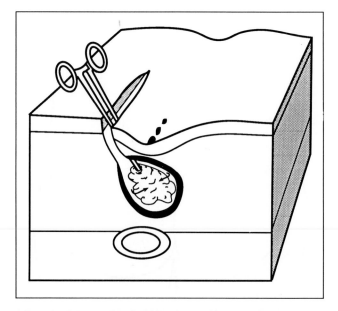

Figure 13-5. Lateral incision and debridement of cavity as described by Bascom.[6]

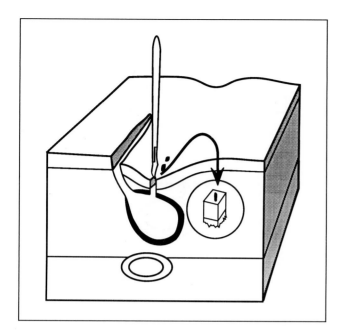

Figure 13-6.   Removal of midline pit a with small incision.

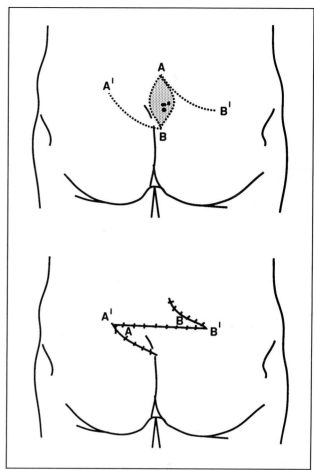

Figure 13-8.   Z-plasty technique for recurrent pilonidal disease.

been described to treat complex or recurrent disease: wide excision and split-thickness skin grafting,[37] cleft closure,[38] excision and Z-plasty[39-41] (Fig. 13-8), modified Z-plasty,[42] gluteus maximus myocutaneous flap[43] (Fig. 13-9), rhomboid fasciocutaneous flap,[44] multiple flaps,[45] and even reverse bandaging.[46] These techniques as a group reportedly achieved primary healing in less than 14 days in 90 percent of cases.[47] There are, however, disadvantages to these aggressive approaches

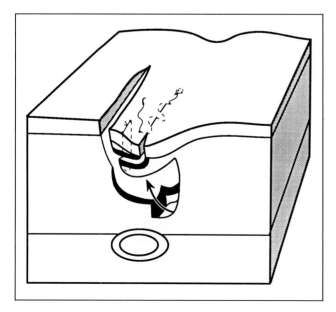

Figure 13-7.   Closure of midline wounds without closure of lateral incision.

(Table 13-2). Nearly all of these techniques require hospitalization and general anesthesia. In addition, up to 50 percent of those procedures requiring skin flaps for wound coverage or closure are associated with a loss of skin sensation or flap tip necrosis.[48]

The problem of the nonhealing midline wound was addressed by Bascom.[49] The technique of "cleft closure" was performed by removing skin from the more damaged side and covering the defect with a flap from the less damaged side (Fig. 13-10). While the wound was open, the base was scrubbed free of debris and granulation tissue. A drain was placed through a separate stab wound and the incision was closed with a removable subcuticular polypropylene suture.

An extremely rare complication of nonhealing pilonidal disease is squamous cell carcinoma arising from the sinus tract.[45]

Summary

Pilonidal disease has three basic presentations: acute abscess, simple sinus, and complex or recurrent disease.

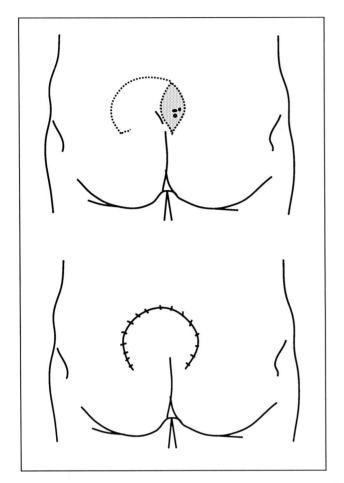

Figure 13-9. Gluteus maximus myocutaneous flap for recurrent disease.

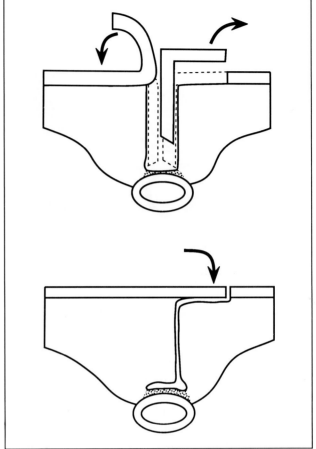

Figure 13-10. U-flap technique as described by Bascom for nonhealing midline wound.[38]

Simple incision and drainage of an acute abscess will bring relief of symptoms for nearly all patients. Additional steps at this point may help reduce recurrence rates. Treatment of a simple pilonidal sinus is eventually effective regardless of surgical techniques. Of the many options, wide excision of the sinus tract to the fascia, without flap coverage or marsupialization, should be avoided. This procedure is associated with prolonged

healing and comparable recurrence rates as compared with less traumatic procedures. Satisfactory treatment of complex or recurrent disease is possible with good results, but often requires an aggressive approach. The use of asymmetric incisions or skin flaps results in reliable primary healing and a low recurrence rate but has a high rate of flap complications.

Table 13-2 Comparison of Techniques Using Primary Wound Closure by Failed Primary Healing and Mean Recurrence Rate Based on Minimum Follow-up in Several Review Articles.

Procedure	Failed Primary Healing, %	Recurrence: < 1-yr Follow-up, %	Recurrence: > 1-yr Follow-up, %
Midline incision	8	8	15
Asymmetric/oblique incision	8	1	3
Skin flap techniques	3	2	8

Modified from: Allen-Mersh TG. *Br J Surg.* 1990;77:123–132.

Hidradenitis Suppurativa

Hidradenitis suppurativa has many similarities to pilonidal disease in terms of age of onset, site of presentation, and high recurrence rate. Most authors note that hidradenitis suppurativa was first described by Velpeau in 1839 and was associated with sweat glands by Verneuil in 1854.[50] The term *hidradenitis suppurativa* is derived from the Greek *hydros* for sweat and *aden* for gland. It is best described as a chronic infection of the apocrine glands and subcutaneous tissue and is primarily confined to areas that contain apocrine glands. The axilla and groin are the most commonly affected areas followed by the perineum in roughly 30 percent of cases. It is also reported to be found in the areola of the nipple and the perianal and periumbilical regions.

The most common age of presentation is after puberty, generally between ages 16 and 40. Hidradenitis suppurativa tends to have a 2 to 1 male predominance although there are contradictory data in the literature.[51] The exact etiology of hidradenitis suppurativa is not certain. Many authors believe that plugging of the apocrine ducts leads the ducts to rupture into surrounding dermis with secondary bacterial infection and then scarring. Predominant organisms cultured from the wounds are staphylococci and streptococci but may include *E. coli, Klebsiella,* and *Proteus* in the perineal region.[52] Hidradenitis has been associated with obesity, poor hygiene, and hyperhidrosis. There are some who believe that depilatories, deodorants, acne, and diabetes are also associated with the disease.

The presentation of hidradenitis suppurativa is similar to other cutaneous infections. Patients often present with an abscess with or without cellulitis. The abscess may subside after a few days spontaneously or with treatment, only to flare up again later. The end result of chronic disease are multiple painful nodules and surrounding fibrosis with cellulitis (Figs. 13-11 and 13-12). Treatment of hidradenitis suppurativa depends on the stage of presentation of the disease.

Early or Acute Disease

Prior to the antibiotic era, low dose radiation therapy was used to treat hidradenitis suppurativa. Conservative treatment of mild cases currently includes improved hygiene, warm compresses, and broad spectrum antibiotic therapy. Treatment with medications designed to treat acne, such as 13 cis-retinoic acid, has not achieved great success. Pain is often the presenting complaint and simple incision and drainage will provide relief in most patients. At this point the most important element is making the correct diagnosis and distinguishing hidradenitis suppurativa from a simple abscess. If the diagnosis

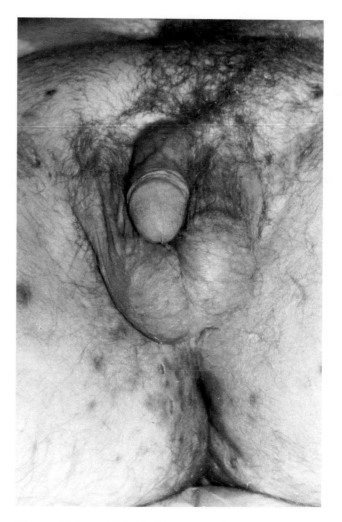

Figure 13-11.   Hidradenitis suppurativa.

is in question, a biopsy specimen of the abscess wall can be taken during the incision and drainage procedure. Histologic evidence of the apocrine gland involvement is diagnostic of hidradenitis. After treatment of the acute infection, patients with limited hidradenitis suppurativa may be cured with excision and primary closure. Early excision of diseased tissue will limit the involvement of surrounding skin by inflammation and scarring.

Late or Chronic Disease

Hidradenitis suppurativa may progress to chronic or recurrent disease despite appropriate treatment. It will usually not respond to conservative medical management at this point. After treatment of any acute infection, the next appropriate treatment includes radical excision of all affected tissue. Treatment of the wound may involve packing the wound and secondary healing, marsupialization of the wound, or coverage with split-thickness skin grafts or skin flaps. Other authors report

190   Fundamentals of Anorectal Surgery

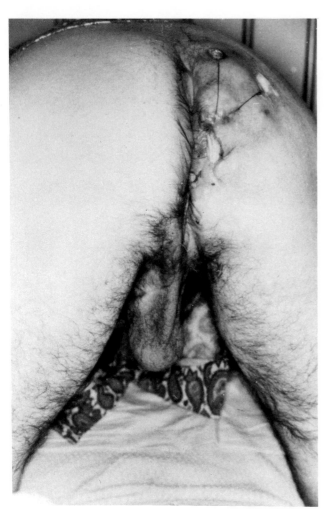

Figure 13-12.   Hidradenitis suppurativa.

success with a "deroofing procedure" which may be used in place of wide local excision.[53] Diverting colostomies are rarely required.[54] Treatment must be individually adjusted to the requirements of the patient.

Complications of longstanding hidradenitis suppurativa include formation of fistulas between the involved skin and the anus or rectum and rare cases of squamous cell carcinoma.

Summary

Hidradenitis suppurativa is a chronic acneiform infection of the apocrine glands and commonly presents in the axilla, groin, and perineum. Recurrence is high with simple incision and drainage. Patients in whom conservative therapy fails will require radical excision of all affected tissues. Conventional treatment of the remaining wound may involve packing the wound and secondary healing or coverage with split-thickness skin grafts.

References

1. Anderson AW. Hair extracted from an ulcer. *Boston Med Surg J.* 1847;36:74.
2. Warren JM. Abscess, containing hair, on the nates. *Am J Med Sci.* 1854;28:112.
3. Hodges RM. Pilo-nidal sinus. *Boston Med Surg J.* 1880;103:485–486.
4. Klass AA. The so-called pilo-nidal sinus. *Can Med Assoc J.* 1956;75:737–742.
5. Franckowiak JJ, Jackman RJ. The etiology of pilonidal sinus. *Dis Colon Rectum.* 1962;5:28–36.
6. Bascom J. Pilonidal disease: long-term results of follicle removal. *Dis Colon Rectum.* 1983;26:800–807.
7. Goligher JC. Pilonidal sinus. In: Goligher JC. *Surgery of the Anus, Rectum and Colon.* 4th ed. London: Bailliere Tindall; 1980:200–214.
8. Powell KR, Cherry JD, Hougen TJ, et al. A pro-spective search for congenital dermal abnormalities of the cerebrospinal axis. *J Paediatr.* 1975;87:744–750.
9. Patey DH, Scarff RW. Pathology of postanal pilonidal sinus: its bearing on treatment. *Lancet.* 1946;2:484–6.
10. Patey DH, Scarff RW. Pilonidal sinus in a barber's hand: with observations on postanal pilonidal sinus. *Lancet.* 1948;2:13.
11. Currie AR, Gibson T, Goodall AL. Interdigital sinuses of barbers' hands. *Br J Surg.* 1953;41:278–286.
12. Gannon MX, Crowson MC, Fielding JWL. Peri-areolar pilonidal abscess in a hairdresser. *Br Med J.* 1988;297:1641–1642.
13. Infection of the breast. In: Hughes LE, Mansel RE, Webster DJT, Gravelle IH, eds. *Benign Disorders and*

Diseases of the Breast: Concepts and Clinical Management. London: Bailliere Tindall; 1989:149.

14. Griffin SM, McEvilly W, Cole, TP. Pilonidal sinus of the penis. *Br J Urol.* 1990;65:422–424.

15. Sroujieh AS, Dawoud A. Umbilical sepsis. *Br J Surg.* 1989;76:687–688.

16. Banerjee A. Pilonidal sinus of nipple in a canine beautician. *Br Med J.* 1985;291:1787.

17. Bowers PW. Roustabouts and barbers' breasts. *Clin Exp Dermatol.* 1982;7:445–448.

18. Elliott D, Quyumi S. A pennanidal sinus. *J R Soc Med.* 1981;74:847–848.

19. Patey DH, Scarff RW. Pathology of postanal pilonidal sinus. Its bearing on treatment. *Lancet.* 1946; 2:484–486.

20. Bascom J. Pilonidal disease: origin from follicles of hairs and results of follicle removal as treatment. *Surgery.* 1980;87:567–572.

21. Buie LA, Curtiss RK. Pilonidal disease. *Surg Clin North Am.* 1952;32:1247–1259.

22. Klass AA. The so-called pilo-nidal sinus. *Can Med Assoc J.* 1956;75:737–742.

23. Dwight RW, Maloy JK. Pilonidal sinus—experience with 449 cases. *N Engl J Med.* 1953;249: 926–930.

24. US Navy. *Statistics of Navy Medicine: Pilonidal Cysts: 1950–1955.* 1956;12:3.

25. Sebrechts PH. A significant diagnostic sign of pilonidal disease. *Dis Colon Rectum.* 1961;4:56–59.

26. Buie LA. Jeep disease. *South Med J.* 1944;37: 103–109.

27. Jensen SL, Harling H. Prognosis after simple incision and drainage for a first-episode acute pilonidal abscess. *Br J Surg.* 1988;75:60–61.

28. Hanley PH. Acute pilonidal abscess. *Surg Gynecol Obstet.* 1980;150:9–11.

29. O'Connor JJ. Surgery plus freezing as a technique for treating pilonidal disease. *Dis Colon Rectum.* 1979;22:306–307.

30. Bascom J. Pilonidal disease: origin from follicles of hairs and results of follicle removal as treatment. *Surgery.* 1980;87:567–572.

31. McLaren LA. Partial closure and other techniques in pilonidal surgery: an assessment of 157 cases. *Br J Surg.* 1984;71:561–562.

32. Brook I. Microbiology of infected pilonidal sinuses. *J Clin Pathol.* 1989;42:1140–1142.

33. Buie LA, Curtiss RK. Pilonidal disease. *Surg Clin North Am.* 1952;32:1247–1259.

34. Feit HL. The use of thorium X in treatment of pilonidal cyst: a preliminary report. *Dis Colon Rectum.* 1960;3:61–64.

35. Allen-Mersh TG. Pilonidal sinus: finding the right track for treatment. *Br J Surg.* 1990;77:123–132.

36. Bascom J. Pilonidal disease: origin from follicles of hairs and results of follicle removal as treatment. *Surgery.* 1980;87:567–572.

37. Guyuron B, Dinner MI, Dowden RV. Excision and grafting in treatment of recurrent pilonidal sinus disease. *Surg Gynecol Obstet.* 1983;156: 201–204.

38. Bascom JU. Repeat pilonidal operations. *Am J Surg.* 1987;154:118–122.

39. Monro RS. A consideration of some factors in the causation of pilonidal sinus and its treatment by Z-plasty. *Am J Proctol.* 1967;18:215–225.

40. McDermott FT. Pilonidal sinus treated by Z-plasty. *Aust N Z J Surg.* 1967;37:64–69.

41. Middleton MD. Treatment of pilonidal sinus by Z-plasty. *Br J Surg.* 1968;55:516–518.

42. Toubanakis G. Treatment of pilonidal sinus disease with the Z-plasty procedure (Modified). *Am Surg.* 1986;52:611–612.

43. Perez-Gurri JA, Temple WJ, Ketcham AS. Gluteus maximus myocutaneous flap for the treatment of recalcitrant pilonidal disease. *Dis Colon Rectum.* 1984;27:262–264.

44. Sherief A, Kamal MS, El Bassyoni F. The rationale of using the rhomboid fasciocutaneous transposition flap for the radical cure of pilonidal sinus. *Dermatol Surg Oncol.* 1986;12:1295–1299.

45. Fasching MC, Meland NB, Woods JE, Wolff BG. Recurrent squamous-cell carcinoma arising in pilonidal sinus tract—multiple flap reconstructions: report of a case. *Dis Colon Rectum.* 1989;32: 153–158.

46. Rosenberg I. The dilemma of pilonidal disease: reverse bandaging for cure of the reluctant pilonidal wound. *Dis Colon Rectum.* 1977;20:290–291.

47. Allen-Mersh TG. Pilonidal sinus: finding the right track for treatment. *Br J Surg.* 1990;77:123–132.

48. Middleton MD. Treatment of pilonidal sinus by Z-plasty. *Br J Surg.* 1968;55:516–518.

49. Bascom J. Pilonidal sinus. In: Fazio V, ed. *Current Therapy in Colon and Rectal Surgery.* Toronto: BC Decker; 1990:32–39.

50. Velpeau A, Verneuil A. Quoted by: Palenta C, Jurkiewicz MJ. Hidradenitis suppurativa. *Clin Plast Surg.* 1987;14:383–390.

51. Masson JK. Surgical treatment for hidradenitis suppurativa. *Surg Clin North Am.* 1969;49:1043–1051.

52. Paletta C, Jurkiewicz MJ. Hidradenitis suppurativa. *Clin Plast Surg.* 1987;14:383–390.

53. Brown SCW, Kazzazi N, Lord PH. Surgical treatment of perineal hidradenitis suppurativa with special reference to recognition of the perianal form. *Br J Surg.* 1986;73:978–980.

54. Thornton JP, Abcarian H. Surgical treatment of perianal and perineal hidradenitis suppurativa. *Dis Colon Rectum.* 1978;21:573–577.

CHAPTER 14

HEMORRHOIDAL DISEASE

Jeffrey W. Milsom

Hemorrhoids have accompanied humans as an important source of suffering since the earliest of recorded times. In the Bible, the Old Testament of I Samuel, Chapters 5 and 6 describes the Philistines after taking the Ark of the Covenant from the Israelis as being smitten by God with *aphelim* or *techorim*. Both words are believed by scholars to relate to hemorrhoids.[1,2] Many centuries ago Maimonides described a variety of soothing medications, ointments, and even suppositories for the treatment of hemorrhoids and argued against surgery as a treatment for the condition.[3]

The term *hemorrhoid* has, from the patient perspective, always signified a variety of anal complaints varying from minor itching to acute disabling pain. Since hemorrhoidal tissue is present in nonpathologic conditions, hemorrhoidal disease should be thought of as hemorrhoidal tissue that causes significant symptomatology.

Anatomy

Hemorrhoids are generally cutaneous and subcutaneous swellings located in the anal canal. They principally lie above the dentate line but may also lie below it. Hemorrhoidal tissue receives its *blood supply* from three directions: (1) superiorly from the superior rectal artery, a branch of the inferior mesenteric artery; (2) laterally from the middle rectal arteries, which arise from the internal iliac arteries; and (3) inferiorly from the inferior rectal arteries, branches of the pudendal arteries. These "vessels" anastomose freely in the anal canal and drain through the respective veins accompanying the arteries.[4] Consequently, the internal hemorrhoidal veins drain into the portal venous system through the superior rectal and inferior mesenteric veins.

Cutaneous *sensation* in this area is mediated through the pudendal nerve and the sacral plexus, both arising from nerve roots 2 through 4, as described in Chapter 1. Some of the pressure sensation in this area may also be mediated by sacral nerve endings (S-2 to S-4) located in the lower rectum and pelvic floor.

Hemorrhoidal tissue is actually a normal part of the anatomy of the anal canal, described as "vascular cushions" in 1975 by Thomson.[5] Bundles of blood vessels seen microscopically to be interspersed with muscle fibers in the submucosa (a "muscularis submucosa") were thought by Thomson to contribute to the "fine tuning" of anal continence. When the submucosal muscle fibers become attenuated and detached from the internal sphincter and the lower rectum, a process associated with aging, the mucosa and submucosa may become freely mobile and prolapse out of the anal orifice.[5] This, in turn, probably leads to the symptoms commonly attributed to hemorrhoids. Hemorrhoidal tissue contains vascular structures or arteriovenous fistulas (Fig. 14-1A)[5-7] whose walls do not contain muscle. Thus, the vessels are sinusoides, not veins (which have muscular walls).

Recent studies have also demonstrated that hemorrhoidal bleeding is arterial and not venous. When hemorrhoidal sinusoides are injured (disrupted), hemorrhage occurs from presinusoidal arterioles.[8] The arterial nature of the bleeding explains why hemorrhoidal bleeding is bright red and has an arterial pH. Hemorrhoids are not related to portal hypertension. With increased portal venous pressure, the body develops portosystemic communications in several locations. In the pelvis, communications enlarge between the superior and middle hemorrhoidal veins, which leads to the development of rectal varices. These varices are located in the lower rectum, not the anus. Because of the rectum's large capacity, they rarely bleed. Older literature[9,10] suggested a relationship between portal hypertension and hemorrhoids—in part because hemorrhoids are common and therefore many portal hypertensive patients have them. Jacobs and colleagues found the incidence of hemorrhoids in patients with portal hypertension is not increased above that expected in the population at large.[11] If hemorrhoidal bleeding were related to portal–systemic connections, then hemorrhoidal bleeding would be venous as in esophageal variceal bleeding rather than the arterial bleeding as described. Hemorrhoidal symptoms may be difficult to manage in these patients because their liver disease frequently is associated with coagulation and platelet problems.

Classification

A standard nomenclature for the location and extent of hemorrhoidal disease has been in use for many years. Although occasionally arbitrary, this schema is extremely useful.

External hemorrhoids are located *below* the dentate line and are covered by anoderm—modified squamous epithelium that bears no skin appendages (Fig. 14-1). They usually have a purplish hue and may swell or enlarge with attempted defecation. They are to be distinguished from external *tags*, which are skin-colored appendages of tissue that may lie anywhere about the perianal area and are believed to be residual swollen or thrombosed external hemorrhoids.

Internal hemorrhoids generally arise *above* the dentate line, are covered by transitional or columnar epithelium and often have visible vessels beneath their delicate mucosal surface. They may extend into the squamous-lined epithelium of the lower anal canal, or they may be continuous with an external hemorrhoidal complex forming a *combined* internal–external complex (Fig. 14-1).

The bundles of hemorrhoids form remarkably consistent complexes in the right anterior and posterior quadrants and in the left lateral position. Minor variations may of course exist. The position of the hemorrhoids bears no relationship to the terminal branching of their arterial supply.

The term **degrees** applies to different stages of descent of *internal* hemorrhoids:

Figure 14-1. (A) Arteriovenous anastomoses (AV shunts) forming hemorrhoidal plexus. (B) Fourth degree internal hemorrhoids. (C) Usual position of the hemorrhoids. Separate external and internal hemorrhoids are seen on the left and a combined internal-external hemorrhoidal complex is seen on the right.

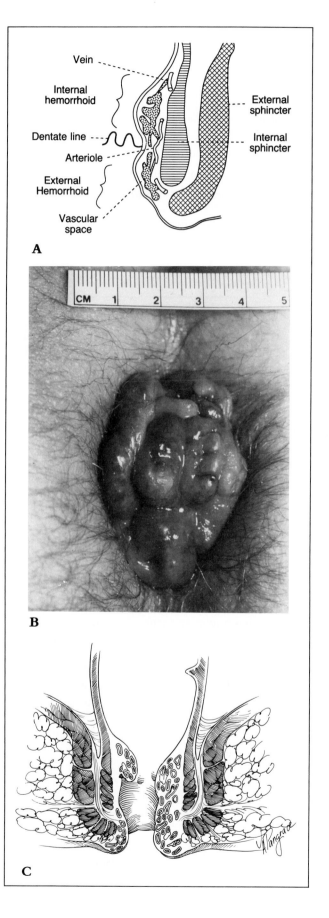

First degree hemorrhoids bulge into the lumen of the anal canal and may cause bleeding during defecation.

Second degree hemorrhoids protrude to the outside only during bowel movements but reduce spontaneously.

Third degree hemorrhoids protrude to the outside either spontaneously or during a bowel movement and require manual replacement.

Fourth degree hemorrhoids (Fig. 14-1B) are permanently prolapsed; attempts at manual reduction are futile.

This classification schema is used later to describe appropriate therapy.

Etiology

Many theories have been proposed to explain this common anal ailment, and it is highly likely that hemorrhoidal disease is multifactorial.

Major Factors

The **"vascular cushion" theory**, proposed by Thomson in his master's thesis on hemorrhoidal disease, entails the concept that normal hemorrhoidal tissues represent discrete masses of thickened submucosa that slide caudally with defecation. The "cushions" fill with blood during defecation and protect the anal canal. Over time, the supporting structures of the hemorrhoids, the "muscularis submucosa," may weaken and lead to prolapse, bleeding, and other symptoms. Haas and others noted that the supporting tissues demonstrate deterioration even by the third decade of life.[6]

Stelzner and others proposed that the anorectal swollen tissues might represent a "**corpus cavernosum recti**," and they demonstrated numerous arteriovenous communications in the anal region.[8]

Dysfunction of the internal anal sphincter (IAS) has also been proposed as a possible cause of hemorrhoidal disease. It has been demonstrated that patients with hemorrhoidal disease have increased activity of the IAS.[12-14] This phenomenon may lead to venous outflow obstruction and congestion, followed by the symptoms related to the hemorrhoids.

Burkitt and Graham-Stewart strongly believe that increased straining with defecation is related to a Western-style low residue diet. Hemorrhoidal disease occurs because of venous backflow related to the **chronic straining**.[15] They supported their theory by the observation that rural Africans, who consume a high fiber diet and thus have soft stools, rarely have hemorrhoidal problems. They and others noted that the defeat of

Napoleon may actually have been precipitated by his low fiber diet, leading to straining and an exacerbation of long-standing hemorrhoidal disease. This then caused the general to falter before the great battle of Waterloo.[16]

Although definitive conclusions about the etiology of hemorrhoids cannot be drawn, most authorities believe that hemorrhoids are *not* varicosities, since this tissue is normally present and only becomes important when the fibromuscular supporting tissue degenerates.[17]

Contributory Factors

Factors that contribute to hemorrhoidal disease include heredity, erect posture, any condition that leads to chronically increased intraabdominal pressure (e.g., ascites, obesity, pregnancy), hormonal changes that occur during pregnancy, chronic diarrheal states associated with inflammatory bowel disease, and possibly the irritable bowel syndrome.

Symptoms

Although a gamut of complaints may ensue from hemorrhoidal disease, most often the symptoms relate to the location and degree of the hemorrhoids. Since hemorrhoidal disease most often leads to *functional* difficulties, a careful history is crucial in understanding how to proceed with therapy.

External Hemorrhoids

In an acute phase, external hemorrhoids may cause severe pain, usually accompanied by a swelling or pressure feeling of recent onset. These symptoms are associated with thrombosis of the hemorrhoidal veins and some bleeding into the tissues of the area. Several days after onset of the pain, the overlying skin may ulcerate or slough with subsequent bleeding from the underlying tissue (dark or "old" blood) or vessels (bright blood).

Over several weeks, the thrombosed area resolves and may leave redundant skin. These "skin tags" may be associated with irritation, itching, feeling of a lump in the area, or problems in cleansing the perianal skin after defecation, but the majority of patients with skin tags are probably asymptomatic.

Internal Hemorrhoids

Acutely, internal hemorrhoids may bleed, prolapse, or cause severe constant pain and swelling. Bleeding is the most common symptom associated with hemorrhoids and per se is characteristically bright red, often dripping into the toilet upon completion of defecation. The bright-colored blood is also frequently smeared on the toilet tissue after the bowel movement. Patients may state that the blood is *not* mixed with the stools, although this is unreliable.

Although the bleeding may be episodic, with time it may become a chronic condition. In rare instances it may lead to significant anemia.

Pain is seen acutely when internal hemorrhoids prolapse irreducibly (fourth degree), usually leading to thrombosis and possibly gangrene (Fig. 14-2). When such conditions are not present, other etiologies for the pain should be entertained (Table 14-1). The pain associated with prolapsed hemorrhoids usually begins after a bowel movement, is constant and throbbing in nature, and may sometimes be relieved by manual reduction.

Protrusion of the internal hemorrhoids may also lead to various degrees of a pressure or swollen feeling in the anal area. Itching related to irritation and subsequent mucous discharge from the columnar epithelium of the internal hemorrhoids may also occur, and patients may complain of moistness in the anal area associated with the protruding hemorrhoids.

Evaluation

The initial phase of patient evaluation must consist of a thorough history, focusing on disorders that may lead to hemorrhoidal bleeding as well as other potential causes for the symptoms. General disorders of bowel function, such as diarrhea and constipation, and associated disorders such as bleeding problems and portal hypertension, should be considered; a dietary history should always be taken. "Hemorrhoids" are nearly always felt *by the patient* to be the cause of anal discomfort or bleeding, but must always, in a sense, be a diagnosis of *exclusion*.

Examination of the anal area is usually undertaken with the patient in a prone position on a special proctologic table. If the patient is elderly or uncomfortable in this position, however, the left lateral decubitus position is an acceptable alternative.

Inspection of the anus should be done slowly, with calm reassurance by the examiner. Patients are often apprehensive and embarrassed, particularly at the first office visit. The skin about the perianum, genitalia, and sacrococcygeal areas should be scrutinized. Gentle, steady spreading of the buttocks will allow for close inspection of the majority of the squamous portion of the anal canal.

Digital examination gives the examiner an appreciation for the amount and location of pain in the anal

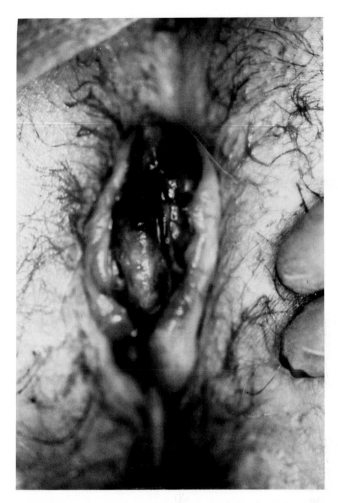

Figure 14-2. Prolapsed thrombosed internal hemorrhoids that have caused swelling of the external hemorrhoids as well.

canal. It enables assessment of sphincter tone and helps exclude other diseases such as palpable tumors and abscesses in the lower rectum and anal canal. Hemorrhoids are not generally palpable unless quite large.

Anoscopy, usually done with a side-viewing instrument, permits a glimpse of the condition of the anoderm and internal hemorrhoidal complexes. As the patient strains the hemorrhoids bulge into the lumen of the anoscope. The degree of prolapse may be assessed by gently withdrawing the anoscope as the patient strains.

Rigid proctosigmoidoscopy and flexible sigmoidoscopy form an important part of the initial examination and are done to exclude more proximal disease. Other tests, such as colonoscopy or barium enema should be performed in patients at risk for polyps or colorectal cancer if bleeding or a change in bowel habits are symptoms. Generally, this complete colonic evaluation is warranted in patients over 50 years of age—or

Table 14-1   Differential Diagnoses in Hemorrhoidal Disease

Symptoms	Other diseases	Hemorrhoidal problems
Acute pain	Fissure Abscess/fistula	Thrombosed Prolapsed thrombosed
Chronic pain	Fissure Abscess/fistula Perianal Crohn's disease	
Bleeding	Fissure Colorectal polyp Colorectal cancer	Internal hemorrhoid Thrombosed external hemorrhoid
Itching/discharge	Hypertrophic anal papilla Fistula Condyloma (anal warts) Rectal mucosal prolapse Rectal prolapse Anal incontinence	Prolapse
Lump or mass	Hypertrophic anal papilla Abscess Anal tag Crohn's disease	Thrombosed prolapsed
Unusual	Anal or rectal tumor (benign or malignant) Ulcerative colitis	

those over 40 who have a higher than average risk of colorectal neoplasia.

Differential Diagnosis

Since patients almost invariably attribute anal pain to hemorrhoids, it is important to recall that acute anal pain is almost always caused by either anal fissure or anorectal abscess. Pain from hemorrhoids is far less common and occurs only in association with thrombosis or prolapse.

If initial external inspection of the anal area is unrevealing, gentle spreading of the buttocks will often reveal a fissure in the posterior or anterior midline, which is usually tender to palpation. An anal or perianal abscess may present as a reddened, fluctuant, tender mass. Thrombosed hemorrhoids are generally visible or palpable on examination.

It is extremely important that other causes of bleeding, itching, or discharge be considered as listed in Table 14-1. Unusual causes of hemorrhoid-like symptoms should be considered when physical examination reveals no sign of significant hemorrhoidal disease.

Treatment: Techniques, Results, and Complications

General Principles

Underlying disorders of gastrointestinal function should be corrected medically or through dietary measures in all patients with hemorrhoidal disease. If constipation and straining with defecation are present, then a diet high in fiber is prescribed, striving for reliably soft stools. This usually requires the ingestion of at least 20 to 30 grams of fiber per day. A prospective double-blind trial published in 1982 demonstrated that psyllium fiber, added to the diet of patients with anal bleeding and pain with defecation, improved symptoms over a 6-week period.[18]

Patients with diarrhea and hemorrhoidal disease, after undergoing appropriate evaluation for the underlying cause of their loose stools, are treated with dietary management and antidiarrheals as appropriate.

Other general supportive measures include use of sitz baths to soothe the acutely painful anal area, and mild oral analgesics such as propoxyphene. A study by Dodi and associates in 1986 showed that significant reductions in anal canal pressures occured in patients with anorectal disorders after soaking in warm (40°C) water.[19] Occasionally, patients use local application of ice packs and, if they prefer this, there is no contraindication.

Topical creams and ointments, while appealing to the patient because their use allows a medicament to be directly applied to the ailing anal region, have never been shown to shrink hemorrhoids or promote healing. One study compared healing rates of a rectal mucosal ulceration using a proprietary hemorrhoid cream versus placebo and found no significant difference.[20] Although the U.S. population spends millions of dollars yearly on over-the-counter anal creams, ointments, and suppositories, there is no evidence that they work better than simple petroleum jelly or any other topical cream. It is highly likely that short-term use of certain hydrocortisone (1 or 2%) creams will ameliorate pruritic symptoms just as they do elsewhere on the skin. Long-term use of corticosteriods is to be avoided because of the thinning and atrophy of the perianal skin that ensues. Pramoxine hydrochloride, a topical antipruritic used effectively for the itching of healing skin in burn patients,[21] has also been used effectively in relieving the itching associated with hemorrhoids and other anal diseases.

External Hemorrhoids

Acute thrombosis of external hemorrhoids generally causes moderate to severe constant external anal pain. Patients generally seek out medical care during the acute phase of pain (first 2–3 days), and if they appear uncomfortable at presentation excision under local anesthesia is advised. If the patient's symptoms are resolving (usually within 48–72 hours), the nonoperative measures outlined earlier are recommended, since symptoms generally resolve quickly after this point.[1]

Excision, not incision, is recommended because the thrombosed area usually involves a plexus of vessels. Incision may not fully evacuate the clot and may cause further swelling and bleeding by lacerating subcutaneous vessels. Incision also is more likely than excision to lead to a skin tag.

Figure 14-3 illustrates the recommended approach to surgical treatment of the thrombosed hemorrhoid, which nearly always can be done in the office setting. Local anesthetic (0.25% bupivicaine with epinephrine 1:200,000) is infiltrated around the thrombosed area. An elliptical area is then removed down to the underlying subcutaneous external sphincter muscle. Care is taken to extend the incision only minimally into the anal canal, since a painful fissure may ensue. Recently, a limited circumferential incision with a small wound has been described as equally effective in evacuating clot from the thrombosed hemorrhoid, but no results were given in

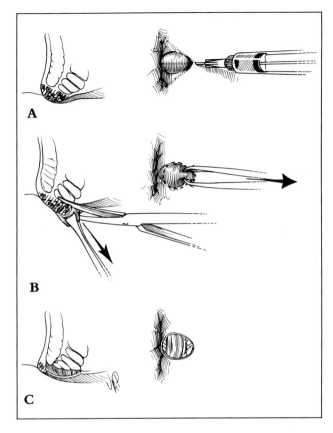

Figure 14-3. Ambulatory treatment of the thrombosed external hemorrhoid: (A) local anesthetic infiltration of the thrombosed area using a 26-gauge needle. (B) *Excision* of the area. (C) The cephalad aspect of the excision is kept out of the anal canal to lessen pain and avoid a fissure. The wound can be left open after hemostasis has been achieved.

the study.[22] After hemostasis has been obtained, the wound can be closed with an absorbable suture or, alternatively, left open. A pressure dressing is applied and the patient is instructed about general dietary measures to keep stools reliably soft. In addition, sitz baths should be taken two or three times daily. A mild oral analgesic may be prescribed but is usually not needed beyond the first 24 hours after the procedure. Healing of the incision occurs within 7 to 10 days, and a follow-up visit should be carried out to assess healing and to reemphasize the importance of diet over the long term.

If an untreated thrombosed hemorrhoid is allowed to progress, ulceration and occasionally bleeding ensue.

Skin tags, or tabs, usually the end result of a resolved external hemorrhoid, are generally asymptomatic and thus should be left alone. If a tag causes troublesome irritation or problems in cleansing the anal area, a conservative excision under local anesthesia can generally be done in the office.

When multiple tags, tags combined with hemorrhoids, or other anal pathology are present and cause significant symptoms, a formal surgical approach may be considered.

Internal Hemorrhoids

Nonsurgical Noninvasive Treatment

Skillful surgical judgment is especially important in managing patients with internal hemorrhoids. An accurate history guides the surgeon as to the severity of disease and impact on the patient's life. Since hemorrhoids are nearly always a functional problem, treatment must proceed cautiously with restoration of function through the least invasive means being the goal. Dietary measures should *always* form an important part of management, regardless of additional strategies. If symptoms consist of only minor intermittent bleeding or protrusion associated with firm stools, a high fiber diet is all that may be needed once more serious underlying etiologies are excluded. Topical creams may be recommended for amelioration of local symptoms such as itching or irritation.

If bleeding or discomfort attributable to hemorrhoids persists despite these measures, of if significant prolapse (second degree or more) is present, then some type of further therapy may be indicated (Table 14-2).

Table 14-2   Treatment of Internal Hemorrhoids by Degree of Prolapse

Severity	Treatment
First degree (no prolapse)	Medical Sclerotherapy; infrared coagulation or banding if symptoms persist
Second degree (spontaneously reducible)	Medical plus Banding with or without sclerotherapy Infrared coagulation
Third degree (manual reduction necessary)	Medical plus Banding and sclerotherapy Possibly excisional hemorrhoidectomy
Fourth degree Irreducible	Excisional hemorrhoidectomy Rarely, multiple rubber band ligations
Acutely prolapsed and thrombosed	Emergency hemorrhoidectomy

Ambulatory Treatment

Sclerotherapy.   One of the oldest treatments for internal hemorrhoids, sclerotherapy aims to cause scarring and eventual shrinking of the hemorrhoidal tissues. Theoretically, sclerotherapy works by obliterating some of the vascularity of hemorrhoids, fixing them to adjacent anorectal muscularis propria to prevent prolapse. John Morgan, in 1869, described injection of iron persulphate into external hemorrhoids.[23] Injection of various substances into the internal pile has been described over the ensuing century, with quinine and urea (5% solution) and phenol (5% in almond oil) being the most popular agents today.[24,25]

The first degree bleeding internal hemorrhoid is most suited for this type of treatment, once dietary measures have failed or have been deemed inadequate as sole therapy. The patient is assisted to the examination position, an anoscope is inserted, and the hemorrhoids are inspected for lack of inflammation, thrombosis, or infection. Again, only internal hemorrhoids are suitable for this form of therapy. Three to five milliliters of 5% phenol in almond oil are injected submucosally into each pile, 1 cm or more above the dentate line, using a 25-gauge spinal needle or a specialized hemorrhoid (Gabriel) needle that is thin at its tip over the last centimeter but is a wide bore needle more proximally. A visible swelling and paling of the surface of the hemorrhoid should be seen during injection. Pain during the injection should alert the surgeon that the needle is either too deep or too distal in the anal canal.

Contraindications to the use of sclerotherapy include inflammatory bowel disease, portal hypertension, known immunocompromised states, presence of anorectal infection, or prolapsed thrombosed hemorrhoids.

Complications of sclerotherapy are related to incorrect placement of the solution or excessive dosing at one site. The most common complication is superficial sloughing of the hemorrhoidal mucosa, which generally will resolve with expectant management. Long-term scarring with stricture formation may result, although this is rare. A tendency toward significant scar formation should be noted in individual patients and cause the surgeon to consider alternative treatments.

Thrombosis of the adjacent hemorrhoid complex (internal and external) may be precipitated by sclerotherapy. In severe thrombosis, excisional hemorrhoidectomy may be required, but generally sitz baths, a high fiber diet, and local measures will allow resolution.

Although unusual, an abscess or *oleoma* may result from sclerotherapy, the latter representing a granulomatous reaction to oil-based sclerotherapy.[26] These complications should be borne in mind in subsequent follow-up.

Results of sclerotherapy have been sparsely reported and difficult to compare with other forms of treatment. Alexander-Williams and Crapp compared injection to freezing and rubber band ligation and found it "satisfactory" over short-term follow-up in first degree hemorrhoids.[27] Denckner and associates compared it to a variety of other treatments and found it to be satisfactory in only 21 percent of patients.[28]

The author and editors believe that sclerotherapy is generally innocuous when used properly but find its value is probably limited to small bleeding areas of internal hemorrhoids not suitable (generally, too small) for banding. It may have a role in the treatment of the small superficial vessels that continue to bleed after treatment by another method. Repetitive use of this technique is to be condemned because of concern over scarring and ineffectiveness.

Infrared Coagulation. The use of infrared coagulation as an office mode of treatment for hemorrhoids was first described by Neiger,[29] then later compared with rubber band ligation and sclerotherapy by Leicester and colleagues.[30] The technology (Redfield Corporation, Montvale, NJ) involves infrared radiation generated by a tungsten–halogen lamp which is focused onto the hemorrhoidal tissue from a gold-plated reflector housing through a specially made polymer tubing using technology similar to laser devices. The infrared coagulator (IRC) light penetrates tissue to the submucosal level and is converted to heat, leading to inflammation, destruction, and eventual scarring of the treated area.[31] The instrument, which looks somewhat like a ray gun, is set at a 1.0-or 1.5-s pulse. Its tip is then applied directly onto the internal hemorrhoid and the trigger fired. The entire process takes only a few seconds. An area of coagulation of 3 to 4 mm^2 generally appears immediately, then leads to the ulceration and scar over 1 to 2 weeks. Depending on the size of the hemorrhoid, up to four spots on each hemorrhoid complex may be treated. Although only one or two areas are treated during one office visit, repeated treatments can be performed every 3 or 4 weeks as needed. Indications for treatment generally include first and second degree hemorrhoids, particularly those which have tortuous superficial vessels and appear unsuitable for banding. The area to be coagulated should be infiltrated with a local anesthetic before treatment since heat and pain are occasionally perceived during application of the probe.

Complications are infrequent and are probably related either to inappropriate coagulation of the anoderm or to bleeding of the coagulated site. In one recent study of 51 patients, 3 developed anal fissures after treatment, and no other complications were noted after a median follow-up of 8 months.[32] This same study compared IRC to bipolar diathermy, finding no significant differences between the two treatments. This technique probably is of most value in first or second degree hemorrhoids, again in instances where rubber band ligation is not feasible. It is quite simple and rapid to use, and probably preferable to sclerotherapy if available.

Bipolar Diathermy. The technique of bipolar diathermy uses an electrical current to generate a coagulum of tissue at the end of the cautery-tipped applicator (ACM Bicap, Stamford, CT).[32] Because the current is bipolar, no grounding of the patient is required. The method has been successfully used to treat obstructing esophageal tumors and bleeding peptic ulcers.[33,34] It seems relatively effective in the treatment of third degree or less hemorrhoids. A 2-s pulse is applied to the base of each hemorrhoid, using several applications as needed. One or two treatment sessions were required in one study[34] and minor complications (fissure) were seen in only 2 of 51 patients in another study.[32] If the equipment were readily available and in use by other specialists, this technique might be worth using, since it also seems safe and rapid. It would be hard to justify purchases, since less expensive methods are readily available.

Direct Current Therapy. This method involves a technique whereby a special probe (Ultroid, Microvasive, Boston, MA) is placed onto and then into the symptomatic internal hemorrhoid. An electrical current up to 16 milliamperes is then passed through the probe. Since current must be applied for up to 10 minutes for each hemorrhoid, and results are comparable to other ambulatory forms of treatment, this method is mentioned only for completeness.[34] It is difficult to believe that any patient or physician would want a probe (and anoscope) held in the anal canal for 10 minutes when other ambulatory methods are equally if not more effective.[35]

Cryotherapy. At one time, cryotherapy was heralded as a technique that allowed painless outpatient destruction of internal and external hemorrhoids. The concept was based on rapid freezing and thawing of tissue, which theoretically caused analgesia and concomitant tissue destruction. A visible edge of an "ice ball" that forms about the cryoprobe depicts the extent of tissue destruction. Although initial reports of large series of patients were exuberant about cryosurgical hemorrhoidectomy,[36,37] it has subsequently proved to be quite painful. Additionally, a profuse foul discharge may ensue from the surgical sites, and healing generally requires 6 weeks or more.[38] Smith and colleagues also found that, in a group of 26 patients randomly treated on one side of the anus with cryosurgery and the other by closed hemorrhoidectomy, pain was more prolonged on the cryotherapy side and 6 of the 7 patients who required further treatment needed it at the cryosurgical site.[39]

This procedure requires expensive, cumbersome equipment and leads to a wound that is malodorous, painful, and slow to heal. With so many alternatives, it is difficult to understand the rationale for its use.

Rubber Band Ligation.   Blaisdell initially described this technique of treating internal hemorrhoids in 1958.[40] It was later refined and demonstrated to be effective by Barron in 1963.[41] It is probably the most widely used technique in the United States in treating hemorrhoids owing to its simplicity, safety, and efficacy.

Once other significant underlying anorectal or medical disorders have been ruled out, this is the treatment of choice for most patients with first and second degree hemorrhoids in whom dietary management has failed. Many if not most patients with third degree hemorrhoids are also candidates. The technique has no role in the treatment of external hemorrhoids. Prior to treatment the patient should have, for a minimum of 7 to 10 days, discontinued the use of all medications that predispose to bleeding.

Technique. After a phosphated enema (CB Fleet Co., Lynchburg, VA) is administered in the outpatient department, the patient is assisted to either the knee-chest or the left lateral decubitus position on the proctology table, and anoscopy is carefully performed to visualize the enlarged internal hemorrhoids. The lower edge of the rubber-banding instrument should be placed at least 1 to 1.5 cm above the dentate line so as to avoid the sensitive anoderm during treatment (Fig. 14-4). A McGivney ligator and a modified Allis clamp can be used to draw the hemorrhoid into the ligator. Alternatively, a suction-equipped ligator can be used. This frees one hand and may allow better visualization of the anal canal.

Most surgeons place two bands on the ligator to ensure tissue constriction and to guard against slippage or breakage. If the suction ligator is used, suction is maintained for 3 s after firing the instrument to draw tissue up into the bander. Immediately after banding, sclerosing solution may be injected above and below the band (Fig. 14-4). This inflates the tissue above (rendering it less likely to slip) and may complement the action of the band by increasing the scarring below. Sclerotherapy should be avoided in anyone with an anal

fissure because the sclerosant can migrate caudally and exacerbate this problem. If the McGivney ligator is used, care must be taken to grasp the area intended for ligation with the Allis clamp to ensure that pain does not ensue. Generally, only two sites are banded at one session, and the patient is told that further banding may be necessary if hemorrhoids are extensive. Patients are cautioned to arise slowly after the procedure, since vasovagal reactions may occur. The entire procedure usually lasts less than 5 minutes. A dull ache or tenesmus may be noticed; pain implies that the rubber bands have been placed too close to the dentate line. If this occurs, they should be removed immediately.

The patient is instructed to avoid strenuous activity over the next week, to take sitz baths as needed for the usual mild to moderate pressure sensation that occurs for the first 48 to 72 hours, and to maintain a diet that results in minimal straining with defecation. Psyllium or other bulk agents are prescribed as necessary. Oral analgesics such as propoxyphene are prescribed if pain is anticipated.

As with all invasive outpatient procedures, all patients should be given an instruction sheet listing postoperative suggestions, potential complications, and appropriate office phone numbers should problems arise.

Complications. With these procedures, complications occur infrequently (<2%) but can be dramatic when they appear. Edema and thrombosis may evolve distal to the banded area, heralded by swelling and pain. The most feared complication after rubber band ligation is sepsis, probably related to necrosis of the banded tissue that allows adjacent soft tissue to become infected. First reported in 1980, this rare event seems to occur most commonly in young males. It is associated with fever, perineal or pelvic pain or both, and difficulty urinating.[42,43] Any patient who develops these symptoms following hemorrhoidal banding must be evaluated immediately. An anesthetic may be required to allow complete examination of the anorectal area. Fatalities have occurred when clostridial and other infections have developed at the banded site, and large doses of appropriate antibiotics are immediately given if there is any question regarding this diagnosis. Operative debridement and removal of the bands are also reasonable therapies as deemed necessary. Diverting colostomy has been required in cases of overwhelming infection.

Delayed hemorrhage may also occur, generally after sloughing of the banded area at 7 to 10 days postprocedure. Although this complication is rare, patients should be cautioned about it and should be encouraged to seek medical attention as necessary. Major bleeding from the area may require suture ligation in the operating room. Occasionally, the ulceration left behind by

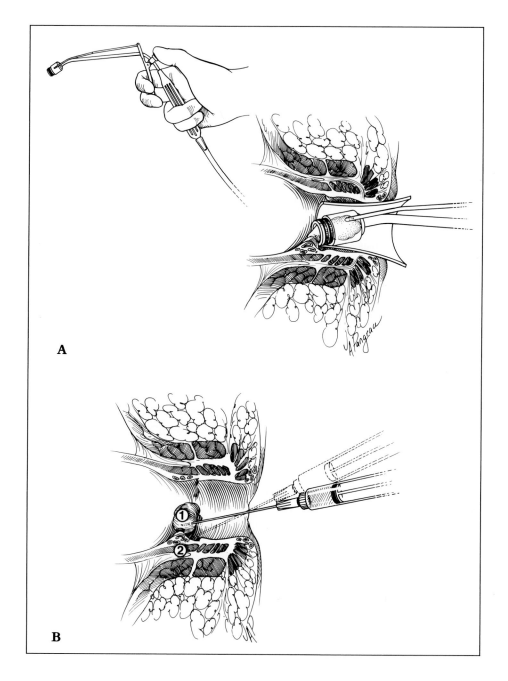

Figure 14-4. (A) A suction rubber band ligator (*inset*) is used to band the internal hemorrhoid 1 to 2 cm above the dentate line. (B) The banded hemorrhoid is first infiltrated with a sclerosing solution to make it larger and less likely to slip, then a small amount of sclerosant is placed beneath the banded area.

the band may extend into the anal canal and lead to a symptomatic fissure. This should be managed conservatively unless symptoms persist over many weeks.

Results. In large series, patient satisfaction has been high (80–91 percent), but probably only 60 to 70 percent of patients are completely cured of symptoms by one session of rubber band ligation.[44-46] If two banding sessions do not ameliorate the symptoms, an alternative form of therapy (hemorrhoidectomy) should be contemplated.

Banding of two or three areas at the same session has

been shown to be safe with a low incidence of complications and pain, and probably leads to more efficient care of the problem.[47,48] A follow-up visit approximately 3 to 4 weeks after banding is advisable to assess results. Use of the technique in immunocompromised patients is discussed later in this chapter.

Overall, the simplicity and good results using rubber band ligation in the management of most uncomplicated hemorrhoidal disease has justified its use as the primary form of ambulatory treatment of hemorrhoids in the United States.

Surgical Approaches to Hemorrhoidal Diseases

Dilation. As a primary treatment for third degree hemorrhoids, dilation was first described in 1968 by P.H. Lord of Great Britain.[49] Both he and, earlier, W.E. Miles,[50] hypothesized that patients with "haemorrhoids" had an abnormal amount of fibrous tissue in the anal canal, especially in the region of the "pecten" (dentate line), which led to stenosis and an obstruction to defecation. Lord thought that dilation relieved this obstruction, thereby reducing the high pressure in the anal canal that might be a cause of hemorrhoids. Hancock and Smith, using anorectal manometry, confirmed that patients with hemorrhoids had higher anal canal pressures, and more frequently than normal controls demonstrated ultraslow waves (0.9–1.6/min).[51]

The *technique* of anal stretch starts with the patient lying in the left lateral position under an intravenous anesthetic. Two lubricated fingers of the surgeon's right hand are inserted into the anorectum and pulled upward toward the ceiling, then two fingers of the left hand are inserted and pulled downward toward the floor. Increasing dilation of *both* the anal canal and lower rectum is carried out to a maximum of eight fingers. The amount of dilation varies: the purpose is to dilate and "iron out" the anorectum until no "constrictions" remain. Lord cautions that it is safer to do too little than too much. A foam sponge is inserted into the anorectum for 1 hour postoperatively to lower the risk of postoperative hematoma formation, and the patient goes home when recovered from anesthesia.

Postoperative care consists of a bulk-forming stool softener and sitz baths. Initially, Lord recommended daily anal dilations with a special grooved dilator. After 2 weeks of this regimen, the patient would be discharged if doing well. Complications of the procedure are less frequent than with standard hemorrhoidectomy. The most troubling one is postoperative incontinence, which occurs in up to 40 percent of patients during the first month after surgery; this is usually minor and resolves.[52]

Although a theoretically frightening procedure, the Lord procedure has demonstrated efficacy in the majority of reported studies, in one achieving results comparable to surgical hemorrhoidectomy in treating prolapsing hemorrhoids.[53] It may be a valued treatment in hemorrhoid patients with severe disease when cost and hospital time are at a premium. It has never gained widespread popularity in North America and is not generally appropriate for elderly patients.

Internal Anal Sphincterotomy. This treatment has been recommended for hemorrhoids for precisely the same theories to which Lord subscribed. Sphincterotomy seems inherently a more controlled technique of lowering anal canal pressures.[54] The techniques may be done under local anesthesia as in the treatment of anal fissure, but in 25 percent of cases, some degree of minor transient incontinence may occur.[55] Sphincterotomy does not address associated tags or external hemorrhoids.

A controlled study by Arabi and colleagues showed no improvement in results compared to rubber band ligation in early hemorrhoids,[56] and Shouten and van-Vroonhoven demonstrated only a 75 percent success rate with sphincterotomy alone.[55]

Although sphincterotomy may be reasonable in the surgical treatment of hemorrhoids with concomitant anal fissure, neither the author nor the editors otherwise recommend its use as the sole treatment for isolated hemorrhoidal disease.

Surgical Hemorrhoidectomy. With the successes of dietary counseling and outpatient procedures such as rubber band ligation, infrared coagulation, and to a lesser extent sclerotherapy, only a small minority of patients suffering with hemorrhoids (probably less than 10 to 20 percent of patients presenting to a colorectal surgeon) require a formal surgical approach. Candidates are those with fourth degree hemorrhoids or rectal mucosal prolapse, those with lesser degrees that have proved refractory to other therapeutic measures, or those in whom concomitant additional anal disease such as fissure, fistula, troublesome tags, or papillae requires surgical management. The urgent or emergent case of prolapsed, thrombosed, and even gangrenous hemorrhoids represents the clearest indication for formal operative intervention.

Although hemorrhoid surgery is filled with much folklore and fear on the part of the patient, an unwavering adherence to certain principles of anal surgery will allow the surgeon to safely relieve the patient of symptoms and minimize complications regardless of technique used.

Preoperative evaluation is undertaken to exclude other significant intestinal problems; sigmoidoscopy and, when indicated, colonoscopy may be performed at the time of hemorrhoidectomy. Active inflammatory bowel disease, immunocompromised states, or bleeding diathesis are all relative contraindications to hemorrhoidectomy.

Unless colonoscopy is contemplated immediately antecedent to hemorrhoidectomy, preparation consists only of a phosphate enema immediately prior to surgery. Perianal shaving is withheld unless the perianal skin is extremely hairy.

Hemorrhoidal Disease   203

General Principles of Hemorrhoid Surgery

First and foremost, anoderm must be conserved during the procedure, and hemorrhoidectomy is never approached as a radical extirpation of all "bulges" into the anoscope or about the perianum. Diseased tissue (internal and external) is removed, but the postoperative scar that ensues from two or three areas will almost certainly anchor the anoderm and lower rectal mucosa so that some bulging hemorrhoidal tissue is safe to leave behind. The sphincter is carefully exposed and left intact during removal of the hemorrhoid. Finally, assurance of adequate hemostasis is attained by careful suture ligation of the apex of the hemorrhoids and by close attention to closure of anoderm in the closed technique.

In the United States, the "closed" technique described by Ferguson and Heaton[57] is most popular because it (1) extirpates diseased tissue, (2) allows for rapid wound healing, (3) seems less uncomfortable than open techniques, and (4) causes minimal postoperative disturbance of continence.[58,59]

Positioning

The patient is assisted to either the prone jackknife or left lateral decubitus position. If the prone position is used, the gluteal area is sprayed with tincture of benzoin or Mastisol solution (Ferndale, Ferndale, MI) and the buttocks are taped apart (Fig. 14-5). This position has the advantage of allowing the first assistant ready access to the operative field, but the left lateral position es-

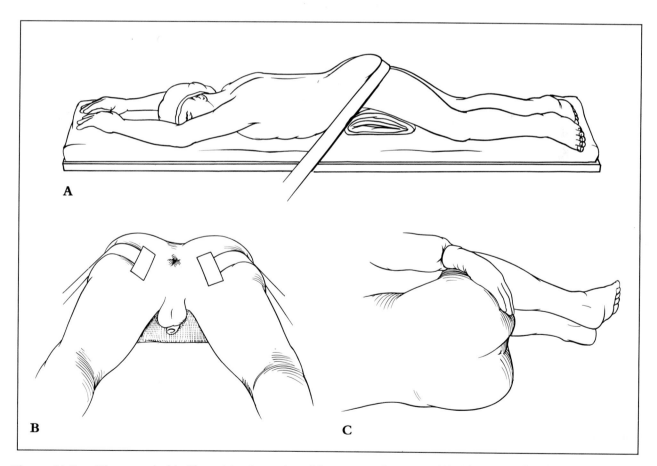

Figure 14-5. The prone jackknife position is employed for most anal surgery. (A) A large towel roll is placed under the pelvis. (B) The buttocks are taped apart and to the sides of the table. (C) The left lateral decubitus position may also be used if, for medical reasons, the patient cannot be placed into the prone position.

poused at the Ferguson Clinic in Grand Rapids, Michigan, is certainly also effective, especially in elderly patients who might not tolerate the prone position unless intubated under a general anesthetic (Fig. 14-5C). Anesthesia may be caudal, spinal, or general, under the discretion of the anesthesiologist, but patients generally do well regardless of anesthetic technique. Patients who prefer minimal anesthesia may have their surgery performed under local anesthesia with only perioperative sedation. Intravenous fluid is given sparingly (<100 ml) and no intravenous antibiotics are indicated unless a specific indication exists. According to the American Heart Association guidelines of March 1991, such indications would be (1) the presence of a mechanical valve, (2) right heart disease, or (3) the presence of endocarditis.

Perianal administration of 0.25% bupivicaine or 0.5% lidocaine and 0.25% bupivicaine mixed with epinephrine 1:200,000 is used to circumferentially infiltrate the anal region subcutaneously, then submucosally up into the anal canal and lower rectum (Fig. 14-6). This usually requires only 10 to 20 ml of anesthetic and will reduce intraoperative bleeding and early postoperative pain.

Sigmoidoscopy can then be carried out as a final check on the condition of the rectum. Anoscopic examination by means of a fiberoptic-lighted Hill-Ferguson retractor is used in planning operative strategy. Alternatively, the Fansler bullet-type retractor works well. A headlight may be used instead of a fiberoptic retractor. The largest hemorrhoid (usually the right posterior) is generally removed first, with the others being removed sequentially according to size. If no significant pile is present in the third quadrant after removal of two hemorrhoids, the area is either left alone or rubber-band ligated well above the dentate line.

The author incises the hemorrhoid in situ with a No. 10 scalpel blade, trying not to completely excise the entire bundle since, again, anoderm is to be conserved at all times (Fig. 14-7). It is simple to remove redundant anoderm as needed after excision of the pile. It is a tragedy to create a stenosis during hemorrhoidectomy by excessively removing anoderm. A relatively narrow V-shaped excision of tissue is performed up to the apex, 1 to 2 cm above the dentate line. The V-shaped wound is important, since if an elliptical wound is created, its widest point is in the mid anal canal where anoderm is most precious.

The subcutaneous external sphincter and the internal sphincter are carefully dissected away from the hemorrhoid (Fig. 14-8). Then, above the dentate line, the pedicle is either tapered to a narrow cephalad point and cut across or clamped and suture-ligated with a 3.0 or 4.0 vicryl or chromic figure-of-eight suture (Fig. 14-9). Downward traction on the pedicle should be avoided so as not to create unsutured dog-ears of the rectal mucosa

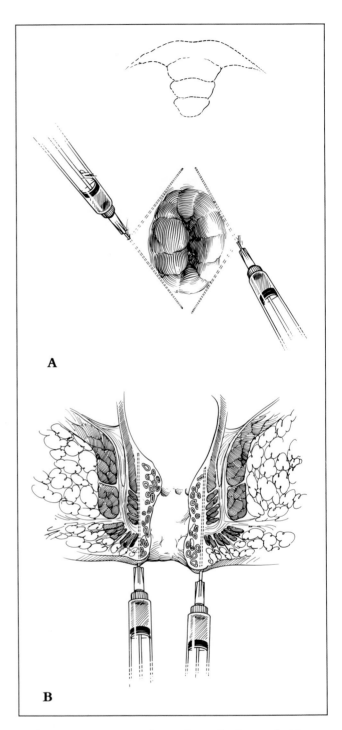

Figure 14-6. (A) Local anesthesia for hemorrhoid surgery begins with subcutaneous infiltration about the lower edge of the sphincter then (B) is completed by circumferential infiltration of the submucosa up to and slightly about the anorectal ring.

which may hemorrhage (Fig. 14-10) after the vasoconstricting effects of the local epinephrine wear off. It is preferable to excise a conservative amount of anoderm and to remove any excessive amount of hemorrhoidal

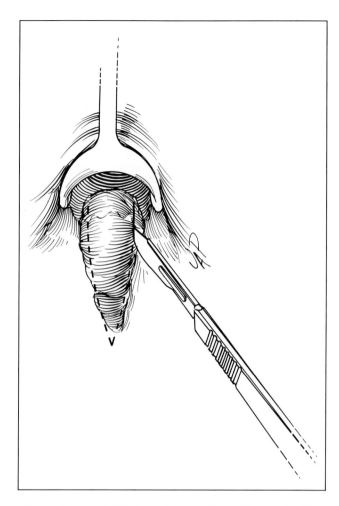

Figure 14-7. Initiation of the excisional hemorrhoidectomy by in situ incision of the complex without grasping the pile. Conservative excision, leaving some of the edges of the pile, is advisable.

tissue by undermining the adjacent mucosa. This permits eradication of the majority of hemorrhoidal tissue and creates flaps that ensure a tension-free wound closure. Hemostasis along the open wound edges can be achieved with electrocautery forceps. Generally, three piles (right anterior and posterior, left lateral) are excised. The wounds are closed in simple running fashion out to the caudal aspect of the wound, which may be partially left open if tension is present (Fig. 14-11). A small anoscope is inserted after conclusion of the case to inspect each wound for hemostasis and to ensure that no stenosis has been created.

If a concomitant anal fissure is discovered at the time of surgery, a left lateral open sphincterotomy is performed by stroking the exposed internal sphincter lightly with the scalpel over the distal half of the sphincter, dividing its superficial fibers.

At the conclusion of the case, if a medium-sized Hill-

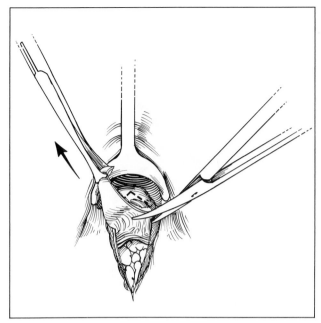

Figure 14-8. The hemorrhoid dissection is carefully continued cephalad by dissecting the sphincter away from the hemorrhoid.

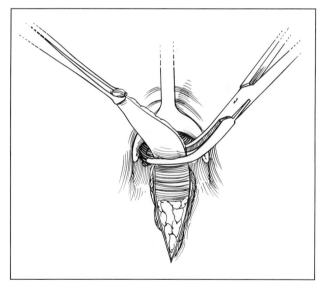

Figure 14-9. After dissection of the hemorrhoid to its pedicle, it is either clamped, secured, or excised; a figure-of-eight suture is then used to secure the pedicle.

Ferguson retractor fits comfortably into the anal canal, it is highly unlikely that postoperative stricture will occur. Small external tags may be excised at the conclusion of surgery if they appear significant. The wounds may be left open. No anal packing is used and a light Telfa® dressing reinforced with gauze is placed over the

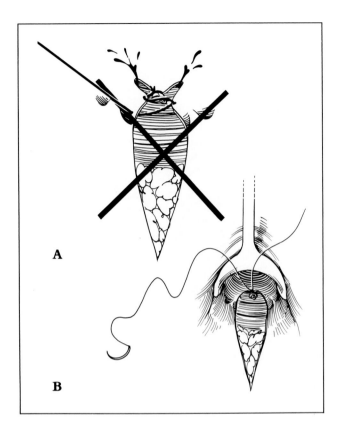

Figure 14-10.   Avoid downward traction on the pedicle (A) which may create unsutured dog-ears of the region leading to postoperative hemorrhage. The pedicle should be sutured without any traction on the wound (B).

wound, held in place with disposable net panties. Even huge hemorrhoidal complexes should be conservatively excised to avoid the chance of postoperative stricture (Fig. 14-12). Packing is avoided because it tends to impede drainage, cause discomfort, and possibly to cause reflex detrusor spasm and difficulty voiding.

Open hemorrhoidectomy, popularized by Milligan, Morgan, and colleagues in 1937,[60] remains the most popular method of surgical treatment of hemorrhoids in Europe, and differs from the Ferguson technique only in that the pedicles are ligated and then the anal canal wounds are left completely open. The purported disadvantage of this technique is the prolonged healing time of the open wounds (4–6 wks), but the operation has proved highly satisfactory in experienced hands.

The *submucosal dissection* of Parks is a closed hemorrhoidectomy procedure but differs from the Ferguson technique in that Parks avoided *any* excision of anoderm. Instead, he made the incision over the piles and dissected out the venous plexi submucosally, then closed the wounds. Results are excellent, but this is perhaps the most tedious and time-consuming of the described procedures.[61]

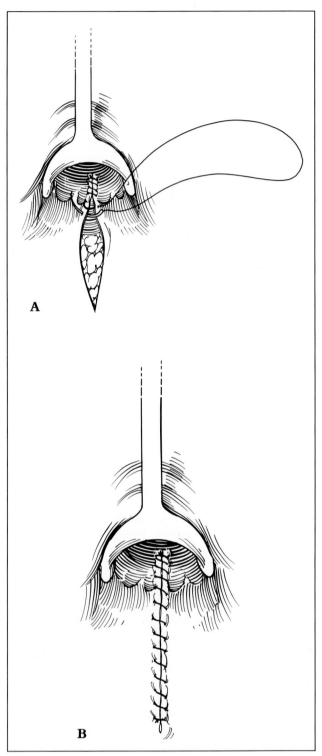

Figure 14-11.   (A) The hemorrhoidectomy wound should be closed in simple running fashion (B) The inferiormost position of the wound may be left open to avoid tension.

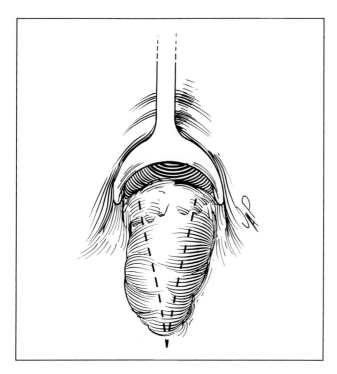

Figure 14-12. A large hemorrhoidal complex should be conservatively excised as well, preserving as much anoderm as possible without leaving redundancy.

The *Whitehead hemorrhoidectomy* has been unjustly maligned because when incorrectly performed, it may lead to rectal mucosal ectropion. Properly performed, however, this operation involves circumferential excision of hemorrhoids and often anoderm with anchoring of perianal skin and rectal mucosa to a region at or above the previous dentate line.[62] This type of approach is rarely needed, but there are occasional patients with circumferential disease who may undergo a "proper" Whitehead hemorrhoidectomy and achieve an excellent result. In Wolff and Culp's review of over 500 patients who underwent a modified type of Whitehead hemorrhoidectomy at the Mayo Clinic, there were *no* instances of anal ectropion.[63]

Laser hemorrhoidectomy still represents a technique in search of validation. Wang and colleagues recently reported a randomized trial comparing neodymium:YAG laser hemorrhoidectomy (plus CO_2 laser for external hemorrhoids) to the closed (Ferguson) technique in 88 patients. Although the laser-treated group required less postoperative pain medication and had a lower incidence of urinary retention (7 percent vs 39 percent), overall complications were similar and prolonged wound healing was noted in the laser-treated group.[64] The expense and potential operating room hazards of the laser equipment mitigate against its use. Nicholson and colleagues conducted a similar prospective ran-

domized trial and found no advantage of any sort with the use of the laser.[65] The Standards of Practice Task Force of the American Society of Colon and Rectal Surgeons summarizes its position as follows[66]:

> No controlled trials have yet been completed to demonstrate superiority or even equivalence of the laser to more traditional treatment methods. Isolated reports suggest that the laser can be used with success, but there is as yet no reason to believe that results will be superior to current techniques.

The popularity of this technique lies in patients' perception that laser technology somehow renders the procedure more effective or less painful.

General Postoperative Care

After hemorrhoidectomy, the intravenous catheter is discontinued in the recovery room to minimize bladder distention and the risk of urinary retention. The patient is told to attempt to void soon after surgery. An adequate dose of the parasympathomimetic drug bethanecol (10 mg subcutaneously) has been shown to increase the likelihood of spontaneous voiding.[67] A small number of patients who live close to the medical facility and are extremely reliable may be discharged within 4 to 6 hours after surgery and instructed to return if bleeding or urinary retention occurs. A strong, preferably nonconstipating, oral narcotic is given for outpatient pain control. Bulking agents and thrice-daily sitz baths are also prescribed.

The majority of postoperative patients will remain in the hospital for 48 to 72 hours, until pain is well controlled, voiding is spontaneous, and wound healing appears uneventful. Reliable patients who live close to the health care facility need not evacuate their bowels prior to discharge. A 500-ml warm tapwater enema administered through a soft latex tube may be given if a spontaneous movement has not occurred in the first 48 to 72 hours. Alternatively, a gentle laxative, such as milk of magnesia, may be administered.

Posthemorrhoidectomy Complications

Postoperative complications are unusual (Table 14-3), with hemorrhage, usually at one of the pedicles, representing the most serious acute problem. Hemorrhage occurred in 4 percent of 500 patients in a study by Buls and Goldberg,[59] with a 1 percent incidence of bleeding severe enough to warrant a return trip to the operating room for suture ligation of a vessel. This is an agreement with a study from the Ferguson Clinic in which over 2000 hemorrhoidectomies were reviewed.[68]

Table 14-3   Posthemorrhoidectomy Complications

	Incidence, %[59,68,69]
Acute (first 48 h)	
Bleeding	2 to 4
Bleeding requiring reoperation	0.8 to 1.3
Urinary retention	10 to 32
Early (first wk)	
Fecal impaction	< 1
Wound infection	< 1
Thrombosed hemorrhoid	< 1
Late	
Skin tags	6
Anal stenosis	1
Anal fissure	1 to 2.6
Incontinence	< 0.4
Anal fistula	< 0.5
"Recurrent" hemorrhoids	< 1

* over 2500 patients

Sepsis related to the wound itself is extremely rare. It is not unusual, however, to see some erythema and drainage from the wound edges. If there is suspicion of infection (fever, increased pain, difficulty voiding) and no obvious other source, the patient should be empirically started on antibiotics and watched carefully. Outpatient observation is acceptable if the patient manifests no signs of toxicity, but severe pain or worsening symptoms should prompt consideration for in-hospital management and careful examination, under anesthesia if necessary.

Postoperative pain is generally moderate in the first 24 to 48 hours, and controllable by parenteral meperidine or morphine sulphate. Patients are encouraged to take oral medication such as oxycodone or propoxyphene and can generally be weaned off stronger medications by the second postoperative day. A psychological incentive is supplied by informing the patient that bowel movements will come easier and sooner once only oral medications are used.

Fecal impaction may occur in the first week to 10 days after hemorrhoidectomy and should be suspected if the patient reports watery feculant discharge, rectal pressure, and constipation during the early postoperative period. This problem is best avoided by giving the patient a high fiber diet with added psyllium or another bulking agent two or three times per day for the first several weeks after surgery. An added mild laxative such as 15 to 30 ml of milk of magnesia per day can be offered to help stimulate the first evacuation. Treatment of an impaction should consist of two or three gentle, warm, 500-ml tapwater enemas given through a soft latex catheter until the impaction is cleared. Anal pain or inability to clear the impaction by these methods may require manual disimpaction under anesthesia.

If *external thrombosis* or swelling of the external hemorrhoids occurs subsequent to hemorrhoidectomy, the usual cause is a subcutaneous bleeding vessel. Gentle compression should be applied to the wound for 10 minutes if it appears to be enlarging. Comfort measures such as sitz baths, analgesics, and local application of a topical soothing cream may then be used. The area will generally resolve spontaneously, and only rarely should any additional therapy be required. Tense edema and swelling may require excision of the external hemorrhoid as described earlier, again erring on very conservative removal of anoderm.

Edematous skin tags, often of concern to patients, should be left alone for 3 to 4 months since they usually shrink significantly over that time and usually require no treatment beyond reassurance.

Anal stenosis, although rare, may be the most troublesome long-term complication and should nearly always be preventable by conservative removal of anoderm at hemorrhoidectomy. Fortunately, anal stenosis may nearly always be treated by simple anal sphincterotomy,[69] leaving the longitudinally oriented wound open if scarring is so severe that a closed-type procedure is not possible.

In unusual instances, when stenosis is severe (will not allow insertion of lubricated index finger or small Hill-Ferguson anoscope at surgery), a plastic surgical correction of the stenosis may be required. A Y-V advancement flap (Fig. 14-13; see treatment of ectropion) may be used when only a section of the anoderm is scarred, performing a partial sphincterotomy in the bed of anoderm excised as needed to widen the anal canal. The anal canal should be augmented such that a medium Hill-Ferguson anoscope fits comfortably into the canal. When the entire anoderm is scarred and narrowed, either two Y-V flaps can be used (Fig. 14-14), or an S-anoplasty may be contemplated (see treatment of ectropion), which attempts to re-line the entire anal canal with unscarred epithelium.[70] The treatment of stenosis is discussed in depth in Chapter 12.

Ectropion may occur by inadvertent removal of anoderm and subsequent caudal displacement of rectal mucosa into the anal canal (Fig. 14-15). This can be avoided by remembering the rule that anoderm may always be safely advanced above the dentate line, but rectal mucosa should rarely be advanced below it. If ectropion does occur postoperatively, the patient may report wetness, itching, and irritation.[71] Most patients, unless entirely asymptomatic, require surgical correction. Treatment, if confined to only one half or less of the anal circumference, may be performed by merely excising the ectopic rectal mucosa, but I believe it is

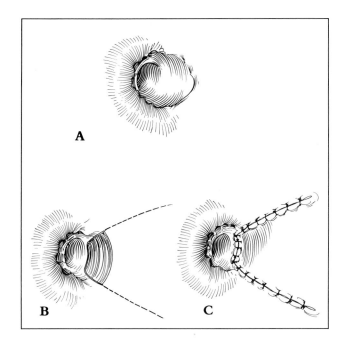

Figure 14-13.   Partial anal ectropion (A) may be treated with excision of the columnar epithelum (B), then advancement of a broad-based full-thickness skin flap over the defect (C).

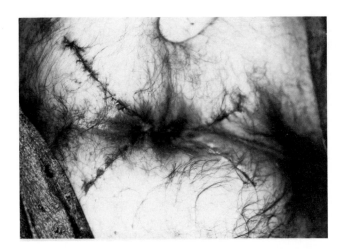

Figure 14-14.   Large areas or nearly circumferential anal ectropion may be treated by bilateral **Y-V** advancement of flaps.

nearly always preferable to perform an anoplasty. The **Y-V** advancement flap is simple and effective (see Fig. 14-13). After a complete mechanical bowel preparation, the rectal mucosa is excised down to sphincter muscle, a broad based **V-** or **U-**shaped flap is mobilized and placed cephalad in the anal canal and sutured to the dentate line and anal canal by interrupted or running 3-0 vicryl sutures. The caudal edges of the flap may be left

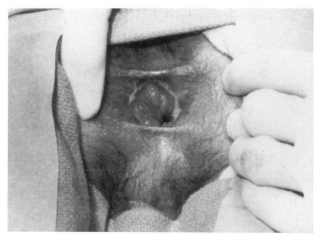

Figure 14-15.   Completely circumferential anal ectropion (classic "Whitehead" deformity).

open to relieve tension. The patient is kept in-hospital for 3 to 5 days and given broad spectrum intravenous antibiotics to minimize the risk of infection and maximize success of the flap. The bowels are confined postoperatively for the 3 to 5 days by a combination of 60 mg codeine and 4 mg loperamide given orally every 6 hours. Bulk agents and gentle laxatives are then given to promote a bowel action following the regimen after hemorrhoidectomy.

In cases of circumferential mucosal ectropion, the classic "Whitehead deformity," or in cases where more than 50 percent of the circumference is involved, the S-anoplasty (Fig. 14-16) remains the procedure of choice.[70] It may be performed on one or both sides of the anus. After complete mechanical bowel preparation, the patient is placed in the prone jackknife or left lateral position and the entire area of ectropion is carefully excised down to underlying anal sphincteric musculature, then cephalad to the dentate line area. Any scarred or thickened squamous mucosa is excised as well. Curvilinear flaps arching back toward the greater trochanter are then taken in an S shape so that one flap arches around anteriorly and the other posteriorly. After skin and superficial subcutaneous tissues have been dissected carefully away from the anus, these broadbased flaps are rotated up into the anal canal and sutured carefully to the internal sphincter *and* the rectal mucosa in the upper anal canal. Any concomitant anal surgery is done before suturing in the flaps, which is done using interrupted 2-0 absorbable sutures in the anal canal and running sutures on the flaps. The wound may be left open laterally to minimize tension. Again, intravenous antibiotics are recommended for 3 to 5 days. A bowel-confining regimen of minimal clear liquids and 4 mg loperamide and 60 mg codeine given orally every 6 hours for 5 to 7 days is recommended. Showers may

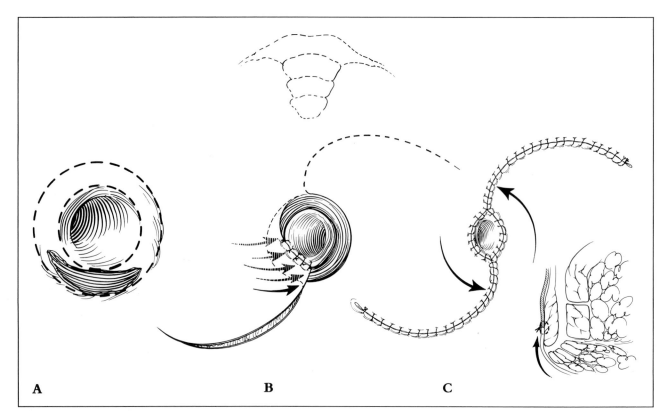

Figure 14-16.   Steps in the performance of an S-anoplasty: (A) Surgery begins with complete excision of all scar and abnormally placed columnar epithelium up to the dentate line region. (B) An S-shaped configuration of the perianal and buttock skin is then mobilized (including a small amount of subcutaneous fat) and advanced up into the anal canal. (C) The bilateral flaps are joined anteriorly and posteriorly and sutured at the dentate line region to the underlying sphincter muscles (*inset*).

be started after the first day, but sitting or lying on the flaps is avoided until discharge from the hospital.

Rarely, anal fissure may develop in the postoperative period, heralded by pain or burning following bowel movements. Often, a degree of stenosis is an associated finding. If fissures occur in the first 3 to 4 weeks following surgery and are of mild to moderate severity conservative measures such as sitz baths, dietary regimen to keep the stools soft, and anal cream should be adopted. The patient must be reassured and advised that soft, bulky stools are necessary to dilate the anal passage naturally and that watery, loose stools can contribute to narrowing of the area. If symptoms are severe, or if conservative measures are not helpful, a careful examination under anesthesia with a planned sphincterotomy or possibly with excision of the fissure and Y-V anoplasty, may be needed.

Fecal incontinence is an unusual but potentially disastrous complication after hemorrhoidectomy and may occur more frequently than reported in the literature (<1 percent). Certain categories of patients should be scrutinized extremely carefully before being considered

candidates for hemorrhoidectomy. This includes elderly patients, especially women, and patients who have had prior anal surgery. These patients require a detailed, careful inquiry regarding anal continence. Digital rectal examination should be performed at rest and during maximum voluntary squeeze to ascertain sphincter tone, and anal manometry should be used to quantify anal pressures. Patients should be counseled about goals of the surgery, and nonoperative measures reconsidered if bowel control is impaired. At surgery, it is entirely acceptable to perform only a one- or two-quadrant hemorrhoidectomy, conserving anoderm, and to rubber-band ligate the other quadrants or leave them alone. The underlying sphincter should be carefully protected. This conservative approach may lead to a slightly greater chance for recurrence, but patients will understand your concern about protecting their continence.

Major incontinence rarely occurs following hemorrhoidectomy, but minor imperfections can occur, especially when open sphincterotomy is done concomitant with hemorrhoidectomy as a "pain relieving" measure. The only time that sphincterotomy should be done is when some degree of stenosis is present or when a concomitant fissure is present.

Recurrence of significant hemorrhoidal disease following the closed hemorrhoidectomy is unusual—only 1 percent in the 2038 patients surveyed by Ganchrow and colleagues.[68] Most symptoms that patients equate with recurrence are either skin tags or small external hemorrhoids, or are related to bleeding of small superficial veins near the healed hemorrhoidectomy wounds. Tags may be excised in the office under local anesthesia if they cause significant irritation. Bleeding from the internal hemorrhoids is nearly always treatable with either rubber band ligation, infrared coagulation, or sclerotherapy.

Special Considerations

Pregnancy

Hemorrhoidal symptoms often first appear or worsen during pregnancy because of increased constipation, generalized engorgement of the pelvic tissues, increased venous pressures related to the enlarged uterus, and a variety of other factors. Straining with childbirth may lead to acute hemorrhoidal symptoms as well, but most symptoms rapidly resolve in the postpartum period.

A conservative approach to hemorrhoids during pregnancy should be followed, especially in the first trimester, with dietary counseling, sitz baths, and topical creams being used to soothe the anal region.

If prolapse and thrombosis occur, hemorrhoidectomy using intravenous sedation and local anesthesia should be considered if the pregnancy seems uncomplicated otherwise. The left lateral decubitus position should be preferentially used in the second and third trimesters. In one study of 25 women, 22 required hemorrhoidectomy during their third trimester, and all except one experienced relief of their symptoms by 1 day postoperatively. There were no complications to the mother or fetus.[72]

If the prolapse and thrombosis occur during delivery, then one study has demonstrated good results with hemorrhoidectomy immediately postpartum. Additionally, if a patient has had significant symptoms *before and* during pregnancy, then consideration should be given to immediate postpartum hemorrhoidectomy, since most of these patients will have long-term symptoms.[73]

Inflammatory Bowel Disease

All inflammatory conditions in the rectum or anus may lead to symptoms that may be confused with hemor-

rhoids. A careful history to exclude mucosal ulcerative colitis or Crohn's disease should therefore be undertaken, especially searching for diarrheal symptoms, weight loss, and abdominal pains.

In Jeffery and colleagues' review of 20 patients with Crohn's disease and 42 patients with ulcerative colitis, the complication rate was high in Crohn's disease (11 complications after 26 courses of treatment), and relatively lower in the ulcerative colitis group (4 complications after 58 courses).[74] One patient in 42 with ulcerative colitis and 6 of the 20 with Crohn's disease ultimately required proctectomy for complications apparently related to hemorrhoidectomy. One might conclude that treatment of hemorrhoids is relatively safe in mucosal ulcerative colitis but contraindicated whenever there is suspicion of Crohn's disease.

Whenever either disease is suspected, a full gastrointestinal evaluation should be undertaken. Finally, whenever active rectal inflammatory disease is present, only conservative measures should be used, and even sclerotherapy and banding should be avoided.

Portal Hypertension

Fortunately, even though the hemorrhoidal plexus represents a portosystemic connection, bleeding from this area is rare in portal hypertension. Rectal varices are occasionally seen in these patients and may also be the cause of bleeding.[75,76] In the event that a patient with portal hypertension presents with massive anorectal bleeding, the patient should be admitted to the intensive care unit, coagulation factors administered as necessary, and a careful anorectal examination carried out to visualize the bleeding area. If necessary, the examination should be done in the operating room to visualize the area accurately with the aid of good assistance as well as proper instrumentation and lighting. Bleeding should be controlled by oversewing of the bleeding hemorrhoidal complex, using polyglactin or any other long-lasting absorbable suture.

Once the patient has been stabilized, a long-lasting method of portal decompression should be considered if the bleeding has been significant.

Immunocompromised States

Leukemia or Lymphoma

Patients with these malignancies often manifest some disorder related to the anorectal region, and both patient and medical consultant may call the ailment "hemorrhoids."[77,78] It is incumbent upon the colorectal specialist to perform an accurate examination at the outset in these patients, again even if this requires an anesthetic in the operating room.

During the acute phase of the leukemic illness, minimal therapy beyond diagnosis and symptomatic treatment of hemorrhoids should be undertaken. Lesions similar to hemorrhoids may actually represent lymphomatous or leukemic tissues, and biopsy is therefore all that should be contemplated under these circumstances.

When the hematologic disorder is quiescent and hemorrhoidal disease flares, conservative therapy may include small excisions of prolapsed thrombosed hemorrhoids with oral antibiotic coverage for 5 to 7 days.

HIV-positive Patients

The fear of prolonged wound healing has very definitely influenced the care of patients infected with the acquired immune deficiency syndrome (AIDS) virus who present with anorectal lesions. Any patient who has developed the syndrome of AIDS (overwhelming opportunistic infection, pneumocystic pneumonia, Kaposi's sarcoma) should undergo only palliative measures for treatment of hemorrhoidal disease, since life expectancy is measured only in months in these patients.

On the other hand, there are significant numbers of HIV-positive patients who are asymptomatic (Centers for Disease Control group II).[79] In these patients, healing may be uneventful or only slightly prolonged. Thus in the asymptomatic HIV-positive patient who otherwise seems healthy, treatment of hemorrhoids has been shown to be safe.[80] Caveats to be observed include:

Band, rather than excise, the hemorrhoids whenever possible.

Treat only one quadrant at a time.

Administer oral antibiotics for approximately 5 days (250 mg metronidazole P.O. orally t.i.d. *or* 500 mg Ciprofloxacin® orally B.I.D.) and preferably have the patient take azidothymidine (AZT) under the direction of a specialist in infectious diseases. These issues are discussed in more detail in Chapter 21.

The patient must be reliable and available for close follow-up.

Specialists from both Great Britain and the United States report that the HIV-positive, asymptomatic patient can do well postoperatively.[81-83]

References

1. Madoff RD. Biblical management of anorectal disease. Presented at the Midwest Society of Colorectal Surgeons Meeting; March 1991; Breckenridge, CO.
2. Dirckx JH. The biblical plague of "hemorrhoids." *Am J Dermatopathol.* 1985;7:341–346.
3. Maimonides M. *Treatise on Hemorrhoids.* Rosner F, Munter S, trans. Philadelphia; JB Lippincott; 1969.
4. Parnand E, Guntz M, Bernard A, et al. Anatomie normal macroscopique et microscopique du resean vasculaire hemorrhoidal. *Arch Fr Mal.* 1976; 65:501–514.
5. Thompson WHF. The nature of haemorrhoids. *Br J Surg.* 1975;62:529–552.
6. Haas PA, Fox TA, Haas GP. The pathogenesis of hemorrhoids. *Dis Colon Rectum.* 1984;27:442–450.
7. Stelzner F, Staubesand J, Machleidt H. Das cavernosum recti—die Grundlage der Inneren Haemarrhoiden. *Langenbecks Arch Klin Chur.* 1962;299:302–312.
8. Thulesius O, Gjores JE. Arterio-venous anastomoses in the anal region with reference to the pathogenesis and treatment of hemorrhoides. *Acta Chir Scand.* 1973;139:476–478.
9. Ackerman LV, Butcher HR. *Surgical Pathology* 3rd ed. St Louis:CV Mosby; 1969.
10. Anderson WA. *Pathology.* 5th ed. St Louis: CV Mosby;1966.
11. Jacobs DM, Bubrick MP, Onstad GR, Hitchock CR. The relationship of hemorrhoids to portal hypertension. *Dis Colon Rectum.* 1980;23:567–569.
12. Hancock BD. Internal sphincter and the nature of hemorrhoids. *Gut.* 1977;18:651–655.
13. Arabi Y, Alexander-Williams J, Keighley MRB. Anal pressures in hemorrhoids and anal fissure. *Am J Surg.* 1977;134:608–610.
14. Kerremans R. In: Arscia SA, ed. *Morphological and Physiological Aspects of Anal Continence and Defacation.* Part III, ch. 1. Bruxelles: Presses Academiques Europeenes, SC; 1969:150–151.
15. Burkitt DP, Graham-Stewart CW. Haemorrhoids—postulated pathogenesis and proposed prevention. *Postgrad Med J.* 1975;51:631–636.
16. Welling DR, Wolff BG, Dozois RR. Piles of defeat:

Napolean at Waterloo. *Dis Colon Rectum.* 1988; 31:303–305.

17. Bernstein WC. What are hemorrhoids and what is their relationship to the portal venous system. *Dis Colon Rectum.* 1983;26:829–834. Guest Editoral.

18. Moesgaard F, Nielsen ML, Hansen JB, Knudsen JT. High fiber diet reduces bleeding and pain in patients with hemorrhoids. *Dis Colon Rectum.* 1982; 25:454–456.

19. Dodi G, Bogoni F, Infantino A, et al. Hot or cold in anal pain? A study of the changes in internal sphincter pressure profiles. *Dis Colon Rectum.* 1986; 29:248–251.

20. Subramanyam K, Patterson M, Gourley WK. Effects of Preparation-H on wound healing in the rectum of man. *Dig Dis Sci.* 1984;29:829–832.

21. Peal L, Karp M. A new surface anesthetic agent: Tronothane. *Anesthesiology.* 1954;15:637–643.

22. Grosz CR. A surgical treatment of thrombosed external hemorrhoids. *Dis Colon Rectum.* 1990; 33:249–251.

23. Morgan J. Varicose state of saphenous haemorrhoids treated successfully by the injection of tincture of persulphate of iron. *Medical Press and Circular.* 1869:29–30.

24. Andrews E. The treatment of hemorrhoids by injection. *Medical Record.* 1879;15:451.

25. Corman ME. Hemorrhoids. In: *Colon and Rectal Surgery.* 2nd ed. Philadelphia: JB Lippincott; 1989:49–105.

26. Gabriel WB. *The Principles and Practice of Rectal Surgery.* London: Lewis; 1963:131.

27. Alexander-Williams J, Crapp AR. Conservative management of haemorrhoids, I: injection, freezing, and ligation. *Clin Gastroenterol.* 1975;4:595–601.

28. Denckner H, Hjorth N, Norryd C, et al. Comparison of results with different methods of treatment of internal haemorrhoids. *Acta Chir Scand.* 1973;139:742–745.

29. Neiger S. Hemorrhoids in everyday practice. *Proctology.* 1979;2:22–28.

30. Leicester RJ, Nicholls RJ, Mann CV. Comparison of infrared coagulation with conventional methods and the treatment of hemorrhoids. *Coloproctology.* 1981;5:313–315.

31. O'Connor JJ. Infrared coagulation of hemorrhoids. *Pract Gastroenterol.* 1986;10:8–14.

32. Dennison A, Whiston J, Rooney S, et al. A randomized comparison of infrared photocoagulation with bipolar diathermy for the outpatient treatment of hemorrhoids. *Dis Colon Rectum.* 1990;33:32–34.

33. Fleischer D. Bicap therapy, cancer. *Endosc Rev.* March/April 1988;10–12.

34. O'Brien JD, Day SJ, Burnham WR. Controlled trial of small bipolar probe in bleeding peptic ulcers. *Lancet.* 1986;1:464–467.

35. Hinton CP, Morris Dl. A randomized trial comparing direct current therapy and bipolar diathermy in the outpatient treatment of third degree hemorrhoids. *Dis Colon Rectum.* 1990;33:931–932.

36. Wilson MC, Schoefield P. Cryosurgical haemorrhoidectomy. *Br J Surg.* 1976;63:497–498.

37. Savin S. Hemorrhoidectomy—how I do it: results of 444 cryorectal surgical operations. *Dis Colon Rectum.* 1977;20:189–196.

38. Goligher JC. Cryosurgery of hemorrhoids. *Dis Colon Rectum.* 1976;19:213–218.

39. Smith LE, Goudreau JJ, Fonty J. Management of hemorrhoids: operative hemorrhoidectomy versus cryosurgery. *Dis Colon Rectum.* 1979;22:10–16.

40. Blaisdell PC. Prevention of massive hemorrhage secondary to hemorrhoidectomy. *Surg Gynecol Obstet.* 1958;106:485–488.

41. Barron J. Office ligation treatment of hemorrhoids. *Dis Colon Rectum.* 1963;6:109–113.

42. O'Hara VS. Fatal clostridial infection following hemorrhoidal banding. *Dis Colon Rectum.* 1980;23:570–571.

43. Russell TR, Donahue JH. Hemorrhoidal banding: a warning. *Dis Colon Rectum.* 1985;28:291–293.

44. Bartizol J, Slosberg P. An alternative to hemorrhoidectomy. *Arch Surg.* 1977;112:534–535.

45. Steinberg DM, Liegois H, Alexander-Williams J. Long term review of the results of rubber band ligation of haemorrhoids. *Br J Surg.* 1975; 62:144–146.

46. Wrobleski DE, Corman L, Veidenheiner MC, Coller JA. Long-term evaluation of rubber ring ligation in hemorrhoidal disease. *Dis Colon Rectum.* 1980;23:478–482.

47. Lau WY, Chow HP, Dorn GP, Wong SH. Rubber band ligation of three primary hemorrhoids in a single session. *Dis Colon Rectum.* 1982;25:331–339.

48. Khubchandani IT. A randomized comparison of single and multiple rubber band ligations. *Dis Colon Rectum.* 1983;26:705–708.

49. Lord PH. A new regime for the treatment of hemorrhoids. *Proc R Soc Med.* 1968;61:935–936.

50. Miles WE. Observations on internal piles. *Surg Gynecol Obstet.* 1919;29:497–506.

51. Hancock BD, Smith K. The internal sphincter and Lord's procedure of haemorrhoids. *Br J Surg.* 1975; 62:833–836.

52. McCaffrey J. Lord treatment of hemorrhoids: four year follow-up of fifty patients. *Lancet.* 1975; 1:133–134.

53. Lewis AAM, Rogers HS, Leighton M. Trial of maximal anal dilatation cryotherapy and elastic band ligation as alternatives to haemorrhoidectomy in the treatment of large prolapsing hemorrhoids. *Br J Surg.* 1983;70:54–56.

54. Allgower M. Conservative management of haemorrhoids, III: partial internal sphincterotomy. *Clin Gastroenterol.* 1975;4:608–618.

55. Shouten WR, vanVroonhoven TJ. Lateral internal sphincterotomy in the treatment of hemorrhoids—a clinical and manometric study. *Dis Colon Rectum.* 1986;29:869–872.

56. Arabi Y, Gatehouse D, Alexander-Williams J, et al. Rubber band ligation of lateral subcutaneous sphincterotomy for treatment of haemorrhoids. *Br J Surg.* 1977;64:737–740.

57. Ferguson JA, Heaton JR. Closed hemorrhoidectomy. *Dis Colon Rectum.* 1959;2:176–179.

58. Ferguson JA, Mazier WP, Ganchrow MI, et al. The closed technique of hemorrhoidectomy. *Surgery.* 1971;70:480–484.

59. Buls JG, Goldberg SM. Modern management of hemorrhoids. *Surg Clin North Am.* 1978;58:469–478.

60. Milligan ETC, Morgan CN, Jones LE, et al. Surgical anatomy of the anal canal, and operative treatment of haemorrhoids. *Lancet.* 1937;2:1119–1124.

61. Parks AG. Surgical treatment of haemorrhoids. *Br J Surg.* 1956;43:337–351.

62. Whitehead W. The surgical treatment of haemorrhoids. *Br Med J.* 1882;1:148–150.

63. Wolff BG, Culp CE. The Whitehead hemorrhoidectomy: an unjustly maligned procedure. *Dis Colon Rectum.* 1988;31:587–590.

64. Wang JY, Chang-Chien CR, Chen JS, et al. The role of lasers in hemorrhoidectomy. *Dis Colon Rectum.* 1991;34:78–82.

65. Nicholsen J, Halleran D. Laser hemorrhoidectomy: a prospective randomized trial. Presented at the American Society of Colon and Rectal Surgeons, 87th Annual Convention; June 12–17, 1988 (unpublished); Anaheim, CA.

66. Standards Task Force. American Society of Colon and Rectal Surgeons. Practice parameters for the treatment of hemorrhoids. *Dis Colon Rectum.* 1990;33(4);7A–8A.

67. Gottesman L, Milsom JW, Mazier WP. Postoperative urinary retention treated with Urecholine: a prospective, randomized, blinded study. *Dis Colon Rectum.* 1989;32:867–880.

68. Ganchrow MI, Mazier WP, Friend WG, et al. Hemorrhoidectomy revisited—a computer analysis of 2038 cases. *Dis Colon Rectum.* 1971;14:128–133.

69. Milsom JW, Mazier WP. Classification and management of postsurgical anal stenosis. *Surg Gynecol Obstet.* 1986;163:60–64.

70. Ferguson JA. Repair of "Whitehead deformity" of the anus. *Surg Gynecol Obstet.* 1959;115–116.

71. Granet E. Hemorrhoidectomy failures: causes, prevention, and management. *Dis Colon Rectum.* 1968;11:45–48.

72. Saleeby RG, Rosen L, Stasik JJ, et al. Hemorrhoidectomy during pregnancy: risk or relief? *Dis Colon Rectum.* 1991;34:260–261.

73. Schottler JL, Balcos EG, Goldberg SM. Postpartum hemorrhoidectomy. *Dis Colon Rectum.* 1973;16:395–396.

74. Jeffery PJ, Ritchie JK, Parks AG. Treatment of hemorrhoids in patients with inflammatory bowel disease. *Lancet.* 1977;1:1084–1085.

75. Weinshel E, Chen W, Falkenstein DB, et al. Hemorrhoids or rectal varices: defining the cause of massive rectal hemorrhage in patients with portal hypertension. *Gastroenterology.* 1986;90:744–747.

76. Hsieh JS, Huang CJ, Huang YS, Huang TJ. Demonstration of rectal varices by transhepatic inferior mesenteric venography. *Dis Colon Rectum.* 1986;29:459–461.

77. Vanheuverzwyn R, Delannoy A, Michaux JL, et al. Anal lesions in hematologic diseases. *Dis Colon Rectum.* 1980;23:310–312.

78. Barnes SG, Sattler FR, Ballard JO. Perirectal infections in acute leukemia. *Ann Intern Med.* 1984;100:515–518.

79. Centers for Disease Control, US Department of Health and Human Services. Classification system for human T-lymphotrophic virus type III/lymphadenopathy–associated with virus infections. *Ann Intern Med.* 1986;105:234–237.

80. Miles AJG, Mellor CH, Gassard BG, et al. The surgical treatment of anorectal disease in HIV-positive males. *Br J Surg.* 1990;77:869–871.

81. Allen-Mersh TG (Moderator), Gothesman LG, Miles AJG, et al. Symposium: The management of anorectal disease in HIV-positive patients. *Int J Colorectal Dis.* 1990;5:61–72.

82. Wexner SD. Anorectal surgery in HIV-seropositive patients. *J R Soc Med.* 1991;84:191–192.

83. Wexner SD, AIDS: What the colorectal surgeon needs to know. *Perspect Colorectal Surg.* 1989;2(2):19–54.

CHAPTER 15

PROCTALGIA FUGAX, LEVATOR SYNDROME, AND PELVIC PAIN

Gregory C. Oliver

In 1859, Sir J.Y. Simpson[1] published his observations on the relationship between coccygeal trauma and the subsequent clinical syndrome which we know as *coccygodynia*. From this time until the present, authors have tended to lump vague perineal complaints of pain into this clearly defined category of coccygeal posttraumatic syndrome. In 1935, Thaysen[2] recognized a pelvic pain syndrome whose clinical characteristics differed from those attributed to coccygodynia and termed this *proctalgia fugax*. He reported two men and one woman who complained to him of sudden attacks of pain without antecedent injury or illness. Episodes were unpredictable and relief occurred spontaneously usually within minutes of the onset. The location of the pain was difficult to characterize, but it was thought to be of rectal origin. Karras and Angelo[3] added 12 new cases of proctalgia and attributed the cause of the pain to muscle spasm of the nonstriated sphincter mechanism. In their patients, they believed nitroglycerin provided relief from spasm. In 1961, Ibrahim[4] added 24 patients with this syndrome. He disagreed with preceding authors on the cause and proposed a mechanism similar to that causing migraine headaches: sudden pelvic vascular congestion. He found nothing to be medically helpful but thought that because of the short duration of symptoms, reassurance of the nonmalignant nature of the problem provided adequate therapy. In 1980, Thompson and Heaton[5] related proctalgia fugax to irritable bowel syndrome and postulated it to be a clinical variant of the latter condition.

In a parallel vein, George Thiele of Missouri published a number of papers[6-11] on a condition he called coccygodynia but attributed the pain to spasm of the levator ani muscles. He recognized that the coccygeal pain was secondary to pelvic muscle spasm causing traction on the insertion sites along the coccyx. In 1958, William T. Smith of Minneapolis, Minnesota, addressed the Minneapolis Academy of Medicine.[12] Smith was able to integrate Thiele's published work with his own patient observations and termed this condition *levator syndrome*. Under this heading, he included both organic causes of levator sling spasm and functional causes. Today his description of the syndrome is essentially unchanged. It is the etiology of the spasm that we have continued to redefine. The author[13,14] reserves the term levator syndrome to describe idiopathic or functional spasm of the levator mechanism and seeks to exclude organic causes of this malady, which may be treated specifically according to the cause.

Pelvic pain is a frequent complaint in my practice. Usually the correct diagnosis is easily discerned after a brief history and physical examination. Many common anorectal conditions present initially with this complaint, and the preceding and subsequent chapters of this text deal with many of these conditions in depth. However, it is not uncommon to see a patient with this complaint in whom all of the common causes of perineal pain can be readily excluded while the cause of the patient's discomfort remains obscure. It is at this point that a methodical evaluation of the history and a careful examination of the pelvic viscera will usually suggest the correct diagnosis. A number of these originally obscure causes will eventually be shown to be of organic origin. Occasionally, computed tomography (CT), magnetic resonance imaging (MRI), electromyography (EMG), or laparoscopy will be necessary to arrive conclusively at a diagnosis for pelvic pain.

After all organic causes of pelvic pain have been excluded, there will remain a group of patients in whom no discernible physical cause of pain can be discovered.

This pain appears to arise from functional causes and can present as several different syndromes. In the clinical practice of colorectal surgery, this type of patient is regularly encountered. Over a 15-year period Grant and associates[15] identified 316 such cases of functional perineal pain. In most large series reported,[11,15-18] females strongly predominate. An awareness of this condition and its varying presentations is critical to the clinician faced with the evaluation of perineal pain. This overview of the organic and functional causes of the complaint as well as the pertinent anatomic considerations is presented as a framework on which an understanding of the diagnosis and treatment of these often obscure syndromes can be built.

Anatomic Considerations

One significant difficulty in our understanding of pelvic pain is the anatomic complexity of the region. The proximity of structures that belong to different organ systems mandates an organized approach to the differential diagnosis of pelvic pain. Added to this has been the relative lack of interest in the study of this area until quite recently. Interestingly, the development of physiologic testing has driven the study of structure within the pelvis. Several current texts[19-21] provide a detailed discussion of the anatomic complexities of this region. Herein, emphasis is on the structures and organs that must be considered in the evaluation of pelvic pain. Each of the following organs or organ systems can cause severe pelvic pain. A complete assessment should exclude each of these as potential etiologies.

Spine and Bony Pelvis

Primary and secondary diseases of the pelvic girdle and the lower axial skeleton may present as pelvic pain. Major considerations are traumatic injury as well as primary and metastatic tumors in the region. The term *coccygodynia* is reserved for primary coccygeal injury that causes pain localized to the coccyx. Used in this specific fashion, the term denotes a coccyx that is tender to touch.

Pelvic Musculature

The major portion of the pelvic musculature consists of striated skeletal muscle. The pelvic floor or pelvic diaphragm is generally synonymous with the levator ani muscles. From medial to lateral, the levator ani consist of the puborectalis, the pubococcygeus, the ileococcygeus, and the ishiococcygeus. Inferiorly, the external

sphincter complex encircles both the anal canal and the internal sphincter. The internal sphincter is a smooth-muscle specialized adaptation of the circular layer of bowel wall.

Reproductive Organs

The prostate and seminal vesicles may be the source of infection or malignancy which can give rise to pelvic pain complaints. Their evaluation is important in the assessment of the complaint in males of any age.

Any disease process affecting the vagina, cervix, uterus, fallopian tubes, or ovaries may present as pelvic pain complaints. Therefore, careful inspection and bimanual examination of the female patient is critical to an accurate assessment of pelvic pain. Endometrial implants within the pelvic cul du sac not infrequently present in this fashion.

Lower Alimentary Tract

Disease of the cecum, appendix, sigmoid colon, rectum, and anus can present as pelvic pain. Direct assessment may include palpation, endoscopic observation, or indirect imaging techniques. Depending upon the historical data gathered, appropriate assessment can be selected and carried out.

Nervous System

Primary and secondary diseases affecting the pelvic innervation may cause pelvic pain. Any condition affecting the cauda equina, S-2 through S-4 nerve roots, and the pudenal nerve may cause this problem. Degenerative disease of the spine, primary or metastatic tumors, cysts, and local trauma must all be considered. Specific physiologic testing is now available in most centers to assess for these conditions. These tests are discussed in Chapter 2.

Conditions Causing Pelvic Pain

Many diseases and syndromes may present with a chief complaint of pelvic pain. For the purposes of this review, these processes are broken down according to their origin in organic or functional causes. Undoubtedly, overlap does exist among these classifications. The intent herein is to offer the clinician faced with a patient who has pelvic pain a rational approach to the differential diagnosis of these conditions. The classification system we favor is based upon Rubin's[14] and appears as Table 15-1.

Table 15-1   Classification of the Causes of Pelvic Pain

ORGANIC CAUSES

Inflammatory diseases of the pelvis and anorectum

Cryptoglandular abscess	Infectious proctitis
Fistula in ano	Prostatitis
Crohn's disease	Tuboovarian abscess
Ulcerative colitis	Endometriitis
Ulcerative proctitis	Diverticulitis
Radiation proctitis	Pelvic appendicitis
Endometriosis	Ectopic pregnancy

MECHANICAL CAUSES

Incomplete rectal prolapse	Fissure
Descending perineum syndrome	Pelvic surgery
Torsed ovary	

NEOPLASTIC CAUSES

Nonmalignant tumors

Nerve	Bone
Muscle	Endometriosis

Malignant Tumors: Primary and Recurrent

Rectum	Uterus	Muscle
Prostate	Bladder	Bone
Ovary	Nerve	Metastatic gastric

NEUROLOGIC CAUSES

Multiple sclerosis

Peripheral neuritic/degenerative disease

ORTHOPEDIC CAUSES

Coccygeal trauma—Coccygodynia

Degenerative disease of the lumbosacral spine

Osteogenic tumors

FUNCTIONAL/IDIOPATHIC CAUSES

LEVATOR SYNDROME/PROCTALGIA FUGAX

DEPRESSION

Organic Causes

Inflammatory Diseases Affecting the Pelvis

Common anorectal disorders that present as perineal or pelvic pain readily lend themselves to diagnosis. These include abscesses (cryptoglandular, intramuscular), fistulas, Crohn's disease, and ulcerative proctitides. These conditions are covered elsewhere in this text and so will not be further discussed here.

In the male patient, chronic or acute prostatitis may present as rectal or pelvic pain. Urinary symptoms are often present and should be elicited in questioning. Digital rectal examination in males should always include careful prostatic palpation to exclude these conditions. When indicated, seminal evaluation after prostatic massage may prove helpful. I have occasionally found transrectal ultrasound examination of the prostate to be helpful in the assessment of pelvic pain.

In the female patient, tuboovarian infections, ectopic pregnancy, and both endometriosis and endometriitis should be considered as a source of pelvic pain. A routine bimanual pelvic examination and a careful speculum examination of the cervix will generally suffice to exclude these sources.

Occasionally, complicated diverticular disease of the sigmoid colon and complicated appendicitis may present as pelvic pain. A careful historical review of the symptoms will generally direct the examiner to a more comprehensive abdominal evaluation. Contrast enema examination of the colon, ultrasonic study, or CT may be helpful in evaluating these less common causes of this complaint.

Mechanical Causes

Rubin[22] points out that an incomplete rectal prolapse may result in rectal pain. One finding that may point to this condition as the cause is a solitary rectal ulcer noted on proctoscopy. Anal fissures are very common conditions which present as perineal or anal pain. Generally, simple mechanical trauma initiates this condition which is then exacerbated by a secondary inflamatory response. Together, these lesions cause muscular spasm and if the problem becomes chronic, hypertrophy of the internal sphincter.

Parks and associates[23] observed that in a population of patients chronically straining during defecation, perineal descent could often be observed. Patients complained of a dull aching pain in the pelvic region after attempts at defecation. Abnormal anal sphincter response and function were observed in this group of patients. More recently, Kiff and associates[24] were able to demonstrate pudendal neuropathy caused by chronic straining, which helped explain the descending perineum syndrome. The pelvic pain associated with this condition is most likely ischemic and is due to disordered sphincter function and secondary neurologic injury.

Lastly, Rubin[14] pointed out that there is a group of patients who complain of pelvic pain after very low anterior resections of the rectum. This may be described as rectal pressure or discomfort in the coccygeal or buttock region. This is presumably due to mechanical trauma of the pelvic floor which occurs during these very low resections. We have noted that it commonly requires 6 to 12 months for these symptoms to subside postoperatively if they subside at all.

Neoplastic Causes

Nonmalignant tumors causing this syndrome are rare but are occasionally encountered. Their effect is related to their sheer mass, which impinges on adjacent structures. Neurogenic benign tumors and cysts have been described[25,26] and should be sought when preliminary tests are suggestive or when an obvious cause is lacking. Rhabdomyomas and leiomyomas of the pelvic musculature are also occasionally found.

Pelvic endometriosis is a nonmalignant condition that causes pain through its ectopic growth pattern and sclerotic tissue reaction to this growth. The cyclic nature of the pain and bleeding should alert the clinician to this consideration. Although endometriosis itself is a common condition, it is uncommon as a cause of isolated pelvic pain.

Both primary and recurrent pelvic malignant tumors can cause pain by direct extension and involvement of the sensory pathways of this region. Most commonly, advanced rectal, prostate, ovarian, uterine, or bladder cancer is the cause of malignant pelvic pain syndromes. Less commonly, malignant bone, muscle, or nerve tumors are the cause. The chronic, progressive, and persistent nature of pain due to malignant disease suggests its consideration in the evaluation of this complaint. A history of pelvic organ malignancy should provoke a thorough search for recurrent disease in any patient who complains of pelvic or perineal pain. Occasionally, pelvic metastases from gastric carcinoma may be the cause of this syndrome as well.

Neurologic Causes

Generally an uncommon primary cause of pelvic pain, several neurologic conditions may include rectal pain among their manifestations. Multiple sclerosis, peripheral neuritis, and degenerative conditions affecting the cauda equina are known to cause pelvic pain symptoms. Degenerative disease of the lumbosacral spine not infrequently may cause pain complaints although pain related to such disorders is generally manifested in the buttock or thigh region. Radicular symptoms should prompt a search for a reversible neurologic process. Such an evaluation may necessitate CT, MRI, myelography, or EMG testing.

Orthopedic Causes

The classic orthopedic condition associated with this complaint is coccygodynia.[1] Traumatic injury to the coccyx may result in degenerative joint disease, arachnoiditis and/or secondary spasm of the muscles with insertions or origins on the coccyx. This diagnosis should only be made when direct manipulation of the

coccyx results in painful complaints. Radiologic confirmation of coccygeal trauma reinforces the diagnosis. Postacchine and Massobrio[27] argue that anatomic variations in coccygeal shape and configuration are responsible for a condition they term idiopathic coccygodynia. They advocate surgical coccygectomy, partial or complete, based upon the radiologic configuration noted. Overall, the treatment of any form of coccygodynia by coccygectomy is a questionable practice. For all cases of coccygodynia not due to direct trauma, a thorough search for the precipitating cause will provide a rational approach to therapy.

Rarely, osteogenic tumors may arise in the spine, sacrum, or pelvis and produce a pelvic pain syndrome. Generally, the chronic persistent nature of this pain prompts a thorough evaluation of this complaint which will lead to a correct diagnosis.

Functional Causes

Up until this point, organic causes of pelvic pain syndromes have been emphasized. The reason for this emphasis is that most clinicians are adept at physical diagnosis and, by being aware of the possible secondary causes of pelvic pain, will formulate a plan to diagnose or exclude these possibilities. Unfortunately, functional or idiopathic causes of pelvic pain occur with disturbing frequency. Two studies, one American[28] and one British,[5] surveyed groups of apparently healthy workers and asked them if they experienced episodic rectal pain. Nineteen percent of the 165 American hospital workers surveyed and 41 of the 301 British counterparts (13.6 percent) responded affirmatively to this question. In the American study, only 4 of the 32 respondees had brought their symptoms to the attention of a physician. Likewise, Thompson and Heaton commented that few if any of those they surveyed had consulted a physician. What is apparent from these studies is that the syndrome of paroxysmal rectal pain is quite common while presentation to the physician is less common. As previously noted, in one busy colorectal surgical practice,[15] 316 cases were seen in a 15-year period. It is the common occurence of this idiopathic condition and the frustration of the patients who suffer from it that mandate our efforts to understand, treat, and hopefully cure this vexing condition.

The Levator Syndrome and Its Varients

Levator syndrome is characterized by episodic pain that occurs internally in the region generally described by most patients as the rectum. The term *levator syndrome* refers to the clinical finding in this group of patients of levator sling tenderness on transanal palpation. *Proc-*

talgia fugax, as a term, denotes a condition of fleeting rectal pain. Douthwaite,[29] in his analysis of proctalgia fugax, ascribed its origins not to the rectum but to a segmental cramp of the pubococcygeus muscle. For the purpose of this discussion, proctalgia fugax is considered a variant of levator syndrome. The perpetual confusion surrounding the use of these terms is clear. A recent major medical text[30] cautioned physicians not to mistake proctalgia fugax for levator syndrome in that the latter is characterized by the physical finding of tenderness of the levator mechanism on physical examination. Immediately preceding this admonition, the author described palpable spasm of the levator ani as a component of proctalgia fugax. True coccygodynia is a secondary condition of the coccyx and so is *not* considered a variant of this syndrome.

The clinical presentation of this syndrome has been well described.[12-14,31-33] Pain is generally dull and aching with its focus seemingly in the rectum. Often patients describe feeling as if they were sitting on a ball. At times the pain is sharp or stabbing and may radiate to the coccyx, buttock, or posterior thigh. Pain may be unilateral or bilateral. Thiele[6] postulated that this radiation of pain is secondary to transient compression or traction on the sciatic and superior gluteal nerves where they pass adjacent to a spastic piriformis muscle on exiting the pelvis. Episodes are usually sudden in onset and brief in duration, generally lasting less than 3 minutes in 91 percent of patients.[31] In this same series, 12 percent of patients experienced pain only at night while 22 percent had pain occur both day and night. Forty percent of patients claimed that passing a stool precipitated their attack of pain. The syndrome affects all ages, with reported incidences extending from 6 to 90 years of age.[15] Generally, it is thought that frequency and severity of symptoms diminish in a given patient with increasing age. In most large clinical series,[12,15,31] women outnumber male sufferers by 3 to 1. However, in the random surveys previously cited,[5,28] males slightly outnumber females in the acknowledgment of having experienced fleeting rectal pain. This finding may represent societal factors which may allow women to complain of this pain to a physician while men find it more difficult to discuss or less troublesome to tolerate. In most instances, pain of functional origin is intermittent while pain from organic sources is more constant.

The clinical assessment of these patients is directed at exclusion of those conditions previously set forth as organic in nature. The hallmark of levator syndrome is tenderness or firmness on palpation of the levator ani mechanism which mimics the patient's symptoms. Most often the tenderness is left sided.[12,15] Typically, the levator mechanism on the affected side is taut and often described as "violin" or "bowstring" in tension. Absence of tenderness on palpation does not exclude

levator syndrome but pressures the clinician to exclude all possible organic causes of symptoms.

The etiology of idiopathic levator syndrome is unknown. Authors have implicated prolonged sitting, cold, heat, sexual activity, and both physical and emotional stress as precipitating factors. Several authors have linked levator syndrome to clinical depression,[34,35] noting that sufferers are typically perfectionists and overanxious by standardized psychological testing. Additionally, cultural tendencies to somatasize depressive disorders do exist and are frequently associated with anal complaints. Clearly, many patients suffering from levator syndrome are depressed. What is less than clear is whether depression is the cause of levator syndrome or vice versa. In the absence of a resolution to this dilemma, an effective therapeutic approach may be all we have to offer these troubled patients.

Attempts to categorize levator syndrome and its variants according to the results of manometric and EMG testing have been to no avail.[16] This, of course, reinforces the application of the term *idiopathic* to this syndrome. No identifiable abnormality of the pelvic floor or its innervation has been detected, even with the most precise physiologic assessments. Lastly, the elusiveness of this diagnosis is nowhere more pronounced than by the common history of surgical procedures performed upon this group of patients in misguided attempts to alleviate their symptoms. Typical procedures noted in our series have been hemorrhoidectomy, lateral internal sphincterotomy, hysterectomy, rectal procidentia repairs, bladder suspensions, rectocele repair, and lumbar laminectomy. As noted earlier in this chapter, levator spasm can be secondary to low pelvic surgery presumably due to a local inflammatory response. Therefore, these operations may exacerbate rather than ameliorate the pain.

The treatment of levator syndrome is empiric and seeks to relieve symptoms. Patients should be reassured that they do not have a malignancy, as cancerphobia is common among them. Therefore, when the diagnosis of levator syndrome is secure, patient reassurance is of major therapeutic value. Large population studies[5,28] demonstrate that most affected patients will be symptomatic six or fewer times per year. Discussion with the patient concerning precipitating factors (e.g., stressful situations) will often allow insight into the causes of a given patient's complaints.

The next level of therapy for levator syndrome sufferers not relieved by reassurance is local massage. The tender, affected levator sling should be vigorously massaged with the examiner's index finger. This will produce patient discomfort as would the massage of any spastic muscle group elsewhere in the body. We attempt to massage the spastic area about 50 times each session or to the tolerance of the patient, which may well be less. This takes about 2 minutes. If symptoms persist, we repeat the massage again every 7 to 14 days. Patients are instructed to soak in a hot tub several times daily between treatments to provide deep heat to the spastic area.

For patients whose symptoms are more protracted, consideration may be given to adding a muscle relaxant, an oral analgesic agent, or both. Because of the frequently associated anxiety found in this group, a short course of diazepam (2 to 5 mg) given two to three times daily may be beneficial. In levator sufferers with prolonged bouts of pain, nonnarcotic analgesics form the bulwark of therapy. Indeed, nonsteroidal antinflammatory analgesics (NSAIDs), such as diflunisal also inhibit prostaglandin synthesis thereby helping to prevent further muscle spasm.

In our own patient population, 87 percent of levator syndrome patients were adequately relieved or cured of their symptoms with the regimen described. The 13 percent for whom this conservative course failed formed the basis of a group we treated with electrogalvanic stimulation,[17] a regimen first reported on by Sohn and associates.[36] The rationale for this therapy is that low frequency oscillating current, when applied to spastic muscles, induces fasciculation and fatigue, thus interrupting the spastic cycle. We treated 102 patients in three 1-hour sessions over a 10-day period using either a hand-held or a self-retaining transanal probe applied to the tender levator sling. Of this most difficult group of patients, 77 percent when surveyed stated that their symptoms were either eradicated or significantly improved by this regimen. In an unselected group of levator syndrome patients, Nicosia and associates[18] treated 45 patients in this fashion and reported this treatment relieved symptoms in 90 percent. Since this earlier work, we have been experimenting with altering the galvanic stimulation sessions, notably shortening the treatment time while increasing the frequency of treatments. We have not yet analyzed the results of this option on treatment outcome.

Finally, anxiety and depression are commonly seen in patients suffering with levator syndrome. Whether this psychiatric state is a coexisting, separate illness or secondary to the chronic painful state engendered by the most extreme forms of levator syndrome, expert psychiatric help may be mandatory. The clinician treating levator syndrome must be alert to the more serious signs of these psychiatric conditions. With this in mind, it is ill-advised to prescribe antianxiety agents or narcotic analgesics for long periods to patients with levator syndrome. Although the vast majority of our patients do very well with a conservative regimen for this condition, the few with serious psychological problems will be helped only with an appropriate referral to competent psychiatric care.

References

1. Simpson JY. Coccygodynia and diseases and deformities of the coccyx. *M Times Gazette*. 1859;40: 1009–1010.
2. Thaysen H. Proctalgia fugax. A little known form of pain in the rectum. *Lancet*. 1935;2:243–246.
3. Karras JD, Angelo G. Proctalgia fugax. *Am J Surg*. 1951;82:616–625.
4. Ibrahim H. Proctalgia fugax. *Gut*. 1961;2:137–140.
5. Thompson WG, Heaton KW. Proctalgia fugax. *J Coll Physicians*. 1980;14:247–248.
6. Thiele GH. Tonic spasm of the levator ani, coccygeus and piraformis muscle: relationship to coccygodynia and pain in the region of the hip and down the leg. *Trans Am Proc Soc*. 1936;37:145–155.
7. Thiele GH. The management of the patient with painful coccyx. *Kansas City Med J*. 1937;13:21–22.
8. Thiele GH. Coccygodynia and pain in the superior gluteal region and down the back of the thigh. *JAMA*. 1939;109:1271–1274.
9. Thiele GH. The painful coccyx: Its cause and treatment. *Kans City Med J*. 1948;24:16–20.
10. Thiele GH. Coccygodynia: the mechanism of its production and its relationship to anorectal disease. *Am J Surg*. 1950;79:110–116.
11. Thiele GH. Coccygodynia: cause and treatment. *Dis Colon Rectum*. 1963;6:422–434.
12. Smith WT. Levator spasm syndrome. *Minn Med*. 1959;42:1076–1079.
13. Salvati EP. The levator syndrome and its variant. *Gastroenterol Clin North Am*. 1987;16:71–78.
14. Rubin RJ. Proctalgia fugax. In: Fazio V, ed. *Current Therapy in Colon and Rectal Surgery*. Philadelphia: BC Decker; 1990:68–71.
15. Grant SR, Salvati EP, Rubin RJ. Levator syndrome: an analysis of 316 cases. *Dis Colon Rectum*. 1975;18:161–163.
16. Neill ME, Swash M. Chronic perianal pain: an unsolved problem. *J R Soc Med*. 1982;75:96–101.
17. Oliver GC, Rubin RJ, Salvati EP, et al. Electrogalvanic stimulation in the treatment of levator syndrome. *Dis Colon Rectum*. 1985;28:662–663.
18. Nicosia JF, Abcarian H. Levator syndrome: a

treatment that works. *Dis Colon Rectum*. 1985;28: 406–408.

19. Wood BA. Anatomy of the anal sphincters and pelvic floor. In: Henry MM, Swash M, eds. *Coloproctology and the Pelvic Floor, Pathophysiology and Management*. London: Butterworths; 1985:3–21.

20. Goldberg SM, Gordon PH, Nivatvongs S, eds. *Essentials of Anorectal Surgery*. Philadelphia: JB Lippincott; 1980:1–16.

21. Goligher JC, Duthie HL. Surgical anatomy of the colon, rectum and anus. In: Goligher JC, ed. *Surgery of the Anus, Rectum and Colon*. London: Bailliere Tindall; 1980:1–47.

22. Rubin RJ. Solitary rectal ulcer syndrome. In: Cameron J, ed. *Current Surgical Therapy*, 3rd ed. Philadelphia: BC Decker; 1989:135–138.

23. Parks AG, Porter NH, Hardcastle J. The syndrome of the descending perineum. *Proc R Soc Med*. 1966; 59:477–482.

24. Kiff ES, Barnes PRH, Swash M. Evidence of pudendal neuropathy in patients with perineal descent and chronic straining at stool. *Gut*. 1984;25: 1279–1282.

25. Ziegler DK, Batnitzky S. Coccygodynia caused by a perineural cyst. *Neurology*. 1984;34:829–830.

26. Kinnett JG, Root L. An obscure cause of coccygodynia. *J Bone Joint Surg*. 1979;61A:299.

27. Postacchine F, Massobrio M. Idiopathic coccygodynia: analysis of 51 operative cases and a radiographic study of the normal coccyx. *J Bone Joint Surg*. 1983;65A:1116–1124.

28. Panitch NM, Schofferman JA. Proctalgia fugax revisited. *Gastroenterology*. 1975;68:1061.

29. Douthwaite AH. Proctalgia fugax. *Br Med J*. 1962; 2:164–165.

30. Kisner JB, Shorter RG, eds. *Diseases of the Colon, Rectum and Anal Canal*. Baltimore: Williams & Wilkins; 1988:573–574.

31. McGivney JQ, Cleveland BR. The levator syndrome and its treatment. *South Med J*. 1965;58: 505–510.

32. Thompson WG. Proctalgia fugax. *Dig Dis Sci*. 1981;26:1121–1124.

33. Swash M. Chronic perianal pain. In: Henry MM, Swash M, eds. *Coloproctology and the Pelvic Floor. Pathophysiology and Management*. London: Butterworths; 1985:388–392.

34. Pilling LF, Swenson WM, Hill JR. The psychologic aspects of proctalgia fugax. *Dis Colon Rectum*. 1965; 8:372–376.

35. Maroy B. Spontaneous and evoked coccygeal pain in depression. *Dis Colon Rectum*. 1988;31:210–215.

36. Sohn N, Weinstein MA, Robbins RD. The levator syndrome and its treatment with high-voltage electrogalvanic stimulation. *Am J Surg*. 1982;144: 580–582.

CHAPTER 16

ANAL NEOPLASMS

David E. Beck and
Steven D. Wexner

Although malignancies of the lower gastrointestinal tract comprise a large portion of the practice of colorectal surgery, anal neoplasms are uncommon. These lesions have an incidence 1/20 that of rectal adenocarcinoma and comprise 1.5 to 4 percent of large-bowel cancers.[1] Current statistics indicate that this incidence is increasing, and the management of these lesions has recently undergone significant alterations. This chapter describes methods of diagnosis and treatment of common malignant and premalignant lesions of the anus.

Anatomy

Knowledge of anal anatomy is essential to understanding the lesions encountered in this area. Confusion has been caused by disagreements concerning terminology and the relative importance of anatomic structures in this complex area. For clinical purposes, the anus can be divided into two areas: the anal canal and the anal margin (Fig. 16-1). In surgical terms the anal canal is related to the sphincter muscles and runs from the anorectal junction (superior portion of the anal sphincter muscles) to the intersphincteric groove (approximately 2 cm distal to the dentate line).[2] Thus the canal relates directly to the internal anal sphincter.

The lining of the anal canal is endodermal in origin and, in the adult, consists of several types of epithelium. At the superior or proximal edge columnar mucosa is

found. Moving distally toward the dentate line a transitional epithelium is encountered. It contains elements of both columnar and squamous epithelium above the dentate line and squamous epithelium distal to it. The proximity of the anal mucosa to the anal sphincters, the extensive blood supply, and lymphatic drainage in this area are important oncologic considerations.[3] Lymphatic spread of anal canal lesions occurs in three different directions; superiorly to the pararectal and superior hemorrhoidal nodes, laterally to the internal iliac nodes, and inferiorly to the inguinal and external iliac nodes.

The anal margin runs from the intersphincteric groove to approximately 5 cm on the perineum. This doughnut-shaped area is covered by nonkeratinized squamous epithelium of ectodermal origin which changes to keratinized squamous epithelium at its outer border at the perineal skin. These differences in epithelial type and in their relaltionship to the sphincter muscle explain the differing characteristics of lesions in each area. Metastatic anal margin lesions usually spread to the inguinal lymph nodes.

Anal Canal

Malignant neoplasms of the anal canal are rare. They include epidermoid carcinoma, melanoma, sarcoma, and adenocarcinoma of the anal glands (Table 16-1).

Epidermoid Carcinoma

Epidermoid or squamous cell carcinoma is the most common anal neoplasm. Additional names for these

The opinions expressed in this chapter are those of the authors and do not reflect the opinions of the United States Air Force or the Department of Defense.

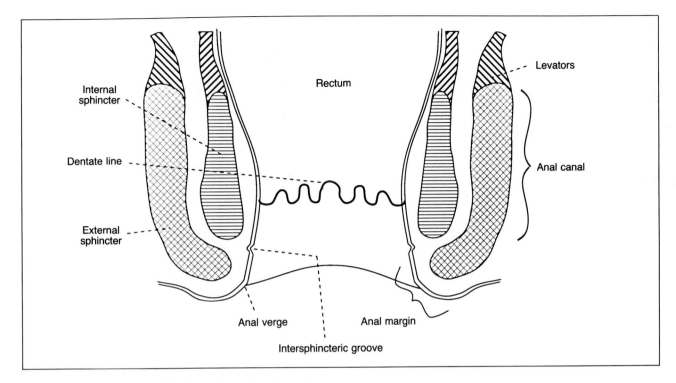

Figure 16-1.   Anatomy of the anal canal and margin.

Table 16-1   Anal Neoplasms

ANAL CANAL	ANAL MARGIN
Epidermoid carcinoma	Premalignant lesions
Squamous	Bowen's disease
Basaloid	Paget's disease
Cloacogenic	Bowenoid papulosis
Basosquamous	Leukoplakia
Epitheloid	Condylomata acuminata*
Transitional	
Mucoepidermoid	Malignant lesions
	Squamous cell carcinoma
Melanoma	Basal cell carcinoma
	Verrucous carcinoma
Adenocarcinoma	Kaposi's sarcoma*
Sarcoma	

* See Chapters 21 and 22

lesions include transitional cell, cloacogenic carcinoma, and others (Table 16-1). Although these lesions have different histologic appearances, their evaluation, treatment, and prognosis are similar and will be discussed together. This decision is not a capricious one, but is instead based upon the identical response of these various lesions to the newer forms of curative chemoradiotherapy.

Diagnosis

The majority of patients with anal cancer are women in their seventh decade of life who present with bright red rectal bleeding and pain. Bleeding occurs in 27 to 74 percent of patients[4] and is usually more constant than that associated with hemorrhoids. Moreover, the bleeding often precedes other symptoms. Of patients with epidermoid carcinoma, 21 to 39 percent have discomfort or pain,[5] which is less severe but more constant than is the pain of an acute fissure. Patients may also occasionally complain of an ulcerated or mass lesion of the anus. The nonspecific nature of complaints may explain delays in diagnosis. However, appropriate questioning will help exclude other differential diagnoses.

The physical examination is helpful in diagnosis and is essential to determine the clinical stage of disease. Anal cancers are either visible or are easily within reach of the examining finger. They tend to be hard, irregular, and usually ulcerated (Figs. 16-2 and 16-3). Most lesions remain undiagnosed until they have grown to between 1 and 5 cm in diameter, but an occasional early lesion may be diagnosed serendipitously upon pathologic review of an operative specimen (Fig. 16-4). This most commonly occurs after hemorrhoidectomy. For this reason, the authors prefer to label each hemorrhoid separately and submit it to the pathologist. The exact location and size of the lesion must be documented

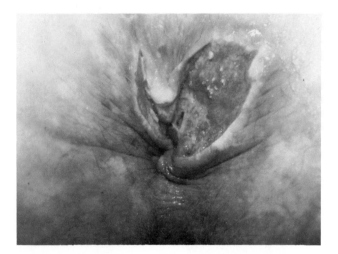

Figure 16-2.   Squamous cell carcinoma of the anus.

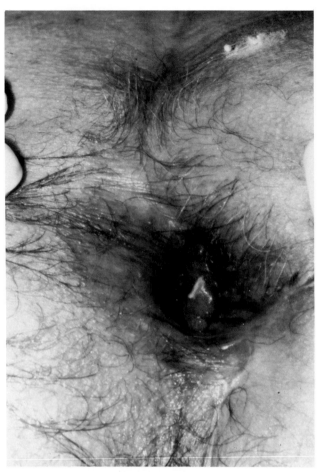

Figure 16-4.   Squamous cell carcinoma of the anus presenting as a prolapsed internal hemorrhoid.

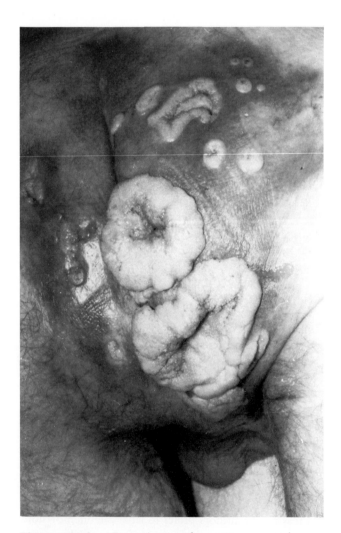

Figure 16-3.   Extensive anal squamous carcinoma. (Courtesy of P. Ronan O'Connor, M.D., Mater Hospital, Dublin, Ireland.)

before initiating treatment. This includes the vertical and horizontal diameter of the lesion, the location relative to the anal verge or dentate line, and position in the anus (e.g., anterior vs posterior and right or left). An assessment of the lesion's fixation, its relation to other structures, and the status of the patient's sphincteric muscles completes the perineal examination. In addition to evaluating the lesion, the clinician should examine the patient for the presence of inguinal adenopathy.

Direct visualization of the anus and rectum is essential to exclude other lesions and to allow biopsy of the lesion to confirm the diagnosis. Anoscopy provides good exposure and is the least expensive method for these purposes. After identification, the lesion should be biopsied by taking several specimens from the edges of the lesion. A local anesthetic is not usually required. Histologically, approximately 70 percent of lesions are found to be squamous cell neoplasms, 25 percent are basaloid neoplasms, and 5 percent are mucoepidermoid.[2] The majority of reports demonstrate that the different histologic types act in a similar clinical manner.

To assist in the clinical staging of these lesions, several methods are currently available. In order of decreasing sensitivity these include intrarectal ultrasonography, CT scanning, and MRI. The details of these diagnostic procedures have been discussed in Chapter 2.

Staging systems for anal carcinoma provide prognostic information and allow comparisons of patient groups. Several systems have been described and subsequently modified, but none has been universally accepted. Limitations of current systems include the inability to stage patients accurately by clinical means alone, alterations in specimens due to therapy, and the frequent lack of tissue for complete evaluation if the therapy does not include surgery. Currently used staging systems vary from simple ones like the Roswell Park Classification (Table 16-2) to the more complex TNM system (Table 16-3). Patients with late stage disease do worse than those with early disease, but most reports do not contain adequate information for appropriate comparisons. The available survival data is discussed below.

Treatment

Anal cancer has been treated by surgery, radiation, chemotherapy, and combinations of these methods. Surgical options include abdominoperineal resection (APR) and transanal (local) excision.

Abdominoperineal Resection. An APR was the standard surgical therapy for anal cancer in the United States prior to 1974, and the reported experience is summarized in Table 16-4. An APR performed for anal cancer is similar to that used for rectal cancer with the exception that a slightly wider margin of perineal skin is removed and a posterior vaginectomy is added for rectovaginal septal involvement. The 5-year survival after this form of treatment averages 50 percent with a published range of 27 to 71 percent.[1,3,26] The wide range in results is explained by the relatively small numbers in some series, differences in reporting, and case selection.[2] Bowman and associates at the Mayo Clinic[7] treated 118 anal canal carcinoma patients over a 26-year period with APR. The 5-year survival was 71 percent, but 40 percent of the patients had recurrent local or metastatic disease. Greenall and colleagues[8] at the Memorial Sloan-Kettering Cancer Center reported on 103 patients with epidermoid carcinoma of the anal canal managed with APR. The absolute 5-year survival was 55 percent and the local recurrence rate was 21 percent.

Abdominoperineal resection is associated with significant morbidity and mortality rates which range from 2 to 14 percent and average 6 percent.[2] Morbidity derives from the major intraabdominal operation required to remove the rectum as well as from the permanent stoma. The local (pelvic) recurrence rate after APR has ranged from 11 to 40 percent,[1,3,26] and such recurrences have rarely been curable.[2] Nodal recurrences in the inguinal regions have been identified in 10 to 25 percent of patients. Distant metastases have been found on presentation in 10 to 15 percent of patients.[7] Many patients subsequently developed distant metastases; these are usually accompanied by pelvic recurrence. At the present time an APR is indicated only after failure of the chemoradiotherapy regimens discussed below.

Local (Transanal) Excision. Local excision should be reserved for lesions that are well differentiated, less than 2 cm in diameter, and located in the distal anal canal. The procedure is similar to that described for early rectal cancers and is described in more detail in Chapter 18. When this procedure was used in selected patients, the reported 5-year survival has ranged from 45 to 100 percent and the local recurrence rate has varied

Table 16-2 Roswell Park Classification for Anal Canal Carcinomas[6]

Stage	Description
0	Carcinoma in situ
1	Sphincter muscle not involved
2	Sphincter muscle not involved
3	Regional metastasis
	A. Perirectal nodes only
	B. Inguinal nodes
4	Distant metastases

Table 16-3 TNM Staging System for Anal Carcinoma

Primary	Tumor
T0	No evidence of primary tumor
T1	Tumor occupying less than ⅓ circumference or length of canal and not infiltrating the external sphincter
T2	Tumor occupying more than ⅓ circumference or length of canal and not infiltrating the external sphincter
T3	Tumor extension to rectum or skin
T4	Tumor extension to neighboring structures
N	Regional lymph nodes
M	Distant metastases

Table 16-4 Outcomes of Abdominoperineal Resection for Anal Canal Carcinoma

Author Year	No. patients	Female, %	Age, mean in yr	Size, < 5, cm%	Recurrence, %		5-year survival, %	Operative Mortality, %
					Local	Distal		
Morson[10] 1960	79	57	58	ns	ns	ns	49	ns
Kuehn, et al[11] 1964	65	55	60	ns	18	69	37	5.0
Klotz et al[12] 1967	194	67	60	66	26	19	50	8.4
Hardcastle and Bussey[13] 1968	83	ns	ns	ns	27	21	48	ns
McConnell[14] 1970	21	49	63	ns	ns	ns	38	14.0
Stearns and Quan[9] 1970	59	58	56	ns	ns	ns	58	ns
Bears and Wilson[15] 1976	80	69	58	74	19	ns	61	3.2
Golden and Horsley[16] 1976	21	69	57	ns	11	10	67	4.8
Sawyers[17] 1977	40	ns	ns	ns	ns	ns	52	ns
Welch and Malt[18] 1977	53	66	ns	3.2*	15	36	42	3.8
Key and Whitehead[19] 1980	25	84	62	ns	16	ns	64	ns
Singh et al[20] 1981	49	65	58	ns	61	27	47	ns
O'Brien et al[21] 1982	21	77	58	ns	ns	24	38	4.8
Schraut et al[22] 1983	26	63	ns	69	35	42	59	3.8
Bowman et al[7] 1984	118	73	59	ns	40	16	71	2.5
Greenall et al[8] 1985	103	69	60	78	21	10	55	ns
Dougherty and Evans[23] 1985	77	82	59	ns	44	18	43	ns
Pillay et al[24] 1987	27	54	58	4.5*	26	ns	50	ns
Brown et al[25] 1988	23	62	59	33†	50	ns	46	9.0
Summary	1129	59	59		28	27	50	5.9

* Mean diameter in cm
† < 4 cm
ns = not specified.

from 8 to 63 percent.[1,26] Bowman and colleagues[7] managed 19 patients with tumors confined to the anal epithelium or internal sphincter by local excision. The group had an overall 5-year survival of 100 percent. One patient had a local recurrence which was treated with an APR; subsequent survival was in excess of 5 years without additional recurrence. Stearns and Quan[9] reported on 30 patients with lesions of the anal canal and perianal area managed by local excision. The 5-year survival was 66 percent and the local recurrence rate was 63 percent. The studies listed in Table 16-5 are neither controlled nor randomized. However, these data support treating selected patients who have early lesions with local excision.

Prophylactic inguinal lymph node excision was considered in the past but is not currently recommended due to a lack of clear indications and demonstrated survival benefit.[3] Clinically involved nodes should be sampled by fine needle aspiration or excisional biopsy for prognostic and staging procedures. Therapeutic lymphadenectomy for clinically detectable lymph node metastases present at the time of APR results in 5-year survival of 10 to 20 percent.[2]

Radiotherapy. Anal carcinomas are radiosensitive tumors, and the role of radiotherapy continues to evolve. Although this method is widely accepted in Europe, its use in the United States has only recently become widespread. The advantages of radiotherapy include treatment of the tumor and its lymphatic drainage with preservation of the anus. Radiation therapy can be administered as external beam therapy, as intraluminal (contact) therapy, or by implants (interstitially). Modern high voltage external beam therapy (1–4 MeV) delivers more energy to the tumor with less damage to the skin than older and lower-voltage external methods. Different techniques and combinations of methods have been described. Each method has advantages and disadvantages, but no prospective comparisons are available.

The reported 5-year survival after external beam radiotherapy ranges from 46 to 92 percent with an average of 68 percent (Table 16-6). The local recurrence rate ranges from 12 to 77 percent. The wide variation in these results is due to differences in technique and patient selection. Some of the poorer results, especially in the American studies, can be attributed to the selection of patients with large tumors for radiotherapy.

Some patients have radiation-associated complications such as skin burns, cystitis, and proctitis; 5 to 15 percent of patients suffer complications severe enough to require rectal excision. This latter group of complications includes incontinence, anal stricture, and mucosal necrosis.[26] Other potential major complications associated with radiotherapy include urethral and

Table 16-5   Outcomes of Local Surgical Therapy for Anal Carcinoma

Author Year	No. patients	Female, %	Age, mean in yr	Size, < 2 cm, %	Recurrence, % Local	Recurrence, % Distal	5-year survival, %
Kuehn, et al[11] 1964	26	55	60	85	8	15	75
Klotz et al[12] 1967	33	67	60	54	33	ns	61
Stearns and Quan[9] 1970	30	58	56	ns	63	23	66
Shraut et al[22] 1983	7	63	ns	86	29	29	71
Bowman et al[7] 1984	14	73	59	92	8	0	100
Greenall et al[8] 1985	11	69	60	73	27	73	45
Goldman et al[27] 1985	17	68	66	ns	ns	ns	80
Summary	138	63	60	78	28	28	71

ns = not specified.

Table 16-6 Outcomes of Radiation Therapy for Anal Canal Cancer

Author Year	No. patients	Female, %	Age, mean in yr	Size, < 5 cm, %	Radiotherapy Dosage (Gy)	Recurrence, % Local	Recurrence, % Distal	5-year survival, %	Continence, %	Major complications, %
EXTERNAL										
Green et al[28] 1980	17	58	65	100	60	6	24	81	100	0
Cummings et al[29] 1982	51	73	63	10	45–50	27	ns	71	77	6
Cantril et al[30] 1983	47	51	64	90*	66	20	ns	80	92	28
Eschwege et al[31] 1985	64	83	62	24†	60–65	19	ns	46	74	14
Doggett et al[32] 1988	35	57	59	3.1cm	64	77	6	92	80	6
Dobrowsky[33] 1989	14	57	72	73†	60	14	ns	57	93	0
EXTERNAL AND/OR INTERSTITIAL										
Salmon et al[34] 1984	158	77	67	36	45–60	33	8	59	80	7
Ying Kin et al[35] 1988	32	75	71	36	64	25	25	61	69	13
Papillon and Montbarbon[36] 1987	222	83	66	69	45–62	12	21	65	80	3
Summary	640	68	58			26	17	68	73	9

* < 4 cm
† T1
ns = not specified.

228

vaginal strictures or fistulas, enterocolitis, and lower extremity edema.

The largest experience is that of Papillon and Montbarbon[36]: 243 patients received a split course of therapy. During the first course, a minimum tumor dose of 30 gray was administered in 19 days using high energy x-rays to a target volume that included the anal area and the presacral and posterior pelvic nodes. Two months later a second course of 15 to 20 gray was given to the bed of the primary tumor with a single-plane [192] iridium implant using five to seven wires placed in steel needles fixed to a plastic template sutured to the perineal skin. Therapy was generally well tolerated, although most patients had a short period of mild proctitis and perianal irritation. There was no perianal fibrosis, but 2.2 percent of patients developed severe anal radionecrosis which required a colostomy with or without rectal excision. All patients had a follow-up of at least 3 years with a 64.4 percent survival; 173 followed for 5 years had a similar 64.1 percent survival. Approximately 20 percent developed local or distal recurrences and subsequently died of cancer.

Overall results of this and other series are comparable to those obtained after an abdominoperineal resection. The major advantage of radiotherapy is that 75 percent of patients retain a functional anus.[3] Additional studies using modern radiotherapeutic techniques are necessary to determine the appropriate role of modern radiotherapy alone.

Multimodality Approach. Because of the inadequate results from surgery or radiotherapy available by the 1970s, additional alternatives were sought. Dr. Nigro, at Wayne State University, proposed a multimodality approach with initial chemotherapy and radiotherapy followed by abdominoperineal resection. In 1974, Nigro reported his initial results in three patients using 5-fluorouracil, mitomycin-C, and radiotherapy (30 gray) followed by an APR in two of the patients.[37] The operative specimens had no residual tumor and the third patient (who refused surgery) was clinically free of tumor at 14-month follow-up.

Additional experience and longer follow-up was reported by the same group in 1983 and again in 1987[38,39]: 104 patients with squamous cell carcinoma of the anal canal were treated at several institutions between 1971 to 1983. Gross tumor disappeared in 97 patients after the initial chemoradiotherapic regimen described above. A radical operation was performed routinely in 24 patients (22 of whom had no residual tumor in the specimens) and for residual disease in 7. Biopsy specimens of the posttreatment scar were obtained from 62 patients after chemoradiotherapy and there was no tumor in 61 of these patients. Toxicity from the chemoradiation was reported to be mild or moderate in 99 of the 104 patients; 5 patients developed toxicity requiring hospitalization but had no long-term complications. Follow-up in this study ranged from 2 to 11 years after treatment: 7 patients had APRs for recurrent disease and 84 patients were alive and free of disease at last follow-up. The authors calculated a 5-year survival of 83 percent. Patients with large (6–8 cm) primary cancers were more likely to have persistent tumors after chemoradiotherapy. These patients and those with recurrent lesions were managed with additional chemoradiation therapy, abdominoperineal resection, or both.

The experience with combination therapy at Wilford Hall USAF Medical Center includes 31 patients treated from 1981 to 1990. Mitomycin-C and 5-fluorouracil were administered as suggested by Nigro and associates.[37-39] The radiotherapy was delivered in 2 gray doses in apposed fields and averaged 38 gray. In our initial 7 patients, an abdominoperineal resection was performed after the combined therapy. In the first 4 patients treated by this method, no residual tumor was found in the pathologic specimens. Based on this and reports of Nigro and other authors, the later 24 patients were examined 4 to 6 weeks after completing chemoradiotherapy. If any residual tumor was suspected a biopsy of the tumor site was performed. Only one patient had persistent tumor which required an abdominoperineal resection. In the overall group, two patients developed hepatic recurrence and one developed metastases to the lumbar spine (12.5 percent). One patient also developed a local recurrence (2 years after initial combination therapy) which was treated with an APR. Compared to historical controls, this is a significantly lower recurrence rate ($P < 0.02$). Since adopting combined chemotherapy and radiotherapy as our primary treatment of anal cancer we have achieved survival rates as good as our previous methods, and there is a trend toward improved survival. In addition, the local recurrence rate has been significantly improved.

The reported experience with multimodality treatment for anal carcinoma continues to expand (Table 16-7). Summarizing the published results shows a local recurrence rate of 3 to 29 percent and a toxicity of 20 to 30 percent.[3] However, the reported follow-up after combination therapy remains short and results of controlled trials are not currently available. Because of the significantly better results obtained with multimodality therapy compared to historical experience with other treatment methods, it seems doubtful that controlled trials comparing radiotherapy with APR will be conducted. The exact role of chemotherapy and radiotherapy in tumor destruction also remains to be fully evaluated. Each technique has a toxicity which is enhanced when the methods are combined. The low inci-

Table 16-7 Outcomes of Multimodality Therapy for Anal Canal Carcinoma

Author Year	No. patients	Female, %	Age mean in yr.	Size >6 cm, %	Radiotherapy Dosage (Gy)	Radiotherapy Chemotherapy	Recurrence, % Local	Recurrence, % Distal	Continence, %	Survival, %	Follow-up	Persistent Tumor, %
Nigro[37-39] (Wayne State) 1984*	104	73	(32–80)	19	30	F,M	7	13	64	83	2–11 yrs	11
Cummings et al[40] (Princess Margaret) 1984	30	66	56	50	50	F,M	6	6	87	93	25 mo (8–50 mo)	7
Sischy[41] (Memorial Sloan-Kettering) 1985	33	56	71	ns	45	F,M	11	7	88	78	51 mo (5–74 mo)	9
Leichman et al[42] 1985	45	64	58	22	30	F,M	4	16	60	89	50 mo (18–124 mo)	16
Enker et al[43] (Memorial Sloan-Kettering) 1986	44	66	55	30	30	F,M	23	0	56	82	42 mo (1–89 mo)	41
Meeker et al[44] 1986	19	89	56	42‡	30	F,M	5	5	47	87	30 mo	12
Pillay et al[24] 1987	18	78	61	ns			19				21 mo	
Flam et al (UCSF)[45] 1987	30	77	61	ns	41	F,M	3	0	100	90	9–79 mo	13
Glimelius and Pahlman[46] 1987	23	93	64	50	40–65	B	9	4	86	79	45 mo	4
John et al[47] (Fresno) 1987	22	ns	61	65‡	41–45	F,M	5	0	100	100	17–62 mo	14
Habr–Gama et al[48] (San Paulo) 1989	30	70	60	47	30–45	F,M	13	7	80	70	36 mo (6–72 mo)	27
Sischy et al[49] (RTOG) 1989	79	65	ns	63†	40	F,M	29	11	90	73	36 mo (20–55 mo)	10
Beck[3] (WHMC) 1990	31	71	59		30–45	F,M	3	10		94	48 mo (1–108 mo)	3
Summary	463	66	55				11	6	80	84		14

* Collected series
† > 3 cm diameter
‡ T3 or T4
F = 5-Fluorouracil.
M = Mitomycin-C.
B = Bleomycin.
ns = not specified.

dence of epidermoid cancer necessitates multicenter prospective controlled trials to study these issues.

Based on current experience, multimodality therapy for anal cancer has become the primary treatment of choice. The authors currently recommend combined therapy as initial treatment for patients with epidermoid anal cancer. The radiotherapy entails 30 to 40 gray given over 3 to 4 weeks using apposed fields. Chemotherapy is given at the same time as the radiotherapy according to the following scheme: intravenous 5-fluorouracil (1000 mg/m^2/day) on days 1 to 5 and days 31 to 35 and mitomycin-C (15 mg/m^2) on day 1. Our patients undergo an evaluation to include a biopsy at the lesion site 1 month after completion of the radiotherapy. An APR is offered to those patients with residual disease following combined therapy.

Melanoma

Anorectal melanomas are rare, accounting for 1 percent of all melanomas and 0.25 to 1 percent of anorectal tumors.[50] The mean age of occurrence is in the fifth decade, and females are affected more frequently than males. The most frequent presenting symptom is bleeding, followed by an anal mass or pain. The lesions are usually elevated, and 34 to 75 percent are pigmented.[51] Small lesions that are pigmented have been mistaken for thrombosed hemorrhoids.

In a large collective review of the histologic features of anorectal melanomas, Cooper and colleagues found that 77 percent of tumors contained melanin pigment microscopically.[51] This finding, along with junctional changes (present in 75% of Cooper's cases) and a nesting growth pattern (even if subtle or focal) is helpful in making a diagnosis of melanoma. Both immunohistochemistry and electron microscopy can demonstrate melanosomes, which helps to confirm the diagnosis. Although most melanomas of the anorectum are thought to arise from melanocytes in the anoderm, primary melanoma of the rectum may occur.[52] This lesion, if it exists, originates from a melanocyte-like cell within the rectal mucosa.[53]

Melanomas are locally invasive and have a high metastatic potential. Patients treated in a curative fashion have a survival of 6 to 20 percent,[54] while series including all patients have reported 5-year survival rates that range from 0 to 12 percent.[51,55] Prognosis is related to tumor size, thickness, and clinical stage. Evaluation should include a biopsy of the lesion and a search for metastatic disease (CT scans of the abdomen, pelvis, and chest; liver function tests; chest x-ray, and bone scans).

Surgery provides the only hope for cure, but none of the published series demonstrated a statistically significant difference in survival between patients treated with local excision and those treated with APR. Most series did, however, demonstrate improved local control with APR. Unfortunately, local recurrence in these cases was often accompanied by the appearance of distal or regional metastases as well.

There is some indication that survival is linked to the depth or thickness of the tumor, but data relating to tumor thickness is lacking in most of the literature.[56] The choice of surgical therapy remains controversial. Some investigators recommend APR for lesions less than 3.0 mm in depth, as they believe these tumors are the only lesions that are potentially curable.[57] Others have concluded that the majority of patients eventually succumb to distal metastases.[56,58] These authors have recommended a local resection when technically feasible. The same authors have reserved abdominoperineal resections for lesions that cannot be locally resected and those which have recurred after local excision.[56,58] An APR has a significant morbidity and mortality, but long-term survival occurred only in patients treated with an APR. Prophylactic lymphadenectomy is not indicated for clinically negative nodes but is helpful for clinically suspicious nodes. Radiotherapy and chemotherapy have demonstrated little benefit in this disease.

Adenocarcinoma

Adenocarcinomas of the anal canal are very rare and are thought to arise in the ducts of anal glands or in long-standing fistulas.[59] These neoplasms affect older age groups and have no sexual predominance.[60] Most of these lesions are slow growing, are locally aggressive, and rarely metastasize. Accurate diagnosis requires a deep biopsy because the lesions have a low grade histologic appearance and readily invade local tissue. The abundant mucin production of these tumors may explain their tendency to dissect soft tissue planes.

These lesions can be treated similarly to rectal carcinomas. Small well-differentiated carcinomas not involving the sphincter mechanism may be managed with a wide local excision. However, older studies identified a high recurrence rate after local excision.[59] If the anorectal musculature is involved an APR is indicated.[26]

Sarcoma

Anorectal sarcomas are very rare and produce symptoms similar to those related to other anal lesions. The lesions may be intra- or extraluminal and may show differentiation resembling any tissue of mesodermal origin. These tumors therefore include leiomyosarcoma, fibrosarcoma, liposarcoma, and others. These tumors are all radioresistant, and APR is the treatment of choice.[61]

Anal Margin

Premalignant Lesions

Premalignant lesions of the anal margin are uncommon. They include Bowen's and Paget's diseases, Bowenoid papulosis, and leukoplakia (see Table 16-1).

Bowen's Disease

Bowen's disease is an uncommon intraepithelial squamous cell carcinoma, named after John T. Bowen, who in 1912 described two patients with atypical epithelial proliferation of the skin.[62] The first perianal case of Bowen's disease was reported by Vickers in 1939,[63] and to date slightly over 150 cases have been reported.[64]

Patients with perianal Bowen's disease commonly present with nonspecific complaints of anal itching, burning, or bleeding. They are usually age 40 to 50 years of age and the majority of patients are female.[64]

Examination of the perineum in symptomatic patients usually reveals raised, irregular, scaly brownish-red plaques with eczematoid features. These lesions may have a gross appearance similar to other diseases such as leukoplakia, squamous cell cancer, condylomata acuminata, dermatitis, or eczema. A significant percentage of lesions are diagnosed after pathologic evaluation of operative specimens.[65] Such diagnosis occurs most frequently after operative hemorrhoidectomy, again emphasizing the benefit of separately labeling and submitting each excised hemorrhoid.

The microscopic appearance of these perianal lesions is characteristic and readily confirms the diagnosis. Bowen's disease demonstrates a disordered epidermal hyperplasia with parakeratosis and hyperkeratosis in the superficial surface layers. The malpighian cells also reveal a disordered hyperplasia, with atypism and malignant dyskeratotic cells. Large atypical cells with haloed large hyperchromatic nuclei (Bowenoid cells) are present and are negative for a periodic acid–Schiff (PAS) stain; mitotic figures are present in all layers (Fig. 16-5).

An accurate diagnosis is important for both prognostic and therapeutic reasons. The clinical course of Bowen's disease has been relatively benign with progression toward invasive carcinoma in 2 to 6 percent of cases.[65] In addition to concern about progression to an invasive cancer, a relationship between these epithelial lesions and nonepithelial malignancies has been proposed.[66] Early reports described such a relationship, but a recent reexamination of the methods and analysis used in these published studies demonstrated several flaws. The authors concluded that the evidence was insufficient to confirm a relationship between Bowen's disease and the subsequent development of internal malignancies.[67] In addition, a recent collective survey of experi-

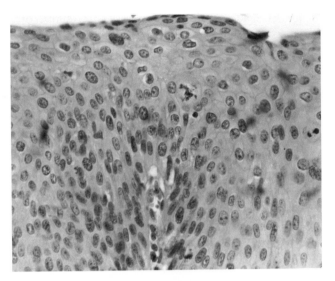

Figure 16-5.   Perianal Bowen's disease (Hematoxylin and eosin, ×240).

ence with perianal Bowen's disease found the incidence of subsequent nonsquamous malignancy to be low, at 4.7 percent.[68]

Patients with anal lesions that appear suspicious or fail to respond to conventional therapy within a month should undergo an evaluation to exclude an associated invasive cancer.[69]

If evaluation demonstrates an invasive carcinoma without metastases, an aggressive approach is warranted to improve the historically poor prognosis associated with these diseases. For adenocarcinoma of the lower rectum the authors recommend an abdominoperineal resection, and for epidermoid anal cancer the authors currently use combination chemoradiotherapy. In the absence of invasive cancer, the authors prefer local excision. Adequate microscopically normal margins are very important, as both Bowen's and Paget's cells may extend beyond the gross margins of the lesion.[64] To ensure a complete excision the authors currently use "lesion mapping." Biopsies are obtained 1 cm from the edge of the lesion and in all four quadrants of the perineum. Specimens 2 to 3 mm in diameter are taken as shown in Fig. 16-6 at the dentate line, anal verge, and the perineum (approximately 2 to 3 cm from the anal verge). This mapping is used to guide a wide local excision of the lesion.[70] After removal of the specimen, the margins of resection are examined by frozen section techniques to ensure complete excision. The wound defect is closed primarily if the wounds encompass less than 30 percent of the anal circumference. Wounds greater than 30 percent are covered with a split-thickness skin graft either at the initial operation or 3 or 4 days later. Alternatively, they may be left to heal by secondary intention. The low recurrence rate in patients

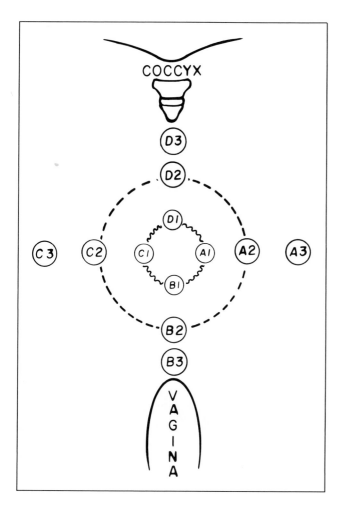

Figure 16-6.   Anal mapping. 1 = Dentate line. 2 = Anal verge. 3 = Perineum (2–3 cm from anal verge).

treated by wide local excision supports this therapy as the appropriate method.

Long-term follow-up is recommended to help limit recurrence of perianal Bowen's disease.[65] However, the limited experience with this disease has hindered the development of a standardized follow-up regimen. An annual complete physical examination, proctosigmoidoscopy, punch biopsy of any new lesions, and random biopsies at the edges of the split-thickness skin graft are recommended.[65] Colonoscopy is also performed at intervals of 2 to 3 years. If a recurrence is found, it is excised with adequate clear margins using the methods already described.

Paget's Disease

Paget's disease is an even rarer intraepithelial adenocarcinoma. The lesion was named for Sir James Paget, who described 15 patients with a characteristic breast lesion in 1874.[71] The extramammary variety can be found

wherever apocrine glands are located. A case of perianal disease was first reported in 1893 by Darier and Coulillaud.[72] Since then over 100 cases of perianal disease have been reported in the surgical literature.[52,73,74]

Patients with perianal Paget's disease average 65 years of age, and the sex distribution is equal.[73] They present with nonspecific complaints of anal itching, burning, or bleeding. The perianal lesions are well demarcated eczematoid plaques that are either ulcerative and crusty or papillary. Less commonly these lesions may have a gross appearance similar to other diseases as described in Bowen's disease.

The origin of Paget's cells has been debated for many years. Theories included primitive multipotential epidermal cells or elements of glandular cells.[74] Recent work supports a glandular origin as these cells contain low molecular weight cytokeratins and carcinoembryonic antigen (CEA). In addition they express the gross cystic disease fluid protein (GCDFP).[74]

On pathologic evaluation perianal Paget's disease is characterized by large, faintly basophilic or vacuolated cells located in the epidermis (Fig. 16-7). The nuclei are vesicular and demonstrate little mitotic activity. In contrast to Bowenoid cells, the Paget cells become highlighted with a periodic acid–Schiff (PAS) stain owing to their high mucin content. Since they contain CEA, they also can be visualized by CEA immunofluorescence techniques.[73]

In Paget's disease, progression of the lesion into an invasive carcinoma has been reported to be as high as 40 percent in untreated lesions.[52] However, the small number of reported patients with these perianal lesions has limited our understanding about prognosis. The association of Paget's disease with other cancers has been much stronger than is the association for Bowen's disease. The incidence of associated malignancies with

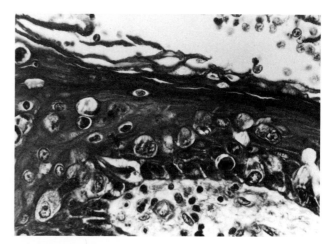

Figure 16-7.   Perianal Paget's disease (Hematoxylin and eosin, ×210).

234 Fundamentals of Anorectal Surgery

Paget's disease in reported series ranges from 38 to 86 percent, and the mortality was high from this cancer despite aggressive therapy.[52,74,75]

In the absence of invasive malignancies, wide local excision is adequate therapy.[73] Currettage and radiotherapy have no place; patients treated with these modalities have had high recurrence rates. In the series reported by Jensen and colleagues, all 7 patients managed with curettage or radiotherapy developed recurrent disease within 6 months.[52]

If an associated malignancy is diagnosed, an aggressive approach is warranted to alter the historically poor prognosis. Long-term survivals have been reported after abdominoperineal resections in patients without metastatic disease at presentation.

Long-term follow-up is essential as 61 percent of the patients in Jensen's series developed recurrent disease up to 8 years after primary treatment. This high figure may be due to inadequate initial treatment.

Bowenoid Papulosis

Bowenoid papulosis is also a rare squamous premalignant lesion. It is histologically similar to Bowen's disease but has several significant clinical differences.[76] The findings are usually numerous 2- to 10-mm diameter lesions on the perineum. The lesions are flat, slightly elevated, and discrete. They are slightly pigmented, generally reddish to violaceous and somewhat scaley. Occasionally the lesions are continuous, forming plaquelike lesions.[77] Ulcers are not present. Histologically they are indistinguishable from Bowen's disease.

These lesions occur in young patients (most are in their late twenties or early thirties) and have been reported more often in males. There has been a high incidence of prior viral infection—herpes simplex virus (HSV) or human papillomavirus (HPV). Hybridization studies have demonstrated HPV-16 DNA in 80 percent of examined lesions.[78] The significance of this is discussed further in Chapters 21 and 22. Basically, however, HPV-16 and HPV-18 are associated both with anal malignancies and with condylomata acuminata. Therefore, condylomata may precede Bowenoid papulosis or anal cancer, especially in patients who practice anal receptive intercourse. Clinically these lesions have a benign course. Patients are usually treated for symptomatic relief. Eradication of these lesions has been accomplished by excision or destruction as described for condylomata. A recent report of low-dose treatment with recombinant interferon-2c has shown promise.[79]

Leukoplakia

Leukoplakia is a whitish thickening of the mucous membranes that may represent a precancerous dermatosis. Patients commonly complain of itching, bleeding, and discharge. Microscopically the lesions appear as hyperkeratosis and squamous metaplasia.[80] Patients should be treated symptomatically, and regular follow-up is indicated because of the questionable malignant potential. Any suspicious lesion should be biopsied to exclude a malignant lesion.

Malignant Lesions

Malignant lesions of the anal margin include squamous cell carcinoma, basal cell carcinoma, and Kaposi's sarcoma. These lesions generally tend to behave in a less invasive manner and have a better prognosis than malignant lesions of the anal canal.

Squamous Cell Cancer

Squamous cell cancer of the anal margin acts in a manner similar to lesions that occur in other cutaneous areas of the body. The lesions appear as raised and flat masses

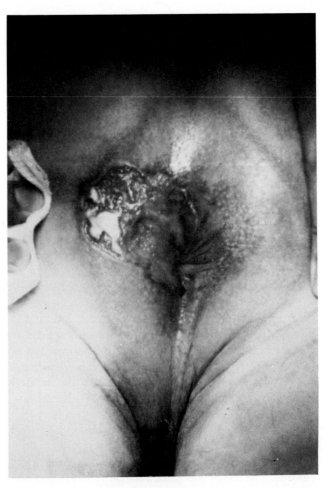

Figure 16-8. Basal cell cancer of the anus. (Courtesy of Frank Harford, M.D.)

that may ulcerate. Appropriate therapy is wide local excision with clear margins.[1]

Basal Cell Cancers

Basal cell cancers of the anal margin are rare and appear as ulcerated masses. They are more frequent in men and usually occur in the sixth decade of life.[26] Nonspecific complaints include bleeding and pruritus. The lesions are similar to other basal cell cancers of the skin and usually have a central ulceration with a raised pearly border (Fig. 16-8). Nielson and Jensen reported on 34 patients collected from the Danish Registry of Cancer.[81] Nineteen patients (59 percent) has tumors less than 3 cm in diameter, but 1 percent of the lesions were 5 to 10 cm in size. The larger lesions required an APR and the smaller ones were treated by wide excision. The importance of adequate margins is stressed by the 29 percent recurrence rate experienced by patients in this series. These lesions are slow growing and rarely metastasize, which explains why no patient in this series died of the disease. A wide local excision with clear margins is the treatment of choice. Incomplete excision leads to a recurrence rate of up to 50 percent.[81] An APR is necessary when lesions extend into the anal canal or surrounding tissues.[82] The role of radiotherapy has not been determined. The 5-year survival of reported patients exceeds 73 percent.[81]

Verrucous Carcinoma

Verrocous carcinomas are well-differentiated squamous cell cancers that are locally aggressive but rarely metastasize. In appearance they resemble large anal condylomata and can only be distinguished by invasion into local tissue.[83] Hence the terms "giant condylomata acuminata" or "Buschke-Lowenstein tumor." Excision with an adequate margin is required to reduce the incidence of local recurrence. For large lesions an APR may be required.

Kaposi's Sarcoma

Kaposi's sarcoma is an uncommon malignancy that occurs in four forms. Most recently a form of this lesion associated with the acquired immunodeficiency syndrome has been described. The lesion is radioresponsive and is discussed in Chapter 22.

References

1. Localio SA, Eng K, Coppa GF. Anorectal presacral and sacral tumors. Philadelphia: WB Saunders; 1987:46–67.
2. Cummings BJ. Current management of epidermoid carcinoma of the anal canal. *Gastroenterol Clin North Am.* 1987;16:125–142.
3. Beck DE. Anal neoplasms. In: Beck DE, Welling DG, eds. *Patient Care in Colorectal Surgery.* Boston: Little, Brown; 1991.
4. Montague ED. Squamous cell carcinoma of the anus. In: Fletcher GH, ed. *Textbook of Radiotherapy.* 3rd ed. Philadelphia: Lee & Febiger; 1982.
5. Mitchel EP. Carcinoma of the anal region. *Semin Oncol.* 1988;15:146–153.
6. Paradis P, Douglas HO, Holyoke ED. The clinical implications of a staging system for carcinoma of the anus. *Surg Gynecol Obstet.* 1975;141:411–416.
7. Bowman BM, Moertel CG, O'Connell MJ, et al. Carcinoma of the anal canal: a clinical and pathologic study of 188 cases. *Cancer.* 1984;54:114–125.
8. Greenall MJ, Quan SHQ, Urmacher C, DeCosse JJ. Treatment of epidermoid carcinoma of the anal canal. *Surg Gynecol Obstet.* 1985;161:509–517.
9. Stearns MW, Quan SHQ. Epidermoid carcinoma of the anorectum. *Surg Gynecol. Obstet.* 1970;131:953–957.
10. Morson BC. Discussion on squamous cell carcinoma of the anus and anal canal. *Proc R Soc Med.* 1960;53:416–419.
11. Kuehn PG, Beckett R, Eisenberg H, Reed JF. Epidermoid carcinoma of the perianal skin and anal canal: a review of 157 cases. *N Engl J Med.* 1964;270:614–616.
12. Klotz RG, Pamukcoglu T, Souilliard DH. Transitional cloacogenic carcinoma of the anal canal. *Cancer.* 1967;20:1727–1745.
13. Hardcastle JD, Bussey HJR. Results of surgical treatment of squamous cell carcinoma of the anal canal and the anal margin. *Proc R Soc Med.* 1968;61:629.
14. McConnel EM. Squamous carcinoma of the anus—a review of 96 cases. *Br J Surg.* 1970;57:89.
15. Bears OH, Wilson SM. Carcinoma of the anus. *Ann Surg.* 1976;184:422–428.
16. Golden GT, Horsley JS. Surgical management of epidermoid carcinoma of the anus. *Am J Surg.* 1976;131:275–280.
17. Sawyers JL. Current management of carcinoma of the anus and perianus. *Am Surg.* 1977;43:424–429.
18. Welch JP, Malt RA. Appraisal of the treatment of carcinoma of the anus and anal canal. *Surg Gynecol Obstet.* 1977;145:837–841.

19. Key JC, Whitehead WA. Surgical treatment of carcinoma of the anus. *South Med J.* 1980;73: 1311–1313.

20. Singh R. Nimme F, Mittelman A. Malignant epithelial tumors of the anal canal. *Cancer.* 1981;48:411–415.

21. O'Brien PH, Jenrette JM, Wallace KM, Metcalf JS. Epidermoid carcinoma of the anus. *Surg Gynecol Obstet.* 1982;155:745–751.

22. Schraut WH, Wang CH, Dawson PJ, Block GE. Depth of invasion, location, and size of cancer of the anus dictate operative treatment. *Cancer.* 1983;51:1291–1296.

23. Dougherty BG, Evans HL. Carcinoma of the anal canal: a study of 79 cases. *Am J Clin Pathol.* 1985;83:159–164.

24. Pillay SP, Watson R, Wynne C, et al. Carcinoma of the anal canal. *Med J Aust.* 1987;147:438–441.

25. Brown DK, Oglesby AB, Scott DH, Dayton MT. Squamous cell carcinoma of the anus: a twenty-five year retrospective. *Am Surg.* 1988;54:337–342.

26. Gordon PH. Current status—perianal and anal canal neoplasms. *Dis Colon Rectum.* 1990;33:799–808.

27. Goldman S, Ihre TH, Seligson U. Squamous-cell carcinoma of the anus: a follow-up study of 65 patients. *Dis Colon Rectum.* 1985;28:143–146.

28. Green JP, Schaupp WC, Cantril ST, Schall G. Anal carcinoma: current therapeutic concepts. *Am J Surg.* 1980;140:151–155.

29. Cummings BJ, Thomas GM, Keane TJ, Harwood AR, Rider WD. Primary radiation therapy in the treatment of anal canal carcinoma. *Dis Colon Rectum.* 1982;25:778–782.

30. Cantril ST, Green JP, Schall GL, Schaupp WC. Primary radiation therapy in the treatment of anal carcinoma. *Int J Radiat Oncol Biol Phys.* 1983; 9:1271–1278.

31. Eschwege F, Lasser A, Chary P, Wibault KJ, Rougler P, Bognel C. Squamous cell carcinoma of the anal canal: treatment by external beam irradiation. *Radiother Oncol.* 1985;3:145–150.

32. Doggett SW, Green JP, Cantril ST. Efficacy of radiation therapy alone for limited squamous cell carcinoma of the anal canal. *Int J Radiat Oncol Biol Phys.* 1988;15:1069–1072.

33. Dobrowsky W. Radiotherapy of epidermoid anal canal cancer. *Br J Radiol.* 1989;62:53–58.

34. Salmon RJ, Fenton J, Asselain B, et al. Treatment of epidermoid anal canal cancer. *Am J Surg.* 1984;147:43–48.

35. Ng Ying Kin NYK, Pigneux J, Auvray H, et al. Our experience of conservative treatment of anal canal carcinoma combining external irradiation and interstitial implant: 32 cases treated between 1973

and 1982. *Int J Radiat Oncol Biol Phys.* 1988;14: 253–259.

36. Papillon J, Montbarbon JF. Epidermoid carcinoma of the anal canal: a series of 276 cases. *Dis Colon Rectum.* 1987;30:324–333.

37. Nigro ND, Vaitkenicius VK. Combined therapy for cancer of the anal canal. *Dis Colon Rectum.* 1974;17:354–356.

38. Nigro ND, Seydel M, Considine B, et al. Combined preoperative radiation and chemotherapy for squamous cell carcinoma of the anal canal. *Cancer.* 1983;51:1826–1829.

39. Nigro ND. Multidisciplinary management of cancer of the anus. *World J Surg.* 1987;11:1–6.

40. Cummings B, Keane T, Thomas G, et al. Results and toxicity of the treatment of anal canal carcinoma by radiation therapy or radiation therapy and chemotherapy. *Cancer.* 1984;54:2062–2068.

41. Sischy B. The use of radiation therapy combined with chemotherapy in the management of squamous cell carcinoma of the anus and marginally resectable adenocarcinoma of the rectum. *Int J Radiat Oncol Biol Phys.* 1985;11:1587–1593.

42. Leichman L, Nigro N, Vaitkevicius VK, et al. Cancer of the anal canal. Model for preoperative adjuvant combined modality therapy. *Am J Med.* 1985;78:211–215.

43. Enker WE, Hellwell M, Janov AJ, et al. Improved survival in epidermoid carcinoma of the anus in association with preoperative multidisciplinary therapy. *Arch Surg.* 1986;121:1386–1390.

44. Meeker WR, Sickle-Santanello BJ, Philpott G, et al. Combined chemotherapy, radiation, and surgery for epithelial cancer of the anal canal. *Cancer.* 1986;57:525–529.

45. Flam MS, John MJ, Mowry PA, et al. Definitive combined modality therapy of carcinoma of the anus. *Dis Colon Rectum.* 1987;30:495–502.

46. Glimelius B, Pahlman L. Radiation therapy of anal epidermoid carcinoma. *Int J Radiat Oncol Biol Phys.* 1987;13:305–312.

47. John MJ, Flam M, Lovalvo L, Mowry PA. Feasibility of nonsurgical definitive management of anal canal carcinoma. *Int J Radiat Oncol Biol Phys.* 1987; 13:299–303.

48. Habr-Gama A, da Silva e Sousa AH, Nadalin W, et al. Epidermoid carcinoma of the anal canal: results of treatment by combined chemotherapy and radiation therapy. *Dis Colon Rectum.* 1989;32:773–777.

49. Sischy B, Scotte Doggett RL, Krall JM, et al. Definitive irradiation and chemotherapy for radiosensitization in management of anal carcinoma: interim report on radiation therapy oncology group study no. 8314. *J Natl Cancer Inst.* 1989;81:850–856.

50. Siegal B, Cohen D, Jacob ET. Surgical treatment of anorectal melanomas. *Am J Surg*. 1983;146:336–338.

51. Cooper PH, Mills SE, Allen MS. Malignant melanoma of the anus—report of 12 patients and analysis of 225 additional cases. *Dis Colon Rectum*. 1982;25:693–703.

52. Jensen SL, Sjolin KE, Shokouh-Amir I MH, Hagen K, Harling H. Paget's disease of the anal margin. *Br J Surg*. 1988;75:1089–1092.

53. Werdin C, Limas C, Knodell RG. Primary malignant melanoma of the rectum. *Cancer*. 1988;61:1364–1370.

54. Bolivar JC, Haris JW, Branch W, Sherman RT. Melanoma of the anorectal region. *Surg Gynecol Obstet*. 1982;154:337–341.

55. NcNamara MJ. Melanoma and basal cell cancer. In: Fazio VW, ed. *Current Therapy in Colon and Rectal Surgery*. Philadelphia:BC Decker; 1990.

56. Ross M, Pezzi C, Pezzi T, et al. Patterns of failure in anorectal melanoma: a guide to surgical therapy. *Arch Surg*. 1990;125:313–316.

57. Wanebo HJ, Woodruff JM, Farr GH, Guan SH. Anorectal melanoma. *Cancer*. 1981;47:1891.

58. Ward MWN, Romano G, Nichols RJ. The surgical treatment of anorectal malignant melanoma. *Br J Surg*. 1986;73:68–69.

59. Parks TG. Mucus-secreting adenocarcinoma of the anal gland origin. *Br J Surg*. 1970;57:434–436.

60. Lee SH, Zucker M, Sato TS. Primary adenocarcinoma of an anal gland with secondary perianal fistulas. *Hum Pathol*. 1981;12:1034–1037.

61. Molnar L, Brezsnvak I, Daubner K, Horak E, Svastits E. Anorectal sarcomas. *Acta Chir Hung*. 1985;26:85–91.

62. Bowen JT. Precancerous dermatoses: a study of 2 cases of chronic atypical epithelial proliferation. *J Cutan Dis*. 1912;30:142–155.

63. Vickers PM, Jackman RJ, McDonald JR. Anal carcinoma in situ: report of three cases. *South Surg*. 1939;8:503–507.

64. Beck DE, Fazio VW. Premalignant lesions of the anal margin. *South Med J*. 1989;82:470–474.

65. Beck DE, Fazio VW, Jagelman DG, Lavery IC. Perianal Bowen's disease. *Dis Colon Rectum*. 1989;32:252–255.

66. Graham JH, Helwig EB. Bowen's disease and its relationship to systemic cancer. *Arch Dermatol*. 1961:88:738–751.

67. Marfig TE, Abel ME, Galligher DM. Perianal Bowen's disease and associated malignancies: results of a survey. *Dis Colon Rectum*. 1987;30:782–785.

68. Arbesman H, Ransohoff DF. Is Bowen's disease a predictor for the development of internal malignancy? A methodological critique of the literature. *JAMA*. 1987;257:516–518.

69. Beck DE, Harford FJ, Bagnall D, et al. Perianal Bowen's disease associated with Crohn's colitis: a case report. *Dis Colon Rectum*. 1989;32:252–255.

70. Beck DE, Fazio VW. Premalignant lesions of the anal margin. *South Med J*. 1989;82:470–474.

71. Paget J. On disease of the mammary areola preceding cancer of the mammary gland. *St Bartholomew's Hospital Report*. 1874;10:87–89.

72. Darier J, Coulillaud P. Sur un case maladie de Paget de la region perineo-anal et scrotale. *Annales de Dermatolgie et Syphiligraphie*. 1893;4:33.

73. Beck DE, Fazio VW. Perianal Paget's disease. *Dis Colon Rectum*. 1987;30:263–266.

74. Armitage NC, Jass JR, Richman PI, Thomson JPS, Phillips RKS. Paget's disease of the anus: a clinicopathologic study. *Br J Surg*. 1989;76:60–63.

75. Helwig EB, Graham JH. Anogenital (extramammary) Paget's disease. A clinopathological study. *Cancer*. 1963;16:387–403.

76. Gross G, Ikenberg H, Grosshans E, et al. Bowenoid papulosis. Presence of human papillomavirus (HPV) structural antigens and of HPV-16 related DNA sequences. *Arch Dermatol*. 1985;121:858–863.

77. Wade TR, Kopf AW, Ackerman B. Bowenoid papulosis of the genitalia. *Arch Dermatol*. 1979; 115:306–308.

78. Ikenberg H, Gissmann L, Gross G, et al. Human papillomavirus type-16-related DNA in genital Bowen's disease and in Bowenoid papulosis. *Int J Cancer*. 1983;32:563–565.

79. Gross G, Roussaki A, Schopf E. Successful treatment of condylomata acuminata and Bowenoid papulosis with subcutaneous injections of low-dose recombinant interferon∝. *Arch Dermatol*. 1986;22:749–750.

80. Corman ML. *Colon and Rectal Surgery*. Philadelphia: JB Lippincott;1984: 214–215.

81. Nielson OV, Jensen SL. Basal cell carcinoma of the anus: a clinical study of 34 cases. *Br J Surg*. 1981:68;856–857.

82. Armitage G, Smith I. Rodent ulcer of the anus. *Br J Surg*. 1954;42:395–398.

83. Shackelford RT, Zuidema GD. Surgery of the alimentary tract. In: *Colon Anorectal Tract*, 3. 2nd ed. Philadelphia: WB Saunders; 1982.

CHAPTER 17

RECTAL CARCINOMA: ETIOLOGY AND EVALUATION

W. Douglas Wong and Ronald Bleday

Approximately 44,000 patients per year in the United States are diagnosed with rectal cancer, half of whom will ultimately die of their disease. Despite this grim overall outlook, and although the cause of this malignancy remains ill-defined, a high survival rate can be achieved with early diagnosis and treatment. Determining the cause of this cancer, improving early detection methods, and optimizing the evaluation and treatment are at the center of improving survival. In this chapter, we discuss current thoughts on the etiology of rectal cancer, as well as the current methods of staging and evaluation of this disease.

Etiology

Epidemiology

Cancer of the large bowel, including rectal cancer, is a disease of western developed countries.[1] For example, in the developing countries of Africa the incidence of large bowel cancer as a percentage of the number of cases of cancer is approximately 2 percent,[1] while in western countries the incidence is approximately 10 times greater. Denmark, Czechoslovakia, the United States, Great Britain, Ireland, Canada, New Zealand, and certain parts of Argentina have the highest incidence[5] of rectal cancer in the world. Black populations in sub-Saharan Africa, white populations in Cali Colombia, and the indigenous population of Greece have the lowest incidence.[2,5] In general, high-risk communities (developed countries) have a predominance of left-sided and rectal cancers, whereas low-risk communities have a preponderance of right-sided cancers.[3] It is

difficult to say whether the incidence of rectal cancer is decreasing or increasing because differences in the definition of the anatomic location of a rectal, sigmoid, or rectosigmoid cancer make it difficult to compare studies. One study[4] reported an increase in the incidence of high rectal cancers in a New York population, with a decreased incidence of cancers within reach of the examining finger. In a recent New Zealand study, however, the incidence of rectal cancer has not shown any significant decrease over a 10-year period between 1974 and 1983.[5]

The differences in the epidemiologic patterns of rectal cancers among various populations strongly point to an environmental or dietary etiologic agent. One study suggests there may be differences in the etiologic agent between right-sided and left-sided colorectal cancers since different carcinogens produced cancers in different parts of the large bowel in experimental animals.[2] With respect to dietary factors, Burkitt,[1] among others,[6,7] has examined the differences in diet between high-risk western populations and developing nations. The studies suggest that differences in the consumption of refined versus unrefined carbohydrates, dietary fiber, and dietary fat contribute to this increased incidence of colon and rectal neoplasms in the western developed countries.

Dietary Fat, Bile Acids, Dietary Fiber

The mechanism by which increased dietary fat causes colorectal cancer is thought to be associated with an increase in the amount of bile and the resultant bile acids in the gastrointestinal tract. Researchers have long suspected that bile acids have carcinogenic potential because of the structural similarities between bile acids and carcinogenic polycyclic aromatic hydrocarbons.[8] High concentrations of fecal bile acids have been observed in people who ingest diets high in fat. Higher concentrations of bile acids in turn cause colonic bacteria to produce increased amounts of secondary bile acids and other metabolic by-products, and it is these compounds that are associated with the high risk of large bowel cancer.[7]

Dietary fiber may play an important role in protecting against colorectal cancer by diluting the concentration of fecal mutagens and bile acids, and by altering the large intestinal luminal environment. In an experiment on human volunteers consuming a high fat western diet, Reddy and associates[9] showed a 2.5 to 4.5 times decrease in the mean fecal mutagenic activity associated with a total increase in stool bulk of only 35 percent from supplementary fiber. Further work has shown that the type of dietary fiber may be important in reducing the fecal mutagenic activity.[10] In a study on humans, wheat bran and cellulose, as opposed to oat bran, were associated with decreases in fecal mutagenic activity as measured by a bacteriologic mutagenic assay.[10]

The luminal environment may also be modified with oral supplements of the bacterium *Lactobacillus acidophilus*. In an animal model, fecal mutagens were decreased in beef-fed rats with supplements of bacteria.[11] The researchers concluded that the *Lactobacillus acidophilus* reduced the amount of fecal mutagens by modifying the intestinal luminal pH. This alteration reduced the activity of the enzymes that metabolize procarcinogens to carcinogens.[12,13] The potentially protective effects of increased dietary fiber, and possibly those of *Lactobacillus acidophilus,* are supported by epidemiologic studies from Finland.[14] Although the Finnish study population had a high intake of dietary fat, particularly in the form of dairy products, it had a very low rate of large intestinal cancer when compared with other industrialized countries.[15] In addition to high levels of dietary fat, however, the study group consumed a large amount of dietary fiber compared to a U.S. population. The effect was a much lower concentration of fecal mutagens in the stool.[15] Although conclusive data must still be produced to confirm the correlation between dietary fiber and a decreased incidence of colonic cancer, the overwhelming metabolic, animal, and epidemiologic data to date seem to indicate that some types of dietary fiber, when ingested in increased amounts, are associated with a decreased incidence of colon and rectal tumors.

Additional Dietary Factors

Although no specific carcinogen has been found to cause colon or rectal cancer in humans, some data have been accumulated regarding an increased risk of rectal cancer in persons who consume large amounts of alcoholic beverages, particularly beer. Studies from Australia and Europe have shown a correlation between increased beer consumption and a high rate of rectal cancer.[16-18] In contrast, increased amounts of vitamin C intake may be protective against rectal cancer.[17] Payne[19] hypothesizes that this beer–vitamin C–rectal cancer relationship may be related to the production or inhibition of carcinogens such as nitroso compounds in the stomach.

Intestinal Microflora

The intestinal microflora influence the development of carcinogens within the intestinal lumen. Experimental animal studies have compared the carcinogenic effects of certain compounds in germ-free rats versus normal rats. Animals were fed high fat diets. The germ-free animals had significantly fewer large intestinal tumors.[20] In a similar experiment, the administration of oral antibiotics that suppressed the intestinal flora of rats also led to a decrease in colonic and rectal tumors.[21] Several studies suggest that intestinal bacteria may be involved with both the initiation and promotion of colorectal cancer. Bacteria may be involved in the production of initiating mutagens via their metabolism of certain dietary factors such as the potentially mutagenic nitroso compounds.[22] Others have found that the intestinal microflora, along with bile and cholesterol, may also promote the production of fecal mutagens when incubated with anaerobic bacteria such as Bacteroides.[23,24] Although there are as yet no conclusive data to link changes in the human intestinal microflora to an increase in the risk of colorectal cancer, there is, as stated by Gorbach and Goldin,[7] substantial evidence that "the intestinal microflora is capable of engaging in reactions that can generate carcinogens, mutagens, or tumor promoters in the large bowel."

Adenoma to Carcinoma Sequence

The etiology of rectal cancer was originally suggested to be related to the production of carcinogens in the intestine by gut bacteria and bile acids.[1,8,25] In 1978, however, Hill and his colleagues reviewed the St. Mark's histologic experience on colorectal cancer and that of others, and concluded that most carcinomas arise in preexisting adenomas (Fig. 17-1).[25,26] They hypothesized that an environmental agent causes adenomas to develop in susceptible individuals, and then other factors encourage these adenomas to grow and occasionally degenerate into carcinomas. They pointed out that the malignancy rate for large adenomas was similar in several different cultural groups. They concluded that the factors that promote these large adenomas to degen-

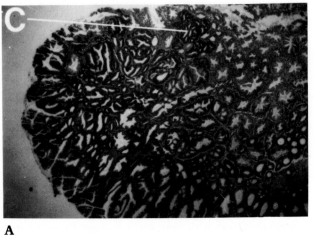

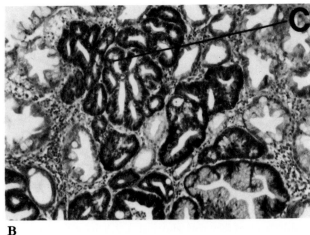

A   B

Figure 17-1.   (A) Small focus of cancer cells is seen arising within a tubulovillous adenoma. (B) Higher power magnification (×290, hematoxylin and eosin) reveals the severely dysplastic cells.

erate into carcinomas are not the factors responsible for the varying differences in the incidence of large bowel cancer seen in different parts of the world: instead, the differences could be attributed to the initiating or adenoma-producing factors related to regional diet. Once a population manifested adenomas, then carcinomas would follow.

Still more recently, a vast quantity of data on the genetics and molecular biology of colorectal cancer has been amassed. As will be discussed, current research suggests that there are a number of genetic factors that increase the susceptibility of an individual to developing colorectal cancer. Although an adenoma to carcinoma sequence is probable in most cases of colorectal carcinoma,[27,28] the etiology is probably multifactorial and not solely related to a dietary or environmental agent.

Genetic Susceptibility

The most obvious case of a genetic susceptibility to colorectal cancer occurs in patients with familial adenomatous polyposis. This disease shows a dominant inheritance pattern with a high degree of penetrance. The specific gene associated with familial adenomatous polyposis has been linked to a genetic deletion or mutation on the long arm of chromosome 5.[29] The specific gene has recently been characterized and termed *MCC* (mutated in colon cancer).[30] A mutation or rearrangement of this gene, however, is seen in only a small percentage (3 percent) of sporadically arising tumors, and the actual gene product has yet to be defined. On a clinical level, if an individual manifests colon or rectal polyps, that individual's adenomas will degenerate into carcinomas in 100 percent of cases.[28] The average age for the diagnosis of cancer in patients with familial

adenomatous polyposis is 35, with the onset of polyps usually seen in the midteens.[28]

Other examples of an inherent susceptibility to colorectal cancer unrelated to familial adenomatous polyposis have been described in recent reviews.[31,32] These studies show that individuals who have two primary relatives with colorectal cancer, or a family history of a variety of other cancers, have an increased risk of developing colorectal cancer. Lynch classified patients into different syndromes based upon their family history and has made recommendations for their surveillance and treatment.[31] Most of the colorectal cancers seen with these Lynch syndromes occur proximal to the sigmoid colon. In contrast, "sporadic" or nonfamilial cancers are primarily seen distal to the descending colon.[33] These studies suggest that most rectal cancers are probably of the sporadic type, even though the final common molecular biologic pathway from normal mucosa to a carcinoma may be the same for both sporadic cancers and cancers that manifest in patients with either the Lynch syndromes or familial adenomatous polyposis.

Overall, it has been estimated that patients with the Lynch syndromes comprise approximately 5 to 6 percent of all colorectal cancer patients.[34] For at least one of these syndromes (cancer family syndrome), a tumor-specific genetic defect has been found to be associated with the long arm of chromosome 18.[35]

With respect to most sporadic colorectal cancers, a tumor-specific allele has not been consistently found. However, as described by Wildrick,[36] a "two hit" phenomenon, which was initially conceived by Knudson for the retinal blastoma gene,[37] may be at work in the initiation of colorectal cancer as well. The "two hit" theory supposes that two genetic events occur at each of the two specific alleles that code for a critical gene in preventing carcinogenesis, such as an antioncogene. In a patient with an inherited predisposition for colorectal cancer, there may already be a congenital mutation or loss of one allele while the second allele eventually mutates sporadically, causing an adenoma and carcinoma. With noninherited or sporadic disease, both alleles lost their function through somatic events.

Again, with either the inherited types of colorectal cancer, which tend to occur on the right side of the large intestine, or with sporadic cancers, as is probably the situation for most rectal lesions, the final molecular events leading to a cancer are probably the same. Although specific familial syndromes for colorectal cancer comprise approximately 5 to 6 percent of all large intestinal cancers as already stated, Cannon-Albright and associates[38] suggested that overall, 19 percent of the total population may have cancer susceptibility genes that are most likely dominantly inherited. It is these susceptibility genes, along with environmental factors, that lead to the formation of adenomas and subsequent carcinomas. If it can be shown that there is a consistent predilection for colorectal cancer within certain families or populations, then there may be the potential to screen these susceptible groups. Although we do not as yet have the practical techniques to mass screen for genetic susceptibility to colorectal cancer, Lynch suggests that individuals with two primary relatives with colorectal cancer be endoscopically screened for colorectal tumors.[31] Cannon-Albright[38] and others[39] even suggest that patients with colon cancer found in only one primary relative be considered at a higher risk for the development of colorectal tumors and, therefore, screened more aggressively.

Tumor Suppressor Genes and Oncogenes

Although the specific genetic mechanisms involved with sporadic-type cancers have not been completely identified, recent research suggests that changes or deletions on three particular chromosomes—5, 17, and 18—may be involved. Genetic analysis of colorectal tumors has revealed a high incidence of genetic deletions on the short arm of chromosome 17 and on the long arm of chromosome 18.[40] Genetic deletions or mutations in these regions appear to lead to a loss in the function of the P53 and DCC tumor suppressor gene products, respectively.[41,42] The function of these gene products appears to be related to either DNA binding (P53) or cell–cell interactions and adhesions (DCC).

Originally, oncogenes were described in virally induced tumors, but they have since been demonstrated in the genetic material of all vertebrates. In humans and other vertebrates, these oncogenes exist as protooncogenes and require a mutation or change in their expression to induce or promote a malignancy.[33] With colorectal cancer, two oncogene families have been the most extensively studied: *myc* and *ras*.

The *myc* oncogene family contains several members, but it is the *C-myc* oncogene that has been found to be associated with colorectal cancers. The *C-myc* oncogene encodes for a nuclear protein that has a role in cell proliferation. Increased expression of the *C-myc*-associated RNA is seen in tubular adenomas and villous adenomas, as compared with normal colorectal mucosa.[43] Increased expression is also found in colorectal cancers, but this expression does not correlate with differentiation. Others have found increased levels of *C-myc* expression in cancers from the left side of the colon.[44]

The *ras* oncogene family encodes for membrane-associated proteins that are involved in signal transduction across the cell membrane. Mutant *K-ras* and *N-ras* oncogenes have been found in human villous adenomas and in carcinomas originating from villous adenomas.[45] In a survey of over 170 colorectal cancer specimens, 40 percent contained mutated forms of the *ras* oncogene; these mutations were most common in adenomas greater than 1 cm as compared with adenomas smaller than 1 cm.[40] Interestingly, *ras* mutations have not been associated with premalignant changes seen in the colorectal mucosa of ulcerative colitis patients. This implies that a different mechanism of carcinogenesis is involved with chronic ulcerative colitis.[46]

Overall, it is not clear exactly where oncogene mutations and tumor suppressor alterations fit into the colorectal tumorigenic process. It may be that a number of mutations and allele losses are necessary for the carcinogenic progression of normal mucosa to a carcinoma. Fearon and Vogelstein have proposed a schematic model (Fig. 17-2)[47] for colorectal carcinogenesis that incorporates both oncogene mutations and loss of tumor suppressor alleles, but further work will be needed to define the precise role of all these genetic events.

Inflammatory Bowel Disease

Ulcerative colitis and Crohn's disease have both been associated with an increased risk of colorectal cancer.[28,48] The risk of carcinoma is related to both the extent and the duration of disease.[28,49,50] The risk of developing a colorectal cancer in a patient with pancolitis from chronic ulcerative colitis (CUC) is about 12 percent after 20 years of disease and 25 percent after 30 years.[49] Rates vary, however, depending upon the patient population of the reporting institutions.[51] The risk of developing a synchronous cancer is also increased in patients with ulcerative colitis. Approximately 12 percent of patients develop multiple colorectal carcinomas compared to a synchronous cancer rate of 3 percent in patients who do not have inflammatory bowel disease.[50]

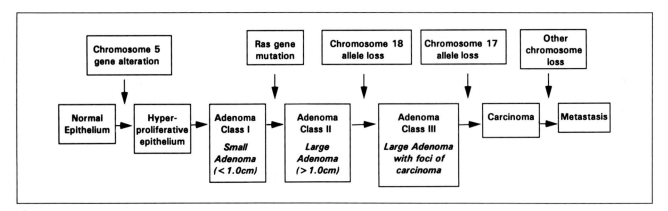

Figure 17-2. A model for the possible molecular events in colorectal tumorogenesis. (*Adapted from:* Vogelstein B, Fearon ER, Hamilton SR, et al. Genetic alterations during colorectal-tumor development. *N Engl J Med.* 319:525–532, 1988.)

The question of a step-wise adenoma to carcinoma sequence in colorectal cancer associated with inflammatory bowel disease is controversial. The fact that certain oncogenes show a different pattern of expression compared with carcinomas arising from adenomas in non-CUC patients has already been discussed. This fact along with the increased rate of multiple cancers in CUC patients points to a different biologic mechanism in the transformation of the CUC mucosa into carcinoma. In other studies, however, a majority of CUC patients with carcinoma of the colon or rectum had adenomatous polyps at the time of resection.[52] Despite the conflicting evidence, it is generally thought that adenomatous changes in CUC patients are not a predictive marker of an ensuing cancer.[28]

Mucosal dysplasia appears to be the histologic marker for an increased risk of developing colorectal cancer in CUC patients.[53] Mucosal dysplasia was associated with an increased risk of cancer in the retained rectum after ileorectal anastomosis. In one study, 42 percent of those patients who developed moderate to severe mucosal dysplasia in their retained rectum developed cancers.[54] Several surveillance studies have found an increased incidence of colorectal cancer in patients with mucosal dysplasia, whereas carcinomas were not found in patients without dysplasia.[55-57] Such surveillance programs were, however, not 100 percent reliable for the early detection of colorectal cancer. In the study from St. Mark's,[55] several advanced cancers developed undetected even with a screening interval of 6 to 12 months.

In conclusion, the ideal surveillance interval in patients with longstanding CUC has not yet been determined. A shorter interval (3–6 mo) would markedly increase the rate of negative findings, and possibly lead to increased complications secondary to the screening process. Some investigators argue that it may not even change the overall survival rate in patients with longstanding CUC.[58] Until such time as a more accurate marker for premalignant changes is found for longstanding CUC, colonoscopic surveillance with biopsies should be done in the range of every 6 to 24 months and possibly more often if dysplasia develops or persists. Since no study has found an increased incidence of cancer in patients with disease of less than 10 years, colonoscopic surveillance should not begin until after at least 10 years of disease.

Patients with Crohn's disease also carry an increased risk of developing colorectal cancer. The risk is not as great as with patients with pancolitis from CUC; the latter patients have about a tenfold increase in incidence of colorectal cancer,[59] while the overall increased risk of colorectal cancer in patients with Crohn's disease is thought to be approximately fourfold.[59] The increased risk of colorectal cancer in Crohn's patients approximates that of patients with longstanding *left-sided* CUC.[50] If only the subset of patients with isolated Crohn's colitis is considered, then the relative risk of developing a malignancy is somewhat higher and probably approximates that of patients with longstanding pancolitis from CUC.[60,61]

Multifactorial Hypothesis

A complete elucidation of how bacteria, bile acids, fiber, and oncogenes collectively cause rectal cancers is unavailable. Some baseline rate of colorectal cancer is probably unavoidable in any population, even those consuming a "perfect" diet.[62] This baseline rate is most closely manifested in very low risk populations such as sub-Saharan blacks. Factors within the "western" diet—related to the increased consumption of fat, cholesterol, and calories and the decreased consumption of fiber—may then lead to a series of changes in the intestinal lumen. These changes might include increases in the bile acid pool, changes in the biochemical milieu, and changes in the number and metabolism of anaerobic bacteria in the colon and rectum. The result is an increase in carcinogens and tumor-promoting factors within the large intestine. Genetic mechanisms may then influence the susceptibility of an individual to these increased carcinogens and tumor-promoting factors. The result is the high rate of colon and rectal cancer seen in most developed countries. As this summary suggests, however, more research is required to clearly define the multiple factors involved in this complicated tumorigenic process. Although the current biochemical and molecular research have thus far proved exciting, early detection with standard methods, complete evaluation of the rectal lesion, and surgical removal remain the cornerstones of treatment.

Evaluation

History

The clinical presentation of a patient with rectal cancer as elicited by a careful history, and the review of systems is varied. Many such cancers do not produce symptoms until moderately advanced, hence a certain number will be detected early only by routine digital and proctosigmoidoscopic examination. Bleeding is the most common presenting symptom of a rectal cancer and unfortunately is often attributed to hemorrhoidal disease, especially in younger patients. The bleeding is characteristically red to maroon and mixed with the stool. It usually occurs in small but persistent amounts and is rarely profuse. Anemia is an unusual early finding. The passage of increased mucus mixed with blood warrants careful examination. The patient may relate a change in bowel habits with increased stool frequency of a looser type of stool. Some patients may note diminished caliber of the stool, describing the stool to be "pencil thin." The patient may report a sensation of incomplete evacuation and may complain of being constipated. Urgency and tenesmus are frequent findings in advanced cases. Complete obstruction by a rectal cancer is rare. Rectal pain is an unusual presenting feature of rectal cancer unless the tumor is invading the sphincter musculature or sacrum or is involving major nerves by direct invasion or pressure. Abdominal pain manifested by mild cramping and bloating may be present. If a history of one or more of these symptoms is elicited, a very careful examination is warranted. In patients eventually found to have a rectal cancer, symptoms have

often been present for several months prior to presentation.

Examination

General

Extensive preoperative evaluation of the patient with a rectal cancer is essential and guides the surgeon in selecting appropriate therapy (Table 17-1).[63] A complete general physical examination with appropriate ancillary testing is performed. Such evaluation should define the extent of the local disease, assess for possible metastatic spread, and determine the operative risk of the individual patient with particular attention addressed to nutritional, cardiopulmonary, and renal status. The medical condition of high-risk patients should be optimized, because the choice of therapy may well be determined by a careful risk assessment. For example, in managing patients with a great operative risk, the surgeon may need to be more flexible in using tumor selection criteria for local therapy.

In this general physical examination any special situations should be noted. For example, patients who are blind, have severe arthritis, or are mentally incapacitated may be poor candidates for a stoma procedure and an alternative to traditional management may have to be found. Similarly, patients with severe anal sphincter dysfunction and problems with continence, those with chronic diarrheal states, and those with paralysis may not be good candidates for a low anastomosis. These important parameters, which can be determined by a complete physical examination, must be carefully sought so as to optimize the treatment for the individual patient with rectal cancer.

Table 17-1 Preoperative Assessment

Spectrum of operative risk	Spectrum of disease	Spectrum of therapy
Better than normal	Confined	Local therapy
Normal	"Garden variety"	Major resection
Worse than normal	Advanced	Adjuvant therapy and major resection
Excessive	Metastatic	Palliative

Note: The goal of preoperative assessment of a patient with rectal cancer is to find the ideal match of the spectrums of operative risk, disease, and therapy to ensure minimum morbidity and mortality while maximizing curability.

Modified from: Rothenberger DA, Wong WD. Preoperative assessment of patients with rectal cancer. *Semin Colon Rectal Surg.* 1990;1:2–10.

Staging the Disease

Staging of a rectal cancer consists of determining the extent of a primary tumor and assessing for the presence or absence of regional and distant metastases. Once determined, the extent of disease can be matched to the patient's risk factors so that the clinician can plan therapy that maximizes the potential for curability while minimizing morbidity and mortality. Accurate preoperative staging is also very important in the selection of patients for controlled trials that may involve preoperative adjuvant therapies. It is important, therefore, that the clinician distinguish as accurately as possible which cancers are confined to the rectal wall and potentially amenable to local therapy, which cancers are so extensive that cure is not feasible even with radical surgery, which cancers might potentially benefit from adjuvant preoperative therapies, and which cancers are best treated by abdominoperineal excision or a sphincter-saving procedure without preoperative adjuvant therapy. The following sections discuss clinical assessment together with the use of imaging technologies to define the depth of invasion and extent of a primary tumor, the presence or absence of perirectal lymphadenopathy, and the presence of adjacent organ invasion or distant metastases.

Clinical Assessment of the Primary Lesion

The examiner can readily determine the size of a rectal cancer, the extent of circumferential involvement, the distance from the anal verge, and a number of macroscopic features by a careful digital rectal examination and rigid proctoscopy. Although these features are important in determining therapy, the depth of invasion is currently the best method that we have for prognostic assessment of a rectal cancer. Lesions confined to the submucosa are associated with nodal or distant metastases in 6 to 11 percent of cases.[64-68] When a rectal cancer extends into the muscularis propria, the risk of metastases increases to 10 to 20 percent.[65,68,69] Furthermore, extension through all layers into the perirectal fat is associated with lymph node metastases in 33 to 58 percent.[68-70] The degree of fixity and the depth of invasion of a rectal cancer are not reliably assessed by clinical examination. Mason[68] reported the reliability of digital examination in assessing pathologic stage to be 75 percent accurate whereas Nicholls and associates[70] were able to determine local disease versus regional disease in 80 percent of instances. Mason proposed a clinical staging system for rectal cancer as seen in Table 17-2.[68]

By using a rigid proctoscope, the clinician can accurately determine the level of the rectal cancer above the anal verge. This is an important determinant in selecting the operative procedure. Similarly, rigid proctoscopy can accurately determine the size of the lesion as well as the macroscopic appearance. Several studies have documented that exophytic polypoid cancers have a better prognosis than do the ulcerative infiltrative neoplasms.[69,71-74] At the time of rigid proctoscopy, a biopsy specimen may be taken to confirm the presence of an invasive malignancy and to determine histopathology and ploidy status.

Biopsy

Histopathology. Biopsy of a rectal cancer to determine the histologic characteristics may have some prognostic value. It is important to note that a 40 percent error rate may occur in grading the degree of tumor differentiation on the basis of a biopsy sample alone. Vascular and lymphatic invasion suggest a poorer prognosis. Well to moderately differentiated cancers have a better prognosis than poorly differentiated cancers, but the inaccuracy in making this determination on the biopsy sample when correlated with the pathologic findings sheds doubt on the reliability of histologic sampling in preoperative staging for treatment planning.

Ploidy Analysis. The normal colon or rectal mucosa usually has cells that carry two types of DNA depending on their phase within the normal cell cycle; a diploid or 2N amount of DNA for the G0/G1 phases and a 4N

Table 17-2   Clinical Staging System for Rectal Cancer

Stage	Definition	Pathological Correlations, %
CSI	Freely movable over muscle indicating confinement to mucosa and submucosa	70
CSII	Mobile but not movable separately from rectal wall indicating absence of transrectal spread	75
CSIII	Mobility of tumor but rectum slightly fixed indicating infiltration of perirectal fat	90
CSIV	Fixed rectal wall indicating infiltration of adjacent structures	

From: Mason AY. Rectal cancer. The spectrum of elective surgery. *Proc R Soc Med.* 1976;69:237–244.

or tetraploid amount of DNA for cells within the synthetic (S) phase. Approximately 94 percent of normal rectal mucosa has a diploid amount of DNA with 6 percent within the S phase of the cell cycle.[75] With abnormal mucosal conditions (tumors, inflammatory diseases, dysplasia), the DNA content of cells can become nondiploid, or "aneuploid." These cells usually contain varying amounts of DNA between the usual 2N or diploid amounts and the 4N or tetraploid amounts. Over the past decade, analysis of the DNA content of colorectal tumors has been investigated to obtain a better objective prognosticating variable.

Approximately 70 percent of human solid tumors have abnormal amounts of cellular DNA, or aneuploidy.[76] For the large intestine, an increased incidence of aneuploidy has been seen with adenomatous polyps and cancers. It is estimated that 10 to 27 percent of polyps[77,78] and 50 to 60 percent of colorectal cancers[77,78] have excessive aneuploid cells. Aneuploidy has not, however, been found to be associated with the degree of differentiation.[77,78]

A recent retrospective study of the ploidy of rectal cancers found ploidy to be a significant prognostic variable.[75] Both the presence of aneuploidy and the relative amount within a tumor were associated with a higher recurrence rate and lower survival. Patients with diploid tumors had a 5-year survival of 64 percent, whereas patients with aneuploid or tetraploid tumors had a 5-year survival of 26 percent. Another study, however, found that increased aneuploidy was only predictive of a worse outcome in Dukes stage B patients.[79] Others have found that increased aneuploidy is merely associated with advanced-stage lesions and is not an independent variable by itself.[80] As Williams and Daly[76] said in a recent review on the subject, "a certain degree of doubt exists as to whether or not DNA ploidy independently acts as a prognostic variable." Certainly all future prospective trials on the treatment of rectal cancer should include an evaluation of the significance of ploidy status.

Besides ploidy, there is some evidence to suggest that proliferative activity, or the number of cells within the colon and rectal mucosa that are within the S or synthesis phase, is an important factor. In a recent study, increased proliferative activity, or cells in the S phase, was found to be associated with a decreased survival in patients with Dukes stage A or B colorectal cancer. The survival rate for low S-phase tumors was 82 percent, whereas survival was 43 percent for high-S-phase tumors.[81] In another study, recurrence of polyps after curative resection of a colorectal cancer was associated with increased rectal mucosal proliferation in the remaining bowel.[82] Again, future trials for the treatment of rectal cancer will need to evaluate this variable.

The clinical use of ploidy status of a tumor, its proliferative activity, or possibly other molecular markers may have more importance in the treatment of rectal cancer than in colon cancer. As clinicians gain experience and confidence with the preoperative staging of rectal cancers by techniques such as endorectal ultrasound, the use of the cellular and molecular markers may help guide the treatment of the more localized lesions (Dukes stages A and B). For instance, a patient with a localized lesion as determined by endorectal ultrasound could undergo local sphincter-saving therapy if the cellular and molecular markers help predict those patients who are apt to have a favorable result. Those patients with unfavorable markers could be directed to more aggressive surgical and adjuvant therapy. At present, however, more study is required for the definitive answers.

Imaging Techniques

Depth of Invasion. Computed tomography (CT) and magnetic resonance imaging (MRI) are reliable for assessing advanced rectal cancers that may be invading adjacent organs or in evaluating complications of the primary tumors such as perforation. However, CT and MRI do not allow visualization of the layers of the rectal wall and are therefore unable to reliably determine the extent of rectal wall invasion of an early cancer. Overall accuracy for CT scanning in determining the depth of invasion of the cancer is in the vicinity of 70 percent (Table 17-3).[83-87] MRI technique is rapidly changing and may prove to be more useful in the future in staging rectal cancer; however, it is currently no better than CT scanning. Neither scanning technique can be relied upon to determine the depth of rectal wall invasion of a cancer.

Endorectal ultrasonography is a relatively new diagnostic modality that has proved highly accurate in preoperatively determining the precise depth of invasion of the rectal cancer. A Bruel and Kjaer 1846 scanner with a 7.0 MHz 8539 transducer separates the layers of the normal bowel wall into five discrete lines and allows discrimination of cancers confined to the submucosa, those extending into the muscularis propria but confined to the bowel wall and those which invade into the perirectal fat.

Beynon and colleagues[89] described a five-layer anatomic model that is most useful in assessing depth of wall invasion (Figs. 17-3 and 17-4). The depth of tumor invasion as determined endosonographically is then used to classify tumors according to a modified TNM classification as proposed by Hildebrandt and Feifel[90] and Hildebrandt and associates.[91] This system categorizes an ultrasound stage T1 lesion (UT$_1$ lesion) as an

Table 17-3   Results of CT Staging of Rectal Carcinoma

Author Year	No. patients	Predicting depth of invasion, %		
		Sensitivity	Specificity	Accuracy
Dixon et al[83] 1981	47	72	89	78
Grabbe et al[84] 1983	154	74	92	79
Adalsteinsson et al[85] 1985	94	62	61	62
Freeny et al[86] 1986	80	61	61	62
Thompson et al[87] 1986	25	77	57	70

Modified from: Wong WD, Orrom WJ, Jensen LL. Preoperative staging of rectal cancer with endorectal ultrasonography. In: Schrock TR, ed. *Perspectives in Colon and Rectal Surgery.* St Louis: Quality Medical Publishing; 1990:315–334.

invasive malignancy confined to the mucosa and submucosa (Fig. 17-5), a UT_2 lesion as one penetrating the muscularis propria but still confined to the rectal wall (Fig. 17-6), a UT_3 lesion as one invading the perirectal fat (Fig. 17-7), and a UT_4 lesion as one that invades an adjacent organ (Fig. 17-8). Comparative analysis between the ultrasonographic diagnosis and the final pathologic confirmation demonstrates an accuracy in the vicinity of 90 percent in many series (Table 17-4).[88,91-97]

A number of comparative studies have been performed to assess the efficacy of endorectal ultrasonography, CT scanning, and digital examination in the preoperative staging of rectal cancer. Some studies have shown a clear superiority for endorectal ultrasonography whereas other studies have shown little difference. The results of these studies are summarized in Table 17-5.[92,95,98-101] It should be noted that in the study by Waizer and associates[100] a 4.0 MHz probe was used compared with a 5.5 or 7.0 MHz probe used by other investigators. This likely accounts for the lesser accuracy attributed to endorectal ultrasonography in this study. It should also be noted that Rifkin and associates[98,101] in 1986 and 1989 and Holdsworth and associates[99] in 1988 compared the accuracies of these methods in determining perirectal fat invasion, not overall tumor stage, mainly in advanced lesions. These studies therefore did not compare the ability of each technique to

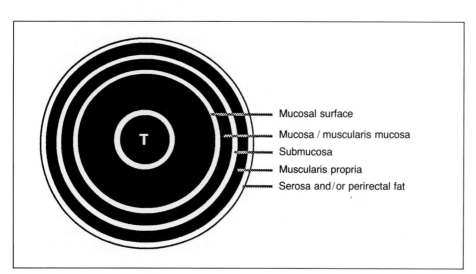

Mucosal surface
Mucosa / muscularis mucosa
Submucosa
Muscularis propria
Serosa and/or perirectal fat

Figure 17-3. Five-layer anatomic model for interpretation of endorectal ultrasonographic scans. Three echogenic (white lines) and two echo-poor (dark lines) layers are visualized. (*From:* Wong WD, Orrom WJ, Rothenberger DA, et al. Preoperative staging of rectal cancer with endorectal ultrasonography. *Dis Colon Rectum.* 33:654–659, 1990.)

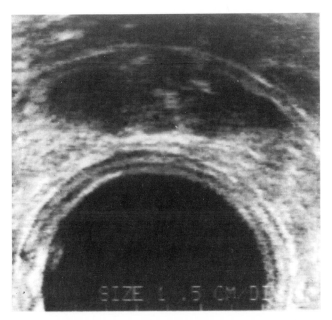

Figure 17-4. Normal rectal wall. The five lines (three hyperechoic, white and two hypoechoic, black) are clearly discernible in ultrasonographic image of rectal wall. (*From:* Wong WD, Orrom WJ, Jensen LL. Preoperative staging of rectal cancer with endorectal ultrasonography. In: Schrock TR, ed. *Perspectives in Colon and Rectal Surgery.* St. Louis: Quality Medical Publishing; 1990:315–334).

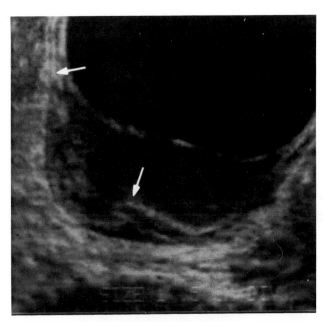

Figure 17-6. uT2 lesion. The submucosal (middle) white line is interrupted between the arrows, with expansion of the outer echo-poor layer (muscularis propria) indicating invasion of the muscle. The outer white line (perirectal fat) is intact, demonstrating that the tumor is confined to the bowel wall. (*From:* Wong WD, Orrom WJ, Jensen LL. Preoperative staging of rectal cancer with endorectal ultrasonography. In: Shrock TR, ed. *Perspectives in Colon and Rectal Surgery.* St. Louis: Quality Medical Publishing; 1990:315–334.)

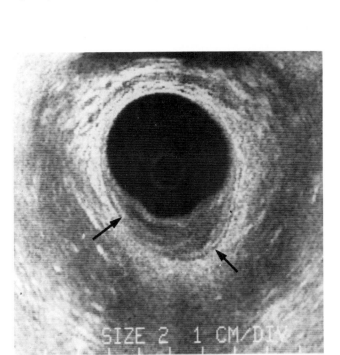

Figure 17-5. uT1 adenocarcinoma of the rectum (invasion into submucosa). The middle white line is interrupted and irregular between the two arrows, indicating invasion of submucosa, but the outer black line (muscularis propria) is not expanded, and the outer white line is intact. (*From:* Wong WD, Orrom WJ, Jensen LL. Preoperative staging of rectal cancer with endorectal ultrasonography. In: Schrock TR, ed. *Perspectives in Colon and Rectal Surgery.* St. Louis: Quality Medical Publishing; 1990:315–334.)

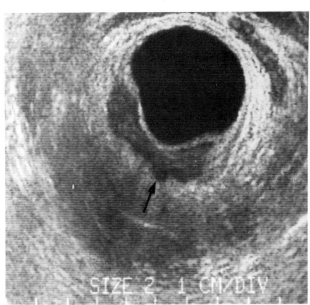

Figure 17-7. uT3 lesion. The outer white line is irregular and interrupted, indicating extension into perirectal fat. (*From:* Wong WD, Orrom WJ, Jensen LL. Preoperative staging of rectal cancer with endorectal ultrasonography. In: Shrock TR, ed. *Perspectives in Colon and Rectal Surgery.* St. Louis: Quality Medical Publishing; 1990:315–334.)

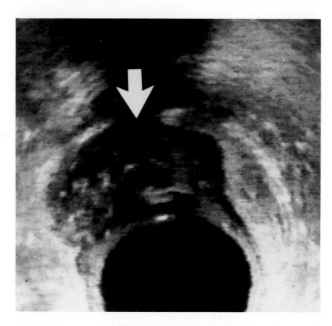

Figure 17-8. uT4 lesion. A large tumor expanding well beyond the rectal wall is seen, with loss of normal tissue between the rectum and vagina (*arrow*). Invasion of the vagina was confirmed at laparotomy. (*From:* Orrom WJ, Wong WD, Rothenberger DA, et al. Endorectal ultrasound in the preoperative staging of rectal tumors: A learning experience. *Dis Colon Rectum.* 33:654–659, 1990.)

assess the depth of invasion of early rectal cancers, in which endorectal ultrasonography has been shown superior because it can distinguish the layers of the rectal wall. Beynon's series[95] includes tumors of all stages and is therefore more representative.

A significant learning curve has been demonstrated by our experience and is graphically demonstrated in Figure 17-9, which compares our early, mid, and more recent experience with the use of endosonography in staging rectal cancers.[88] It can be seen that overall accuracy has steadily improved over the three time periods. Since October 1988, when the turning point was felt to be achieved, our overall accuracy has been 88 percent for determining depth of invasion with a 4 percent undercall and an 8 percent overcall. This compares favorably with other investigators' experience.[91,92-97]

Perirectal Lymph Node Assessment. Perirectal lymph node metastases are rarely identified by the examining clinician except in very advanced cases. A number of investigators have assessed the ability of CT scanning to identify lymph node metastases; reported sensitivities are in the range of 30 percent with overall accuracies of about 45 percent.[83,84,86,87] Dooms and associates[102] report little difference in the ability of CT

Table 17-4   Accuracy of Endorectal Ultrasonography in Determining Depth of Rectal Wall Invasion of Rectal Tumors. A summary of report series.

Author Year	No. patients	Accuracy, %	Overstage, %	Understage, %
Romano et al[92] 1985	23	87	4	9
Boscaini et al[93] 1986	11	91	0	9
Hildebrandt et al[91] 1986	76	88	11	1
Accarpio et al[94] 1987	54	94	4	2
Beynon et al[95] 1989	100	93	5	2
Zainea et al[96] 1989	30	90	3	7
Heintz et al[97] 1989	66	88	6	6
Wong et al[88] 1990	49	88	8	4

Adapted from: Wong WD, Orrom WJ, Jensen LL. Preoperative staging of rectal cancer with endorectal ultrasonography. In: Schrock TR, ed. *Perspectives in Colon and Rectal Surgery.* St Louis: Quality Medical Publishing; 1990:315–334.

Table 17-5 Comparative Studies for Determining Depth of Invasion by Digital Examination, CT Scanning, and Endorectal Ultrasonography

Author Year	No. patients	Accuracy to Depth of Invasion, %		
		Digital examination	Endorectal ultrasonography	CT scanning
Romano et al[92] 1985	23	. . .	87	83
Rifkin et al[98] 1986	59*	. . .	93	69
Holdsworth et al[99] 1988	36*	. . .	86	94
Waizer et al[100] 1989	68†	82.8	76.2	65.5
Beynon[95] 1989	42	61.9	95.2	71.4
Rifkin et al[101] 1989	102(US)* 82(CT)	. . .	72	53

* Compared accuracy for perirectal fat invasion only.

† Used a 4-MHz probe.

From: Wong WD, Orrom WJ, Jensen LL. Preoperative staging of rectal cancer with endorectal ultrasonography. In: Schrock TR, ed. *Perspectives in Colon and Rectal Surgery*. St Louis: Quality Medical Publishing; 1990:315–334.

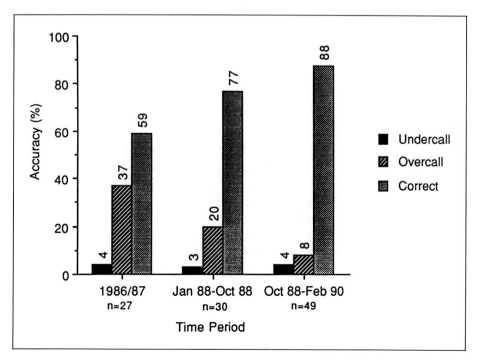

Figure 17-9. Endorectal ultrasonographic learning curve graphically demonstrated by comparison of our early, middle, and recent experience. (*From:* Wong WD, Orrom WJ, Jensen LL. Preoperative staging of rectal cancer with endorectal ultrasonography. In: Shrock TR, ed. *Perspectives in Colon and Rectal Surgery*. St. Louis: Quality Medical Publishing; 1990:315–334.)

or MRI in detecting normal lymph nodes: both modalities rarely identified such nodes. Hodgman and associates[103] reported a slight superiority of CT over MRI in detecting lymph node metastases but neither technique was very accurate in this regard. This inaccuracy is partly explained by the absence of any criteria except size to determine the presence of lymph node metastases as assessed by these imaging modalities.

Endorectal ultrasonography is capable of detecting small perirectal and mesorectal lymph nodes. The difficulty lies in reliably distinguishing the benign nodes from the malignant. However, as experience is gained, accuracies for detecting metastatic lymph nodes by endorectal ultrasonography in the 80 to 85 percent range can be achieved. Endosonographically identified malignant lymph nodes are hypoechoic in a manner similar to primary tumors and tend to be more circular than oval (Fig. 17-10). Beynon[95] stated that because normal nodes and the majority of reactive nodes are not identified by ultrasound, the presence of an echo-poor lesion in the perirectal tissues is indicative of a metastatic node. Beynon[95] compared the accuracy of endorectal ultrasonography with CT scanning in determining lymph

node involvement in 46 patients with carcinoma of the rectum. A clear superiority for endorectal ultrasound was demonstrated: an overall accuracy of 87 percent as compared with 57 percent for CT scanning.[95] Our most recent experience at the University of Minnesota has demonstrated that lymph node status has been accurately predicted in 88 percent of cases with a specificity of 90 percent and a sensitivity of 88 percent.[88] Therefore, endorectal ultrasonography is emerging as a reliable means of determing the presence or absence of lymph node metastases in the presence of a rectal cancer.

Adjacent Organ Invasion. Endorectal ultrasound is useful in determining local invasion of adjacent organs such as the prostate in males and the vagina in females. However, overall these organs are better delineated by CT scanning, particularly when assessing for sacral invasion or for invasion of the base of the bladder or other pelvic organs (Fig. 17-11). MRI is probably equivalent to CT scanning in this regard.

Distant Metastases. A chest x-ray should be obtained to exclude lung metastases, and liver function tests, although nonspecific, may be suggestive of liver metastases. Computed tomography and MR scanning can often identify unsuspected liver metastases and are obtained if such information would alter the operative or therapeutic approach. CT scanning has an accuracy in the 95 to 100 percent range in detecting liver metastases.[86,87,104] Kelvin and Maglinte reported a sensitivity of 95 percent for MRI in detecting metastatic liver disease as compared with 87 percent for CT scanning even with ethiodized oil emulsion-13 (EOE-13) enhancement.[105] MRI may eventually prove to be superior for detecting liver metastases (Fig. 17-12). Abdominal ultrasound is also a useful adjunct for the detection of unsuspected liver metastases. Intraoperative ultrasonography to detect occult hepatic metastases that are not palpable at the time of laparotomy may prove to be an important staging modality in the future.

Diagnostic Recommendations

Routine hematologic and biochemical investigations are performed in those patients for whom surgery is contemplated. A preoperative baseline carcinoembryonic antigen (CEA) level is obtained to serve as a reference for follow-up examinations in the postoperative surveillance period. Abnormalities in liver function studies may suggest occult metastases. A chest x-ray is obtained to rule out pulmonary metastases. We do not routinely advocate CT or MRI unless the finding of a metastatic lesion on such scans would alter the therapeutic approach. These imaging modalities are expensive, and

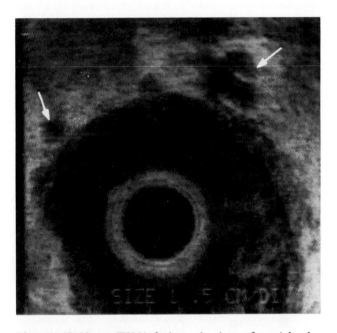

Figure 17-10. uT3N1 lesion. A circumferential adenocarcinoma of the rectum is seen, with invasion into the perirectal fat (irregular outer border). *Left arrow* indicates an enlarged metastatically involved lymph node. *Right arrow* represents an island of tumor adjacent to the extensive neoplasm. (*From:* Wong WD, Orrom WJ, Jensen LL. Preoperative staging of rectal cancer with endorectal ultrasonography. In: Shrock TR, ed. *Perspectives in Colon and Rectal Surgery.* St. Louis: Quality Medical Publishing; 1990:315–334.

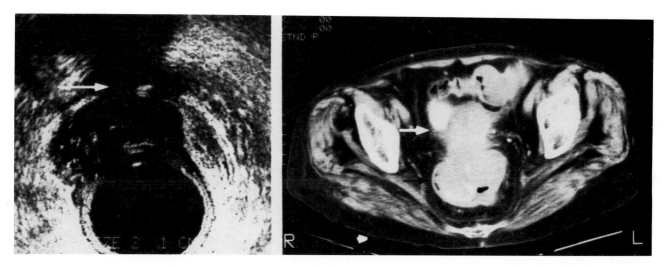

Figure 17-11.   The rectal ultrasound correctly diagnosed this UT4 rectal lesion invading the vagina (*left*). However, the extent of the rectal involvement is better appreciated on the CT scan (right) which shows vaginal and uterine invasion (*upper arrow*). (*From:* Rothenberger DA, Wong WD. Preoperative assessment of patients with rectal cancer. *Semin Colon Rectal Surg.* 1990;1:2–10.)

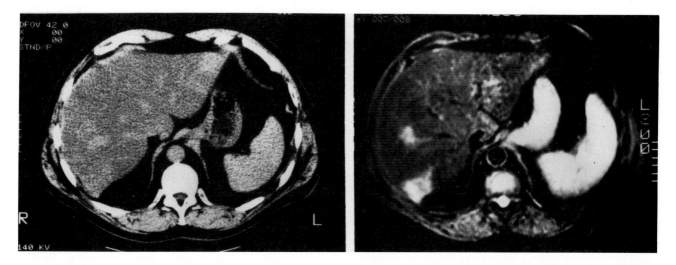

Figure 17-12.   Although CT scanning is very accurate for detecting liver metastases, MRI may prove to be superior. The two large right hepatic lobe metastases seen on the MRI (*right*) were not evident on the CT scan (*left*). (*From:* Rothenberger DA, Wong WD. Preoperative assessment of patients with rectal cancer. *Semin Colon Cancer. Rectal Surg.* 1990;1:2–10.)

unless they have a direct influence on decision making they are usually unnecessary. An intravenous pyelogram examination is not obtained unless there is a significant suspicion of a urologic abnormality.

Patients with large bowel carcinoma are at risk of a synchronous cancer in 2 to 8 percent of cases and a synchronous benign polyp in 12 to 62 percent of cases.[106-111] In the absence of obstruction, a preoperative colonoscopy should be performed. This is the pre-

ferred method over contrast barium enema because of its accuracy and therapeutic advantages. However, in the absence of colonoscopic capability, an air contrast barium enema and proctoscopic or flexible sigmoidoscopic examination can be substitutued. In patients in whom bladder invasion is suspected, a preoperative cystoscopy may be of value. We do not routinely obtain nuclear scans (e.g., bone scan or brain scan) unless the clinical findings suggest metastatic lesions in these areas.

Staging

Macroscopic

The clinician examiner can determine a number of macroscopic features of the rectal cancer that may influence therapeutic options. The majority of rectal cancers fall into two categories: exophytic (fungating) or ulcerating carcinoma. The latter suggests a more aggressive tumor and is less amenable to local therapies. Rarely, a rectal cancer is of the infiltrative type with submucosal extension of several centimeters, making the determination of an adequate margin more difficult. The level of the rectal cancer can be accurately assessed by rigid proctoscopy. This finding may have some influence on the therapeutic surgical options. Similarly, the extent of circumferential rectal involvement of the cancer should be noted and its precise location recorded. An anterior rectal cancer should be evaluated for potential vaginal involvement. The fixity of distal lesions can be assessed by the examining finger. Mason[68] proposed a clinical staging system based on tumor mobility.

Microscopic

In 1925, Broders[112] proposed a grading system for rectal cancer based on microscopic assessment of the degree of differentiation. In 1939, Grinnell[113] proposed the grading system that is currently used worldwide. This grading takes into account the glandular architecture, the nuclear polarity, the degree of mitosis, and the propensity for invasiveness (Table 17-6). Tumor grade was correlated by Grinnell[113] with the risk of lymph node metastases (Table 17-7). Newland and associates[114] showed a significant relationship between stage of colorectal cancer and histologic grade and documented some evidence that histologic grade is related to survival.[114] Dukes and Bussey reported the relation of histology and prognosis in a large number of rectal cancers[115] (Table 17-8).

Table 17-7   Correlation of Tumor Grade and the Incidence of Lymph Node Metastasis in Colorectal Cancer

Grade	No. patients	Lymph node metastases, %
Low	85	6
Average	79	32
High	52	54

Adapted from: Grinnell RS. The grading and prognosis of carcinoma of the colon and rectum. *Ann Surg.* 1939;100(4):500–533.

Table 17-8   Correlation of Tumor Grade and Survival in Rectal Cancer

Grade	No. patients	5-yr survival
Low	407	77.3
Average	1266	60.6
High	424	28.9

Adapted from: Dukes CE, Bussey HJR. The spread of rectal cancer and its effect on prognosis. *Br J Cancer.* 1958;12(3):309–320.

Staging Systems

Staging of rectal cancer has assumed new meaning and importance in recent times. Historically, staging systems were proposed for retrospective evaluation of the treatment of similar cancers and for prognosis. Today, staging is considered critical to the prospective evaluation of the extent of disease and subsequent treatment selection. Although purely pathologic features have a definite bearing on outcome, many clinical features are also important determinants and hence many of the more recent staging systems have stressed a clinical pathological approach.

Table 17-6   Microscopic Grading of Rectal Cancer

Grade	Differentiation	Glandular structure	Nuclear polarity	Invasive tendency	Mitoses
I (low)	Well differentiated	Preserved	Basal	Minimal	Rare
II (avg)	Moderately differentiated	Loose and irregular	Scattered	Moderate	More numerous
III (high)	Poorly differentiated	Absent	Lost	Significant	Frequent

Adapted from: Grinnell RS. The grading and prognosis of carcinoma of the colon and rectum. *Ann Surg.* 1939;100(4):500–533.

Dukes' Classification (1932).[116] Dukes' classification was intended to provide a pathologic basis for prognosis in patients with rectal cancer. He categorized the lesions into three categories as outlined in Table 17-9. Dukes and Bussey[115] reported on the survival of more than 2000 patients undergoing operation for rectal cancer based on Dukes' staging system. These data show the value of this simple pathologic classification in predicting survival. Dukes' classification remains the most commonly used staging system today.

In 1936, Dukes and coworkers modified this staging system by subdividing C cases into a C_1 category, in which regional lymph nodes were involved but did not reach the gland at the apex of the mesenteric ligation, and a C_2 category in which lymph node metastases extended to the apical nodes.[117] This was done to define a category with lymph node metastases that were still encompassable by radical surgery and hence potentially curable.

Kirklin Classification (1949). In 1949, Kirklin and associates[118] from the Mayo Clinic reviewed Broder grade 2 cancer specimens from the rectum and sigmoid and classified them according to a modified Dukes' classification as outlined in Table 17-10. Grade B lesions were divided into two categories depending on whether or not the tumor penetrated through the muscularis propria.

Astler–Coller Classification (1954). Astler and Coller[119] further modified Kirklin's classification by subdividing C cases into those without full-thickness wall penetration and those with complete penetration (Table 17-11). Survival data on 14 C_1 lesions and 125 C_2 lesions showed a 5-year survival of 42.8 percent for C_1 lesions compared to 22.4 percent for C_2 lesions.

Other modifications to Dukes' classification have been put forth, yet whether any are indeed an improvement remains controversial.[120,121]

The Australian Clincopathologic Staging System. The Australian clincopathologic staging system was proposed to include pertinent clinical, operative, and

Table 17-9 Dukes' Classification

Stage	Features
A	Cancer confined to rectal wall. No lymph node metastasis
B	Cancer extends into perirectal tissues; no lymph node metastasis
C	Lymph node metastasis present

Table 17-10 Kirklin Classification

Stage	Features
A	Limited to mucosa
B_1	Into muscularis propria but not penetrating through
B_2	Penetrating through muscularis propria
C	Metastatic lymph nodes

Table 17-11 Astler and Coller Classification

Stage	Features
A	Limited to mucosa
B_1	Into muscularis propria but not penetrating through
B_2	Penetrating through muscularis propria
C_1	Confined to wall with lymph node metastases
C_2	Penetrates wall with lymph node metastases

pathologic information.[115] This method separates patients who are deemed incurable at the time of surgery into a stage D and allows for an anatomically accurate definition of tumor spread. This staging method (Table 17-12)[114] is somewhat complex but may have greater prognostic value than the standard Dukes' or Astler–Coller systems.[122] Chapuis and associates[123] compared the clinicopathologic staging system to the pTNM classification and concluded that the simpler clinicopathologic system provided better prognostic discrimination than the more complex and cumbersome pTNM system.

TNM System. The American Joint Committee on Cancer (AJCC) and the Union Internationale Contre le Cancer (UICC) have developed a universal staging system for all anatomic sites.[124] The system for colorectal cancer staging was modified to correspond to Dukes' 1932 system. However, the TNM system provides both relevant clinical and pathologic information in more detail within each stage group. The TNM system emphasizes the depth of invasion, the number and site of metastatic lymph nodes, and the presence or absence of distant metastases. This system is presented in Tables 17-13 and 17-14.[124]

Table 17-12   Australian Clinicopathological System of Staging Rectal Cancer

Stage	Substage	Spread
A	A1	Mucosa
	A2	Submucosa
	A3	Muscularis propria
B	B1	Beyond muscularis propria
	B2	Free serosa involved
C	C1	Local node metastases
	C2	Apical node metastases
D	D1	Local tumor remaining (histologic)
	D2	Distant metastases (clinical)

From: Newland RC, Chapuis PH, Pheils MT, MacPherson JG. The relationship of survival to staging and grading of colorectal carcinoma: a prospective study of 503 cases. *Cancer.* 1981;47:1424–1429.

Table 17-13   TNM Classification for Cancer of the Colon and Rectum

PRIMARY TUMOR (T)

TX	Primary tumor cannot be assessed
T0	No evidence of primary tumor
Tis	Carcinoma in situ
T1	Tumor invades submucosa
T2	Tumor invades muscularis propria
T3	Tumor invades through the muscularis propria into the subserosa, or into nonperitonealized pericolic or perirectal tissues
T4	Tumor perforates the visceral peritoneum, or directly invades other organs or structures

REGIONAL LYMPH NODES (N)

NX	Regional lymph nodes cannot be assessed
N0	No regional lymph node metastasis
N1	Metastasis in 1 to 3 pericolic or perirectal lymph nodes
N2	Metastasis in 4 or more pericolic or perirectal lymph nodes
N3	Metastasis in any lymph node along the course of a named vascular trunk

DISTANT METASTASIS (M)

MX	Presence of distant metastasis cannot be assessed
M0	No distant metastasis
M1	Distant metastasis

From: American Joint Committee on Cancer. *The Manual for Staging Cancer.* 3rd ed. Philadelphia: JB Lippincott; 1988:75–80, 145–150.

Table 17-14   TNM Stage Grouping for Colorectal Cancer

	T	N	M	Dukes Stage
Stage 0	Tis	N0	M0	
Stage 1	T1	N0	M0	A
	T2	N0	M0	
Stage II	T3	N0	M0	B
	T4	N0	M0	
Stage III	Any T	N1	M0	C
	Any T	N2, N3	M0	
Stage IV	Any T	Any N	M1	

From: American Joint Committee on Cancer. *The Manual for Staging Cancer.* 3rd ed. Philadelphia: JB Lippincott; 1988:75–80, 145–150.

The TNM system has two advantages over the Dukes' classification. First, clinically documented metastases warrant a separate category. Second, the confusion that has arisen because of the various modifications of the alphabetically based Dukes' system is avoided by this new, precise nomenclature.[125] Its main drawback is its complexity, which limits easy application by requiring a reference table.

Ultrasound Staging System.   As previously discussed, endorectal ultrasonography can distinguish the layers of the rectal wall and is an accurate means of assessing for metastatic lymph nodes. For this reason, a useful modification of the TNM (UICC) staging system was proposed by Hildebrandt and Feifel[90] for preoperative ultrasonographic staging of rectal tumors (Table 17-15). An ultrasonographic stage T_1 lesion

Table 17-15   Endorectal Ultrasonographic Staging System

Stage	Tumor Features
uT_1	Confined to mucosa/submucosa
uT_2	Invading into but not through muscularis propria
uT_3	Invading perirectal fat
uT_4	Invading adjacent organ
N_0	Lymph node metastasis absent
N_1	Lymph node metastasis present

Adapted from: Hildebrandt U, Feifel G. Preoperative staging of rectal cancer by intrarectal ultrasound. *Dis Colon Rectum.* 1985;28:42–46.

Table 17-16   Determination of Depth of Wall Invasion by Endorectal Ultrasonography Compared to Definitive Pathologic Staging in 49 Patients Staged Since October 1988

Ultrasonographic diagnosis	No. patients	Pathologic Diagnosis, no. patients					Accuracy by stage, %		
		T0*	T1	T2	T3	T4	Overall accuracy	Overcall	Undercall
T0*	7	7	0	0	0	0	100	. . .	0
T1	9	0	8	1	0	0	89	0	11
T2	8	0	0	7	1	0	88	0	13
T3	22	0	0	4	18	0	82	18	0
T4	3	0	0	0	0	3	100	0	. . .
Summary	49	7	8	12	19	3	88	8	4

* T0 = benign or carcinoma in situ.

From: Wong WD, Orrom WJ, Jensen LL. Preoperative staging of rectal cancer with endorectal ultrasonography. In: Schrock TR, ed. *Perspectives in Colon and Rectal Surgery.* St Louis: Quality Medical Publishing; 1990:315–334.

(UT1) is a malignant lesion confined to the mucosa and submucosa. The UT2 lesion is confined to the rectal wall with invasion into but not through the muscularis propria. A UT3 designation denotes invasion into the perirectal fat whereas a UT4 designation indicates a lesion invading an adjacent organ such as the prostate, vagina, or bladder. N0 denotes no evidence of regional nodal metastases whereas N1 implies involvement of a perirectal node with metastatic disease. The usefulness of this staging classification depends on the accuracy of endorectal ultrasonography. Our results with endorectal ultrasound preoperative staging of rectal tumors is presented in Tables 17-16 and 17-17. These results have been separated into data representing the determination of depth of wall invasion and those identifying the accuracy of endorectal ultrasonography in determining lymph node metastases.

With the evidence at hand of the efficacy of endorectal ultrasound in preoperatively staging rectal cancers with respect to the depth of invasion and the presence or absence of lymph node metastases, the next logical step would be to incorporate this modality into a comprehensive clinicopathologic staging system.

Table 17-17   Accuracy of Endorectal Ultrasonography in Determining Metastases to Regional Lymph Nodes Compared to Final Pathologic Evaluation in 55 Patients Since January 1988

Overall nodal status			
Ultrasonographic		Pathologic, no. patients	
Stage	No. patients	N0	N1
N0	35	31	4
N1	20	4	16

Accuracy = 85%
Sensitivity = 80%
Specificity = 89%

From: Wong WD, Orrom WJ, Jensen LL. Preoperative staging of rectal cancer with endorectal ultrasonography. In: Schrock TR, ed. *Perspectives in Colon and Rectal Surgery.* St Louis: Quality Medical Publishing; 1990:315–334.

Comment

It is clear that there is no single etiologic agent in rectal cancer. Given the progress in identifying genetic defects in familial forms of colorectal cancer, patients at risk for this disease may soon be identifiable by simple genetic studies so that they can be intensively screened and counseled about preventive measures.

Unfortunately, many patients who are at high risk of developing rectal cancer are not identified until a cancer is well established. Once such a tumor is diagnosed, every effort should be made to evaluate the patient clinically for operative risk factors. Identifiable prognostic features related to the biologic behavior of the tumor should be sought to allow accurate staging so that treatment can be planned for optimal survival with minimal morbidity. Clinical evaluation, biological markers, and imaging modalities will enhance the preoperative staging of rectal cancers while the collection and integration of clinical, imaging, and pathologic information will allow further refinements in staging and classification and thereby in treatment of the patient.

References

1. Burkitt DP. Epidemiology of cancer of the colon and rectum. *Cancer.* 1971;28:3–13.
2. Stewart HL. Geographic pathology of cancer of the colon and rectum. *Cancer.* 1971;28:25–28.
3. Haenszel W, Correa P. Cancer of the colon and rectum and adenomatous polyps: a review of epidemiologic findings. *Cancer.* 1971;28:14–24.
4. Berg JW, Howell MA. The geographic pathology of bowel cancer. *Cancer.* 1974;34:807–814.
5. Jass RJ. Subsite distribution and incidence of colorectal cancer in New Zealand 1974–1983. *Dis Colon Rectum.* 1991;34:56–59.
6. Wynder EL, Reddy BS. Dietary fat and fiber and colon cancer. *Semin Oncol.* 1983;10(3):264–272.
7. Gorbach SL, Goldin BR. The intestinal microflora and the colon cancer connection. *Rev Infect Dis.* 1990;12(suppl 2):5252–5261.
8. Weisburger JM. Colon carcinogens: their metabolism and mode of action. *Cancer.* 1971;28:60–70.
9. Reddy BS, Chand S, Simi B, et al. Metabolic epidemiology of colon cancer: effects of dietary fiber on fecal mutagens and bile acids in healthy subjects. *Cancer Res.* 1987;47:644–648.
10. Reddy BS, Engle A, Katsitis S, et al. Biochemical epidemiology of colon cancer: effect of types of dietary fiber on fecal mutagens, acid and neutral sterols in healthy subjects. *Cancer Res.* 1989;49:4629–4635.
11. Goldin B, Gorbach SL. Alterations in fecal microflora enzymes related to diet, age, lactobacillus supplement and dimethylhydrazine. *Cancer.* 1977;40:2421–2426.
12. Edwards CA, Duerden BI, Read NW. The effects of pH on colonic bacteria grown in continuous culture. *J Med Microbiol.* 1985;19:169–180.
13. Goldin BR, Gorbach SL. The effect of milk and lactobacillus feeding on human intestinal bacterial enzyme activity. *Am J Clin Nutr.* 1984;39:756–761.
14. International Agency for Research on Cancer Intestinal Microecology Group. Dietary fibre, transit time, fecal bacteria, steroids and colon cancer in two Scandinavian populations. *Lancet.* 1977;2:207–211.
15. Reddy BS, Hedges AR, Laasko K, Wynder EL. Metabolic epidemiology of large bowel cancer: fecal bulk and constituents of high risk North American and low risk Finnish population. *Cancer.* 1978;42:2832–2838.
16. Kune S, Kune GA, Watson LF. Case control study of alcoholic beverages as etiologic factors: the Melbourne Colorectal Cancer Study. *Nutr. Cancer.* 1987;9:43–56.
17. Potter JD, McMichael AJ. Diet and cancer of the colon and rectum: a case control study. *Natl Cancer Inst.* 1986;76(4):557–569.
18. Dean G, MacLennan R, MacLoughlin H, et al. Causes of death in blue collar workers at a Dublin brewery 1954–73. *Br J Cancer.* 1979;40:581–589.
19. Payne JE. Colorectal carcinogenesis. *Aust N Z J Surg.* 1990;60:11–18.
20. Reddy BS, Watanabe K. Effect of intestinal microflora on 3,2′-dimethyl-4 aminobiphenyl induced carcinogenesis in F344 rats. *J Natl Cancer Inst.* 1978;61:1269–1271.
21. Goldin BR, Gorbach SL. Effect of antibiotics on the incidence of rat intestinal tumors induced by 1,2 dimethylhydrazine dihydrochloride. *J Natl Cancer Inst.* 1981;67:877–880.
22. Hill MJ. Bacterial factors in the aetiology of large bowel cancer. In: Welvaart K, Blumgart LH, Kreuning J, eds. *Colorectal Cancer.* The Hague: Leiden University Press; 1980;vol 18:15–22.
23. VanTassel RL, MacDonald DK, Wilkins TD. Stimulation of mutagen production in human feces by bile and bile acids. *Mutat Res.* 1982;103:233–239.
24. Lederman M, VanTassel RL, West SEH, Ehrich MF, Wilkins TD. In vitro production of human fecal mutagen. *Mutat Res.* 1980;79:115–124.
25. Hill MJ. Bacteria and the aetiology of colon cancer. *Cancer.* 1979;34:815–818.
26. Muto T, Bussey JHR, Morson BC. The evolution of cancer of the colon and rectum. *Cancer.* 1975;36:2251–2270.
27. Hill MJ, Morson BC, Bussey HJR. Aetiology of adenoma-carcinoma sequence in large bowel. *Lancet* 1970;1(8058):245–247.
28. Tierney RP, Ballantyne GH, Modlin IM. The adenoma to carcinoma sequence. *Surg Gynecol Obstet.* 1990;171:81–94.
29. Bodner WF, Barley CJ, Bodner J, et al. Localization of the gene for familial adenomatous polyposis on chromosome 5. *Nature.* 1987;328:614–616.
30. Kinzler KW, Nilbert MC, Vogelstein B, et al. Identification of a gene located at chromosome 5q21 that is mutated in colorectal cancers. *Science.* 1991;251(4999):1366–1370.
31. Lynch HT. The surgeon and colorectal cancer genetics: case identification, surveillance and management strategies. *Arch Surg.* 1990;125:698–701.
32. Lynch P, Winn RJ. Clinical management of hereditary non-polyposis colon cancer: high risk clinics and registries. *Hematol Oncol North Am.* 1989;3(1):75–86.

33. Astin SM, Costanzi C: The molecular genetics of colon cancer. *Semin Oncol.* 1989;16(2):138–147.

34. Mecklin JP. Frequency of hereditary colorectal carcinoma. *Gastroenterology.* 1987;93(6):1021–1025.

35. Boman BM, Lynch HT, Kimberling WJ, Wildrick DM. Reassignment of a cancer family syndrome gene to chromosome 18. *Cancer Genet Cytogenet.* 1988;34:153–154.

36. Wildrick DM. Molecular genetic studies of colon cancer. *Hematol Oncol North Am.* 1989;3(1):1–15.

37. Knudson AG Jr. Mutation and human cancer. *Adv Cancer Res.* 1973;17:317–352.

38. Cannon-Albright LA, Skolnick MH, Bishop T, Lee RG, Burt RW. Common inheritance of susceptibility to colonic adenomatous polyps and associated colorectal cancers. N Engl J Med. 1988;319:533–537.

39. Orrom W, Brzezinski WS, Wiens EW. Heredity and colorectal cancer: a prospective community based endoscopic study. *Dis Colon Rectum.* 1990;33:490–493.

40. Vogelstein B, Fearon ER, Hamilton SR, et al. Genetic alterations during colorectal-tumor development. *N Engl J Med.* 1988;319:525–532.

41. Baker SJ, Preisinger AC, Jessup JM, et al. P53 gene mutations occur in combination with 17p allelic deletions as late events in colorectal tumorigenesis. *Cancer Res.* 1990;50:7717–7722.

42. Fearon ER, Cho KR, Nigro JM, et al. Identification of a chromosome 18q gene that is altered in colorectal cancers. *Science.* 1990;247:49–56.

43. Imaseki H, Hayashi H, Masamor T, et al. Expression of *c-myc* oncogene in colorectal polyps as a biological marker for monitoring malignant potential. *Cancer.* 1989;64:704–709.

44. Rothberg PG, Spandorfer JM, Erisman MD, et al. Evidence that *c-myc* expression defines two genetically distinct forms of colorectal adenocarcinoma. *Br J Cancer.* 1985;52:629–632.

45. Forrester K, Almoguera C, Han K, Grizzle WE, Perucho M. Detection of high incidence of *K-ras* oncogenes during human colon tumorigenesis. *Nature.* 1987;327:298–303.

46. Meltzer SJ, Mane SM, Wood PK, et al. Activation of *C-Ki-ras* in human gastrointestinal dysplasias determined by direct sequencing of polymerase chain reaction products. *Cancer Res.* 1990; 50:3627–3630.

47. Fearon ER, Vogelstein B. A genetic model for colorectal tumorigenesis. *Cell.* 1990;61:759–767.

48. Ballantyne GH. Risk of colorectal cancer in patients with chronic ulcerative colitis and Crohn's disease. *Probl Gen Surg.* 1987;4:154–167.

49. Mir-Madjlessi SH, Farmer RG, Easley KA, Beck GJ. Colorectal and extra-colonic malignancy in ulcerative colitis. *Cancer.* 1986;58:1569–1574.

50. The threat of cancer. In: Banks PA, Present DH, Steiner P, eds. *The Crohn's Disease and Ulcerative Colitis Fact Book.* New York: Charles Scribner and Sons; 1983:97–106.

51. Riddell RH. Why the variation in colitic cancer rates from different centers? In: Rachmilewitz D, Zimmerman J, eds. *Inflammatory Bowel Diseases.* Dordrecht; The Netherlands: Kluwer Academic Publishers; 1990:79–88.

52. Dawson IMP, Pryse-Davies J. The development of carcinoma of the large intestine in ulcerative colitis. *Br J Surg.* 1959;47:113–128.

53. Morson BC, Pang LSG. Rectal biopsy as an aid to cancer control in ulcerative colitis. *Gut.* 1967; 8:423–434.

54. Johnson WR, McDermott FT, Pihl E, et al. Mucosal dysplasia: a major predictor of cancer following ileorectal anastomosis. *Dis Colon Rectum.* 1983;26:697–700.

55. Lennard-Jones JE, Morson BC, Rictchie JK, Williams CB. Cancer surveillance in ulcerative colitis: experience over 15 years. *Lancet.* 1983;2:149–153.

56. Manning AP, Bulgim OR, Dixon MF, Axon ATR. Screening by colonoscopy for colonic epithelial dysplasia in inflammatory bowel disease. *Gut.* 1987;28:1489–1494.

57. Nugent FW, Haggitt RC. Results of a long-term perspective surveillance program for dysplasia in ulcerative colitis. *Gastroenterology.* 1984;86:1197.

58. Gyde SN. Screening for colorectal cancer in ulcerative colitis: dubious benefits and high costs. *Gut.* 1990;31:1089–1092.

59. Prior P, Gyde SN, Macartney JC, et al. Cancer morbidity in ulcerative colitis. *Gut.* 1982; 23:490–497.

60. Gyde SN, Prior P, Macartney JC, et al. Malignancy in Crohn's disease. *Gut.* 1980;21:1024–1029.

61. Weedon D, Shorter RG, Ilstrup DM, et al. Crohn's disease and cancer. *N Engl J Med.* 1973;289:1099–1103.

62. Knudson AG. Hereditary cancer, oncogenes, and anti-oncogenes. *Cancer Res.* 1985;45:1437–1443.

63. Rothenberger DA, Wong WD. Preoperative assessment of patients with rectal cancer. *Semin Colon Rectal Surg.* 1990;1:2–10.

64. Hager T, Gall FP, Hermanek P. Local excision of cancer of the rectum. *Dis Colon Rectum.* 1983; 26:149–151.

65. DeLeon ML, Schoetz DJ, Coller JA, et al. Colorectal cancer: Lahey Clinic experience, 1972–1976. *Dis Colon Rectum.* 1987;30:237–242.

66. Stearns MW, Sternberg SS, DeCosse JJ. Treatment alternatives, localized rectal cancer. *Cancer.* 1984;54:2691–2694.
67. Morson BC. Factors influencing the prognosis of early carcinoma of the rectum. *Proc R Soc Med.* 1966;59:35–36.
68. Mason AY. Rectal cancer. The spectrum of elective surgery. *Proc R Soc Med.* 1976;69:237–244.
69. Morson BC, Bussey HJR, Samoorian S. Policy of local excision for early carcinoma of the colorectum. *Gut.* 1977;18:1045–1050.
70. Nicholls RJ, Mason AY, Morson BC, Dixon AK, Fry IK. The clinical staging of rectal cancer. *Br J Surg.* 1982;69:404–409.
71. Papillon J. rectal and anal cancers. Conservative treatment by irradiation—an alternative to radical surgery. New York: Springer-Verlag; 1982.
72. Greaney MG, Irvin TT. Criteria for selection of rectal cancers for local treatment. *Dis Colon Rectum.* 1977;20;462–466.
73. Michelassi F, Vannucci L, Montag A, et al. Importance of tumor morphology for the long term prognosis of rectal adenocarcinoma. *Am Surg.* 1988;54:376–379.
74. Hughes EP, Veidenheimer MC, Corman ML, et al. Electrocoagulation of rectal cancer. *Dis Colon Rectum.* 1982;25:215–218.
75. Scott NA, Rainwater LM, Wieand HS, et al. The relative prognostic value of flow cytometric DNA analysis and conventional clinical pathologic criteria in patients with operable rectal carcinoma. *Dis Colon Rectum.* 1987;30:513–520.
76. Williams NN, Daly JM. Flow cytometry and prognostic implications in patients with solid tumors. *Surg Gynecol Obstet.* 1990;171:257–266.
77. Fischbach W, Mossner J, Seyschab H, Hohn H. Tissue carcinoembryonic antigen and DNA aneuploidy in pre-cancerous and cancerous colorectal lesions. *Cancer.* 1990;65:1820–1824.
78. Armitage NC, Robins RA, Evans DF, Turner DR, Baldwin RW, Hardcastle JD. Influence of tumor cell DNA abnormalities on survival in colorectal cancer. *Br J Surg.* 1985;72:828–830.
79. Jones DJ, Moore M, Schofield PF. Prognostic significance of DNA ploidy in colorectal cancer: a prospective flow cytometric study. *Br J Surg.* 1988;75:28–33.
80. Banner BF, Thomas-De-La-Vega JE, Rosman DL, Coon JS. Should flow cytometric analysis precede definitive surgery for colon carcinoma? *Ann Surg.* 1985;202:740–744.
81. Bauer KD, Lincoln ST, Vera-Roman JM, et al. Prognostic implications of proliferative activity and DNA ploidy in colonic adenocarcinoma. *Lab Invest.* 1987;57:329–335.
82. Scalmati A, Roncucci L, Ghidini G, Biasco G, Ponz de Leon M. Epithelial cell kinetics in the remaining colorectal mucosa after surgery for cancer of the large bowel. *Cancer Res.* 1990;50:7937–7941.
83. Dixon AK, Fry IK, Morson BC, et al. Pre-operative computed tomography of carcinoma of the rectum. *Br J Radiol.* 1981;54:655–659.
84. Grabbe E, Lierse W, Winkler R. The perirectal fascia: morphology and use in staging of rectal carcinoma. *Radiology.* 1983;149:241–246.
85. Adalsteinsson B, Glimelius B, Graffman S, Hemmingsson A, Pahlman L. Computed tomography in staging of rectal carcinoma. *Acta Radiol Diagn.* 1985;26:45–55.
86. Freeny PC, Marks WM, Ryan JA, Bolen JW. Colorectal carcinoma evaluation with CT: preoperative staging and detection of postoperative recurrence. *Radiology.* 1986;158:347–353.
87. Thompson WM, Halvorsen RA, Foster WL Jr, et al. Preoperative and postoperative CT staging of rectosigmoid carcinoma. *AJR.* 1986;146:703–710.
88. Wong WD, Orrom WJ, Jensen LL. Preoperative staging of rectal cancer with endorectal ultrasonography. In: Schrock TR, ed. *Perspectives in Colon and Rectal Surgery.* St. Louis: Quality Medical Publishing; 1990:315–334.
89. Beynon J, Foy DMA, Roe AM, et al. Endoluminal ultrasound in the assessment of local invasion in rectal cancer. *Br J Surg.* 1986;73:474–477.
90. Hildebrandt U, Feifel G. Preoperative staging of rectal cancer by intrarectal ultrasound. *Dis Colon Rectum.* 1985;28:42–46.
91. Hildebrandt U, Feifel G, Schwarz HP, et al. Endorectal ultrasound: instrumentation and clinical aspects. *Int J Colorectal Dis.* 1986;1:203–207.
92. Romano G, deRosa P, Vallone G, et al. Intrarectal ultrasound and computed tomography in the pre- and postoperative assessment of patients with rectal cancer. *Br J Surg.* 1985;72(suppl):S117–S119.
93. Boscaini M, Masoni L, Montori A. Transrectal ultrasonography: three years' experience. *Int J Colorectal Dis.* 1986;1:208–211.
94. Accarpio G, Scopinara G, Claudiani F, et al. Experience with local rectal cancer excision in light of two recent preoperative diagnostic methods. *Dis Colon Rectum.* 1987;30:296–298.
95. Beynon J. An evaluation of the role of rectal endosonography in rectal cancer. *Ann R Coll Surg Engl.* 1989;71:131–139.
96. Zainea GG, Lee F, McLeary RD, et al. Transrectal ultrasonography in the evaluation of rectal and extrarectal disease. *Surg Gynecol Obstet.* 1989;169:153–156.
97. Heintz A, Bueb G, Frank K, et al. Endoluminal

ultrasonic examination of sessile polyps and early carcinomas of the rectum. *Surg Endosc.* 1989;3:92–95.

98. Rifkin MD, McGlynn ET, Marks G. Endorectal sonographic prospective staging of rectal cancer. *Scand J Gastroenterol.* 1986;21(suppl):S99–S103.

99. Holdsworth PJ, Johnston D, Chalmers AG, et al. Endoluminal ultrasound and computed tomography in the staging of rectal cancer. *Br J Surg.* 1988;75:1019–1022.

100. Waizer A, Zitron S, Ben-Barush D, et al. Comparative study for preoperative staging of rectal cancer. *Dis Colon Rectum.* 1989;32:53–56.

101. Rifkin MD, Ehrlich SM, Marks G. Staging of rectal carcinoma: prospective comparison of endorectal US and CT1. *Radiology.* 1989;170:319–322.

102. Dooms GC, Hricak H, Crooks LE, et al. Magnetic resonance imaging of the lymph nodes: comparison with CT. *Radiology.* 1984; 153:719–728.

103. Hodgman CG, MacCarty RL, Wolff BG, et al. Preoperative staging of rectal carcinoma by computed tomography and 0.15T magnetic resonance imaging: preliminary report. *Dis Colon Rectum.* 1986;29:46–50.

104. Zaunbauer W, Haertel M, Fuchs WA. Computed tomography in carcinoma of the rectum. *Gastrointest Radiol.* 1981;6:79–84.

105. Kelvin FM, Maglinte DDT. Colorectal carcinoma: a radiologic and clinical review. *Radiology.* 1987;164:1–8.

106. Travieso CR, Knoepp LF, Hanley PH. Multiple carcinomas of the large intestine: a review of the literature and a study of 261 cases. *Dis Colon Rectum.* 1972;15:1–16.

107. Reilly JC, Rusin LC, Theuerkauf FJ Jr. Colonoscopy: its role in cancer of the colon and rectum. *Dis Colon Rectum.* 1982;25:532–538.

108. Heald RH, Bussey HJR. Clinical experiences at St. Mark's Hospital with multiple synchronous cancers of the colon and rectum. *Dis Colon Rectum.* 1975;18:6–10.

109. Floyd CE, Stirling CT, Cohn I Jr. Cancer of the colon, rectum, and anus: review of 16,687 cases. *Ann Surg.* 1966;163:829–837.

110. Langevin JM, Nivatvongs S. The true incidence of synchronous cancer of the large bowel: a prospective study. *Am J Surg.* 1984;147:330–333.

111. Brahme F, Ekelund G, Mellner C, et al. Metach-

ronous colorectal polyps: comparison of development of colorectal polyps and carcinomas with and without history of polyps. *Dis Colon Rectum.* 1974;17:166.

112. Broders AC. The grading of carcinoma. *Minn Med.* 1925;8:726–730.

113. Grinnell RS. The grading and prognosis of carcinoma of the colon and rectum. *Ann Surg.* 1939;100(4):500–533.

114. Newland RC, Chapuis PH, Pheils MT, MacPherson JG. The relationship of survival to staging and grading of colorectoral carcinoma: a prospective study of 503 cases. *Cancer.* 1981;47:1424–1429.

115. Dukes CE, Bussey HJR. The spread of rectal cancer and its effect on prognosis. *Br J Cancer.* 1958;12(3):309–320.

116. Dukes CE. THe classification of cancer of the rectum. *J Pathol Bacteriol.* 1932;35:323–332.

117. Gabriel WB, Dukes C, Bussey HJR. Lymphatic spread in cancer of the rectum. *Br J Surg.* 1935–1936;23:395–413.

118. Kirklin JW, Dockert MB, Waugh JM. The role of the peritoneal reflection in the prognosis of carcinoma of the rectum and sigmoid colon. *Surg Gynecol Obstet.* 1949;88:326–331.

119. Astler VB, Coller FA. The prognostic significance of direct extension of carcinoma of the colon and rectum. *Ann Surg.* 1954;139:846–852.

120. Schubert W. Dukes' classification: American chaos versus British order. *Canadian Journal of Surgery.* 1990;33(1):8–11.

121. Beart RW Jr, vanHeerden JA, Beahrs OH. Evolution in the pathologic staging of carcinoma of the colon. *Surg Gynecol Obstet.* 1978;146:257–259.

122. Chapuis PH, Fisher R, Dent OF, et al. The relationship between staging methods and survival in colorectal carcinoma. *Dis Colon Rectum.* 1985; 28:158–161.

123. Chapuis PH, Dent OF, Newland RC, Bokey EL, Pheils MT. An evaluation of the American joint committee (pTNM) staging method for cancer of the colon and rectum. *Dis Colon Rectum.* 1986;29(1):6–10.

124. American Joint Committee on Cancer. *The Manual for Staging of Cancer. 3rd ed.* Philadelphia: JB Lippincott; 1988:75–80,145–150.

125. Fielding LP, Ballantyne GH. Classification systems for staging colorectal cancer. Past, present, and future. *Probl Gen Surg.* 1987;4(1):39–53.

CHAPTER 18

RECTAL CARCINOMA: TREATMENT

Bruce A. Orkin

The treatment of rectal carcinoma remains largely surgical; thus, most of this chapter is devoted to perioperative management and outcome in the surgical patient. Many factors influence the choice of surgical management of a patient with rectal carcinoma: patient fitness, obesity, adequacy of bowel preparation, obstruction, tumor location, adjacent organ fixation or invasion, presence of metastatic disease, and the experience and preferences of the surgeon. One type of treatment is not necessarily the best for each patient. Therefore, a variety of approaches have evolved.

History

Rectal cancer as a disease entity has been known and described at least since the time of John of Arderne in the 14th century.[1] However, surgical treatment was not employed until the 19th century when limited sacral or local perineal excisions were attempted.[2]

The surgical treatment of rectal carcinomas may be divided into three overlapping periods.[3] The first period began with the successful excision of a tumor of the anal canal by Paget in 1739 and lasted until the end of the 19th century.[4] This was a period of primarily palliative tumor excision and debulking from the perineal approach.[4-15] The second period began at the end of the 19th century and continued into the 1940s. During this period curative resection was developed, beginning with the concepts of wide lymphovascular resection and concluding with general acceptance of the abdominoperineal resection as the treatment of choice.[16-30] The third period was notable for the development of sphincter-saving operations for carcinomas of the upper and then the middle third of the rectum. This phase began in the 1940s and continues today. It is based on

the understanding that appropriately selected sphincter preserving procedures do not compromise cure. A variety of techniques including pullthrough procedures, anterior resection, coloanal anastomosis, and combined abdominosacral approaches have been employed with the goal of preserving continence.[31-39] A fourth period may be developing which is marked by selected local treatment of early rectal cancers and possibly by laparoscopic resections.

General Considerations

Surgical treatment may be curative or palliative. Curative treatment is performed with the intention of eradicating all of the tumor and any associated spread. The choice of a specific treatment is based on preoperative staging and the medical condition of the patient along with his or her desires. Radical surgery involves an en bloc resection of the tumor and the rectum along with the perirectal fat, the mesentery, and the local and regional lymph nodes. Palliative treatment may be pursued when complete removal of the tumor is not possible because of unresectable local or distant spread or when the patient is deemed unable to withstand a curative procedure because of poor medical condition.

Preoperative Preparation

General

The preoperative preparation of the patient who is to undergo an operation for the treatment of a rectal cancer is discussed in Chapters 4 and 5. Prophylactic measures should be used to reduce the risks of deep venous

260

thrombosis, pulmonary embolism, and sepsis. If blood transfusions are likely to be needed, autologous donation is a good option prior to elective procedures.

Stoma Marking

Whenever a temporary or permanent stoma is a possibility the preferred site should be marked preoperatively. The patient must be observed in the standing, sitting, and supine positions so that creases, bulges, scars and bony prominences, and the beltline may be identified. These areas should be avoided. The stoma should lie in an area of flat smooth skin that the patient can easily see. Generally, this spot lies to the right or to the left of the umbilicus, over the rectus muscle and below the beltline. The bowel should be brought through the rectus muscle, as this reduces the incidence of parastomal hernias. Prior to surgery, the patient should visit with an enterostomal therapist and, if possible, another patient with a similar stoma.

Physiological Testing

Preoperative evaluation of anal sphincter function in preparation for a sphincter-saving procedure is important to ensure a satisfactory functional outcome. A careful history and physical examination is usually adequate. The patient should be asked about incontinence, urgency, soiling with diarrhea, and prior anorectal surgery. In selected cases, manometric and even electromyographic assessment of sphincter activity may be helpful. These studies are discussed in Chapters 1 and 6.

Synchronous Colorectal Cancers

Preoperative clearance of the entire colon is essential whenever possible because of the high incidence of synchronous carcinomas and polyps. This incidence has been estimated to be 1.7 percent to 7.6 percent for synchronous cancers and 27 percent to 75 percent for synchronous polyps.[40-52] The differences in these rates may be due to (1) the inclusion in some series of patients with ulcerative colitis or familial polyposis, (2) study design and methods used in screening, or (3) the lesions included such as carcinoma in situ and hyperplastic polyps. The majority of synchronous lesions are found outside of the surgical segment in which the index cancer resides and thus would not be included in a standard resection. Therefore, preoperative knowledge of additional colonic pathology will frequently alter the planned procedure.

Total colonoscopy is the preferred method for the identification of synchronous lesions since barium enema studies (both single and double contrast) frequently miss both polyps and cancers.[43,47,48,53] If preoperative assessment is not possible, intraoperative colonoscopy may be performed. Occasionally, screening of the colon is not possible, for example, in patients who present with colonic obstruction. These patients should have careful intraoperative palpation of the colon and should then undergo clearance colonoscopy within 3 to 6 months after their operation.

Curative Management
Rationale

Since Miles' studies at the turn of the century, the major axiom of surgical treatment of colorectal carcinoma has been to remove the lesion with adequate margins along with as much of the attendant lymphatic drainage as possible.

Routes of Spread

Adenocarcinoma of the rectum spreads along four major routes: (1) transmurally with subsequent direct invasion of contiguous structures, (2) via the lymphatic channels, (3) by hematogenous routes, and (4) by implantation of exfoliated cells, primarily at the time of surgery.

Cancers of the rectum are initially confined to the bowel wall. They tend to grow radially around the lumen until they are circumferential, following the bowel wall lymphatics that lie in this direction. The rate of growth around the bowel wall has been estimated to be 25 percent in 6 months. Penetration of the muscular layers of the wall frequently occurs; however, growth in the longitudinal axis of the bowel is generally quite limited. Distal intramural spread rarely occurs beyond 1 cm except when there is extensive proximal obstruction of the lymphatics. Two centimeters is now the acceptable minimal distal margin; no survival benefit has been demonstrated with longer distal margins (see Distal Margins below).

Lymphatic metastases usually occur in a stepwise fashion, involving the lymph nodes adjacent to the lesion before the distant ones.[23] Occasionally the disease may be found in the distant nodes only. In addition, distal mesorectal deposits may occur in the absence of distal intramural spread. This concept is illustrated in Figure 18-1. Nevertheless, spread limited to the lower lymph nodes alone carries a better prognosis. Spread to the lateral lymph nodes in the internal iliac chain may occur, although the reported incidence is quite low.[54] Hojo and associates,[55] however, found metastases to the pelvic side wall nodes in 9 percent of patients with high rectal lesions and in 23 percent of patients with rectal

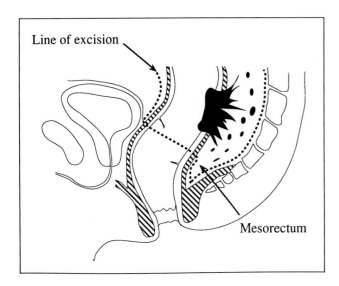

Figure 18-1.   Although a distal margin of only 2 cm may be acceptable, the mesorectal excision must be complete. (Adapted from Heald RJ, Husband EM, Ryall RD. The mesorectum in rectal cancer—the clue to pelvic recurrence? *Br J Surg.* 1982;69;613–616.)

lesions below the peritoneal reflection. The lower rates found in most series may be due to the limited lateral tissue removed and subsequently examined.

Exfoliated tumor cells, theoretically, have the ability to implant on distant surfaces. Thus, cells shed into the bloodstream may cause distant metastases, whereas tumor cells shed from the outer surface of the tumor or from the lumen of the bowel may implant within the pelvis and the peritoneal cavity, causing local recurrence. Fortunately, the process of tumor cell implantation is quite inefficient, and only a very small percentage of the cells that are shed successfully implant. Surgical treatment should address these routes of spread to minimize the dissemination of tumor cells.

Principles of Surgical Treatment and Choice of Operation

The principles of resective surgery include minimal handling of the primary tumor, proximal or high vascular ligation, en bloc resection of any adherent or invaded tissues, and proximal and distal luminal occlusion. Some of these principles are based upon facts, others are founded upon theory or upon restrospective review. Each of these principles is discussed in depth and the available data presented. In addition, preserving anal sphincter function has been an increasingly important goal. However, maintaining anal continence should not compromise the likelihood of cure.

The treatment chosen for a particular patient with a rectal carcinoma depends on several factors. Foremost among these are the location and extent of the tumor and the condition of the patient. The location of the tumor refers to its vertical distance from the anus as well as its radial orientation. The level is usually expressed in centimeters from either the anal verge or the dentate line to the lower edge of the lesion as measured during rigid proctoscopy. This must be interpreted with the length of the individual patient's anal canal in mind. Six cm from the anal verge in a women with a 2-cm anal canal places the tumor 4 cm above the anorectal ring, a location amenable to a sphincter-saving procedure, whereas the same tumor measured in a man with a 4-cm anal canal may not allow an adequate distal margin. Rectal tumors may invade through the wall and involve adjacent structures; this must be considered when planning a resection.

Patient variables often limit the options available. The individual's chronological age may be of less significance than is the physiological age. For this reason, the preoperative medical evaluation should always be considered.

Low Anterior Resection Versus Abdominoperineal Resection

The goal of extirpative surgical therapy is to remove the disease-bearing segment of bowel with an acceptable margin and the relevant lymphatics. In the last few decades, a great deal of attention has been focused on improving functional outcome. Clearly, a patient with a normally functioning sphincter and an intact route of defecation will have a better quality of life than will a patient with a permanent colostomy.[56] Although operations that restore continuity are desirable, the cure rate must not be compromised.

The relative frequency of these operations has changed markedly. During most of the first half of the 20th century an abdominoperineal resection was the preferred procedure for virtually all carcinomas of the rectum and low sigmoid colon. Since Dixon and others popularized the procedure of anterior resection during the 1940s and 1950s there has been an ever increasing effort to extend the limits of sphincter-saving operations.[33,35] These procedures have now replaced abdominoperineal resection for the vast majority of rectal carcinomas.

Several authors have reviewed their personal and institutional experiences with resection for rectal cancers, and all have shown a marked shift toward sphincter-saving procedures.[57] More than 27,000 cases were reviewed in a survey of the members of the American College of Surgeons published in 1980.[58] Before 1973 only 18.6 percent of curative operations for rectal cancer were anterior resections, whereas 28 percent were between 1973 and 1978. Since that time staplers have become fairly standard in many institutions and sphincter-saving operations now account for up to 80 percent of these procedures.[59]

The importance of lymphatic spread was initially demonstrated by Miles, who concluded that tumor cells could be spread through the lymphatic system in three directions: upward along the superior hemorrhoidal vessels to the inferior mesenterics and the periaortic nodes, laterally through the lateral ligaments into the iliac system along the pelvic sidewall, and inferiorly through the sphincter mechanism and perianal skin to the inguinal nodes (Fig. 18-2). Miles believed that a curative operation for cancers of the rectum and sigmoid had to encompass all of these areas.

Proximal Resection Margin.   The proximal resection margin in these operations is not generally a factor since a generous amount of proximal bowel should be removed along with the associated lymphovascular tissues.

Distal Resection Margin.   The length of the distal resection margin is a key question, since there may be very little resectable bowel between a low rectal lesion and the anal sphincters. It is clear that intramural spread beyond 1.5 cm from the raised edge of the lesion is very uncommon.[60-64] In a study of 516 patients in whom margins were measured in the fresh resected specimens, Wilson and Beahrs[65] found that distal margins greater

than 2 cm did not influence survival or local recurrence rates. However, margins of less than 2 cm have been associated with increased failure rates in this and other studies.[62,66] The presence of distal intramural spread greater than 5 mm from the palpable edge of the tumor is almost always associated with extensive lymphatic metastases, poorly differentiated or mucinous histology, and advanced disease.[61,67-70] Therefore, although a 2-cm distal margin is acceptable, if a greater margin can be easily obtained it should be.

Proximal Lymphatic Spread.   Spread to the proximal or cephalad lymph nodes in the bowel mesentery appears to be the major route of lymphatic dissemination. As early as 1925, dye injection studies demonstrated that lymphatic flow from the mid and upper rectum runs almost exclusively into the superior hemorrhoidal–inferior mesenteric complex; while in the rectum below 8 cm, flow may also occur to the inferior and middle hemorrhoidal channels.[71] Dukes[20] and others[27,28] confirmed this upward lymphatic spread. Although initially thought to be uncommon, discontinuous spread or "jumping" was found in up to 30 percent of specimens.[72] High ligation of the inferior mesenteric artery at its origin from the aorta, or just below the left colic branch, allows the sigmoid and rectal mesenteries and their attendant lymph nodes to be removed. The presence or absence of metastases to the lymph nodes as well as the number of lymph nodes involved has repeat-

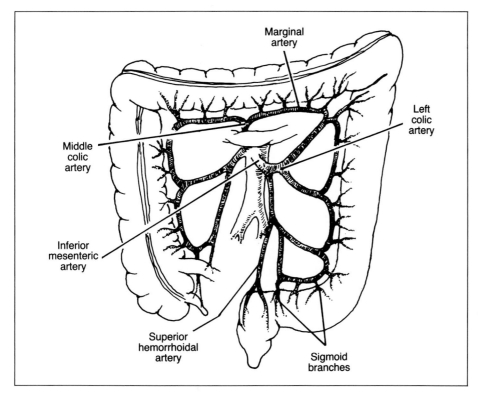

Figure 18-2.   Arterial anatomy of the left colon.

264 Fundamentals of Anorectal Surgery

edly been shown to be important in prognosis. Although some patients with higher nodal involvement may be cured by surgery, this is not universally accepted. However, high ligation is important to ensure a tension-free low rectal anastomosis, and it does assist in obtaining a higher number of lymph nodes. This latter factor is of prognostic significance only.

Lateral Lymphatic Spread. Lateral pelvic lymphatic spread, also emphasized by Miles, occasionally occurs, although most series report very low rates. This may be because most studies are performed on standard resection specimens and little lateral tissue may be present for examination. Studies in which gold was injected submucosally showed that less than 1 percent of the lymph drainage of the upper and mid rectum is directed through the pelvic lymphs nodes.[73] The lower the lesion, it seems, the higher the rate of lateral lymphatic spread. Reported rates of lateral lymph node involvement vary from 0.5 to 9 percent for lesions above the peritoneal reflection and from 16.5 to 28 percent for those below.[55,72,74] Lateral lymph node excision to the pelvic sidewalls is a relatively standard part of a curative resection; however, dissection beyond the iliac vessels is controversial. This is discussed below under Controversies.

Distal Lymphatic Spread. Miles considered distal lymphatic spread to be one of the major routes by which rectal cancer spreads. However, distal spread is seen in only 1 to 2 percent of clinical cases and only with extensive proximal lymphatic blockage by metastatic disease.[63,68,75] Therefore, lymphatic spread is common proximally, is rare distally, and is more common later-

Table 18-1 Five-year Survival After Abdominoperineal Resection (APR) or Low Anterior Resection (LAR)

Author/Year	APR		LAR	
	No. patients	5-yr survival, %	No. patients	5-yr survival, %
Waugh et al[77] 1955	69	52	126	66
Deddish and Stearns[78] 1961	248	65	150	69
Gilbertsen[79] 1962	193	43	17	35
Williams et al[80] 1966	93	46	89	57
Glenn and McSherry[8] 1966	368	40	123	44
Palumbo and Sharpe[81] 1968	67	50	76	57
Zollinger and Sheppard[82] 1971	328	41	401	49
Slanetz et al[83] 1972	277	47	247	56
Stearns[84] 1978	227	48	225	56
Strauss et al[85] 1978	34	44	49	55
Fick et al[86] 1990	29	59	39	72
Summary of studies	*1933*	*47*	*1542*	*55*

Table 18-2   Local Recurrence Rates After Abdominoperineal Resection (APR) or Low Anterior Resection (LAR)

Author/Year	APR		LAR	
	No. patients	Local recurrence, %	No. patients	Local recurrence, %
Wolmark and Fisher[66]* 1986	232	5	181	13
Pheils et al[87] 1983	95	5	98	14
Graf et al[88] 1990	100	17	50	16
Fick et al[86] 1990	27	15	32	13
Amato et al[89] 1991	69	11	78	12
Summary	*523*	*9*	*439*	*13* NS

* Mean follow-up 4 years. All Dukes stages B and C.

ally with lesions lying below the peritoneal reflection. More important than distal lymphatic spread, however, is spread within the mesorectum. Even with distal margins of 1 cm or less, complete mesorectal excision is associated with local recurrence rates of 3 percent or less.[76] For this reason, a complete mesorectal incision is important.

Studies in which survival results after abdominoperineal resection have been compared with those after low anterior resection have failed to show any compromise of cure rates with the latter (Table 18-1). Indeed, in many series, low anterior resection was associated with improved outcome. Also, few reports have documented any differences in local (Table 18-2) or overall recurrence rates.[67,83,90-94] However, there are many problems with these comparisons including tumor variability, unmatched groups, different surgeons, differing techniques, and a natural bias toward performing an abdominoperineal resection for larger and more advanced lesions. Also, because of the routes of lymphatic drainage, more distal lesions may carry a poorer prognosis.

In practice, the major factor to be considered in deciding whether or not to do a sphincter-saving operation is the ability to obtain a distal margin of at least 2 cm without compromising the sphincter muscles. The level at which it is technically possible to do an anastomosis has been progressively lowered. Initially, this was because of the development of innovative approaches to the anastomotic site such as coloanal anastomosis, eversion techniques and transacral exposure.

Recently, however, the use of staplers have made most of these other procedures obsolete. An abdominoperineal resection is now rarely necessary unless the tumor is adherent to the levators or to the sphincter complex, or is within the anorectal ring.

Resection Techniques

Abdominoperineal Resection

For most of the 20th century, abdominoperineal resection (APR) has been the standard operation against which all others were compared. The procedure involves the radical excision of the sigmoid colon, rectum, and anus along with the relevant blood supply and lymphatics (Fig. 18-3). The perineum is closed and a permanent colostomy is constructed in the left lower abdominal quadrant. Most surgeons now perform this operation with the patient in the combined or synchronous Lloyd-Davies position which provides good access to both the abdomen and perineum without repositioning (Fig. 18-4). Some prefer to perform the abdominal phase, complete the colostomy and abdominal closure, and rotate the patient into the jackknife or Kraske position for the perineal phase. This gives excellent exposure of the perineum but requires rolling the intubated patient over and reprepping. The procedure will be described with the patient in the synchronous position.

Preoperatively, the patient should be counseled about and marked for the colostomy. The risks and benefits

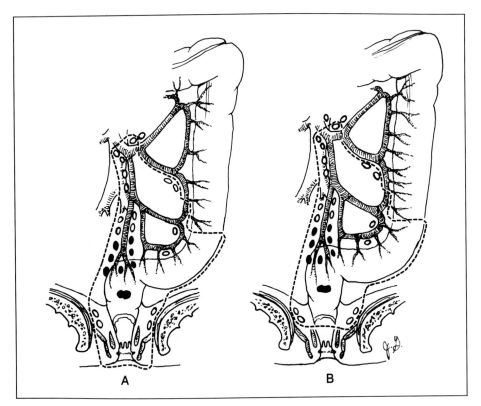

Figure 18-3. Extent of the excision. (A) Abdomino-perineal resection. (B) Low anterior resection.

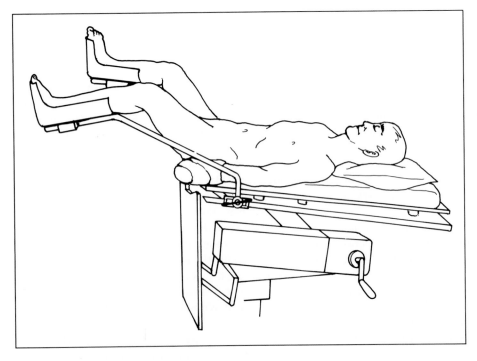

Figure 18-4. Patient position. Combined or synchronous Lloyd–Davies position provides good access to both the abdomen and perineum. Note that the Allen stirrups (Allen Medical Co., Bedford Heights, OH) are bootlike in configuration and therefore avoid pressure on the peroneal nerve.

including the possibility of impotence and retrograde ejaculation should be discussed. Clearly, meticulous technique and hemostasis, careful handling of tissues, sound judgment, and rapid but deliberate work promote a good outcome.

Abdominal Phase

Position. All left colon and rectal resections are performed in the synchronous or lithotomy/Trendelenburg Lloyd-Davies position. This allows access to the abdomen and perineum without repositioning. Anesthesia is induced with the patient in the supine position. A urinary catheter is placed. The legs are supported by Allen stirrups (Allen Medical Co., Bedford Heights, Ohio) with the hips abducted and flexed between 15° and 45°. The calves and feet should be parallel to or slightly above the level of the knees to promote venous drainage during the procedure. Sequential calf compression stockings are used to reduce the incidence of deep venous thrombosis. Low dose subcutaneously administered heparin may be used selectively. The buttocks should hang well over the end of the table with the upper sacrum supported by a cloth roll. If the scrotum hangs down, it may be fixed to a thigh with sutures or tape. Both arms are carefully tucked at the patient's sides with the hands protected by towels. If absolutely necessary, the right arm may be extended for the anesthesiologist.

The rectum is washed out with saline until clear, followed by a final wash of povidone-iodine solution. A pursestring suture of heavy silk is placed around the anus. The abdomen and perineum from nipples to thighs are cleansed and painted with povidone-iodine solution or a similar preparation, and the drapes are placed. The Mayo stand is positioned either over the patient's head and chest or over one of the legs. The large light is centered over the abdomen and is angled slightly down into the pelvis; the smaller light is positioned over the patient's head and is aimed sharply into the pelvis. The surgeon stands on the patient's left with the first assistant across from him or her on the patient's right. The second assistant stands between the patient's legs to provide pelvic retraction.

Incision and Exploration. A midline incision is generally used, although a low transverse incision can be made. The midline incision, however, allows free access to both the pelvis and the splenic flexure and keeps both sides of the anterior abdominal wall free for stoma placement. The incision begins at the pubic symphysis and extends around the umbilicus to midway between the umbilicus and the xiphoid (Fig. 18-5). It may be extended as needed. Care must be taken when dividing

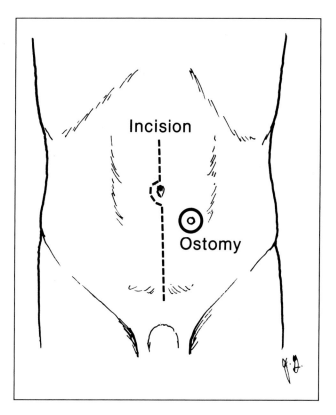

Figure 18-5. Incision from the pubic symphysis to midway between the umbilicus and the xiphoid.

the peritoneum not to enter the bladder. The bladder may be palpated by grasping the preperitoneal tissues at the lower end of the incision between the index finger and the thumb and sliding upward until the edge of the bladder wall is reached. The peritoneum may then be safely divided at this point. The retractors will easily keep the remainder of this tissue out of the way. After any anterior abdominal wall adhesions have been lysed, a plastic wound protector may be inserted, and laparotomy pads are placed between the plastic and the cut surfaces of the wound. A self-retaining Balfour-type retractor is placed. The abdomen is thoroughly explored, with particular attention being paid to the liver and the periaortic lymph nodes. Intraoperative ultrasonography of the liver may be performed at this point.

Exposure. Good visualization of the pelvis is critical in all of these procedures. When necessary, the peritoneal reflections of the cecum and terminal ileum may be divided to allow them to be packed superiorly along with the small bowel. The patient is placed in the Trendelenburg or head-down position. The small bowel and cecum are packed superiorly out of the field by having the first assistant hook an index finger or a retractor under the upper end of the incision to lift the upper

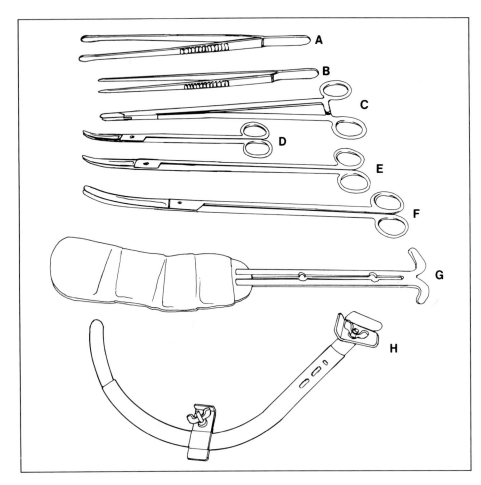

Figure 18-6. Useful instruments for pelvic dissection. (A) Long Russian forceps. (B) Long flat serrated bowel forceps. (C) Long needle holder. (D) Standard Harrington scissors, flat on the curve. (E) Long Harrington scissors. (F) Extralong Goligher design, uterine decapitation scissors. (G) and (H) C-arm extender for the Balfour retractor and attachable malleable blade retractor.

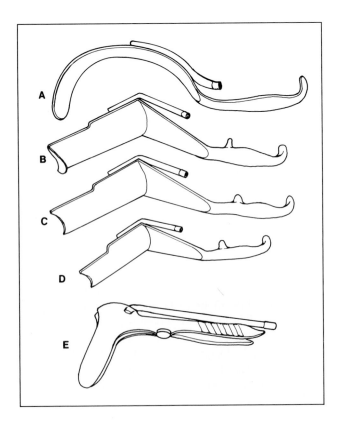

abdominal wall. The bowel is then packed superiorly beneath a flat wet towel. This towel is laid out with its short end stretched from the right to the left gutter across the spine and aorta, extending up over the bowel onto the chest. Rolled wet laparotomy pads are stuffed into each lateral gutter to anchor the corners of the towel. A C-arm extender is connected to the Balfour retractor; the malleable blade attachment is positioned over the aorta to keep the packed bowel in place (Fig. 18-6). The St. Mark's pelvic retractors, the Deavor retractor, and narrow and wide malleable retractors are extremely helpful for retracting anteriorly and exposing the deep pelvis. Good lighting is critical and may be obtained by using retractors that are fitted with fiberoptic lights or with a head light (Fig. 18-7).

Mobilization. The sigmoid colon is released from its peritoneal attachments in the left iliac fossa (Fig. 18-8), with care being taken to peel the left ureter and gonadal

Figure 18-7. Lighted retractors. (A) Deaver, (B) St. Mark's design, long with lip. (C) St. Mark's design, long flat. (D) St. Mark's design, short. (E) Pratt bivalve anal retractor.

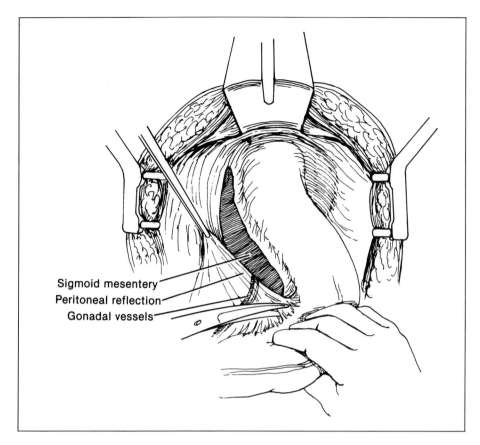

Sigmoid mesentery
Peritoneal reflection
Gonadal vessels

Figure 18-8. Abdominoperineal resection or low anterior resection: mobilization. The sigmoid colon is released from its peritoneal attachments in the left iliac fossa.

vessels posterolaterally. The left ureter must be visualized and protected (Fig. 18-9). The dissection proceeds in the cephalad direction, dividing the peritoneal reflexion along the white line of Toldt. The dissection may be undertaken with either a scissors or electrocautery. The sigmoid colon and its mesentery are completely mobilized to the midline, separating the mesentery from the retroperitoneum. The sigmoid is held up straight and the peritoneal surface is incised posteriorly on the right. A finger is passed beneath the inferior mesenteric artery and vein in the base of the mesentery; these may then be isolated by sharp dissection proceeding superiorly. Fat may be easily removed from this plane by firmly squeezing the tissues between the thumb and forefinger. The inferior mesenteric artery and vein are divided between clamps and doubly ligated. The inferior mesenteric artery may be divided at its origin from the aorta or it may be divided just distal to its first branch, the left colic artery (Fig. 18-10).

The site for proximal transection of the bowel is chosen according to the location of the tumor and the length of proximal bowel needed to construct a healthy, well-vascularized colostomy. This site generally lies at or near the descending colon–sigmoid junction. Greater freedom of the bowel and mesentery must be attained when operating on obese patients with a thick abdominal wall and a bulky mesentery. As much mesentery as is reasonably possible is removed along with the attendant lymphatic drainage. An umbilical tape is passed around the bowel at the chosen point and a second one is placed 10 to 15 cm proximal to it. The proximal tape is tied down with one knot to isolate the lumen. The distal tape is used for gentle traction and as a marker. The remaining mesentery is then divided by cutting the peritoneal surface, separating the fat, and individually ligating the vessels. The bowel is divided either between straight clamps or with a linear stapler. The cut edges are wiped with a swab soaked with povidone-iodine. The proximal end is wrapped in a lap pad and placed in the left upper quadrant beneath the packing.

Pelvic Dissection. The sigmoid colon is held up with moderate tension put on the sigmoid mesentery. The scissors or the electrocautery is used to divide the peritoneal surface, beginning at the upper edge on the right and continuing down over the sacral promontory, laterally over the vessels, and down into the cul-de-sac or pouch of Douglas (Fig. 18-11). Anteriorly, several veins may be encountered and bleeding may be controlled with the electrocautery. The left peritoneum is divided in a similar fashion and the two incisions are joined anteriorly.

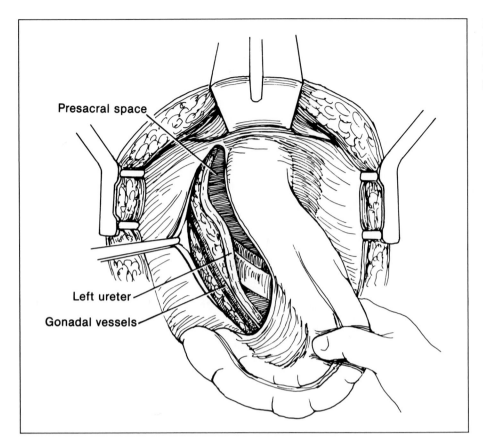

Figure 18-9. Abdomino-perineal resection or low anterior resection: mobilization. Identification of the left gonadal vessels and ureter.

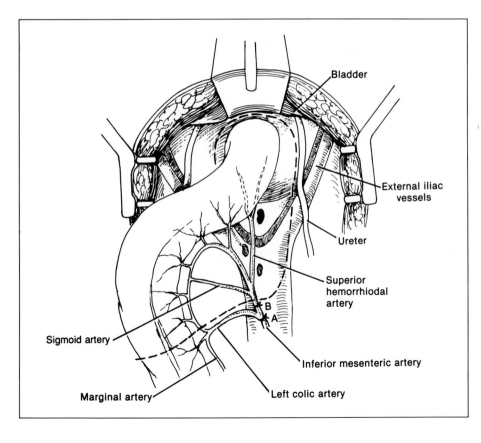

Figure 18-10. Abdomino-perineal resection or low anterior resection: mobilization. The interior mesenteric artery may be divided at its origin from the aorta (A) or just distal to the left colic artery (B). Performance of a tension-free low anastomosis may dictate high ligation (A).

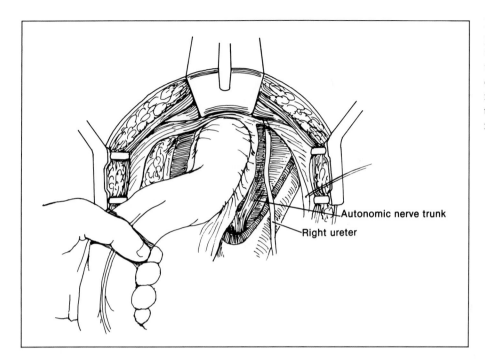

Autonomic nerve trunk
Right ureter

Figure 18-11. Abdomino-perineal resection or low anterior resection: pelvic dissection. Holding up the sigmoid colon and identifying the right gonadal vessels, the ureter, and the sacral autonomic trunk.

The presacral space is entered at the pelvic brim and the sharp dissection is carried down along the sacral curve, posterior to the rectum and its mesentery and anterior to the presacral fascia. The hypogastric neural plexus may be identified and separated from the meso-rectum at the level of the sacral promontory. In most cases, it may be sharply dissected from the mesorectum and preserved.

It is important to enter the correct posterior plane since dissection here is relatively bloodless, preserves much of the neural plexus, avoids injuring the presacral vessels, and sets up the lateral and anterior dissections. Once this plane has been entered, firm upward traction is maintained on the rectum, and the loose areolar attachments in the presacral space may be separated by blunt and sharp dissection. The plane may be quickly opened down to and on either side of the rectosacral ligament. Division of the rectosacral ligament is performed sharply with a long, curved, blunt-tipped scissors, such as the Goligher design (see Fig. 18-6). This may also be accomplished with the electrocautery. It is important to emphasize that there is no role for blunt presacral dissection, as this technique encourages bleeding, autonomic nerve injury, and incomplete dissection.

The posterior dissection curves anteriorly along the coccyx and the levator muscles to the anorectal ring. Once this portion of the procedure has been completed, the rectum will rise up out of the pelvis significantly (Fig. 18-12). The plane is widened on either side by blunt dissection until the "lateral stalks" are defined.

The lateral dissection is performed sharply on either side, staying on the pelvis sidewalls. The rectum is firmly retracted medially with the left hand allowing precise division of these tissues. The course of the ureters must be kept clearly in mind, as they may be pulled down into the upper portion of the dissection field. Mass clamping and ligation of these lateral tissues is to be discouraged since a large amount of the lateral mesorectal tissue and lymph nodes will be left in place. Often no large vessels are found; however, when they are they may be individually ligated.

The anterior dissection is facilitated by angling the lipped St. Mark's retractor inferiorly while pulling up and by countertraction by the operator pushing posteriorly and superiorly on the anterior rectal wall. The fascia of Denonvilliers is cut at the anterior edge of the pouch of Douglas and the plane between this and the anterior structures is followed down.

In women, the rectovaginal septum may be completely separated in this fashion using sharp dissection, frequently repositioning the retractors to keep the plane under traction. If the tumor invades or is adherent to the vaginal wall, a posterior vaginectomy is indicated.

In men, the bladder trigone and seminal vesicles are preserved when there is no evidence of tumor invasion. This may be made easier below the tumor by cutting across the fascia of Denonvilliers down onto the anterior rectal wall, finishing the dissection in this plane.

The pelvic dissection is complete when the anorectal ring is reached on all sides (Fig. 18-13). With very low tumors a wider resection may be desirable and the dissection is completed more laterally on the levators. These will be divided later during the perineal dissection.

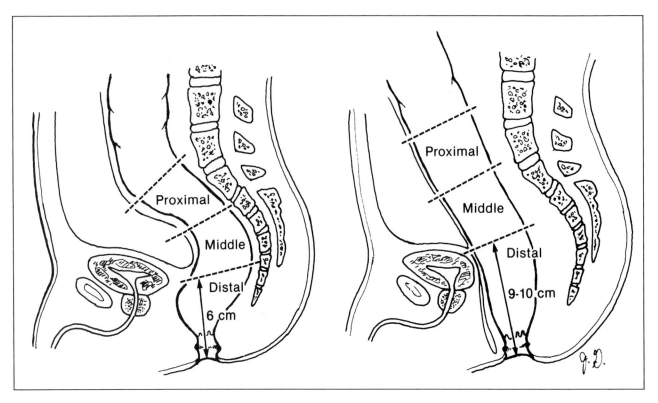

Figure 18-12. Abdominoperineal resection or low anterior resection: After division of the rectosacral ligament and completion of the posterior dissection, the rectum will rise out of the pelvis significantly, increasing the length of rectum available for the distal margin.

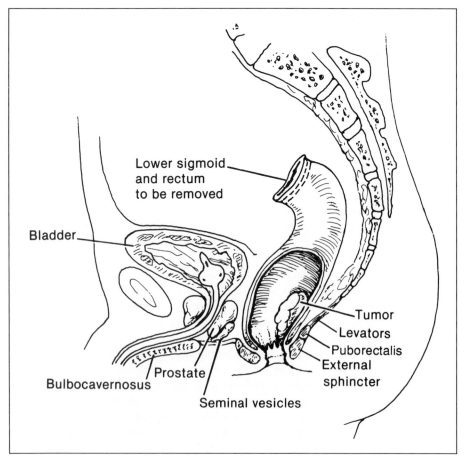

Figure 18-13. Abdominoperineal resection: perineal phase. Lateral view of the pelvis after completion of the abdominal phase.

Perineal Phase.   An elliptical incision is made on the perineum from the middle of the perineal body anteriorly to just below the coccyx posteriorly (Fig. 18-14). Laterally, the incision extends to the ischial tuberosities but should not be so wide as to compromise a tension-free cutaneous closure. As the incision is deepened the medial cut edges on either side are grasped with three or four Allis or Kocher clamps placed in a vertical row, approximating the skin in the midline. These help to keep the anus closed and provide a convenient handle for retraction of the specimen (Fig. 18-15).

The ischiorectal space is divided close to the lateral pelvis walls, taking most of the fat with the specimen. The lateral margins of the wound may be retracted with Gelpi, St. Mark's pattern, Weitlaner perineal, or spring retractors. The pudendal neurovascular bundle is encountered on either side and is ligated or cauterized and then cut.

The dissection is continued up to the coccyx posteriorly and along the levators laterally. The presacral space is entered by cutting the anococcygeal ligament (the median raphe of the leavtors) (Fig. 18-16). A finger is placed through this opening, hooking the levator mus-

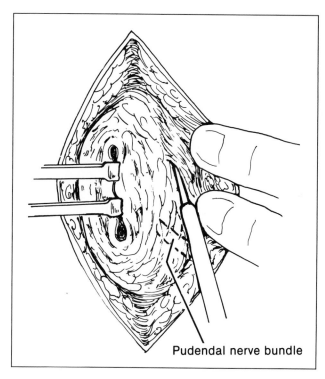

Pudendal nerve bundle

Figure 18-15.   Abdominoperineal resection: perineal phase. Dissection through the ischiorectal fossae, encountering the pudendal neurovascular bundle.

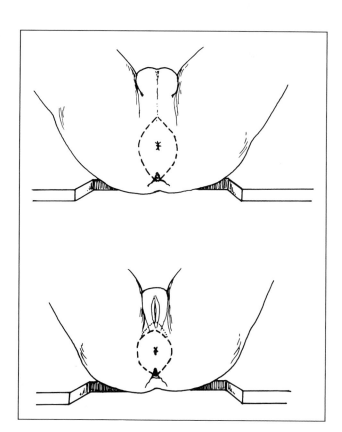

Figure 18-14.   Abdominoperineal resection: perineal phase. Skin incision from the middle of the perineal body anteriorly to just below the coccyx posteriorly and to the ischial tuberosities laterally. In women this incision may be extended anteriorly to include the posterior vagina.

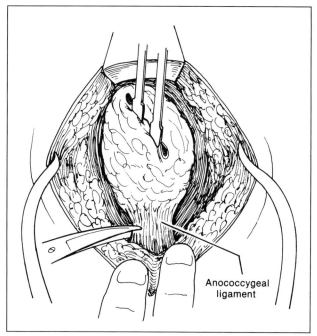

Anococcygeal ligament

Figure 18-16.   Abdominoperineal resection: perineal phase. The levators are exposed laterally, as is the coccyx posteriorly. The anococcygeal ligament (the median raphe of the levators) is cut to allow entry to the presacral space.

cles and dividing them laterally with the cautery, first on one side and then on the other (Fig. 18-17). A clamp or suture may be placed on the lateral cut edges for easier identification and later approximation.

The anterior dissection in the male is the most difficult portion of this phase since the rectum and anal sphincters are closely apposed to the membranous urethra, prostate, and seminal vesicles. The anterior skin is retracted up while the surgeon keeps moderate pressure on the rectum; this reveals the dissection plane (Fig. 18-18). Palpation of the urinary catheter in the urethra helps avoid injuring this structure. This plane is dissected sharply and carefully. With the first finger of the surgeon's left hand hooked around the remaining tissue above and with the thumb pushing down on the lower segment of the specimen, the remaining tissues may be clearly felt, guiding the dissection.

In women the rectovaginal septum is usually dissected fairly easily. In cases of suspected vaginal wall invasion or low anterior tumors, the posterior vagina and perineal body may be resected en bloc.

The specimen is removed from below, hemostatis is obtained with the cautery and suture ligatures as necessary, and the pelvis is copiously irrigated with warm saline from above and below. The perineal wound is closed whenever possible.

The closure is performed in layers, beginning with the levator muscles. It may be possible to bring the

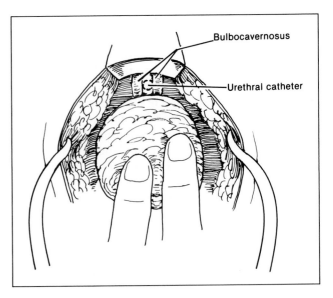

Figure 18-18. Abdominoperineal resection: perineal phase. Anterior dissection in the male, exposing the membranous urethra, prostate, and seminal vesicles.

remaining muscles together in the midline for part or all of the length of the cut edges with large sutures of 0 or 2-0 polyglycolic acid. The ischiorectal fat is approximated with two or three layers of interrupted absorbable sutures and the skin is closed with either a running subcuticular 4-0 absorbable suture or interrupted vertical mattress sutures.

Colostomy Construction. The colostomy is constructed from the cut end of the proximal sigmoid colon or the descending colon and is usually placed in the left lower quadrant. Two Kocher clamps are placed in the incision, one on the cut edge of the fascia and one at the subcuticular level. Holding a folded laparotomy pad in his or her left hand, the surgeon lifts firmly up on the left abdominal wall from within, tenting up the wall by pushing up with the fingers and pulling down on the Kocher clamps. This pressure is maintained until the full thickness of the ostomy aperture has been completed.

A 3-cm diameter circular skin incision is made at the marked site. The fat is entered and the skin plug is removed. Progressively deeper right-angle retractors held in the transverse direction are used to divide the fat longitudinally with the cautery until the anterior rectus fascia is encountered. The middle of the anterior rectus fascia is divided longitudinally. A closed large Kelly clamp is pushed through the muscle against the left hand, which continues to tent the abdominal wall up. The clamp is gently but firmly spread wide in the transverse direction, and the right-angle retractors are repositioned against the posterior fascia, separating the rectus muscle. The posterior fascia and peritoneum are then

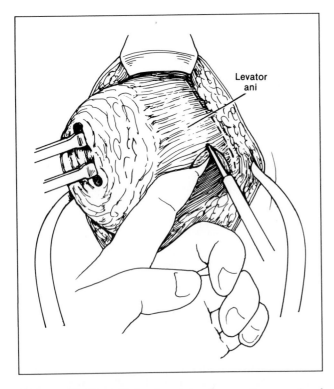

Figure 18-17. Abdominoperineal resection: perineal phase. Dividing the levators laterally.

divided with the cautery, coming down on the laparotomy pad protecting the left hand.

The large Kelly clamp is passed through the opening, which is then dilated to two finger-breadths, taking care to keep a finger or an instrument through the aperture at all times. The bowel is prepared by trimming the mesentery as needed to provide adequate length to traverse the abdominal wall. No more than 2 cm of distal bowel should be completely cleared of mesentery. If necessary, the mesentery may be defatted to allow easier passage through the wall. A good blood supply must be maintained to the ostomy to avoid necrosis.

The bowel is passed through the opening using a Babcock or large Kelly clamp. Two to three centimeters of bowel should sit comfortably above skin level to create the everted stoma (Fig. 18-19). Several interrupted sutures of a 3-0 absorbable material may be placed between the bowel serosa and the peritoneum and the posterior rectus sheath. Several sutures may also be placed from the serosa to the anterior rectus sheath. When feasible, the lateral gutter may be closed to avoid an internal hernia. We do not routinely suture the bowel to either the posterior or the anterior rectus fascia or close the lateral gutter.

Some surgeons use an "extraperitoneal" method of creating the colostomy. This entails tunneling the bowel beneath the lateral peritoneum before bringing it through the abdominal wall. Although this may reduce the risk of internal and paracolostomy herniation, it requires a far greater length of free bowel and much more dissection.

Pelvic Drainage. The pelvis may be a postoperative repository for much fluid and blood. For this reason, pelvic drainage is undertaken. Although Penrose and other drains were used extensively in the past, closed suction drainage is much more effective and reduces the possibility of retrograde migration of bacteria. The practice of bringing drains out of the perineal closure is to be condemned because of the high rate of associated perineal sepsis, persistent sinuses, and patient discomfort. One or two closed suction drains may be placed into the pelvis from above, exiting through a lateral lower abdominal stab wound. If there is a large dead space below the levators that cannot be obliterated by suturing, a small closed suction catheter may be placed and brought out through a stab wound to one side of the perineal closure. This should be removed within 2 days of the operation. The pelvis may be irrigated through a suction drain. However, randomized studies have failed to demonstrate any significant benefit to this technique.[95-97] A mesh sling may be placed to exclude the

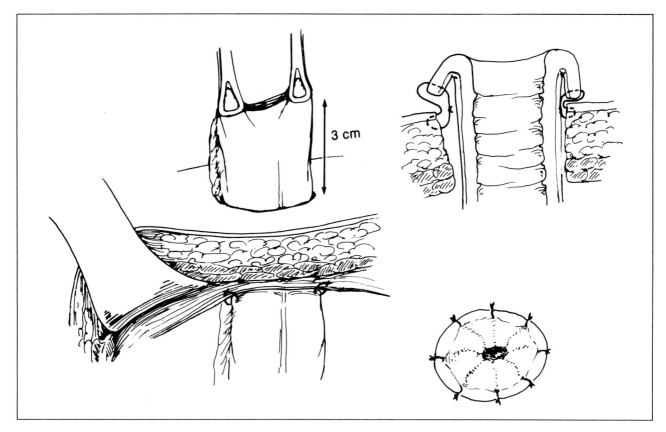

Figure 18-19.   Abdominoperineal resection: creation of the colostomy.

small bowel from the pelvis prior to closing the abdomen if postoperative radiation is contemplated. This is discussed under Radiation Therapy.

Colostomy Maturation. After the abdomen is closed a towel is placed over the wound. There is no role for secondary maturation of stomas now. The staple line is excised or the straight clamp removed and the mucosa is tacked to the skin in eight equidistant locations around its circumference (see Fig. 18-19). The edge of the mucosa is sutured to the subcuticular level of the skin. The stitch should not be placed through the skin since this will encourage implantation of mucosal cells and subsequent severe peristomal skin irritation and breakdown. A stoma appliance is fitted and secured, and an abdominal dressing is applied.

Low Anterior Resection

Low anterior resection (LAR) of the rectum is performed almost entirely from the abdominal approach. The patient is positioned just as for the abdominoperineal resection since access to the perineum allows transanal placement of an end-to-end stapler and, with very low anastomoses, transanal placement of the pursestring suture. In difficult situations, a coloanal anastomosis and loop ileostomy may be performed to salvage a failed or technically impossible intrapelvic anastomosis.

Dissection. The procedure is begun as described above for the abdominoperineal resection. The splenic flexure is routinely mobilized to permit an adequate resection and a subsequent tension-free anastomosis. The proximal level of transection is chosen so that a generous portion of the vascular tree and attendant lymphatics of the rectosigmoid mesentery are removed with the specimen. However, the site must be chosen so that a tension-free and well-vascularized anastomosis may be constructed. This proximal division is generally at about the level of the descending–sigmoid colon junction.

The distal level of transection should be at least 2 cm beyond the palpable edge of the tumor. A 3- to 5-cm margin is preferred if attainable without undue difficulty. Additional length may be obtained by dividing the rectosacral ligament as described above and continuing the posterior dissection down into the anorectal ring. It is important to divide the rectal mesentery well below the line of distal bowel transection. Indeed, when performing a resection of a low or mid-rectal cancer the entire mesorectum should be removed, leaving only a 2- to 3-cm cuff of defatted rectum with which to construct the anastomosis. This segment of bowel will derive an adequate blood supply from its inferior aspect. There is

some convincing evidence that complete mesorectal excision decreases the rate of pelvic recurrence.[98,99]

The surgeon performs the distal transection by pulling up on the rectum with the right hand while the left index and middle fingers are placed across the bowel below the tumor. A right angle bowel clamp, a pursestring device, or a linear stapler is placed below the fingers, marking the lower edge of the distal line of resection (Fig. 18-20). The rectum is washed out from below, again using povidone-iodine. A right-angle bowel clamp is placed across the distal line of resection, just above the fired staple or first clamp, and the bowel is divided in between.

Immediate inspection of the opened specimen for margin of clearance is critical. If an open anastomotic technique is being employed, four long stay sutures are placed around the cut edge of the distal rectum as the bowel is cut. These are very helpful when suturing or placing the pursestring.

Anastomotic Techniques. A well-constructed anastomosis should be tension-free and should have a good blood supply. The calibers of the proximal and distal segments should be equalized, and intestinal contents should not be spilled during its creation. Good serosa-to-serosa apposition has been the hallmark of gastrointestinal anastomoses; however, recent experience with certain stapling techniques suggests that mucosal apposition with a double row of permanent staples is also safe.

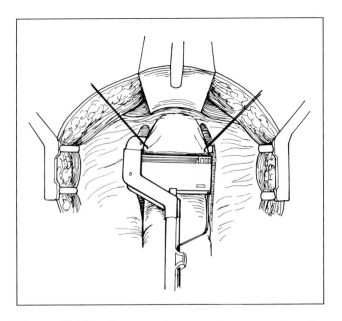

Figure 18-20. Low anterior resection: transecting the bowel distal to the tumor. A right-angle bowel clamp, a pursestring device, or a linear stapler is placed at the lower edge of the distal line of resection.

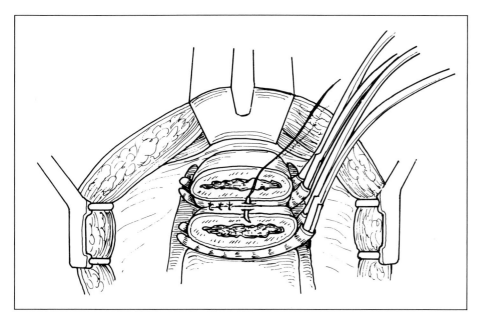

Figure 18-21. Low anterior resection: hand-sutured anastomosis. After placing the posterior row of sutures, the two lumens are positioned side by side while being occluded by the two Foss clamps.

Hand-sutured Anastomosis. A two-layer technique has been traditionally used in many centers and has been clearly described by Oliver Beahrs, M.D., of the Mayo Clinic.[100] A curved Foss clamp (rubber or cloth shod) is placed across the rectum 1 to 2 cm below the line of distal transection. If the distal segment is too short the rectum may be held open by long stay sutures and the anastomosis constructed after cleansing the lumen with povidone-iodine dampened sponges. A second curved Foss clamp is placed across the proximal sigmoid or the distal descending colon just above the chosen level of proximal transection. The two Foss clamps are then positioned side by side to ensure adequate approximation. After placement of a straight clamp, the proximal bowel is cut if this has not already been done, and the specimen is removed. The opened lumen is cleansed.

The Foss clamps are placed side by side with the bowel walls separated by 2 to 3 cm. Seven interrupted sutures of 3-0 silk are placed as a posterior seromuscular layer, working from the right to the left. Each suture is tagged with a straight hemostat. The posterior walls of the rectum and proximal bowel are brought together with the Foss clamps, and the sutures are tied sequentially, cutting the middle five and leaving the lateral two tagged (Fig. 18-21). If the distal end is very deep the posterior row of interrupted sutures may be placed with the proximal end out of the pelvis. The proximal bowel is then run down to lie adjacent to the distal end while gently pulling up on the sutures to remove the slack. A running mucosal suture of 3-0 chromic catgut or polyglycolic acid suture is placed, beginning on the right lateral side. This suture is tied on the outside of the bowel and the short end is tagged. The suture is passed back through the rectal wall into the lumen, and

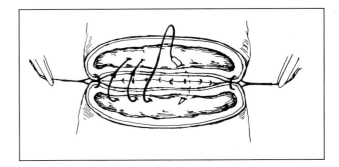

Figure 18-22. Low anterior resection: hand-sutured anastomosis. The mucosa and submucosa of the posterior wall are approximated in a running over-and-over fashion.

the mucosa and submucosa of the posterior wall are approximated in a running over-and-over fashion (Fig. 18-22). When the left lateral wall is reached several stitches are locked to prevent pursestringing. The running over-and-over suture is continued around anteriorly, inverting the layers. The suture is tied to the short tagged end and cut. The Foss clamps are released to allow inversion of the anterior wall. Seven 3-0 silk sutures are then placed as an anterior seromuscular layer to complete the anastomosis. These are tied and cut as they are placed. The anastomosis is inspected and additional silk sutures may be placed, as necessary. The tagged lateral silk sutures are cut last (Fig. 18-23).

Several alternatives to the two-layer technique of sutured anastomoses exist. A one-layer anastomosis may be constructed using either closely placed interrupted sutures of 3-0 silk or a running suture of 2-0 Prolene.[101] At the Cleveland Clinic a posterior row of

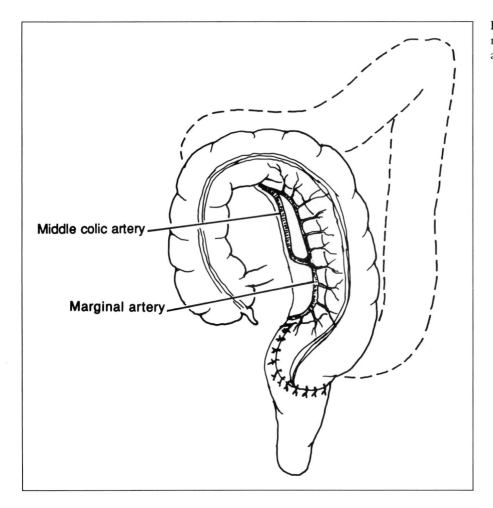

Figure 18-23. Low anterior resection: the completed anastomosis and anatomy.

Middle colic artery

Marginal artery

interrupted mattress sutures of 3-0 polyglycilic acid material is placed and tagged and then tied after sliding the proximal bowel down; a single seromuscular layer is placed anteriorly.[102] A side-to-end anastomosis using the antimesenteric surface of the proximal bowel may occasionally be easier to perform when the mesentery is very bulky or when the lumen sizes are quite disparate.[103,104]

Stapled Anastomosis. Staplers for creating intestinal anastomoses were first successfully developed and used in the Soviet Union. In 1977, the first commercially available instrument was introduced in the United States.[105] Since then these units have rapidly evolved into very reliable and easily used products (Figs. 18-24, 18-25, and 18-26). Their major disadvantage is their high cost. However, because they allow the safe construction of anastomoses deep in the pelvis or in the anal canal, stapling techniques have displaced most of the other pelvic anastomotic methods.

Most rectal stapled anastomoses are constructed in an end-to-end fashion by transanal placement of an intra-luminal circular stapler. Other methods of creating a stapled anastomosis have been described but are used only occasionally. A side-to-side anastomosis may be constructed with a GIA-type stapler, a triangulated anastomosis may be performed, and the intraluminal circular stapler may be placed from above via a colotomy which is closed in turn by a linear stapler. A side-to-end stapled anastomosis may be created with the patient in the supine position. This technique is particularly useful when there is a large discrepancy in size or if the proximal bowel is bulky. No pursestring is required proximally and the anastomosis is made through the antimesenteric border. A potential problem with this method is the risk of ischemia in the antimesenteric segment between the circular staple line and the open end of the proximal bowel.[102]

In operations with curative intent, there should be no compromise of the margins of resection for the sake of an anastomosis. As the distal rectum is transected, four long stay sutures are placed around its circumference and are tagged with straight hemostats. These are important since once the rectum is cut the distal end will

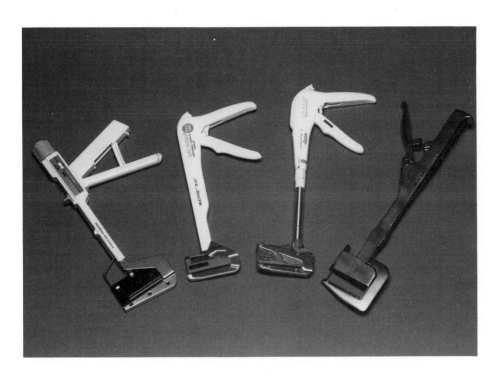

Figure 18-24. Linear staplers. (Left to right) Ethicon Inc. (Sommerville, NJ); United States Surgical Corporation (Norwalk, CT)—standard TA-55, United States Surgical—Roticulator 55, 3-M Medical Surgical Division (St. Paul, MN).

tend to fall deep into the pelvis, where it may be difficult to visualize. Exposure is facilitated by the use of the lighted St. Mark's design and Deaver retractors or a headlight; it is best to have two assistants.

An assistant may push on the perineum with a fist to elevate the distal end within the pelvis.[102] A pursestring suture of 2-0 Prolene is placed in an over-and-over fashion beginning and ending anteriorly (Fig. 18-27). A similar pursestring suture is placed in the proximal end

of the bowel. No more than 2 to 3 mm of full-thickness bowel wall should be included with each bite and most of this should be seromuscular. If more is taken, the gathered tissue may not fit within the diameter of the instrument's circular blade.

Several automated pursestring devices are available and may be used. If the rectum has been transected very low or in the upper anal canal it may be necessary to place the pursestring transanally. The largest possible

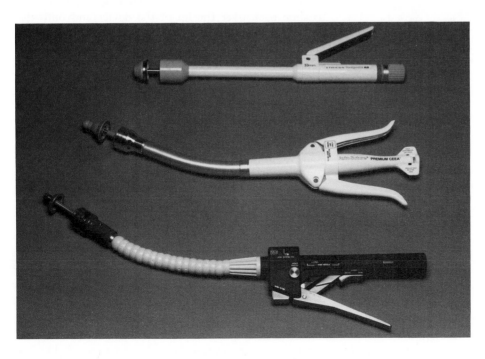

Figure 18-25. Intraluminal circular staplers. (Top to bottom) Ethicon, Inc. (Sommerville, NJ), United States Surgical Corporation (Norwalk, CT), 3-M Medical Surgical Division (St. Paul, MN).

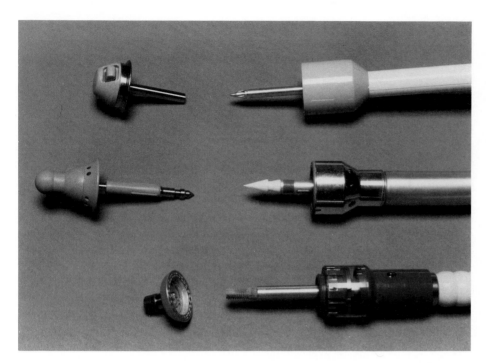

Figure 18-26. Intraluminal circular staplers. Detail of detachable heads and pointed trocar, where available. (Top to bottom) Ethicon, Inc. (Sommerville, NJ), United States Surgical Corporation (Norwalk, CT), 3-M Medical Surgical Division (St. Paul, MN).

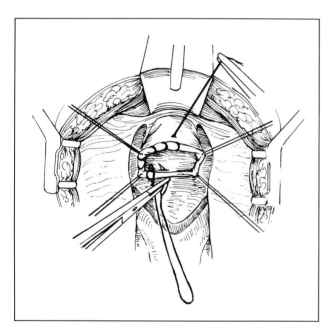

Figure 18-27. Low anterior resection: stapled anastomosis. Placement of the distal pursestring suture using 2-0 Prolene® in an over-and-over fashion beginning and ending anteriorly.

diameter stapler should be used. Most colorectal anastomoses may be constructed with 31- or 33-mm diameter devices.

The stapler is placed through the anus and out the cut distal end of the rectum. This is facilitated by gentle traction on the stay sutures to keep the rectum open. If

the rectal remnant is very long it may be necessary to place a finger into the rectum from above to guide the instrument around the sacral curve. After full insertion, the device is opened as far as possible. If the head or anvil is detachable, it is now removed and placed into the proximal bowel. The proximal pursestring suture is tied down. If the anvil is not detachable, the distal pursestring suture may be tied first.

The instrument is partially withdrawn while holding the stay sutures. This allows the cut edge of the rectum to slide back over the lip of the device and onto the shaft. The distal pursestring suture is tied down snugly taking care to not cut the bowel on the edge of the housing with the taut suture (Fig. 18-28). The proximal bowel is brought down into the pelvis and the shaft from the anvil/head is slid into the lower shaft until it locks (Fig. 18-29). If the head is not detachable the proximal bowel is brought over the head and its pursestring suture is tied down. The instrument is advanced slightly until the rectal wall is gently tented against its edge.

The operator holds the proximal bowel just above the anvil, and the stapler is closed until snug and until the correct anastomotic thickness is indicated on the handle. If the patient is female, just before the stapler is completely closed, the pelvic operator should place a finger in the vagina to ensure that the posterior vaginal wall has not been inadvertently caught in the anastomosis. The stapler is fired and then opened with two complete rotations of the wingnut (Fig. 18-30). It is then removed by rocking carefully to one side and then the other until it comes free from the anastomosis. During

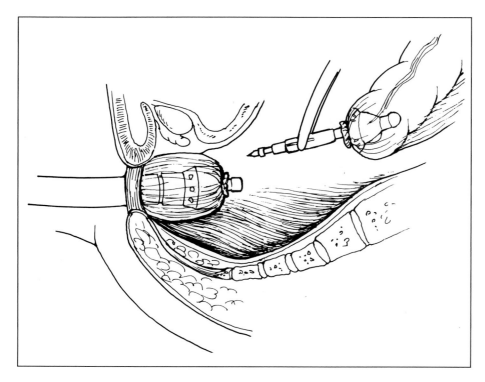

Figure 18-28. Low anterior resection: stapled anastomosis. The distal and proximal pursestring sutures tied.

this process the anastomosis is supported by the abdominal surgeon.

The "doughnuts" created by the circular knife cutting through the bowel proximally and distally are immediately examined for completeness and thickness. Care is taken to keep them oriented so that if a defect is discovered its location may be more easily discovered (Fig. 18-31). The rectum is irrigated with povidone-iodine solution to check for a watertight anastomosis.

Alternatively, the pelvis may be filled with saline and the rectum insufflated with air. Leakage of povidone-iodine or air bubbles, respectively, alerts the surgeon to the presence of an incomplete anastomosis. This may be repaired with interrupted sutures or the anastomosis may need to be revised. All anastomoses should be leak-free at the conclusion of the procedure.

The abdomen and pelvis are copiously irrigated with warm saline. It has been difficult to demonstrate an

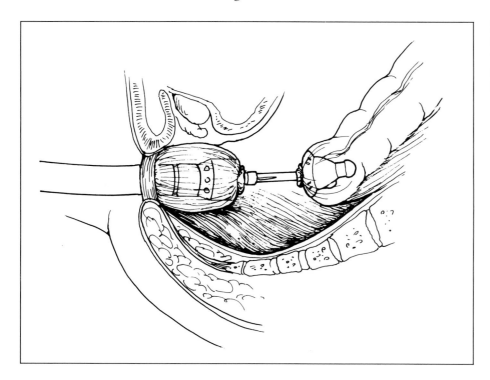

Figure 18-29. Low anterior resection: stapled anastomosis. The shaft of the anvil/head inserted into the instrument shaft.

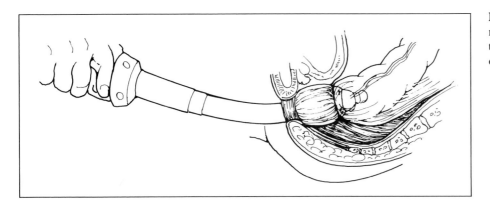

Figure 18-30. Low anterior resection: stapled anastomosis. Firing the stapler to complete the anastomosis.

advantage to adding antibiotics to the irrigant. One or two soft, noncollapsing closed suction drains are placed in the presacral space beneath the anastomosis and brought out through a separate stab wound in the left or right lower quadrant. If the pelvis is extremely dry, these may occasionally be omitted. The omentum may be mobilized and wrapped around the anastomosis or placed into the presacral space when it is long enough. Occasionally, a proximal diverting loop ileostomy or transverse colostomy may be created if there is concern about the bowel preparation or the adequacy of the anastomosis.

Double-stapled anastomosis. This modification of the now-standard stapling technique was first described by Griffen and Knight in 1980. The distal bowel is closed with a linear stapler before the specimen is removed. The anastomosis is constructed with a circular intraluminal instrument either directly through or immediately adjacent to the linear staple line. Both animal studies and subsequent clinical experience have shown this to be a safe and expeditious manner of creating an anastomosis.[106-109] This method is of particular use when attempting to anastomose a large diameter rectum with a smaller diameter proximal bowel. The smaller

lumen dictates the use of a smaller end-to-end stapler or significant adjustments during sewing. It may be difficult to place and tie down the distal pursestring, increasing significantly the risk of an anastomotic leak. However, it may be very difficult to maneuver the linear stapler deep enough into the pelvis since the instrument may be wider than the deep pelvic space. In these instances, a 30 mm-linear stapler may be used instead of the usual 55 or 60 mm type.

The rectal mobilization is performed in the same fashion as for a standard low anterior resection. The linear stapler is placed across the rectum and a right-angle bowel clamp is placed just proximal to it so as to obtain a margin of at least 2 to 3 cm beyond the distal palpable extent of the tumor in the unstretched rectum. The stapler is then fired, and the remaining rectum is irrigated from below with povidone-iodine solution to remove any fecal material and desquamated cells. The rectum is transected with a knife or heavy scissors, and the cut edges of the bowel are wiped with a povidone-iodine dampened gauze sponge.

Before the linear stapler is removed, two lateral stay sutures can be placed to maintain control of the distal segment (see Fig. 18-20). This is particularly useful for

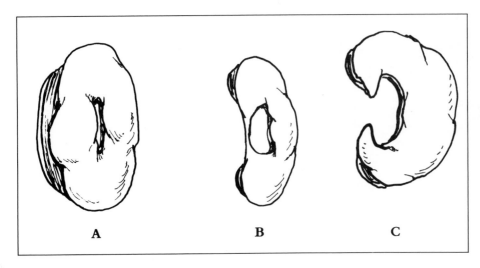

Figure 18-31. Low anterior resection: stapled anastomosis. Tissue "doughnuts" retrieved from the stapler. (A) Complete ring. (B) Mucosa complete but seromuscular layer incomplete. (C) Incomplete ring.

A   B   C

very low anastomoses. The proximal bowel is divided between straight clamps, again wiping the cut edges, and the specimen is removed from the field. The specimen is opened in the operating room on a separate back table to examine the margins.

Continuity is reestablished by means of an intraluminal end-to-end stapler, most of which now come with a sharp-tipped trocar (see Fig. 18-26). The anvil head is removed and passed to the abdominal operator. It is replaced with the trocar (if separate), and the shaft and trocar are retracted all the way into the body of the instrument. The anvil is placed into the proximal bowel and the pursestring is tied down snugly. The stapler is passed to the perineal assistant who places it gently into the rectum, taking care not to traumatize the anal sphincters. The end of the instrument is positioned at the linear staple line in the rectum and the trocar is advanced through the bowel wall immediately adjacent to the staple line (see Fig. 18-20). The anvil and proximal bowel are brought down into the pelvis and shaft of the head is joined to the shaft of the body (after removing the trocar tip, if necessary) (Fig. 18-32). The instrument is closed and fired, creating the anastomosis under the direct vision of the abdominal operator (Fig. 18-33). After the instrument is removed the anastomosis is tested and the "doughnuts" are examined as has been previously discussed.

Drains.   Dissection of the presacral space and pelvis exposes a large nonperitonealized surface. Fluids and blood tend to accumulate here, and the bony pelvis does not collapse to obliterate the space. Pelvic abscesses may occur because this collection is an almost ideal medium for bacterial growth. Theoretically, suction drainage

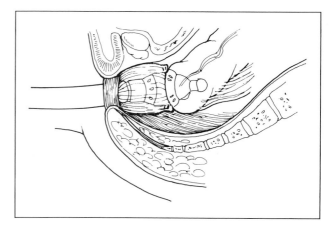

Figure 18-33.   Low anterior resection: double-stapled anastomosis. The completed anastomosis.

helps to evacuate this area and to reduce this risk. Retrospective studies seem to suggest that presacral drainage *is* effective in lowering the rate of pelvic sepsis after anterior resection and in improving primary perineal healing after abdominoperineal resection.[103,110-115] Although multiple Penrose drains and the perineal route of drainage have been used in the past, a closed sterile system is preferable to minimize retrograde bacterial migration.

Despite their apparent usefulness, these drains often become obstructed, and on reoperation large collections may be seen. Continuous irrigation and suction using one or more large-diameter drains has been tried to remove the fluid and hematoma more efficiently and in the hope of reducing the rate of pelvic sepsis.[95] Several prospective randomized trials have failed to support this claim.[96,97] The very low rates of pelvic sepsis in these and other recent studies make it very difficult to demonstrate any significant differences.

Diversion.   A diverting stoma is not a substitute for a technically sound anastomosis but may be used as an adjunct in patients who are thought to be at risk for anastomotic leakage. This group includes patients who have received high-dosage pelvic radiation, immunocompromised patients, and those in whom the anastomosis is to the lower 3 or 4 cm of rectum. Complete mesorectal excision appears to increase the likelihood of low anastomoses leaking. A transverse loop colostomy has been traditionally used, but a loop ileostomy is better tolerated, is easier to manage, is more completely diverting, and is easier to close.

Several studies have been published in which the usefulness of diverting ostomies was examined. They concluded that the presence of a diverting stoma had no protective effect on the development of an anastomotic leak but that it did seem to reduce the clinical con-

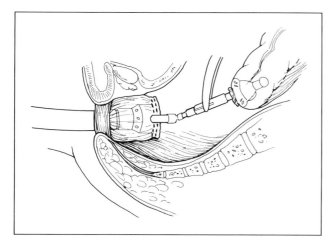

Figure 18-32.   Low anterior resection: double-stapled anastomosis. The shaft with its sharp-tipped trocar has been advanced through the closed end of the rectum. The proximal anvil/head is inserted into the distal shaft.

sequences of a leak.[116,117] Fielding and colleagues reviewed 2056 patients who had an elective colorectal anastomosis.[118] A diverting stoma was used in 15.8 percent of these patients at the preference of the operating surgeon; these patients were compared with those who did not have a stoma. The mortality (7.0 percent versus 6.1 percent respectively) and morbidity rates were quite similar, even though the leakage rate was higher in the diversion group. No conclusions about the relative usefulness of a stoma may be drawn from this nonrandomized study since the patients who received a stoma were selected at the time of surgery. Fielding did recommend that each surgeon review his or her own experience; when the anastomotic leak rate falls below 5 percent an ostomy should rarely be necessary.

There are few reports that compare patients with similar risks who did or did not have a stoma constructed concurrently with an elective anastomosis. Graffner and associates randomized patients who had a stapled low anterior resection early in their experience with this instrument to having or not having a protective colostomy.[119] He concluded that stomas were not necessary on a routine basis and were of questionable value even for the small number of patients in whom a "vulnerable" anastomosis is identified.

Clearly, a stoma is no substitute for a sound, well-constructed, well-vascularized, tension-free anastomosis in bowel that has been adequately prepared.

Coloanal Anastomosis

Coloanal anastomosis (CAA) is a method for reestablishing intestinal continuity after a very low anterior resection. Essentially, the proximal bowel is anastomosed to the anal canal somewhere between the anorectal ring and the anal verge. This operation began as a modification of a number of pullthrough procedures in which the anastomosis was performed to the everted anal canal or low rectum. In the typical coloanal anastomosis the suturing is performed transanally without eversion. There are a variety of ways to create this anastomosis. The anastomotic site may be approached in several ways including eversion of the rectal stump, transsphincteric or transsacral exposures, or endoanal techniques. The endoanal method may involve a direct anastomosis to the cut bowel (mucosa and muscularis propria/internal sphincter), a submucosal dissection with suturing of the proximal bowel to the cut edge of the mucosa within a muscular cuff, or an intersphincteric dissection with anastomosis to the skin at the intersphincteric groove (Fig. 18-34). Thus, the level of the anastomosis may be at the anorectal ring, at the dentate line, or in the anal skin. These anastomoses may be constructed with sutures or with staples.

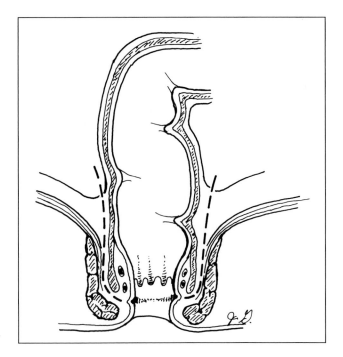

Figure 18-34. Coloanal anastomosis. The dissection plane through the intersphincteric groove is shown as one variation.

This operation was initially described and popularized by the late Sir Alan Parks at the St. Mark's Hospital in London.[120] His technique involved injecting epinephrine 1:300,000 submucosally to assist in identifying the plane of dissection and in hemostasis and then stripping the anal mucosa from the dentate line up to the low rectum. The mid sigmoid colon was brought through the muscle wall sleeve and anastomosed to the cut edge of the dentate line with a single layer of interrupted sutures. Each stitch incorporated the anal mucosa, some internal sphincter, and the full thickness of the colon (Fig. 18-35). A temporary loop transverse colostomy and presacral drains were used in all of his patients.

A stapled coloanal anastomosis may be constructed using similar methods to those described for a low anterior resection. The pursestring suture may be placed transanally or a double-staple method may be used. The rectal dissection may be carried right down into the intersphincteric plane to the level of the dentate line. A 30-mm linear stapler is placed across the anal sleeve and fired. This size stapler is useful at this level since the anal sleeve is much narrower than the low rectum: it may be technically possible to place this narrower instrument into the anal canal dissection through the pelvis. Coloanal anastomosis may also be used to salvage an inadequate rectal anastomosis.

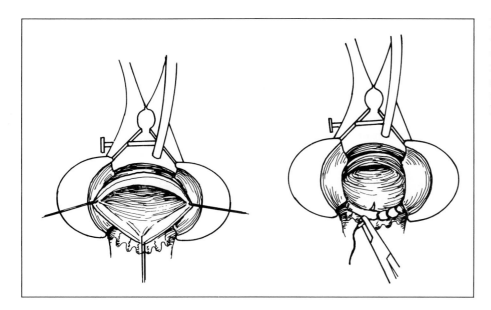

Figure 18-35. Coloanal anastomosis. The descending colon is brought through the muscle wall sleeve and anastomosed to the cut edge of the dentate line with a single layer of interrupted sutures.

Coloanal Anastomosis With a Colonic Pouch. Some workers have suggested that adding a **J**-shaped reservoir above the coloanal anastomosis improves function by decreasing evacuation frequency and urgency. Although patients with a reservoir tend to have fewer stools each day, the results have not been impressive and some patients require enemas or suppositories to evacuate. This technique has not gained general acceptance because of the additional manipulation involved and because of the difficulty getting an adequate length of bowel to do both the pouch and the anastomosis.[121-123] If a coloanal anastomosis with a colonic pouch is undertaken, strong consideration should be given to a diverting loop ileostomy. Several prospective randomized trials are currently underway to assess whether or not a colonic **J** pouch results in significantly improved bowel function.

Posterior Approaches

The transsacral method was first used by Kocher in 1875,[124] but it has been associated with Kraske's name ever since he presented it in 1884.[125] Although the original descriptions include a sacral colostomy, the procedure was soon modified to include anastomosis to the rectal remnant.[126] A few surgeons have tenaciously held to the belief that there is some advantage to these procedures, but with the advent of staplers and of transanal techniques, these procedures have been relegated to the realm of historical interest only. Significant complications are associated with these procedures including incontinence, anastomotic leaks, wound breakdown, and fistula formation. The risk of these complications is further increased in patients who have had radiation

therapy. Fecal diversion, rarely necessary in patients who undergo low anterior resection, is routinely employed with these procedures.

Transsphincteric (York–Mason) Method. Excellent exposure is attained with this method (Fig. 18-36); however, transecting the sphincter carries a significant risk and should be avoided whenever possible. Originally only a low resection was performed through the posterior approach without a concomitant abdominal approach. This limited the extent of proximal lymphatic clearance and was eventually supplemented by a combined abdominal–posterior approach when used for

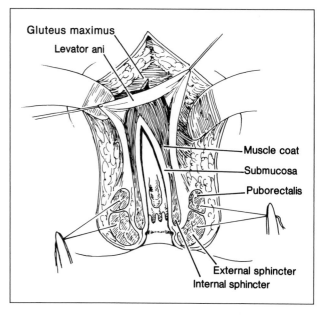

Figure 18-36. Transsphincteric (York–Mason) method.

malignancies.[127] In the series of 65 patients reported by Lazorthes and associates[128,129] there were no operative deaths, but a 9 percent incidence of pelvic sepsis or anastomotic leak was encountered.

Transsacral (Kraske) Resection: Localio Technique. The para- or transsacral approach also affords excellent exposure of the low rectum without sphincter division. Localio at New York University believes that the combined abdomino–sacral procedure is indicated for mid third tumors in obese women and in thin men. He believes that a transsacral resection will lower the level for anastomosis and improve the lateral and distal clearance by allowing dissection under direct vision. This opinion is not widely shared.

The patient is placed in the lateral position with left side up and is draped for simultaneous anterior and posterior access. The abdominal incision is begun midway between the left costal margin and the iliac crest and then extended obliquely down to the suprapubic region and across the midline. The left colon, splenic flexure, and rectum are mobilized, the blood supply is ligated, and the bowel is transected. A transverse incision is made over the sacrococcygeal ligament, the coccyx is removed, and the presacral space is entered. The levator ani muscles are split longitudinally in the direction of their fibers. The rectum is further mobilized laterally and inferiorly in the presacral space behind the retrorectal fascia. The rectosigmoid stump is delivered through the incision, the rectum is freed from the remaining lateral and anterior tissues, and the distal rectum is clamped with a right-angle bowel clamp at least 3 cm below the tumor. The proximal bowel stump is brought down into the posterior wound, and a two-layered inverting anastomosis is created, placing the first row of sutures before transecting the bowel. An omental flap is sutured around the anastomosis and between the bowel and the sacral wound.[128,129]

Transsacral (Kraske) Resection: Marks Technique. Marks[130] combined abdominosacral excision with full-dose preoperative radiation therapy for mid and low rectal cancers, attempting to extend the limits of sphincter preservation and improve local recurrence rates. He performs the procedure in two phases.

The abdominal phase begins with mobilization of the left colon to the mid transverse colon. The proximal resection margin is placed just above the sigmoid–descending colon junction to avoid radiated bowel. A cloth tape is tied just proximal to the level of proximal transection. The rectum is mobilized and transected and the specimen is removed. The proximal end with its tape is placed in the pelvis. A proximal transverse colostomy is always used. The abdomen is closed and the patient is rolled into the modified right lateral Sims' position.

The sacral phase is begun with a slightly curved incision from S-4 to the supraanal region to the left of the midline. The coccyx and possibly one or two segments of the sacrum are removed. The sacrococcygeal ligament and the levators are divided and the pelvis is entered. The cloth tape is grasped, bringing the proximal bowel into the wound. The rectal stump may be lengthened by careful dissection. A single-layered anastomosis is constructed using interrupted sutures of catgut. The deep tissues are closed in layers. The skin closure is delayed. The colostomy is closed 8 weeks later after a contrast study through the distal colostomy limb demonstrates an intact anastomosis.[130]

Localio compared 175 patients who underwent abdominosacral resection with 320 who underwent anterior resection. Although perioperative mortality was 2 percent in both groups, there was a 9.7 percent leakage rate after abdominosacral resection versus only 1 percent after anterior resection. Thirteen of seventeen leaks developed into "well controlled" fistulas.[129] Marks noted only one fistula in 150 surgically treated patients and 1 anastomotic failure in 24 patients having an abdominosacral resection. He stated that "several sacral wounds were slow to heal" but only 1 was "significant."[130] Thus 5 to 10 percent of patients who are subjected to transsacral resection are essentially doomed to sacral colostomies.

Hartmann Operation

The Hartmann operation (named for Henri Hartmann, 1860–1952, professor and chairman of surgery at the Hôtel Dieu in Paris) is performed in the same fashion as the anterior resection except that instead of constructing an anastomosis, the distal rectal is closed either with staples or sutures and the proximal bowel is matured as a colostomy. This procedure is used frequently in cases of acute or complicated diverticular disease, but only occasionally for rectal cancer. It may be appropriately used in the presence of obstruction, perforation, poor patient condition, extensive and unresectable pelvic disease, or intraoperative cardiovascular instability. The advantages are that the perineal phase is avoided, the operation is shortened, and there is no anastomosis at risk. The remaining "Hartmann's pouch" or oversewn rectal stump is well tolerated. Occasionally, patients will pass some mucus or develop a mucus plug. The second stage (colostomy takedown with anastomosis) is a major operation and many elderly patients never have the stoma closed.

Other Techniques

Biofragmentable ring (BAR). Methods of approximating the bowel without suturing have been attempted since antiquity but it was the Murphy "button," introduced in 1892, that was the most successful.[131] Named for its inventor, John B. Murphy, professor of surgery at Northwestern University in Chicago, editor of the journal *Surgery, Gynecology and Obstetrics,* president of the American Medical Association, and a founder and regent of the American College of Surgeons, it was the most accepted method of bowel coaptation for many years.

The biofragmentable ring (BAR) (Valtrac, Davis and Geck) was described by the late Dr. Thomas Hardy of Columbus, Ohio, and his colleagues in 1987.[132] It is made of polyglycolic acid and breaks apart after 2 to 3 weeks. Several sizes are available. Pursestring sutures are placed in each end of the bowel to be apposed. They are then tied down around either end of the ring, and the ring is closed with a palpable and audible click. One of the few advantages of this technique is that the ring is contained entirely within the lumen and no secondary opening is necessary as with some of the stapling techniques. Its use in the low rectum is somewhat limited because of difficulty with placing the ring and tying the pursestrings. In several large reports including a prospective randomized trial the safety of the ring has been clearly demonstrated.[132,133] Nevertheless, it has not enjoyed widespread use.

Pullthrough Procedures. These procedures are primarily of historical interest and today are rarely if ever used in the treatment of rectal carcinoma. They fall into two broad categories: those that rely on eversion of the rectal stump out onto the perineum and those that transect the rectum at the level of the anorectal ring. In addition, the anastomosis may be performed primarily or in a delayed fashion. These techniques were originally developed as alternatives to the posterior (trans-

sphincteric and transsacral) approach, but with the increased popularity of anterior resection and with marked improvements in perioperative care and antimicrobial therapy, they have fallen into disuse.

The first description of a pullthrough procedure is generally attributed to Maunsell in 1892.[134] Weir subsequently amplified the method.[135] The rectal stump is everted, the proximal colon is passed through the everted lumen, the lesion is amputated, and a primary anastomosis is created by the perineal operator. The procedure was modified by Turnbull and Cuthbertson and by Cutait and Figliolini, who left 7 to 8 cm of the pulled-down colon wrapped in gauze outside the everted rectum for 7 days, suturing the everted rectal edge to the seromuscular layer of the pulled-through segment; a delayed amputation and anastomosis was performed after 10 to 14 days (Fig. 18-37).[136,137] This was thought to be safer than the original method, and in their series there were far fewer anastomotic complications with delayed anastomosis than with a primary one.[102,138] The eversion techniques are limited in that they require an extensive proximal mobilization to get enough bowel length to pull through and that at least 6 cm of distal rectum must be retained or the rectum cannot be effectively everted. The delayed anastomotic method, though associated with fewer complications, leaves a foul, necrotic mass protruding from the anus which is uncomfortable for the patient and dilates the sphincters. Also, these procedures all incorporated a diverting colostomy; thus they all necessitated two or three stages. Later, Weakley, working with Turnbull at the Cleveland Clinic, advocated a primary anastomosis of the everted bowel using a circular stapler during the first stage, changing this to a two-stage operation.[102]

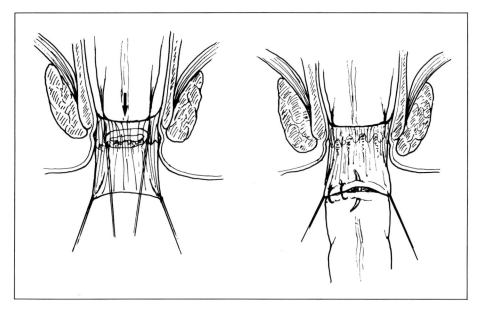

Figure 18-37. Pullthrough procedure. The mobilized proximal bowel is pulled through the everted rectum (arrow). The seromuscular layer is sutured to the everted rectal edge. The pulled-through segment may be transected and the anastomosis may be completed primarily or after 10 to 14 days.

To address lower lesions, Babcock in 1932 and Black in 1955 described techniques in which the bowel was transected at the level of the anorectal ring and then pulled through the anal canal without eversion; this was followed by delayed amputation. Babcock in 1947 published a description of the procedure in which a mucosectomy was performed beginning at the dentate line and carried up into the rectum; the lower rectal dissection was then done from below. The pullthrough was then accomplished with a delayed anastomosis.[36] This left a larger raw surface area for the proximal bowel to adhere to.

Harry E. Bacon at Temple University in Philadelphia began using the pullthrough procedure in the 1940s after performing cadaver trials. In 1945 he presented his method which included a full mobilization of the rectum and left colon with a high ligation of the inferior mesenteric artery. The perineal phase involved a submucosal dissection from just below the dentate line to the levators. The bowel was pulled through and transected 7 cm from the anal verge. At 7 days the excess bowel was trimmed and the colon–anoderm anastomosis was constructed with interrupted catgut. Daily digital dilation and enemas every other day were performed. Anoplasty was required for stenosis in 3.3 percent. In a review of 2849 cases of colorectal carcinoma treated by Bacon, 705 patients were treated with a pullthrough procedure for midrectal (7–12 cm) lesions. Operative mortality and long-term survival were no different when the patients undergoing pullthroughs, abdominoperineal resection, and anterior resection were compared.[38]

Obstruction

Colorectal carcinomas may present with partial or complete obstruction. Most obstructions are due to lesions in the sigmoid colon, the splenic flexure, the transverse colon and, less frequently, the rectum. Symptomatic obstruction of the right side of the colon is a late event because of the liquid nature of the stool on this side of the bowel and its large diameter. Approximately, 4 to 6 percent of patients with a rectal adenocarcinoma present with obstruction.[139,140] Symptoms include progressively narrower stools, constipation or diarrhea or both, abdominal distention, bloating and pain, and nausea and vomiting. The diagnosis of complete obstruction is suspected by history and confirmed by examination and plain x-rays. The etiology and level of the obstruction may be more difficult to establish, but a gentle contrast study with water soluble material or a careful endoscopic procedure will clarify the situation. Low rectal lesions, of course, will be easily defined by digital examination and proctoscopy.

Patients with obstruction require immediate hospitalization, intravenous rehydration, and usually surgery. Although three-stage procedures have been used in the past (proximal colostomy, resection, anastomosis), the standard treatment for patients with acute and complete malignant rectal obstruction is a two-stage procedure with initial resection, Hartmann pouch and colostomy, and subsequent colostomy take-down and anastomosis. Primary anastomoses in the unprepared left colon have been commonly associated with high leakage rates,[140] whereas staged resections have traditionally been shown to have much lower morbidity and mortality rates.[141-147] Unfortunately the multistaged approach often results in a prolonged course including at least two major operations. Many patients will not undergo the second procedure because of their medical condition or progression of their disease and will be left with a permanent colostomy even if there is adequate rectum left to fashion an anastomosis.

A one-stage procedure would be preferable if it could be performed with reasonable risk. There are distinct advantages to a single-stage procedure in that the cumulative hospital stay is much shorter, there is no ostomy with its attendant risk of complications, and only one operation is required. The major problem in these cases is the large fecal and bacterial load in the obstructed colon. Normally, the feces are cleared and the bacterial counts markedly reduced by preoperative bowel preparation. Of course, this is not possible in patients who present with obstruction. Several techniques have been developed recently to address this problem and to permit a one-stage procedure of resection and primary anastomosis. These include a total abdominal colectomy with ileoproctomy and an on-table lavage. Both procedures are discussed below.

Tube Cecostomy

Tube cecostomy may be helpful in very high risk patients. It does help to decompress the proximal colon but does little to reduce the fecal stream and certainly does not defunctionalize the distal bowel.[148,149] For these reasons it has little or no practical application.

Proximal Ostomy

Colostomy or ileostomy may be used alone as an initial procedure in the management of obstruction with the goal of isolating the obstructing lesion from the fecal stream and decompressing the segment above the lesion but below the level of the ostomy. Whenever this procedure is elected, either a loop or a double-barreled ostomy (with mucous fistula) should be performed. A loop transverse colostomy, which is easily performed, has traditionally been employed. However, it may be difficult to manage because of size and location on the abdominal wall, is often incompletely diverting, and is prone to complications such as prolapse and intussusception. A loop ileostomy is much easier to manage[150] but is distant from the site of obstruction and may not adequately decompress the colon, especially if the ileocecal valve is competent. A loop or divided sigmoid colostomy generally works well and decompresses the bowel near the lesion; however, the sigmoid colon requires more mobilization and manipulation to create an acceptable stoma and may get in the way of a subsequent procedure.

Although this seems to be a simple and safe procedure, in reality it carries a significant complication and mortality rate. In a review by Mirelman and coauthors of 271 patients from the Lahey Clinic, colostomy creation was associated with a 21 percent morbidity and a 2.2 mortality rate, while colostomy closure had a 49 percent morbidity and 4.2 percent mortality rate.[151] In a review of the literature by Mitchell and colleagues in 1978, complications were observed in 11 to 49 percent of patients and 0 to 2.8 percent died perioperatively.[152]

Fortunately, the indications for colostomy alone are decreasing and procedures such as resection with ostomy or on-table lavage with primary anastomosis are usually preferred.

Subtotal Colectomy

Subtotal colectomy with ileorectal anastomosis is safe although it is a longer operation and is more appropriately used for obstructing and/or perforating cancers of the left or sigmoid colon.[153-158] It is generally well tolerated in younger patients with good anal sphincter function, but the diarrhea that results is often difficult for elderly patients to manage. There is a very limited role for this procedure in patients with primary rectal tumors since very little bowel would remain and since there are usually other viable options.[159,160]

Preoperative Decompression/Recanalization

The bowel may be decompressed endoscopically, especially if the obstruction is partial. This allows bowel preparation and a single-stage procedure.[161] Recent successes with preoperative recanalization have been reported in small series of patients with obstructing rectal and colonic carcinomas. This may be accomplished with the use of a proctoscope or a flexible sigmoidoscope and either electrocautery or lasers.[162-164] This application of the laser may be one of its most useful

roles in colon and rectal surgery. Eckhauser reported 11 patients in whom laser recanalization was performed. Nine of these lesions were above the peritoneal reflection; all went on to single-stage resections. There were few complications, and decreased hospital stay and cost were noted among the benefits.[165]

Intraoperative Bowel Preparation

On-table lavage preparation of the proximal colon with standard resection and anastomosis has proved to be a safe and useful procedure.[166-169] The risk of prolonging the procedure and of a fecal spill during the preparation must be balanced against the advantage of a single-stage procedure. One's enthusiasm must be tempered with good medical and surgical judgment, and this approach should not be attempted in higher risk patients.

The distal rectum is irrigated with saline followed by povidone-iodine at the beginning of the procedure and again after placement of the distal clamp or staple line. On-table lavage preparation is performed by irrigating 6 to 12 liters of warm saline through the colon with the last few liters containing an antimicrobial agent such as kanamycin, neomycin, or povidone-iodine. Proximal access for instillation of the irrigant is accomplished via a foley catheter placed through a doubled pursestring suture as a cecostomy, appendicostomy, or ileal enterotomy (with the tube passed through the ileocecal valve). Alternatively, a long intestinal tube may be passed from the mouth or nose through the ileocecal valve; this is particularly helpful when there is significant small bowel dilatation. The effluent is collected in a large plastic bag or a suction trap.

The lumen of the bowel is occluded just proximal to the lesion and the resection is performed, mobilizing the splenic flexure and the left transverse colon. The distal colon is draped over the left side and secured in the drainage system. Various methods have been advocated for doing this including the use of large-bore ribbed anesthesia respirator tubing, suturing the bag around the bowel, and open drainage into a bag or basin (Fig. 18-38). A closed technique is preferable. The colon is irrigated initially with 200 to 500 ml at a time and formed fecal matter is broken up manually and carefully milked out into the bag. Once the majority of the stool has been removed, continuous irrigation may be performed, taking care to assure unobstructed flow. Once the irrigation is completed and the bowel is emptied as completely as possible, the distal end is amputated and removed with the bag. A standard anastomosis is then constructed.

The key to success is the avoidance of peritoneal contamination. Spreading peritonitis and perforation are contraindications to the use of this technique. Be-

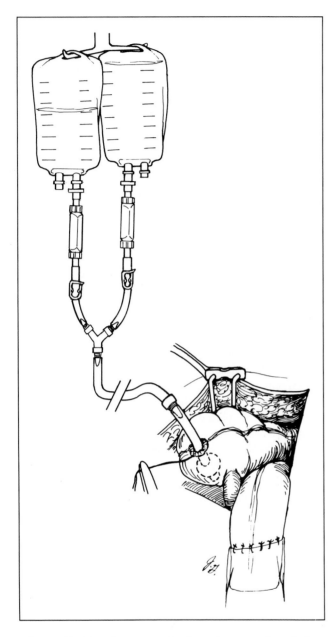

Figure 18-38. Intraoperative bowel preparation. Irrigation through the appendiceal stump and out the cut left colon into a plastic bag.

cause on-table preparation prolongs the operative procedure by 30 to 45 minutes, it should not be used when the patient is unstable or at high anesthetic risk.

Controversies

High Ligation

Ligation of the inferior mesenteric artery may be performed at a point just below the takeoff of the left colic artery or at the inferior mesenteric artery's origin from the aorta, sacrificing the left colic artery (see Fig. 18-10). Clearly, the higher ligation allows removal of additional lymphatic tissue, but whether this confers any survival advantage is equivocal. These highest lymph nodes have been found to have metastatic disease in from 8 to 10 percent of patients.[170-172] In Grinnell's (1965) series[173] those patients who had high ligation of their inferior mesenteric artery had a 5.7 percent improvement in 5-year survival compared with those who did not. This difference was *not,* however, statistically significant, and none of the 19 patients treated with high ligation and having involved high lymph nodes survived free of disease. Several other groups reported no improvement in survival with very high ligation, even in Dukes C patients (involved lymph nodes).[172-176]

There is some concern that high ligation of the inferior mesenteric artery with transection of the left colic artery may compromise the blood supply to the descending colon. In fact, this is rarely the case, and the middle colic and marginal arteries supply this portion of the colon quite well in most cases.[177-179] Therefore, removal of the descending colon is rarely necessary, even when performing a very high ligation. Despite these considerations, knowledge of the status of these nodes may help in planning postoperative therapy; and since little risk is involved, high ligation remains a standard part of the author's resectional treatment of rectal cancer.

Radical Lymphadenectomy

The lateral lymphatic pathways to the iliac vessels may be involved in from 0 to 28 percent of patients depending on the level of the tumor and the study being quoted.[55,72,73,93] Williams and his colleagues found several types of lateral spread in their whole mounted specimens.[64] These included direct extension to the margins of resection, regional lymph node involvement, extranodal deposits of tumor within the mesorectum, and extramural venous, lymphatic, and perineural invasion. The proponents of this technique believe that local recurrence is primarily due to inadequate lateral margins.

The term *radical lymphadenectomy* refers to the wide removal of the lateral and superior lymphatic system. This includes a high ligation of the inferior mesenteric artery flush with the aorta and an extended periaortic and pelvic lymph node dissection beginning at the duodenum and extending down to take the periaortic and lateral iliac nodes. The lateral limits of the dissection are usually the median borders of the iliac vessels, but some authors begin well out on the iliac fossa wall and may even ligate the hypogastric vessels, taking them with the specimen. Clearly, these radical resections carry a significant morbidity with them, and early attempts were abandoned because of high complication rates, es-

Table 18-3 Survival and Local Recurrence Rates for Patients Who Underwent Curative Resections With Extended Lymph Node Dissection Versus Standard Lymph Node Dissection

	Pathologic stage	Extended lymph node dissection	Standard lymph node dissection
No. patients	B	74	94
	C	89	124
5-year survival, %	B	83	64*
	C	53	31*
Local recurrence in 5 years, %	B	26	8*
	C	44	25*

* $P < 0.05$
Table developed from data in Koyama Y, Moriya Y, Hojo K. Effects of extended systematic lymphadenectomy for adenocarcinoma of the rectum—significant improvement of survival rate and decrease of local recurrence. *Jpn J Clinc Oncol.* 1984;14:623–632.

pecially ureteric injury and urinary and sexual dysfunction.[54,78,180]

Recently, interest in this approach has been revived. The surgical group at the National Cancer Center Hospital in Tokyo have been quite aggressive and have presented some compelling supportive data. In 1984 they reported that those patients having an extended lymphadenectomy along with their resection for cure had lower local recurrence rates and improved 5-year survivals (Table 18-3).[181] Although postoperative mortality was the same (1.4 percent), morbidity was much higher after resection with an extended lymph node dissection: urinary dysfunction occurred in 39 percent (versus 9 percent after standard dissection; $P < 0.05$) and impotency in 76 percent (versus 38 percent; $P < 0.05$).[182] Unfortunately, a number of other workers have failed to confirm these impressive results.[183-187] The limited benefit along with the concomitant major morbidity has prevented widespread acceptance of this technique.

En Bloc and Extended Resection

Rectal carcinomas may spread directly beyond the bowel wall to involve other pelvic organs. At the time of surgical exploration involvement of the vagina, uterus, ovaries, bladder, seminal vesicles, prostate, or small bowel may be found in from 5 to 26 percent of patients.[188-194] The pelvic sidewalls, the sacrum, and the coccyx may also be invaded. From 25 to 50 percent of these patients will have disease limited to the pelvis, making resection for cure a real possibility.[195] At the time of exploration, it is often impossible to tell whether this adherence is inflammatory and benign or invasive

and malignant. Roughly 50 to 70 percent of these adhesions will contain tumor cells. To separate these "adhesions" is very tempting but poses a high risk of cutting across tumor and leaving disease in situ or shedding viable tumor cells into the field. Whenever possible, an en bloc excision of part or all of the organ involved should be performed with the goal of complete excision with clear margins. It is likely that there is a subset of patients with tumors that are locally aggressive but metastasize late. These patients, it seems, would be eminently curable.

Generally, good results have been reported with this policy with survival rates approaching or equalling those without local extension so long as the entire tumor is resected.[196-199] En bloc excision of the lower ureters and internal iliac vessels has even been advocated with excellent local control in one small series.[200] Only one group has found significantly poorer survival and local control with pathologically confirmed invasion.[193] Symptomatic involvement of the sciatic notch indicates a situation unlikely to be helped by surgery. Surgical exploration is often necessary to fully establish resectability.

When partial resection of the pelvic organs will not result in adequate margins or in reasonable function, pelvic exenteration is a reasonable alternative in carefully selected patients. This procedure may be performed with acceptable morbidity and mortality (5 to 10 percent) and with 5-year survivals of 40 percent or better.[196,201-204]

Lesions that invade the sacrum may also be resectable when localized. Resection of the sacrum up to the S-3 nerve roots is generally compatible with reasonable function. If one of these roots is left, acceptable urinary function may be retained; however, if both are sacrificed, function will be lost. If the sacrectomy is combined with cystectomy, this concern is of course irrelevant. These operations are difficult and often very bloody. The combined effort of a colorectal surgeon, an orthopedist, and a neurosurgeon is generally best. In one recent series of 20 patients, there were no operative deaths; however, 35 percent of these patients had urinary complications, 25 percent suffered wound disruptions, and the median blood loss was 1600 ml. Long-term survival was rare but long-term control of local disease and palliation of symptoms was achieved in the majority of patients.[205]

Hysterectomy, Posterior Vaginectomy

Though the lymphatic pathways of the low rectum overlap those of the female genital tract, there appears to be no difference in pelvic recurrence by sex nor does prophylactic removal of these structures seem to confer any survival or recurrence benefit.[206,207] Therefore, resection of the uterus and vagina is limited to patients in whom the disease is adherent or very close to these structures.

Oophorectomy

The incidence of occult ovarian metastases in patients operated on for rectosigmoid cancer has been reported to be from 3 to 7 percent, and, in women with Dukes C lesions, the incidence may be as high as 17 percent.[192,208-214] The cause may be related to the shared pelvic lymphatics or to transperitoneal implants.

Although, invasion or spread to the ovaries is a clear indication for therapeutic oophorectomy; the value of prophylactic oophorectomy is not clear. Patients with discernible involvement of the ovaries at operation usually have extensive intraperitoneal disease and a very poor prognosis. There have been sporadic reports of patients with microscopic ovarian spread who were cured by "prophylactic" oophorectomy.[215,216] Blamey and associates reported a 1.4 percent incidence of reoperation for metachronous ovarian spread in 882 women followed after resection of a colorectal cancer.[217]

Perhaps of more significance is the increased risk these women have for developing a primary ovarian malignancy. This risk has been estimated to be approximately five times that which exists in women in the general population.[218] Despite these considerations, there is no strong evidence that prophylactic oophorectomy is of benefit in the treatment of colorectal cancer.[206] Nevertheless, since oophorectomy during colorectal surgery carries little risk and adds little time to the procedure, it seem reasonable in the absence of obvious disease to remove the ovaries prophylactically in postmenopausal women.[219,220]

No-Touch Technique

The no-touch technique attempts to reduce the incidence of distant spread and local recurrence by avoiding dissemination of tumor cells during the operative procedure. That tumor cells may be shed into the venous system was first demonstrated by Cole and his coworkers, who found cancer cells in the venous effluent of a perfused cancer-bearing segment of colon.[221] Soon thereafter Fisher and Turnbull[222] found tumor cells in the portal venous blood of 32 percent of 25 patients being resected. The number of free cancer cells has been shown to increase initially during the induction of anesthesia and to increase further during surgery.[223] Even so, patients who had neoplastic cells in the blood during surgery did not go on to poorer survival. It appears that most of these cells failed to implant or were destroyed by the patients' defenses.

The first description of lymphovascular ligation before right colon mobilization was published in 1952 by Barnes, who hoped to reduce the spread of disease to the liver.[224] Turnbull believed that results could be improved by isolating the tumor as much as possible before manipulating it. Techniques for isolation included lymphovascular isolation accomplished by ligating the mesenteric vascular and lymphatic channels as high as possible before mobilizing the colon and luminal isolation performed by occluding the bowel with tied umbilical tapes above and below the lesion and washing out the retained ends. Impressive improvements in survival were reported in Turnbull's retrospective series; unfortunately his results are difficult to evaluate since he used a different staging system and because his patients were selected.[225] Ligating the arterial supply concurrently or even before the venous drainage is cut may be important, since Ackerman demonstrated that venous occlusion increases lymphatic flow.[226]

Wiggers and his colleagues in the Netherlands conducted a prospective randomized trial of the no-touch technique, evaluating 236 patients with colorectal cancer operated for cure.[227] Patient and tumor factors were very similar in both the no-touch and conventional groups except that there were more males in the no-touch group. Follow-up was longer than 5 years in all patients. These were no statistical differences in outcome in the no-touch versus conventional operation groups when examining the rates of liver metastases (14 versus 22 percent), 5-year survival (60 versus 56 percent), total deaths (40 versus 44 percent), deaths due to recurrent disease (25 versus 31 percent), or deaths of patients with vascular invasion (31 versus 52 percent). In each of these categories, however, there was a distinct *tendency* for improved results with the no-touch technique. It may be that a larger study will have to be performed before any conclusive statement may be made. Nevertheless, once it is learned the no-touch technique is a simple and straightforward method of resection that has no more morbidity or operative mortality than does the standard technique.

Sphincter Reconstruction

Sphincter reconstruction after abdominoperineal resection has been tried intermittently with limited success. Generally, a colostomy that functions well is preferable to the results of direct perineal colostomy.[228] Recently, Williams and colleagues described a technique of reconstruction involving a coloperineal anastomosis and a neosphincter made with a transposed gracilis muscle.[229] A totally implanted stimulator continually stimulated the gracilis muscle, attempting to convert the rapid twitch skeletal muscle to a slow twitch, fatigue-resistant muscle. A loop ileostomy was used during muscle training. A good result was seen in the first patient in whom this technique was applied. Subsequently, Cavina and colleagues reported 47 patients using a similar technique.[230] There were no perioperative deaths but mild, moderate, and severe complications occurred in 62, 27, and 11 percent, respectively. Cavina believed that these complications did not alter the functional results except in two cases of early distal colonic ischemia. Follow-up revealed good function in 56 percent, fair in 22.5 percent, and poor in 12.5 percent. Overall, the group thought their patients enjoyed a better quality of life than comparable patients after an abdominoperineal resection. Whether this technique will become a common alternative to colostomy is doubtful because of the high complication rates and the decreasing indications for colostomy.

Surgery and Intraoperative Pelvic Hyperthermochemotherapy

Intraabdominal hyperthermia has been used in the treatment of various malignancies (pancreatic, gastric) with mixed success. Generally, local recurrence rates may be reduced but most patients go on to die of disseminated disease at the same rate as those without this additional treatment.[231-233] Chemotherapeutic agents may be added to the immersion fluid to potentiate the effect of hyperthermia. Fujimoto and associates tested the effectiveness of this innovative technique in reducing local recurrence of rectal cancer.[234] Patients operated upon for cure were randomized to resection with intraoperative hyperthermochemotherapy (14) versus resection alone (12). All had an extended lymphadenectomy. At the completion of the resection the pelvis was filled with mitomycin C in normal saline which was then heated with a specially designed device to 45°C for 90 minutes. Cytology of pelvic washings before treatment revealed viable tumor cells in 6 of 14 patients; viable cells were not seen in the exudate obtained from the drains postoperatively. There were 2 local recurrences in the 12 control patients and none in the 14 treated patients at a mean follow-up of 17 months. There were no differences in complications. The lack of statistical improvement may be due to the small numbers and short follow-up. Whether this will be a useful technique remains to be seen.

Treatment of Residual Disease

Complete surgical resection remains the most effective treatment for rectal carcinoma. Except in the case of intracavitary radiation of an early tumor, incomplete excision of a rectal cancer generally precludes cure.

Postoperative adjunctive radiotherapy has been given for residual disease with minimal response. Microscopic disease responds better than macroscopic disease. Treatment and tumor response are limited by the intolerance of the surrounding tissues, and most trials have high complication rates.[235] Doses of 45 to 50 gray with local boosts of 10 to 15 gray have been used in a number of studies. Local failure rates were 30 to 70 percent with microscopic disease and 50 to 87 percent with gross disease.[236-238] Radiation combined with chemotherapy has been tried with poor results and quite high complication rates. Median survival in one study in all groups was 17 months.[239]

Preoperative radiotherapy alone or in combination with intraoperative radiation or brachytherapy have been used to shrink tumors thought to be unresectable initially, to reduce rates of local recurrence and spread and to treat locally recurrent disease. These methods are discussed below.

Local Treatment

Rationale

The surgical treatment of rectal cancer is based on the belief that spread occurs through the wall and then via the lymphatics. Wide excision of these tissues should cure these patients if the disease has not spread beyond the limits of the resection and if no tumor cells are implanted during surgery. Early lesions without spread to the nodes and with limited penetration of the bowel wall are fairly uniformly cured by radical procedures. Pathologic studies of early colorectal carcinomas have shown that when invasion was limited to the submucosa the lymph nodes were involved in 5 percent or fewer of patients without other risk factors. The lymph nodes were diseased in 27 percent of these patients with tumors that were poorly differentiated, had mucinous histology, or had invasion of the lymphatic channels or veins. However, when the muscularis propria is invaded the incidence of lymphatic spread rises to 10 percent or more even in the absence of these factors.[240,241]

Local treatment of rectal cancer has a number of significant advantages (Table 18-4). The major disadvantage is that no pathologic staging of the lymph nodes is possible.

The key to successful local treatment of rectal neoplasms is patient selection. Four groups of patients are candidates for local treatment. The first group consists of patients with early, minimally invasive lesions without spread who may be treated for cure. When properly selected these lesions may be cured at a similar rate to that achieved with radical resection. The second includes those patients with extensive disseminated disease who may be treated with palliative intent. The third group is composed of patients who are in very poor general medical condition and who are at high risk for any surgical procedure. The fourth group includes

a relatively small number of patients who are psychologically unable to accept a colostomy when one is a necessary part of the radical approach.

Local Treatment for Cure. The generally accepted criteria for local treatment for cure include the following: The lesion should be mobile by digital examination; this is indicative of confinement of the lesion to the bowel wall. There should be no palpable lymph nodes in the presacral space (this finding is relatively uncommon). Treatment for cure should be limited to those patients who will be compliant with close follow-up since early detection of recurrence is desirable with the possibility of salvage by retreatment or radical resection.

Additional criteria are used by various surgeons and are summarized in Table 18-5.[41,242]

Endorectal ultrasonograph has become the most helpful method of staging these lesions.[243,244] It is very accurate in estimation of the depth of bowel wall penetration; however, it is limited in its ability to detect lymphatic spread (see Chapter 17). Based on these criteria, it is estimated that 3 to 5 percent of patients with a rectal carcinoma are candidates for local treatment.[41,59]

The decision to proceed to a radical resection is based

Table 18-4 Techniques of Local Treatment for Rectal Carcinoma Compared

Method	Advantages	Disadvantages
All	Rare mortality Minimal morbidity Abdominal surgery avoided Little time lost from work and home Avoidance of a stoma Financial savings	No lymphatic staging
Local excision	Complete specimen available for pathologic examination Rare complications Well tolerated with little pain Single procedure	Requires general or regional anesthesia
Electrocoagulation	Viable tumor cells less likely to be seeded Little pain	No specimen available for staging Relies on "feel" for extent of excision Requires repeated procedures and anesthesia Postprocedure fevers Postoperative bleeding
Endocavitary radiation	Outpatient procedure No anesthetic Few side effects No tissue planes opened	Repeated treatments Limited availability No specimen available for staging May be difficult to tell scar from recurrence

Table 18-5 Selection Criteria for Curative Local Treatment of Rectal Carcinoma

Criteria	Indications	Contraindications
Fixation	Mobile	Fixed
Pelvic lymph nodes	Not palpable	Palpable
Technically possible	Yes	No
Good follow-up	Likely, patient compliant	Not likely
Differentiation*	Well- or moderately differentiated	Moderately or poorly differentiated
Morphology*	Exophytic	Ulcerating
Size*	<3–4 cm	>3–4 cm
Radial extent*	<1/3–1/2	>1/3–1/2
Histologic type*	Typical adenocarcinoma	Mucinous; signet cell
Vascular/lymphatic channel invasion*	Absent	Present
Endorectal ultrasound*	Limited to rectal wall or submucosa	Through wall or into muscle

* Relative indications.

on pathologic findings. Low and high risk groups are defined by the completeness of removal, the histologic type and grade, and vascular or lymphatic invasion. Patients with high risk lesions should be seriously considered for radical resection.

Local destruction of a low rectal cancer may be achieved by local excision, electrocautery, cryotherapy, or laser ablation. In addition, endocavitary radiation will be included in this discussion because, even though it is not a surgical technique, it is an effective method of locally treating these specific early lesions for cure.

Local Excision

Essentially, local excision is a wide excisional biopsy. Operating proctoscopes or retractors are used to dilate the anus and the lesion is removed with an adequate margin of normal tissue. The major advantage of this method is that the entire lesion is available for pathologic examination.

Endoscopic Snare Excision. This technique is appropriate for polypoid or pedunculated lesions; complications include hemorrhage and perforation.

Investigators have tried risk estimation for lymphatic metastases based on the level of invasion of a cancer in a polyp. Haggit and colleagues and Nivatvongs and associates have examined this issue closely; they think that if the neoplasm is limited to the mucosa or invades only the head of the polyp then the risk of lymph node metastases is small.[245,246] In this situation, close follow-up with repeated colonoscopies is all that is necessary. Both also agree that if the carcinoma reaches the base of the polyp (level 4) this risk rises dramatically. If the base is invaded or if the resection margin is not clear, they recommend formal resection. Less clear is the risk of spread if the neoplasm invades the neck (level 2) or the stalk (level 3). In Nivatvongs' series, invasion to level 2 or 3 was not associated with lymphatic spread. In Haggit's study, level 2 and 3 invasion was associated with a 20 percent rate of lymphatic metastases. Morson and others are of the opinion that when the tumor is completely removed and is not into the base, resection is not warranted.[247]

Several additional factors are indicative of a higher likelihood of spread. These include lymphovascular channel invasion, location in the rectum, and poor differentiation of mucinous histology. The appropriate treatment of the patient with an invasive carcinoma invading onto the neck or stalk of a polyp remains an area of controversy.

Transanal Excision. Posterior lesions are best treated with the patient in the lithotomy position, whereas anterior lesions are easier to approach with the patient in the prone jackknife position. Lateral lesions may be operated upon with the patient in either position, although some workers prefer a lateral decubitus orientation. A complete bowel preparation is performed preoperatively just as for a transabdominal resection. The dissection plane may be infiltrated with epinephrine solution (1:200,000) although this is not strictly necessary. Submucosal disk excision is acceptable for villous lesions but generally a full thickness of the bowel wall is removed along with an adequate margin of normal mucosa. Stay sutures are useful for traction and orientation (Fig. 18-39). The specimen is pinned out on a cork board by the surgeon and oriented for the pathologist. The wound is closed with interrupted sutures placed through the full thickness of the wall. Transverse closure avoids rectal stenosis. Lesions up to 8 to 10 cm from the anal verge may usually be treated. Occasionally, higher lesions may be brought down or prolapsed with traction. Care must be taken during dissection of anterior lesions because of the pelvic structures here. Opening into the peritoneal cavity is not usually a problem so long as an adequate bowel preparation was performed and a good closure is obtained.[241]

Transanal Endoscopic Microsurgery (TEM). The new technique of transanal endoscopic microsurgery (TEM) allows for local excision of sessile polyps and small cancers from the mid and high rectum.[248-250] These are lesions that are not accessible by means of standard transanal techniques and would otherwise require surgical excision via the abdominal or transsacral approach. The TEM technique relies on specialized equipment (Wolff Company, Chicago, IL; Fig. 18-40) through which the lesion may be clearly visualized and modifications of standard surgical excisions may be performed. The system consists of an operating proctoscope (outside diameter, 4 cm) equipped with a stereoscopic operating microscope and an airtight cap. This cap contains four sealable ports for instrument placement and allows controlled gas insufflation and the use of standard surgical techniques employing specially adapted scissors, electrocautery, forceps, and suture.

A standard surgical bowel preparation is employed. Patients with small polyps may require only regional anesthesia; however, larger lesions mandate general anesthesia because of the longer operating time and the need for prolonged immobilization during the surgery. The lesion must be positioned within the inferior aspect of the operating field because of the angle of the optics and instruments. A 12- or 20-cm operating proctoscope is used, depending on the level of the neoplasm. The lesion is visualized by means of a simple cap with a viewing port and manual gas insufflation. The proctoscope is held in position by an attached double-ball-and-socket joint, which allows frequent adjustments in position during the dissection. The operating head or cap is placed on the end of the proctoscope and the viewing system is inserted. The primary surgeon views the field directly through the stereoscopic lens system while the assistant and others may observe using the attached video camera. The rectum is dilated by pressure-controlled insufflation of CO_2. Available instruments include right- and left-angled scissors and forceps, a needle holder, an injection needle with a protective sleeve, an electrocautery probe, and a com-

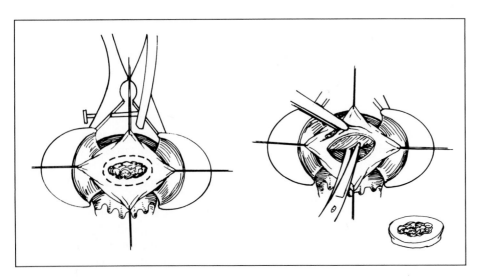

Figure 18-39. Transanal excision.

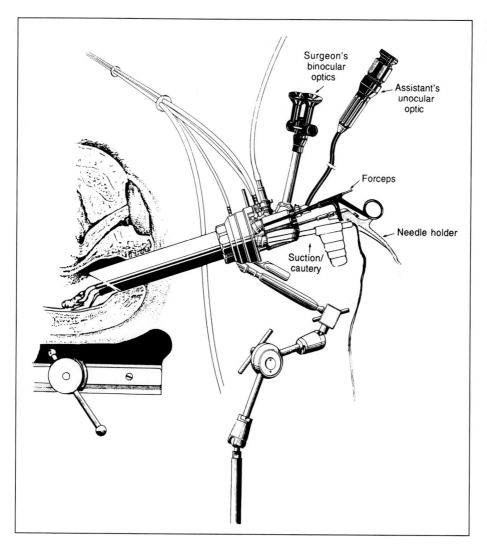

Figure 18-40. Transanal endoscopic microsurgery (TEM).

bined coagulation–cautery instrument. Disk excision of sessile polyps and small cancers may be performed with primary sutured closure of the defect.

Local Excision Through the Posterior Approach. Transsphincteric (York–Mason)[251] and trans- or parasacral (Kraske)[252] approaches have been used for lesions above the reach of standard transanal techniques. These techniques have already been described. Though excellent access may be afforded by these methods, they are rarely necessary any longer. Significant complications including wound breakdown and fistulas occur fairly frequently, and carcinomatous seeding of the rectal enterotomy site and the retrorectal and parasacral tissues is an additional risk.[242,253]

Electrocoagulation

Local treatment by electrocoagulation was first described by Byrne in 1889.[254] Strauss and colleagues in 1913 initially advocated its use for the palliative treatment of rectal cancer but subsequently extended their indications to curative treatment of selected lesions.[255] Although it is not widely applied, several groups including Salvati's in New Jersey and Madden's in New York have become ardent advocates of its use to avoid a permanent colostomy in patients with low rectal cancers. A theoretical advantage of this form of therapy is that it may be less likely to cause seeding of viable tumor cells. Disadvantages include the lack of a pathologic specimen for staging; reliance on visual and tactile evidence of complete eradication of the tumor; the necessity for several procedures, each of which requires hospitalization and anesthesia; and unclear indications for conversion to a radical resection.

The method used by the New Jersey group as published by Eisenstat and associates is reviewed here as a basis for discussion.[254] The lithotomy position is preferred. Because of the length of the procedure and the heat generated, general anesthesia is necessary. It is supplemented with 30 ml of bupivacaine with 1:200,000 epinephrine and 300 turbidity units of hyaluronidase instilled locally. A specially designed 15-cm long operating proctoscope with an external diameter of 4 cm and with a built-in light source, suction, and a distal bevel of 45° is used. Internal sphincterotomy is occasionally employed to allow placement of the scope. The Cameron bipolar electrocautery with a 5-mm ball tip is used to char the tumor surface and a 1- to 2-cm margin of normal tissue. The coagulated material is removed with uterine curettes and biopsy forceps. This sequence is repeated in layers until normal tissue is encountered. Then the base of the wound is heated.

The procedure is extremely tedious and takes an average of 60 to 90 minutes to perform. A great deal of smoke and debris is created which must be suctioned and irrigated out. The patient is discharged after 2 to 5 days, no antibiotics are used, and generally there is minimal pain. The wounds heal by secondary intention.

Monthly follow-up visits are critical. Suspicious areas are biopsied, and residual or recurrent disease is retreated. Abdominoperineal resection is recommended if more than three treatments are required, if satellite lymph nodes are palpable, or if the tumor is not being controlled.

Several variations of the technique have been described by other authors. Crile and Turnbull used a low-intensity cutting current, combing away the tumor with a brass wire loop until muscle was encountered.[256] They believe that, when coagulated, carcinomatous tissue crumbles and may be wiped away; that muscle chars to the consistency of leather; and that fat may be recognized by its color and because it sizzles.

Madden frequently performs the procedure under regional anesthesia. Using a self-retaining retractor with a light source, he is able to treat tumors up to 13 cm. A needlepoint electrode is advocated because its smaller surface allows for greater heat and penetration and better tactile discrimination (very important in his estimation for determining the depth of invasion and completeness of destruction). An electrocautery unit with spark-gap generator (Castle Bovie CSV Electrosurgical Unit, Sybrom Corp., Rochester, NY) is recommended. Intermittently during the procedure, the tip of the cautery is thrust into the base of the wound. Tumor will resist this insertion and normal tissue will bubble or foam with cauterization. The process may require from 1 to 4 hours. After 10 to 12 days the procedure is repeated and biopsies are taken. In Madden and Kandalaft's experience postoperative bleeding was a common complication, usually occurring after 6 to 9 days; operative control was often necessary. The average number of procedures performed on each patient was four, each requiring hospitalization and an anesthetic.[257,258]

Postoperative fevers are very common and generally respond to antipyretic agents alone. Pelvic sepsis occurs rarely; bleeding is very common, both shortly after treatment and 1 to 3 weeks later. This hemorrhage requires transfusion, reoperation, or both for control in between 10 and 22 percent of patients treated with electrocautery.[259,260] Rectal stricture is frequently seen if more than 50 percent of the circumference of the rectum has been treated. The incidence increases with the number of treatments required. Treatment of anterior lesions in women may cause a rectovaginal fistula. Anterior tumor location over or penetrating into the rectovaginal septum is thought to be a relative contraindication to electrocoagulation by many surgeons.

Cryotherapy

Cryosurgical destruction of a variety of lesions including neoplasms and hemorrhoids has been promoted at various times and by various authors. At present, a liquid nitrogen probe is applied, freezing the tissues. The advantages of this technique are that it is easy to apply and does not usually require an anesthetic. Unfortunately, the wounds that result often heal slowly and may drain copious amounts of foul discharge for several weeks. Also, the equipment is costly. Complications are similar to other destructive techniques and included hemorrhage (14 percent), stenosis (26 percent) and others such as peritonitis or fistulas (8 percent) in one series.[261-263] It is rarely employed for the treatment of rectal tumors at this time.

Laser Vaporization

A number of lasers are available for use in surgery, among them the carbon dioxide (CO_2), neodymium yttrium aluminum garnet (Nd:YAG), argon, and tunable dye lasers. These instruments have different penetration and absorption characteristics but are generally used in one of two ways: tissue vaporization or tissue cutting. In tissue vaporization, lesions such as small tumors or condylomata may be treated by vaporization, sucking away the residue in the smoke plume. This is similar in concept to electrocoagulation, as described above. In tissue cutting (laser ablation) the laser may be used as an expensive knife or cutting cautery to perform local excision. There is little new about these approaches except for the equipment used. In patients with rectal cancer, lasers may have their best application in the treatment of obstructing tumors, either for palliation or to achieve decompression and preoperative bowel preparation. These issues are addressed elsewhere in this chapter. Lasers may also be useful in the treatment of bleeding from radiation proctitis.

Endocavitary Irradiation

Adenocarcinoma of the rectum is a relatively radiosensitive tumor. Externally delivered, high-dose radiation has been known to eradicate small tumors occasionally. Unfortunately, since doses above 50 gray are necessary for a significant effect, external beam radiation is usually not curative, and high doses are associated with an increased rate of complications. The pelvis is a large, broad portion of the body, and there is a great deal of tissue between the entry site of the radiation beam and the tumor. Thus, high voltage delivery systems are used to maximize the penetration and minimize the complications of radiation.

As attested to by the many local treatments available for cancers located in the rectum, these lesions are particularly amenable to direct treatment because of their accessibility. Endocavitary radiation was introduced by Papillon in his 1973 report to avoid many of the limitations of external beam therapy.[264] Radiation energy is delivered through a specially designed proctoscope with a *high* output (10–20 gray/minute) and a *low* voltage (50 kV). This is distributed over a 3-cm diameter field with a focal distance of only 6 mm. Thus, only a small rim of normal mucosa is exposed and virtually all of the complications of external beam treatment are avoided. Although some patients will require a local anesthetic or an internal sphincterotomy to allow placement of the treatment proctoscope, the procedure can generally be performed on an outpatient basis (Fig. 18-41). Using a Philips (Philips, Eindhoven, The Netherlands) RT-50 or similar contact radiation machine, 100 to 150 gray may be administered in divided doses at 2- to 4-week intervals. Lesions larger than 3 cm are treated with overlapping fields in some centers. Tumors may be located anteriorly or posteriorly. They should be distal to the peritoneal reflection and should not overlap the dentate line because the anal skin is very sensitive to radiation.[265] In some trials treatment is supplemented by radioactive interstitial implants.

The patient is followed closely with digital and proctoscopic examination. Biopsies are performed when recurrence or incomplete response is suspected. Patients with larger lesions who are not candidates for surgical resection or who refuse surgery are being treated in some institutions with a combination of external beam and endocavitary radiation.[265]

Results of Curative Treatment

Mortality, Morbidity, and Functional Results

Despite major advances in perioperative management and marked decreases in operative mortality, survival after surgical treatment of rectal carcinoma has changed little over the past 50 years.

Operative Mortality

Since the late 19th century, operative mortality has fallen steadily. In 1900 a death rate of 19.7 percent was reported in 881 cases operated upon by the most eminent surgeons of the time.[266] Since the mid-1970s mortality in the first 30 days after surgery has stabilized at about 2 to 3 percent. It is extremely uncommon for a patient to die on the operating table; most postoperative deaths are due to cardiopulmonary complications.

Perioperative Morbidity

Patients who undergo surgical resection of rectal cancers are at risk for a large variety of perioperative complications. It is quite important that, whenever possible, these risks be discussed with the patient and family before surgery.

All patients are at risk for cardiovascular and pulmonary complications including shock, blood loss, myocardial infarction, congestive heart failure, pneumonia, pulmonary insufficiency, edema or embolism, and thromboembolic events. Abdominal morbidity may arise from colonic or anastomotic vascular insufficiency, prolonged ileus, small bowel obstruction, intraperitoneal infection, volvulus, or internal hernia. Specific problems involving intraoperative bleeding, the urinary tract, sexual dysfunction in men and women, perineal hernias and unhealed perineal wounds, anastomotic leaks and stenosis, and stomas are briefly discussed below.

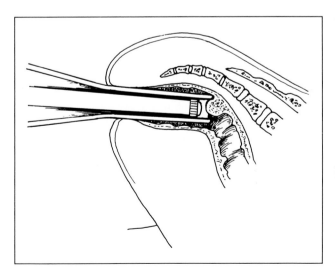

Figure 18-41. Endocavitary irradiation. Position of the treatment proctoscope.

Intraoperative Bleeding.   Blood loss is an accepted part of surgery; however, a goal of good surgical technique is to minimize the amounts lost and to try to avoid unnecessary transfusions. The most difficult hemorrhage that may be encountered during surgical resection of the rectum is from the sacrum. Attempts at suture ligation of bleeding points deep to the presacral fascia are likely to worsen the bleeding. If a bleeding vessel can be clearly seen, ligation or cautery may control it. Unfortunately, the bleeding often emanates from the basivertebral veins and not the presacral venous plexus. The basivertebral veins may be ruptured when the presacral fascia and periosteum are tented up by traction on the rectum prior to opening of the presacral space. When ruptured, they retract into the sacral foramina where they cannot be controlled by the usual measures.[267] This type of bleeding may usually controlled by direct pressure and packing of the pelvis.[268] Often after several minutes of pressure the bleeding ceases. If bleeding continues, a pack may be left in the presacral space exiting the perineal or lower abdominal wound. This pack may be removed several days later under local anesthesia. Control may also be obtained by driving a sterile thumbtack into the foramen.[269] One report even suggests that by fracturing the sacrum the bleeding site may be directly exposed and controlled.[267]

Urinary Tract Complications.   Urinary tract infections, urinary retention, and iatrogenic injury of the ureters are fairly common problems. Roughly 4 percent of patients develop a urinary tract infection during their postoperative course. Patients who undergo rectal surgery are at risk because most have an indwelling urinary catheter for at least several days and many have a preexisting element of urinary stasis. Careful sterile technique when placing the catheter and using a closed drainage system will help reduce this incidence. However, any catheter left in place for an extended period will cause colonization of the urine. Therefore, the urinary catheter should be removed as soon as it is practical. A urinanalysis and culture will reveal the diagnosis. *Escherichia coli*, *Proteus* species, streptococci, and *Pseudomonas* species are the most common infecting organisms. Most of these offending organisms may be successfully controlled with an oral or intravenous course of an antibiotic such as a trimethoprim–sulphamethoxizole combination (Bactrim®, Septra®) or ampicillin.

Urinary dysfunction is quite common after pelvic surgery especially in elderly men. This is frequently due to benign prostatic hypertrophy in this group of patients. In one study of 85 patients from Japan, complete urinary retention was seen in 31 percent at 2 weeks but this decreased to 8 percent by 1 month.[270] It was most common after rectal eversion, pullthrough, and abdom-inoperineal procedures and did not occur in any of the patients having an anterior resection. One half of the men in this series noticed changes in urinary function versus only one third of the women. Although urinary problems are common the majority are resolved within 1 month after surgery. Prostatic size as determined by preoperative palpation does not correlate with postoperative difficulties; however, preoperative symptoms of prostatic hypertrophy such as frequency, nocturia, urgency, difficult initiation, and weak stream, do. Factors associated with an increased incidence of postoperative urinary dysfunction include male sex, tumor less than 9 cm from the anal verge, and wide or radical lymphadenectomy.[271]

Intermittent or continuous catheterization may be necessary for several days to several weeks. This alone resolves urinary dysfunction difficulties 70 percent of the time.[272] Urecholine is rarely helpful. Transurethral resection of the prostate may be necessary in men with benign prostatic hypertrophy who do not improve within 2 to 3 weeks. Urodynamic investigation may be indicated if dysfunction persists after 2 to 3 months. In Aagaard and associates' report of 25 patients followed with serial urodynamic studies postoperatively, 5 patients had persistent problems.[273] Three had benign prostatic hypertrophy and 2 had lower motor neuron injuries, all clearly predicted by these investigations.

Intraoperative injury of the ureters may occur in 0.3 to 6 percent of colorectal operations.[274] Injuries include complete or partial suture ligation, stenosis or obstruction from angulation due to an adjacent suture, complete or partial crush injuries, partial wall incision or complete transection, devascularization, and segmental excision. These injuries should be avoidable in uncomplicated cases, but they may be encountered more frequently when there is pelvic inflammation or extensive malignant disease: the ureters may become involved in the process and may be difficult to find and to separate. Indeed, when there is adherence of the tumor to a ureter, separation is contraindicated since tumor may be transected, shedding tumor cells and leaving disease behind.

If there has been prior pelvic surgery, if there is an inflammatory mass, or if the tumor is large, precautions are in order. Computed tomography with intravenous contrast or an intravenous pyelogram may help to clarify the anatomy including the proximity of the ureters to the tumor; obstruction and hydronephrosis may also be seen. If there is any concern, ureteric stents should be placed cystoscopically at the beginning of the procedure.[272,275] If this was not done and the ureters cannot be identified intraoperatively, stents may be placed through an anterior cystotomy or via the renal pelvis. Although stents do not guarantee the safety of the ureters, they do help the surgeon identify their location and course.

To avoid iatrogenic ureteric injuries, the ureters should be clearly identified in the operative field in all cases so that they may be protected. This does not mean that they should be skeletonized since extensive stripping of the ureters may devascularize them. Instead they should be seen and their course should be understood. This is usually done quickly and easily during the sigmoid and upper rectal mobilization. Peristaltic activity and palpation may aid in their identification.[272] Occasionally, time must be taken to find them and to ensure their safety. It is sometimes nearly impossible to find the ureters because of scarring or the underlying pathologic process. In this situation, the ureters may be found more proximally and traced distally. If there is any question about their integrity, an intraoperative intravenous pyelogram may be of occasional use. Alternatively, methylene blue may be given intravenously to locate a leak. The possibility of ureteral duplication must be kept in mind.

If the ureter is injured, immediate recognition and repair is best. If the ureter is clamped and this is recognized intraoperatively, the clamp is removed and, if the site appears viable then the ureter is stented for 5 to 7 days. Small puncture wounds of the ureter generally require drainage alone, although stents may be placed. When necessary, a short segment of ureter may be resected and the ends anastomosed. The ureter should be mobilized proximally and distally to ensure a tension-free anastomosis. The ends are spatulated and an oblique anastomosis with 5.0 chromic catgut is constructed over stents. When the injury is in the lower ureter, the proximal end is reimplanted into the bladder as a ureteral neocystostomy. When a significant length of the distal ureter is involved with the tumor, it should be resected en bloc. If the remaining ureter is not long enough to reach the bladder, it may be mobilized and brought across and anastomosed to the opposite ureter. In practice this is rarely necessary. Since it also puts the other side at risk if there is a complication, it is not generally done. If it is known that the ipsilateral kidney is nonfunctional, then the ureter may be ligated. If no other method is available or if the patient is unstable, a cutaneous ureterostomy may be performed. This stoma, however, is very prone to stricture and should be avoided whenever possible.[274] When wide pelvic resections or exenterations are performed, an ileal conduit (Bricker) may be created for urinary diversion.[272]

Urethral injury may be primarily repaired and/or stented with a urinary catheter to avoid leakage through the perineal wound or formation of a urinoma. Urethral strictures may be treated secondarily. Bladder wall lacerations are closed with two layers of absorbable suture and urinary catheter drainage is maintained for 7 to 10 days postoperatively.[272]

In the early postoperative period, urinary tract injuries may be recognized by increased drainage from the pelvic or abdominal drains, from the vagina, or through the perineal or abdominal wound. Leg pain that persists or increases in intensity, an increasing abdominal mass, or anuria may all be signs of this complication. The creatinine level of the drainage should be compared with that in the serum and in the urine. Indigo carmine or methylene blue may be given and a diagnosis made if the drainage becomes colored. CT scan and cystoscopy may help to localize the injury.

Sexual Dysfunction: Men.   Erection is initiated and maintained by a complex combination of vascular and neuromuscular phenomena. Rapid filling of the dilated venous sinusoids of the corpora cavernosa along with decreased outflow contribute to the turgidity of the penis. Muscular contraction due to parasympathetic activity adds to the rigidity and decreases venous outflow further. Ejaculation is mediated primarily by sympathetic nerves.

Sexual dysfunction is very common in men after a variety of pelvic surgical procedures including radical prostatectomy, cystoprostatectomy, low anterior resection, and abdominoperineal resection. Impotence may occur in about 15 percent of patients who undergo low anterior resection and in 45 percent after an abdominoperineal resection. Other ejaculatory dysfunction may be seen in 32 and 42 percent of these patients, respectively. The complication rates after surgery for benign conditions such as inflammatory bowel disease are much lower (5 percent impotence and 6 percent ejaculatory dysfunction).[276-279] This is probably because the dissections performed for benign disease are closer to the bowel wall and avoid injuring the nerves.

The sympathetic nerves arise from S-2 to S-4 and run in the hypogastric plexus, which may be identified at the level of the sacral promontory. Below this promontory, the plexus splits into a right and left bundle which progress laterally below the presacral fascia. Anterior traction on the low sigmoid and rectum prior to entering the correct space may stretch or avulse these nerves, leading to bladder or ejaculatory dysfunction. The pelvic plexus may also be injured during the lateral dissection since many of its branches run adjacent to the middle hemorrhoidal vessels, wrapping around the rectum anteriorly at the level of the seminal vesicles. At this point the nerves are intertwined with the capsular vessels of the prostate, which lie within Denonvilliers' fascia. Erectile dysfunction may be caused by damage to the cavernous nerves as they course along the seminal vesicles and prostate. Ligation of the internal iliac arteries may result in vasculogenic impotence, especially when the internal pudendal vessels are also interrupted.[279]

Sexual Dysfunction: Women.   There is little information on sexual dysfunction in women after operations for rectal carcinoma. Cirino and associates questioned 18 women postoperatively and found a number of problems including decreased desire (78 percent), loss of sexual satisfaction (44 percent), dyspareunia (34 percent), and a decreased capacity for orgasm in 1 patient (5 percent).[278] Metcalf and colleagues carefully examined sexual dysfunction after proctectomy for *benign* disease in 100 women. Fifty had undergone an ileal pouch–anal anastomosis and 50 had a continent (Koch) ileostomy. Most had an *increased* frequency of intercourse after operation, presumably due to their improved health after cure of their ulcerative colitis. There were few problems after the ileal pouch operation, but a number of patients complained of dyspareunia after proctectomy with a continent (Koch) ileostomy. This was thought to be due to angulation or stenosis of the vaginal vault or retroversion of the uterus.[280] This is useful information, but it is likely that sexual dysfunction in women is a much more common problem after operation for malignant disease due to both neurologic injury and anatomic changes.

Perineal Hernia.   Infrequently, perineal hernias have been reported to occur after abdominoperineal resection or pelvic exenteration; the rate reported is from 0.1 to 1 percent of these patients.[281,282] Hernias are probably fairly common but only rarely cause symptoms significant enough to attract attention. When these procedures are performed, a large portion of the pelvic floor is removed; often, little is left to provide support. Abdominal contents, principally the small intestine, will fall into the pelvis and may come to rest beneath the level of the pelvic floor on the cutaneous perineal closure. Patients may notice a perineal bulge that increases with coughing. Complications of perineal hernia include skin ulceration, evisceration, persistent perineal wound, and perineal enterocutaneous fistula. Operative repair is a major undertaking and should be performed only for symptoms or complications. Whenever possible, recurrence of disease should be excluded preoperatively. An abdominal approach is recommended so that all of the structures may be adequately seen and to facilitate mobilization of the loops of small bowel. Repair may be performed with a sheet of mesh sewn across the pelvic outlet. If long enough, the omentum should be brought down and placed between the mesh and the small bowel to reduce the risks of sepsis, small bowel erosion, and fistula formation. Any of several muscle flap techniques may also be employed.

Unhealed Perineal Wound.   Among the most chronic and difficult complications of proctectomy are unhealed perineal wounds. Patients operated on for malignancy encounter this problem less frequently than do patients with inflammatory bowel disease.[283] These wounds may have not healed initially or may open subsequently. A wound that has failed to heal after 6 months is considered an unhealed perineal wound. These wounds may continuously drain a foul material, soiling undergarments and causing a great deal of patient discomfort and distress.

After abdominoperineal resection for cancer there is usually little left of the levators to pull together, although occasionally they may be partially apposed. The perineal wound may be managed in one of three ways: 1. Miles closed the peritoneum and packed the open perineal cavity from below. This was often associated with slow healing. 2. Both the peritoneum and the perineal skin may be closed with suction drainage of the resultant dead space. When this is performed it is likely that the peritoneum ends up down in the pelvic cavity or separated as the small bowel descends into the dead space. 3. The perineum alone may be closed, allowing the small bowel to obliterate the pelvic space. This latter method gives the wound the opportunity for primary healing whereas leaving it open mandates secondary healing.[284] Placing a vascularized pedicle of omentum in the pelvic space may also reduce the incidence of complications.[285]

Persistently draining wounds are initially treated with aggressive wound care and repeated curettage. Deeper wounds should be cleansed with peroxide on cotton applicator sticks and, when possible, irrigated with a Waterpik® (Teldyne,™ Fort Collins, CO). Damp-to-dry dressings help to debride nonviable cells and promote healthy granulation. These treatments need to be repeated 2 or 3 times each day. The patient usually cannot see the area well and must be assisted by a family member or a visiting nurse.

If good healing does not occur, the tract should be evaluated for the presence of an enteroperineal fistula, for foreign material, or for recurrent disease. An examination under anesthesia with curettage and trimming of the wound edges is often helpful. A fistulogram and a small bowel series will help to identify a fistula.

Early surgical correction should not be attempted since many of these wounds will heal with conservative management. However, prolonged treatment with packing and curettage, especially of large, high defects, may be very debilitating for the patient and may result in a small-bowel fistula.[286]

A number of methods have been described for closing perineal defects. Since it is contained within the bony pelvis, the space cannot just collapse. For moderately shallow wounds, excision of the fibrous walls of the cavity, converting the space to a wound that is broadest at its base, followed by split-thickness skin grafting is appropriate. Rarely, the coccyx and lower sacral segment may be excised, allowing the posterior perineum to obliterate the wound. Narrow defects have been obliterated with fibrin glue after curettage in a few case reports.

Perhaps the most effective method in use is filling the defect with a muscle or myocutaneous flap. Although this is a major procedure, the chronic abscess cavity will be excised and the pelvis will be filled with well-vascularized normal tissue. In this way, primary healing may be achieved in the presence of sepsis, and any cutaneous defects may be covered. There are many reports extolling the virtues of gracilis, rectus abdominis, and gluteal muscle and myocutaneous flaps, all of which have merit. Good healing may be anticipated in the majority of patients treated with these methods, although patients who have had high-dose radiation therapy seem to do less well.[286-293]

Anastomotic Leakage. Leakage from or dehiscence of a colorectal anastomosis is one of the major complications of surgery for rectal carcinoma. The rates reported vary widely according to a number of variables which include the skill and experience of the surgeon and the method by which leakage is sought (Table 18-6). Akwari and Kelly reported a clinical leak rate of 5 percent in 400 patients who had a two-layered, hand-sewn colorectal anastomosis at the Mayo Clinic between 1975 and 1977.[307] This rate rose to 9 percent for anastomoses within 10 cm of the dentate line. Others have confirmed the higher leak rate with low anastomoses.[102]

Clinically apparent leakage is far less common than that found by routine radiologic examination. In Goligher and associates' report from 1977, 137 patients had a hand-sewn anastomosis; a clinical leak rate of 6.5 percent was found along with a radiographic leak rate of an additional 28.5 percent.[308] Several other studies have confirmed this observation for both sutured and stapled anastomoses (Table 18-7). In most recent series from major centers, clinical leak rates of 4 to 6 percent are quoted.

Anastomotic leaks are most commonly due to technical factors.[315] Constructing an anastomosis low in the pelvis may be very difficult. Incomplete anastomoses may occur with both hand-sewn and stapled techniques, particularly on the posterior side. In 1988, Fazio reported experience with 744 stapled colorectal anastomoses performed at the Cleveland Clinic. Leak rates of 0.6, 3.2, and 5.8 percent were found with high, low, and very low (>5 cm) anastomoses respectively.[102] Other major factors include adequacy of the vascular supply to the anastomosed ends of the bowel and tension on the suture line. In addition, bacterial contamination, drains,

the level of the anastomosis, corticosteroid therapy, prior radiation, and systemic disease such as diabetes, atherosclerotic disease, and anemia may contribute.[116,315,316]

In the early 1980s when staplers had just become available, the leak rate appeared to be higher than that with hand-sewn anastomoses. As additional experience was gained this difference disappeared. Now most workers agree that a safe, reliable anastomosis may be constructed in the low rectum more easily with the circular stapler than by suturing.[298,306,317] In a large prospectively randomized trial of gastrointestinal anastomoses performed in Scotland, 224 of 1004 patients studied had rectal anastomoses.[306] They were well matched for clinical factors and for the level of the anastomosis. No differences were found between sutured and stapled anastomoses in clinical leak rates, sepsis rates, time to return of gastrointestinal function, or hospital stay. However, a significantly higher number of sutured anastomoses had radiographically demonstrated leaks (12.4 versus 4.1 percent). Staplers may reduce operative time, although they are expensive.[298,303,306,317]

"Protecting" a tenuous anastomosis with a proximal diverting colostomy is a time-honored concept. Diverting the fecal stream may allow additional time for a weak anastomosis to heal and gain strength; it makes intuitive sense. Leaks are usually due to technical problems and an incomplete anastomosis. Radiation and tension on the anastomosis also appear to be important. Diverting colostomies do not appear to improve the healing of these anastomoses; however, they do seem to reduce the clinical sequelae.[116,117,304] Heald's group retrospectively reviewed their patients who had undergone a low anterior resection with mesorectal excision and anastomosis. In this nonrandomized comparison, 6 of the 75 patients without a stoma required emergency laparotomy for peritonitis while only 1 of the 125 patients with a diversion was explored.[318] It is prudent to consider a protective diverting ostomy when there is concern regarding the healing of the anastomosis. Either a colostomy or an ileostomy may be used.

Several recent randomized trials have attempted to determine the usefulness of intraoperative testing of anastomoses.[314,319,320] Two main methods have been described: (1) filling the pelvis with saline and transanally insufflating air with a proctoscope, or a bulb syringe, and (2) instilling povidone-iodine into the rectum under mild pressure. Localized leaks are then repaired. Beard and associates published a prospective, randomized trial of 143 patients; air testing of the anastomosis was performed in one half of them.[314] Eighteen leaks were identified by the test and were repaired. The postoperative clinical leak rate was reduced significantly from 14 percent in the no-test group to 4 percent in the

Table 18-6   Clinical Anastomotic Leakage Rates Using Sutures or Staplers for Rectal Anastomoses

Author/Year	Sutured		Stapled		Comments
	No. patients	Leak, %	No. patients	Leak, %	
Goligher et al[294] 1979			62	3.2	
Adloff et al[295] 1980	25	16	26	8	
Bolton and Britton[296] 1980	10	10	20	5	
Smith[297] 1981			3594	9.8*	
Beart and Kelley[298] 1981	35	3	35	3	
Dorsey and Stone[299] 1981			40	25	
Heald and Leicester[300] 1981			100	13	Very low anastomoses
Detry and Kestens[301] 1981			100	11	
Fazio et al[302] 1985			125	0.8	
McGinn et al[303] 1985	60	3	58	12	
Feinberg et al[106] 1986			79	8	Double stapled
Antonsen and Fronborg[304] 1987			178	15	
Belli et al[305] 1988			74	4	
Griffen et al[107] 1990			75	2.7	
WSHASG†[306] 1991	113	4.4	111	8.6	

* Pooled results from polled members of the American Society of Colon and Rectal Surgeons.
† From the West of Scotland and Highland Anastomosis Study Group.

tested group; similarly, the radiologic leak rate was reduced from 29 percent to 11 percent. It should be noted that the gastrograffin contrast study was not a benign procedure and was complicated by pain and tenderness in 2 patients and gram-negative sepsis in another 2; 1 of these 4 patients died as a result.

Detection of incomplete anastomoses and potential sites of leakage would seem to be a logical and prudent goal. Some anastomotic defects will be suspected because incomplete "doughnut" rings are retrieved from the circular stapler. Others will be identified and repaired intraoperatively by routine use of these insufflation and irrigation techniques; however, this does not guarantee a leak-proof anastomosis.[320]

The management of anastomotic leakage depends on the clinical condition of the patient. A subclinical leak

Table 18-7 Stapled Anastomotic Leakage Rates by Clinical Suspicion and Radiographic Examination

Author/Year	No. patients	X-ray leak, %	Clinical leak, %	X-ray leaks clinically suspected, %
Goligher et al[294] 1979	24	25	8.3	33
Ling et al[309] 1979	21	43	14	33
Dorricott et al[310] 1980	50	26.7	4	23
Kirkegaard et al[311] 1981	30	16.7	6.7	40
Marti et al[312] 1981	79	8.8	3.8	43
Brennan et al[313] 1982	10	50	40	80
McGinn et al[303] 1985	58	24	12	50
Fazio et al[302] 1985	79	3.8	1.2	33
Beard et al[314] 1990	70	29	14	48

that is detected radiographically in an otherwise asymptomatic patient requires no treatment but does require close follow-up. A patient who has fever, leukocytosis, and local pain may have a pelvic abscess; such abscesses are often due to a posterior anastomotic leak. These usually present within the first 5 to 10 days postoperatively. In the absence of systemic toxicity or peritonitis, antibiotics and supportive measures may allow resolution of small infections. If larger, these collections are often successfully drained transanally through the anastomosis. A drain may be left in place for several days to weeks. If an abscess presents later, CT-guided placement of a drainage catheter may avoid an operation. If the patient does not respond to these measures or presents with significant systemic toxicity or peritonitis, then exploration of the abdomen is necessary. Most major anastomotic leaks and dehiscences will require resection of the region with a Hartmann pouch and proximal end colostomy. Attempts to repair the defect, even if protected with a proximal colostomy, are doomed to failure because the inflamed tissues will not hold sutures. Simple drainage and proximal colostomy is a less satisfactory method of management since the source of infection is not removed and the fecal column between the ostomy and the leak remains to contaminate the site. This method has been all but

abandoned in the treatment of complicated diverticular disease, as it should be here. After 3 to 6 months, continuity may be reestablished. The double-stapled technique or a coloanal anastomosis may be particularly useful in this setting.

Anastomotic Stenosis. The true incidence of anastomotic stenosis is unknown, since most are not clinically relevant. They may be related to the technique of construction because most are made with an inverting method, to vascular insufficiency caused by overzealous clearing of the mesentery from the ends of the bowel, to overaggressive tightening of the stapler, or to the use of small diameter staplers.[102,321] Rates of anastomotic stenosis range from 5 to 20 percent and depend somewhat upon the definition and the aggressiveness with which they are sought. Some authors only describe symptomatic lesions which are usually less than 12 mm in diameter, whereas others state that the inability to pass a 19-mm proctoscope or a finger is significant.[102] There is some evidence that stenosis is a more common problem with stapled anastomoses.[297] Most stenoses dilate over the first few months after surgery as the tissues heal and remodel and as formed stools pass through. Killingback has observed that stenoses after stapled anastomoses tend to occur early and to resolve with time; clinically significant stenoses occur later and may progress.[322] Proximal diversion may increase the rate of anastomotic stenosis since no stools are passing through and helping to dilate the lumen.[323] Probably only 1 to 2 percent need treatment. Indications for intervention include constipation or obstipation, repeated or severe impaction, and the inability to perform colonoscopy on the patient. Treatment may consist of dilation by means of a finger, graduated dilators, or a balloon.[324] Rarely, an anastomosis must be surgically revised.[102,105,297] Transabdominal resection with reanastomosis is the standard approach, although transanal stricturoplasty is a good alternative for low rectal stenoses. A novel approach involves concurrent transanal resection and reanastomosis of the strictured area using an intraluminal circular stapler.[325-327]

Colostomy Complications. When a colostomy is necessary, most problems may be avoided by creating a well-constructed stoma in a well-informed patient. Since the patient will generally have to live with this new route of evacuation for the rest of his or her life, early education and support will help to avoid many psychosocial and physical problems before they occur. The assistance of well-trained enterostomal nurses and interaction with individuals with similar ostomies (available through the United Ostomy Association and other national and local support groups) are invaluable aids for the patient with a new colostomy.

Postoperatively, the stoma is observed for color, evidence of inadequate blood supply, bleeding, mucocutaneous separation, and peristomal infection and drainage. Observation is facilitated by the application of a transparent, disposable, two-piece appliance at the time of surgery. The stoma may be observed through the clear plastic or the pouch may be removed, leaving the faceplate in place.

Prior to discharge, the new ostomate must be taught the technical skills necessary for care of the colostomy. Most patients learn these rather quickly but some are unable to do so because of physical limitations or because of denial or rejection of the stoma. A visiting nurse with enterostomal training may have to come to the patient's home regularly for a time, and consultation with the enterostomal therapist at each clinic visit is very useful. The diet is usually unrestricted although some foods may cause a bad odor, a high output, or increased flatus. Occasionally, a blockage may occur at the level of the fascial outlet. This is generally due to bulky, fibrous food. These blockages often improve spontaneously but may require irrigation or endoscopic decompression to resolve.

A colostomy may be allowed to drain constantly or may be "trained" to empty only when irrigated.[328] If a regulated colostomy is preferred, the patient is taught to irrigate the stoma with 250 to 500 ml of tap water using a cone tip and an enema bag with tubing. Gradually, the volume may be increased to as much as 1000 ml. Irrigation may be performed once a day, once every other day, or once every third day. Between irrigations a well-regulated colostomy does not generally require a pouch; a small stoma covering may suffice.

Psychosocial adaptation to a new ostomy is a complex issue and may be very difficult or even impossible for some patients.[329,330] Concerns regarding body image, sexuality, limitations of activities, and soiling must be addressed for most patients to thrive.

Though one of the simplest procedures to perform, creation of a colostomy is associated with complications in up to 30 percent of patients.[331-335] These problems may occur early in the perioperative period or many years later. Early complications include hemorrhage, ischemia, infection, recession, high ostomy output, and peristomal skin irritation. Stenosis may be caused by a narrow outlet or by edema and swelling. Late complications include these problems as well as ulcers, pseudopolyps, hernias, prolapse, obstruction, fistulas, trauma, and perforation. Peristomal skin irritation and breakdown may be due to a poorly fitted or poorly adherent appliance, poor placement on the abdominal wall, or allergy to a component of the faceplate. Many of these problems may be avoided by strict attention to the details of stoma construction and placement and by proper appliance use.

Functional and Physiological Results After Low Anterior Resection

The stated goal of a low anterior resection is to cure the cancer and to reestablish continuity so that the patient may function normally. Although major incontinence is uncommon, minor leakage is frequent.[336] In this operation, most if not all of the rectum is removed and replaced by the descending colon. The rectum is noted for its capacitance and compliance (the ability to accommodate increasing volumes with minimal increases in pressure). Bringing the relatively noncompliant descending colon down to replace the normally compliant rectum reduces the reservoir function above the sphincters and predisposes these patients to frequent evacuation.[337,338] Additionally, the left colon may be denervated during this procedure, leading to more frequent bowel movements because of reduced motor activity, reduced segmental relaxation, and consequent faster colonic transit.[339]

The activity of the anal sphincter muscles may also be compromised by this operation. Usually this is a modest change, but in some patients major damage may occur, especially to the internal sphincter.[326,340-342] Stretching during transanal placement of a stapler or pursestring may result in decreased resting pressures.[342] Generally, the external sphincter is not physically injured.[342-344] There may, however, be a component of neurologic injury of both sphincters due to hypogastric nerve injury during the pelvic dissection, pudendal nerve stretch, or transection of the intramural neural plexus. The lower the anastomosis, the more likely is sphincter damage.[338,345]

Fortunately, over time the neorectum dilates and is able to assume more of a reservoir function. The anal sphincters also tend to improve, although this is variable, and the frequency of evacuation slows. These changes may take up to 6 to 12 months to occur and may be assisted by judicious use of bulking agents and motility-slowing medications.[340,341]

Long-Term Survival

Patients who develop rectal carcinoma rarely survive 5 years without treatment. Approximately 4 percent of patients in whom resection or diversion is performed for palliation will be alive after 5 years and virtually all go on to die of their disease.[346] Overall survival after curative resection averages about 50 to 55 percent at 5 years in a large number of series (Table 18-8). In the first half of the 20th century, survival improved because of better operative techniques and earlier aggressive surgical management which included lymphovascular resection. However, since the adoption of these methods, survival by stage of disease has improved relatively little.[69,94,186,346,348]

The only recent improvement in radical surgical treatment has been the extension of lymphatic clearance. Heald and associates have followed a policy of complete mesorectal dissection and excision in all patients with rectal carcinoma. They believe that most pelvic recurrences arise from tumor rests left behind at the time of resection in the lymphatic tissues that remain. If these are removed, then results should be improved. They reported their initial 115 patients operated on for cure in 1986,[99] noting that their rate of abdominoperineal resection had dropped to only 11 percent. After a mean follow-up of 4.2 years there were 3 pelvic recurrences. The corrected probability of survival at 5 years was 87 percent, and tumor-free survival by Dukes stage was 94 percent for A lesions, 87 percent for B lesions, and 58 percent for C lesions. In 1990, they reported 57 patients who had undergone a curative "ultra-low" anterior resection for lesions within 7 cm of the anal verge, some of whom actually had a stapled coloanal anastomosis.[187] The distal margins ranged from 2 to 35 mm, but these differences were not associated with any difference in outcome.[366] Although overall survival was 80 percent, a 17 percent rate of serious complications was noted. Moreover, 15 percent of patients were in-

continent 2 years after colostomy closure. Local recurrence was only 3.5 percent.

Recurrence After Major Resections

Most patients with recurrence die of distant disease. A smaller number die primarily because of local recurrence or carcinomatosis. Recurrence rates vary somewhat between studies; however, overall recurrence remains around 50 percent. Approximately 80 percent of recurrences are discovered within 2 years of surgery, but 3 to 5 percent occur after 5 years.[92,367,368] Therefore, the longer the follow-up, the higher the recurrence rates. The median interval to recurrence was 22 ± 4 months in a collected series reported by Devesa and colleagues.[369] Distant recurrence develops in 40 to 50 percent of patients while local recurrence is found in from 10 to 25 percent of patients.[353,370-378] The liver is the most common site of initial distant recurrence; the lungs hold a distant second place. Initial isolated recurrence in the lungs may be more common with rectal cancers than with colonic ones, although this has not been clearly established. This is possible, in theory, because of greater vascular communication between the rectum and the systemic circulation via the middle and inferior hemorrhoidal veins.

The site of initial recurrence was examined in a study of 412 patients resected for cure at the Memorial Sloan-Kettering Institute in New York City; 44.2 percent developed a recurrence. The initial recurrence was at a single site in 25 percent and in several locations in 19 percent. Sites of initial recurrence included the pelvis in 36.3 percent, the liver in 23.9 percent, other viscera in 28.3 percent, and other intraabdominal or retroperitoneal locations in 11.4 percent.[358]

Gerard and his colleagues in the EORTC in 1988 published their results from 341 surgically treated patients.[379] With a mean follow-up of 6.3 years, 15 percent of these patients had an isolated local recurrence while 15 percent had isolated distant recurrences; 8 percent had both. Of the initial distant recurrences, 73 percent were in the liver, 15 percent were in the lungs, 6 percent in bone, and 3 percent in the peritoneum. These numbers are fairly representative of the distributions found in other reports. However in a series from the University of Chicago, only 30 percent of initial recurrences were found in the liver and 46 percent in the lungs.[186] The initial site of recurrence is somewhat contingent upon the Dukes stage of the index lesion. Rosen and colleagues reported local and distant recurrence rates of 0 percent and 15 percent in patients with Dukes A lesions, 16 percent and 24 percent in patients with Dukes B lesions, and 10 percent and 58 percent in patients with Dukes C lesions, respectively.[356] Local recurrence rates are quite low in colon

Table 18-8   Review of 5-year Survival Rates (%) After Resection of Rectal Carcinomas, Overall and by Dukes Stage

Author/Year	No. patients	Overall	A	B	C	Comments
Dukes[347] 1940			93	65	23	
Grinnell[171] 1953		53		65	35	
Mayo and Fly[348] 1956	689	52				APR
Gilbertsen[349] 1960			80	50	23	
Lloyd-Davies[350]* 1969		55		66	35	
Zollinger and Sheppard[82] 1971	328	41				APR
Slanetz et al[83] 1972	277	31	81	52	33	APR
Stearns[84] 1974	227	48				APR
Whittaker and Goligher[351] 1976	407	49	80	62	33	
Patel et al[352] 1977	435	54	65	63	30	
Strauss[85] 1978	83	51	86	42	26	
Corman et al[353] 1979			81	62	33	
Enker et al[354] 1979	216	65	. . .	87	50	
Heberer et al[355] 1982			86	80	59	
Rosen et al[356] 1982	180		86	65	33	
Localio[128] 1983	646	61	89	57	36	ASR
Williams and Johnston[357] 1984			82	77	56	
Pilipshen et al[358] 1984	412		84	64	39	
Ohman[359] 1985			83	48	22	
Glass et al[183] 1985	75		100	78	27	*
Isbister and Fraser[360] 1985			78	73	39	
Hojo[361] 1986	273		93	73	49	
Danzi et al[362] 1986	93		86	62	31	APR

Table 18-8 (Continued)

Author/Year	No. patients	Overall,	A	B	C	Comments
McDermott et al[59] 1986	1144	48	93	71	41	
Enker et al[184] 1986	412	54	81	48	36	
Davis et al[363] 1987	235	42	75	55	31	
Michelassi et al[186] 1988	154	53		56	43	
Kune et al[364] 1990	467	33	65	46	28	
Dixon et al[365] 1991	303	52	100	66	45	APR
		64	100	71	53	AR

APR = combined abdominoperineal resection. AR = anterior resection with anastomosis. ASR = abdominosacral resection.
* Maingot R, ed. *Abdominal Operations.* 5th ed. New York: Appleton-Century-Crofts; 1969: 1750–1751.
† Extended abdominoiliac lymphadenectomy.

cancer, whereas they are relatively high after surgery for rectal cancer.

Factors Influencing Survival

Many factors have been examined to determine which are of the greatest significance in predicting survival and recurrence. Predicting outcome allows patients to plan ahead and also allows the design and subsequent evaluation of follow-up programs and adjuvant treatment trials. The most significant factors in virtually all studies are the depth of penetration of the bowel wall and the presence and extent of lymph node and distant metastases.[55,57,65,73,353,356,371,380-388] This was recognized and incorporated into the first really useful staging system for rectal cancer by Cuthbert Dukes and his colleagues at the St. Mark's Hospital in London.[389] This method of staging and the confirmation of a pathologically complete resection are clearly the most important predictors of outcome.[390] The Dukes staging system and several others are discussed in Chapter 17 and reviewed in Tables 17-9 to 17-15.

Devesa and associates reviewed the literature on prognostic factors in colorectal cancer and divided them into four categories: (1) tumor-dependent variables, (2) host-dependent variables, (3) biochemical variables, and (4) surgeon-dependent variables (Table 18-9).[369] The tumor-dependent variables have been the factors most carefully studied. Host-dependent variables attempt to quantify the patient's cellular response against tumor growth. Lymphoplasmocytic and eosinophilic tumor infiltration have been examined in particular.[391-394] Biochemical variables may reflect tumor growth or host reaction. Aside from carcinoembryonic antigen (CEA), biochemical studies have not yet yielded any convincing marker of biologic aggressiveness.[391] Elevated serum levels of acute phase reactant proteins (APRP) (e.g., α-acid glycoprotein, α-antitrypsin, transferrin, haptoglobin, C-reactive protein, cathespin B) may be found in a high proportion of patients with disseminated or locally extensive tumor but have little sensitivity or specificity and therefore are of little use. Liver enzymes are late indicators of hepatic disease since a large tumor load is usually necessary before they become significantly elevated. If they are elevated in the *absence* of demonstrable hepatic lesions, the incidence of recurrence is higher. Variability between surgeons may be the least significant of these factors but does seem to play a role. After all these factors have been considered, the Dukes stages are still the most accurate and reproducible predictors of outcome.

Lymph Node Metastases. Adenocarcinomas seem to preferentially spread into lymphatic channels and usually establish metastatic deposits in the regional lymph nodes before they reach the central system. There is a clear tendency for nodes directly adjacent to the lesion to be involved prior to more proximal nodes.[75,76] Although this tendency has been often noted, skipped nodes and isolated deposits in higher nodes are well known to occur.[72] Nevertheless, staging systems that differentiate between the involvement of

Table 18-9   Factors Affecting Prognosis in Rectal
Carcinoma

_____

TUMOR-DEPENDENT VARIABLES
Probably significant
   Lymph node status
   Depth of wall penetration
   Tumor mobility
   Obstruction
   Total number of symptoms
   Preoperative tumor perforation
   Intraoperative perforation
   Mucinous and signet-cell histology
   Malignant fixation
   Venous and perineural invasion
   Lateral and mesorectal spread
   Rate of growth
   DNA ploidy

Questionable significance
   Age
   Sex
   Interval between onset of symptoms and treatment
   Rectovesical or rectovaginal fistula
   Concurrent adenomas or carcinomas
   Macroscopic morphology
   Degree of differentiation
   Number of involved quadrants
   Distance from the anal verge

HOST-DEPENDENT VARIABLES
Regional lymph node activity
In vitro tests of lymphocyte activity
Delayed cutaneous sensitivity testing

BIOCHEMICAL VARIABLES
Preoperative carcinoembryonic antigen (CEA) level
Elevated serum levels of acute phase reactant proteins
Liver enzymes

SURGEON-DEPENDENT VARIABLES
Selection and performance of operation/treatment
Use of adjuvant therapy
Completeness of extirpation

_____

low and high lymph nodes have some prognostic significance. Also, the more lymph nodes involved the higher the risk; patients with one to four positive lymph nodes have a 55 to 60 percent cure rate as opposed to those with 5 or more involved lymph nodes who have a cure rate of only 33 percent.[384,395,396] Involvement of the highest regional lymph nodes such as those at the base of the inferior mesenteric artery is a grave finding and denotes fairly certain systemic spread of the disease. In Grinnell's (1965) report[173] none of the 19 patients

with high ligation of the interior mesenteric artery and involved high lymph nodes attained prolonged survival.

Obstruction. Many studies confirm that patients who present with obstruction have a much poorer prognosis than those who do not.[397-399] Some of these patients may progress to perforation; therefore the initial treatment of the patient with obstruction must be planned to avoid this often catastrophic complication. Certainly, these tumors are generally more advanced, are usually circumferential, and have penetrated the muscularis of the bowel wall. Many of these lesions will not be resectable for cure.

Symptoms. Asymptomatic patients seem to have an overall better survival, because these tumors tend to be found while in an earlier stage.[400-404] Stage for stage, their progress is similar to that noted for symptomatic patients. Patients presenting with bleeding probably have a slightly better outlook than those with other symptoms such as change in stool habits or obstruction, since bleeding may be an early sign whereas changes in stool are generally associated with larger, annular lesions.[405]

Perforation. Perforation may occur in one of three ways. First, direct growth of the tumor through the bowel wall may be complicated by necrosis. Perforation of the tumor through the bowel wall may result in free communication with the peritoneal cavity and peritonitis or may be walled off by adjacent tissues and the omentum and thus contained. This type of perforation may also be complicated by a rectovaginal or rectovesical fistula. Free perforation may allow viable cells to implant on distant peritoneal surfaces, while a contained perforation may lead to local recurrence. The contained type of perforation may occur in the cecum because of retrograde pressure and the higher wall tension found in this largest-diameter area of the bowel. This will only occur if there is a competent ileocecal valve. The third form of perforation occurs intraoperatively. The rectum may be entered during either sharp or blunt dissection. The bowel wall adjacent to the tumor may be opened or the tumor itself may be entered. Cutting through the lesion is probably associated with a greater decrease in local and distant control rates.[406-411]

It is a common practice to irrigate the rectum below the distal clamp or staple line before opening it to wash out or fix free tumor cells and thereby to avoid local dissemination, but the available data do not clearly support this practice. Long and Edwards irrigated the bowel lumen with formalin in 40 of 185 patients and found lower local recurrence rates in these patients (2.6 versus 14.3 percent).[412] Irrigation of the pelvis to prevent implantation of free-floating cells has been advocated by a number of authors. Several agents such as povidone-iodine, antibiotics, Dakin's solution, mercuric chloride, nitrogen mustard, Lugol's solution, ethyl alcohol, saline, and sterile water, have all been suggested and used, but the evidence supporting or refuting their effectiveness in reducing local recurrence has been unconvincing.[413,414]

Differentiation. The majority of rectal adenocarcinomas are classified as moderately differentiated. The few that are labeled "well differentiated" tend to be less aggressive and often present as Dukes A lesions. Conversely, poorly differentiated tumors have a poorer prognosis and usually behave much more aggressively, metastasizing earlier and recurring more frequently.[381,395,415] Lesions that demonstrate mucinous and signet-cell histologies are also associated with poorer outcomes.[416,417]

Vascular and Neural Invasion. Pathologic evidence of vascular and neural invasion is thought to be indication a poor prognosis.[418,419] It is difficult to estimate the actual significance of such findings, because the rates of invasion reported vary widely and are often related to how aggressively the evidence is sought by busy surgical pathologists. For example, venous invasion has been reported to occur in from 10 to 60 percent of specimens.[420-426] Using special stains and multiple sections, Talbot and associates found venous invasion in 52 percent of their patients.[427] These patients appeared to have more advanced disease by Dukes stage, had poorer 5-year survival rates, and had higher rates of hepatic metastases.[421,422] Talbot and associates also found that invasion of *extramural* veins was associated with much poorer survival than was invasion of intramural veins. Spread into thick-walled extramural veins was particularly ominous, and 5-year survival was only 8 percent in patients with this finding and Dukes C lesions. Host reaction and inflammation around the site of invasion seemed to improve the outlook somewhat.[428]

Lateral and Mesorectal Spread. Both the extent of mesorectal spread and the involvement of lateral resection margins have recently been confirmed as prognostic factors. Cawthorn and associates[429] found that patients with "slight" mesorectal spread (≤ 4 mm) had a 5-year survival rate of 55 percent, whereas patients with greater mesorectal spread only had a survival rate of 25 percent. This factor seemed to be independent of the lymph node status and Dukes stage in their analysis. Heald and associates have found a significant improvement in local recurrence rates when rectal resection included complete mesorectal excision, as already noted above.[76,98,99,430] This includes a local recurrence rate of 3.6 percent after a 10-year follow-up of 110 rectal carcinomas in which the margin of resection was greater than 1 cm.[76] Because of the data from Heald and from Cawthorn and associates, the editorial board of The Lancet has recommended that "the number of millimetres of mesorectal spread should become part of the standard histopathology reporting."[431]

Age. Fewer than 10 percent of colorectal cancers occur in patients below the age of 40 years, and fewer than 1 percent are in those below age 20. These tumors tend to present at a more advanced stage and are more likely to have a mucinous histology. For these and other reasons, colorectal carcinoma in the young may represent a separate type of malignancy. Nevertheless, stage for stage these patients have the same prognosis as those of any age.[431-434]

Elderly patients with rectal carcinoma also do just as well as their younger, "middle-aged" counterparts. In fact, patients in their eighties and nineties seem to tolerate surgery remarkably well. This may be a reflection of their innately good constitution which has allowed them to live to an advanced age. When correction is made for cardiovascular deaths, the elderly also have the same prognosis as all other patients with colorectal cancer.[435,436]

Gender. Although gender is mentioned in a number of studies, no definitive statement may be made about any difference in prognosis between men and women. Any slight differences are probably of little practical significance since treatment regimens using hormonal manipulations have never been proved of benefit in colorectal malignancies.

Tumor Size. The calculated volume of the primary tumor does not appear to have a direct effect on prognosis.[437-439] Surprisingly, size also has no direct relationship with penetration of the bowel wall, incidence of local recurrence, or lymph node involvement.[85,440,441] Some less aggressive tumors may grow to large sizes and remain localized, whereas many small lesions may demonstrate more aggressive behavior and cause early metastases, perforation, or both.[196]

Direct Spread. When all types of direct invasion are considered together, most reports indicate that involvement of adjacent structures is associated with a poorer prognosis for the patient; however, this is quite dependent on the tissue invaded and the extent of extrarectal spread.[395,439,442] Clearly, patients with tumors that invade the sacrum and pelvic wall will do less well than patients without such invasion. Tumors that invade adjacent structures do not necessarily have a poorer outlook.[196] However, en bloc resection is required so as not to obviate the curative intent of the resection.

Morphology. Exophytic tumors have a better prognosis than do endophytic ones. This seems reasonable since exophytic tumors tend to grow into the lumen of the bowel rather than through the bowel wall.[186,391,399,443,444]

DNA Ploidy. Flow cytometry is an analytical tool that allows the measurement of cellular and subcellular particles. Although developed in the 1970s, it has only recently become a useful clinical tool because of refinements in instrumentation including electronics, computer control, and laser light sources. Flow cytometry analysis is based on hydrodynamic focusing. The tissue to be examined is processed into a suspension of cells that may be run past a light beam in single file order. The scatter of light is measured and interpreted. Forward-angle light scatter and 90° light scatter are read separately and give information about the cell size and its internal structure. In addition, stains and immunohistologic labels may be used to look at specific attributes of the cells and their contents.

DNA analysis of colorectal tumor cells has been studied fairly extensively in the last few years. Two parameters seem to correlate with poorer prognosis: increased aneuploid DNA content and increased S-phase percentage[445-450] (Table 18-10). Aneuploidy is a sensitive indicator of malignancy in colorectal cells; however, only 50 to 70 percent of these neoplasms demonstrate significant aneuploid peaks on the histograms, whereas the remainder show a primarily diploid profile. Aneuploid tumors tend to be found in higher stages and are associated with poorer histologic grades. S-phase analysis indicates the percentage of cells that are actively proliferating and thus have a higher DNA concentration. Analysis of normal mucosa reveals an S phase of 4 to 10 percent whereas malignant lesions generally have an S-phase reading of 10 to 20 percent. There is a moderate overlap between these ranges in most series. An increased S-phase fraction is also often correlated with poorer survival and histology. It is critical that each laboratory have its own normal values and that the technique be well controlled. Poor technique will yield falsely aneuploid results.

Most studies suggest that (1) higher stage tumors have a greater proportion of aneuploid cells, (2) aneuploid tumors tend to have a higher growth rate (S-phase fraction) and poorer survival than do diploid tumors, (3) aneuploid tumors are associated with other histologic parameters indicative of a poor prognosis such as vascular invasion.

Thus, DNA analysis may be a helpful independent predictor of tumor behavior and patient prognosis, especially in early lesions where decisions regarding further treatment must be made. However, there is great variability between studies which may be related to definitions and technical problems.[465] The overall role of flow cytometry and DNA analysis in the assessment and treatment of rectal carcinoma has yet to be defined.

Coloanal Anastomosis

Parks and Percy's classic report included 76 patients with rectal cancer; nearly half of the lesions began between 4 and 8 cm from the anal verge. Mortality was 4 percent, all from pulmonary embolism. There were two anastomotic leaks with pelvic sepsis, and 8 patients with pelvic sepsis but without a demonstrable leak. Function after 3 months was normal in 39 of 70 patients evaluated, while 30 patients were continent but had some irregularity and three to four bowel movements per day. Only 1 patient was incontinent. The patients operated upon for cure did as well as similarly staged patients who underwent abdominoperineal or low anterior resection.[466]

Hautefeuille and colleagues from Paris reported in 1988 their experience with 35 patients treated with coloanal anastomosis for adenocarcinoma of the mid third of the rectum.[467] They used a technique similar to Parks' including a left lower quadrant protective colostomy. There were no operative deaths, and 74 percent of these patients had an uncomplicated course with closure of the colostomy and good function. A gastrograffin enema was performed after 2 months and this demonstrated 7 leaks (11 percent of patients), 3 of which were asymptomatic. None of the 4 patients with symptomatic leaks required reoperation, and 6 of these 7 patients had their colostomy closed with 2 failures. Three patients did not have their colostomy closed because of early recurrence. No strictures were found and only 1 of the 31 restored patients had poor function (3.2 percent); this was due to a persistent vaginal leak. The 24 patients with long-term follow-up had a 5-year survival rate of 64 percent.

Even high-dose radiation therapy is not necessarily a contraindication to coloanal anastomosis. Cohen and his associates described their series of 8 patients who received high-dose preoperative radiotherapy and underwent resection with coloanal anastomosis after 4 to 6 weeks.[195] There were no anastomotic complications and 6 of 8 patients had excellent functional results. Others have reported similar results with coloanal anastomosis for a variety of indications.[468-471]

Pappalardo and associates in Rome attempted to evaluate the physiological results of coloanal anastomosis.[472] Twenty patients with carcinomas between 5

Table 18-10   Significance of DNA Flow Cytometry Analysis in Colorectal Cancer

Author/Year	No. patients	Aneuploid, %	Independent factor, +/−	5-year survival, %[a]	SPF[b]
Armitage et al[451] 1985	134	55	+	19 vs 43	
Kokal et al[452] 1986	77	69	+		
Melamed et al[453] 1986	33	52	−		
Bauer et al[454] 1987	60	81	−		+
Rognum et al[455] 1987	100	63		64 vs 49	
Emdin et al[456] 1987	37	62	+		
Scott et al[457] 1987	121	51	+	64 vs 50	
Schutte et al[458] 1987	279	62	+		+
Borkje et al[459] 1987	17	53			
Bosquillon et al[460] 1989	117	>70	+		
Fausel et al[461] 1990	27	56		53 vs 67	
Kouri et al[462] 1990	157	68	+[c]		
Yamaguchi et al[463] 1990	52	52		21 vs 71	
Schillaci et al[464] 1990	70	75	−		

[a] Aneuploid/nondiploid vs diploid.
[b] Increased S-phase fraction correlates with poorer prognosis.
[c] When stage D tumors were excluded.

and 8 cm from the anal verge were entered into the study. Seventeen underwent coloanal anastomosis after curative resection of the rectum, while 3 patients who were incontinent preoperatively underwent abdominoperineal resection. They were compared with 20 matched control subjects. These authors used an intersphincteric dissection and everted the bowel to construct their anastomosis. Patients and subjects were evaluated preoperatively and then the patients were retested at 3 and 12 months postoperatively. One patient developed a pelvic recurrence and underwent an ab-

dominoperineal resection, and 1 died with metastases. This left 15 patients available for postoperative testing. Anal canal manometric pressures measured in the control subjects and in the patients preoperatively were the same. Postoperatively, resting pressures fell modestly (70 mm Hg to 57 mm Hg, mean); however, squeeze pressures dropped to about half their preoperative levels (40 mm Hg to 22 mm Hg, mean). By 12 months postoperatively, both the resting and squeeze pressures had returned to about 90 percent of their preoperative levels. Interestingly, reservoir compliance had dropped after surgery to less than one half of the preoperative levels but returned to 86 percent of these levels by 12 months. This seems reasonable since the compliant and accommodating rectum has been replaced by the more muscular and contractile sigmoid or descending colon. Evacuation frequency, up to four to five per day postoperatively, also improved to two or three per day at 1 year. Thus, both anal sphincter and neorectal function improved during the year of evaluation.

Coloanal anastomosis is a useful approach when a standard low anterior anastomosis is not possible. Equivalent survival should be expected when the tenets of cancer surgery are adhered to. The chance of cure should not be compromised to save function. In experienced hands, this is a safe and viable operation. The coloanal anastomosis is also a valuable option if reoperation is necessary after a low anterior resection has failed because of leakage or stenosis. As has been mentioned earlier in this chapter, the coloanal anastomosis may be combined with a colonic J reservoir.[122]

Local Treatment

Local methods have become acceptable as the definitive treatment for large adenomas and carefully selected early carcinomas of the rectum. Evaluation of the results of these methods is difficult because there are no prospectively randomized studies. All the available data are based on reports of groups of patients treated by one technique or another. The outcome in these groups of patients may then be compared only with historical controls or the results from patients with nonequivalent lesions who underwent more radical treatment. A major issue is that the classic staging systems are based upon pathologic examination of the resected specimen and the associated lymph nodes. Of course, this is not available after local treatment. There appears to be a group of patients with early lesions that will do well no matter what type of local treatment is performed so long as the primary tumor is destroyed. The goal is to identify that group as accurately as possible.

Local Excision.   Polypoid carcinomas uniformly do well with 5-year survivals approaching 100 percent after complete snare or disk excision.[247,473-475] Sessile carcinomas do not appear to be adequately treated by snare excision since 5-year survivals average only 40 percent.[251] Those patients with neoplasms that are excised with a rim of normal tissue and are limited to the submucosa (Dukes A; TNM-T1) do quite well with 5-year survivals of 90 percent or better and local recurrence rates of 3 to 21 percent (Table 18-11). At least half of those patients with local recurrence may be cured by radical surgery.

Biggers and his colleagues at the Mayo Clinic reported the largest series to date of patients who underwent local therapy.[479] Of the 234 patients in this group, 188 had a local excision of the tumor. The rest had either electrocoagulation, cryosurgery, laser ablation, or intracavitary radiation. More than one tumor was found in the rectum in 14 percent of patients. The 93 patients with in situ cancers had normal survival. Well-differentiated lesions that were less than 3 cm in diameter had a 5-year survival of 58 percent versus 13 percent in all the others. Patients with well-differentiated cancers did better than those with moderately or poorly differentiated ones. Local recurrence was seen in 49 patients, while 5 developed distant disease. The probability of recurrence at 5 years was 11 percent after excision of in situ lesions and 27 percent after excision of invasive ones. Ten patients died of their cancer, 46 died of other causes, and 19 died of unknown causes. Although Biggers' results appear to be poorer than most of those reported by other groups, these investigators concluded that local treatment was quite justified in selected patients.

Complications with transanal excision occur relatively infrequently. The most common postoperative problem is hemorrhage. This may stop spontaneously or may, on occasion, require electrocoagulation or suture ligation. Wound dehiscence may occur but usually is well tolerated and heals spontaneously. Sepsis is rare but may require drainage. Perforation into the peritoneal cavity is extremely rare with low rectal lesions but may be possible, especially in women with a very low cul-de-sac.

Although the rate of lymph node metastases in patients with tumors limited to the submucosa is relatively low, 3 to 21 percent develop recurrences. If local treatments are extended to include larger lesions and those that penetrate the muscularis propria, these rates will undoubtedly increase. Some workers are attempting to improve these results by adding radiation therapy to their protocols. These trials may also include patients with lesions not usually thought to be well treated by local methods but who are too frail to undergo resection or who refuse a colostomy. The theoretical advantages of the addition of radiation to local treatment are to treat lymphatic disease, to shrink the primary lesion, and to limit local recurrence due to implantation of viable cells during the excision.

Ellis and his group at the University of Florida reported 9 patients who underwent local excision followed by 45 to 60 gray of external beam radiation.[481] All of the lesions treated were exophytic adenocarcinomas measuring 3 cm or less. Clear margins were confirmed in 8 of the 9 patients, and invasion was limited to the submucosa in 8 of the 9 patients as well.

Table 18-11 Results of Local Excision for Rectal Carcinoma

Author/Year	No. patients	5-yr survival, %	Local recurrence, %	Salvaged after local recurrence
Morson et al[473a] 1977	91	82	3	
Hagar et al[476] 1983	33[b]	90	3	
	20[c]	78	17	
Stearns et al[253] 1984	31	84	26	
Killingback[477] 1985	39	82	23	5/9
Cuthbertson and Simpson[478] 1986	28	79	21	6/6
Biggers et al[479] 1986	188[d]		21	
DeCosse et al[480] 1989	57	83		
LOCAL EXCISION PLUS RADIATION THERAPY				
Ellis et al[481] 1988	9	89	0	. . .
Horn et al[475e] 1989	17[b]	100	0[e]	
	14[c]	83	43	3/6
Despretz et al[482] 1990	25		20	3/5

[a] Includes malignant polyps and colotomy for excision with transanal local excision.
[b] with invasion limited to the submucosa.
[c] with invasion of the muscularis.
[d] 188/234 with an adenocarcinoma had a local excision.
[e] 3 of 17 had recurrence of villous adenoma but no carcinoma.

There was no operative mortality and minimal morbidity. After a mean follow-up of 64 months there were no recurrences. One patient died of pneumonia at 12 months.

Despretz and associates in Créteil, France, treated 25 patients preoperatively with 35 gray of external beam radiation.[482] The median size of these tumors was 4 cm. Each patient underwent local excision with placement of plastic tube loop for postoperative brachytherapy (20–25 gray). Six of these 25 excisions were incomplete, and 2 of these patients went on to develop local recurrences. With a mean follow-up of 40 months, 5 (20 percent) patients had a local recurrence. Three were salvaged with abdominoperineal excision, 2 for cure and one with distant disease for palliation. One of the 20 patients with local cure subsequently developed distant metastases. Although these studies are small and have

limited follow-up, the results are encouraging enough that additional investigations seem warranted.

Some authors have advocated "local excision" using a parasacral or transsphincteric approach.[251,483–488] Complications including impotence, bladder dysfunction, wound infections, and fecal fistulas are common, and most of these lesions may now be addressed transanally.[489] Therefore, these methods are not advocated for the majority of cases.

When the muscularis propria is invaded the rate of lymphatic metastases increases from less than 10 percent to the 20 to 30 percent range. In addition, the local recurrence rate is much higher in these patients. Therefore, most authors advocate conversion to a radical resection when this invasion is found on pathologic examination. This situation should occur less often now with the benefit of preoperative staging using endorectal ultrasonography. Other relative indications for radical resection or the addition of radiation after local excision are poorly differentiated histology, lymphatic or venous infiltration, and an inadequate resection margin.[475,490]

In conclusion by careful selection of patients with invasion limited to the submucosa, lesions less than 3 cm in size, and favorable histologic findings, very high cure rates may be obtained.[41,247,253,473,475,490,491]

Transanal Endoscopic Microsurgery (TEM). The early results using transanal endoscopic microsurgery (TEM) have been very encouraging. In 1988, Professor Buess and his colleagues reported their first 140 patients. Excisions were performed for adenomas in 110 patients and for early carcinomas in 30. The average operating time was 1.5 hours. In 6 cases the peritoneum was opened during resection of lesions in the intraperitoneal rectum. All were closed; one patient required a sigmoid resection. The procedure was well tolerated by all patients. Complications occurred in 7 patients (5 percent). They included hemorrhage requiring suturing; suture line dehiscence (3 of 5 required a temporary colostomy), rectovaginal fistula (2), and pulmonary embolism (1—the only death). Buess and colleagues thought that lesions invading beyond the submucosa (T2 or T3) should be treated with radical surgery.[249]

In a more recent unpublished analysis of 274 patients, 74 had a malignancy while 191 had an adenoma.[492] Most were located from 8 to 11 cm above the anal verge, but 4 adenomas and 2 carcinomas lay in the 20- to 23-cm range. Of the 74 patients with cancer, 22 were subjected to radical operations after TEM excision; this was based on the depth of penetration and completeness of excision. Follow-up was only an average of 10 months in this recent series. Of the 191 patients with adenomas, 7 experienced recurrence. Snare procedures or hot biopsies were used in 5, 1 underwent an anterior resection, and 1 had TEM excision. Fifteen new polyps were found, 13 of which were snared or electrocauterized and 2 removed by TEM. Thus, only 4 of these 191 patients (2 percent) required a second operation. Recurrence after excision of a carcinoma was staged by the depth of penetration of the bowel wall. Lesions that were limited to the submucosa (T1) and that were well or moderately well differentiated had a recurrence rate of 3 percent (1/29); however, patients who were at higher risk with poor differentiation or with lymphovascular invasion had a 40 percent recurrence rate (2/5). Lesions that invaded into the muscularis (T2) had a 7 percent recurrence (1/15), and those that penetrated through the muscularis (T3) had a 33 percent recurrence rate (1/3). Though the numbers are small when grouped in this fashion, the trend for higher recurrence with deepening invasion of the rectal wall is again seen. The investigators' recommendations include TEM as definitive treatment only in those patients with

completely excised adenomas and carcinomas limited to the submucosa (Dukes A, T1). Patients with lesions invading the muscle are treated with radical resection unless they are poor surgical candidates.

This technology extends our ability to apply precise local surgical treatment to lesions in the mid and high rectum that have previously been out of reach. The risks are small and the potential benefits are great; however, this method requires a great deal of practice, the procedure may be quite tedious and time-consuming, and the equipment is expensive. Furthermore, there are relatively few patients who will be candidates for the procedure. Therefore, at least for now, this technique may be limited to the larger referral centers that can afford the equipment and that see or will be referred enough patients to make this approach worthwhile.

Electrocoagulation.   Electrocoagulation as a method of primary treatment of small rectal cancers has not gained widespread popularity for several reasons. First, the procedure is often long and tedious and creates much smoke and heat. For these reasons, the procedure is usually performed under a general anesthetic. Second, multiple procedures are the rule rather than the exception and this requires time and energy from both the surgeon and the patient. Third, no definitive pathologic specimen is obtained for staging purposes. And last, relatively high complication rates have been associated with its use (Table 18-12).

Operative mortality remains low in all series, although complications have been reported in from 8 to 28 percent of patients. Hemorrhage, either immediately postoperatively or after 1 to 2 weeks, is quite common. Although hemorrhage is usually self-limited, occasionally a patient must be transfused, returned to the operating room for coagulation or suture ligation, or both. Stricture of the rectum, abscess formation, and perforation also may occur. Treatment of an anterior lesion in a woman is particularly likely to result in a rectovaginal fistula.

Factors that appear to improve prognosis are treatment of lesions that are less than 3 cm in diameter and less than one-third the circumference of the rectum.[254] Some authors report better results with exophytic (polypoid) tumors versus endophytic (ulcerated) ones,[256,260] while others have obtained almost equivalent outcomes.[496]

Overall survival rates are remarkably consistent between studies and lie in the 60 to 70 percent range. It is difficult to compare these results with those of radical surgery because there is no pathologic staging. The stated goal of this procedure is to avoid abdominoperineal resection and colostomy. Local failure (20 to 30 percent of patients) generally mandates a radical resection, leading to the very anatomic arrangement one

Table 18-12   Outcome After Curative Electrocoagulation

Author/Year	No. patients	Outcomes, %				
		Operative mortality	Compli-cations	5-yr survival	Local failure	Salvage rate
Madden and Kandalaft[259] 1971	52	0	28	71	23	33
Crile and Turnbull[256] 1972	62	0	0(?)	68	13	87
Culp and Jackman[493] 1974	59				30	33
van Slooten and Van Dobbenburg[494] 1980	43	0	27		28	50
Hughes et al[495] 1982	39	4	21	69	30	43
Madden and Kandalaft[496] 1983	156	0	23	71*	33(?)	
Hoekstra et al[497] 1985	33	0	8	71	6	100
DeGraaf et al[498] 1985	49	0	14	61	31	38
Salvati et al[499] 1988	91	2	21	47	38	29†

* 62% disease free.
† Five-year survival of 58% in those patients not requiring salvage APR versus 29% after APR conversion.

hoped to avoid. Unfortunately, "salvage" by abdominoperineal resection does not achieve very good survival.

Electrocoagulation may have a role in the palliative treatment of patients with rectal cancer. Generally good local control and low morbidity has been reported with repeated procedures.[500]

Endocavitary Irradiation.   Studies of external beam radiation alone for the treatment of rectal cancer have shown poor response rates. Although these tumors are relatively radiosensitive, the amount of radiation the tumor receives when delivered externally is severely limited by injury to surrounding normal structures and the higher energy needed to penetrate the body to reach the tumor. In addition, the dose–time relationship reduces the effectiveness of the method. Typically, 40 to 50 gray of orthovoltage radiation are given to a fairly large tissue volume in 1.8- to 2-gray fractions over 4 to 6 weeks. In contrast, endocavitary radiation is delivered directly to the tumor, treating a small volume of tissue with 30 to 40 gray of minimally penetrating radiation

over 3 to 4 minutes. This is repeated at 1- to 3-week intervals until a dosage of 120 to 160 gray is reached. Because of the nature of the radiation and its delivery, complications are rare. Localized proctitis may develop and a few rectovaginal fistulas have been reported when treating anterior lesions. Occasional minor bleeding or discharge may occur.

With fairly large series, Papillon in France and Sischy in Canada have both reported excellent results with selected patients. Papillon followed 245 treated with endocavitary irradiation for more than 5 years.[500] All lesions were less than 4.5 cm and were well or moderately well differentiated. Patients were treated with 100 to 160 gray in four treatments over 6 weeks. Some also had iridium implants placed. A disease-free survival of 76.3 percent was found; normal anal function was documented in 181 patients. Six required a colostomy because of treatment failure. Cancer-related deaths occurred in 8.9 percent of patients, whereas 13.2 percent died of intercurrent disease. The cancer death rate after 10 years was 9.1 percent. Local failure occurred in 13 (5.3 percent) of these patients; 3 of these 13 were salvaged by abdominoperineal resection. Nine patients with local failure died of carcinoma, and there was 1 operative death. Nodal failure occurred in 12 (4.9 percent) patients; 3 of these 12 were salvaged by radical surgery. Eight patients with nodal failure died of their cancer, and there was 1 operative death in this group. Papillon recommends treatment for cure of patients with lesions that are well to moderately well differentiated, that are less than 4.5 cm, and that are confirmed by digital examination or ultrasonography to be confined to the bowel wall.

Sischy and colleagues reported a 95 percent local control rate in 192 patients treated for cure.[265] Cancer recurred in 9 of these patients; 3 died, 5 were salvaged by abdominoperineal resection, and 1 was alive with disease at the time of his publication. Five-year survival could be assessed in 80 patients, and 93 percent were disease-free.

Lavery and his colleagues at the Cleveland Clinic treated 62 patients, some of whom had an excisional biopsy.[501] With a mean follow-up of 31 months, 56 (76 percent) were free of disease; 10 patients died of unrelated causes; 15 (24 percent) developed a recurrence of whom 9 could be salvaged by additional treatment. The remaining 6 had distant disease. The recurrence rate was higher when the initial lesion was ulcerated.

The advantages of this mode of treatment are easily recognized. Radical surgery and a colostomy are avoided, general anesthesia is not required, no hospital stay is necessary, there is no loss of work or home time, a significant financial saving is likely, there is no systemic morbidity, and the complication rate is low. The key to success is careful selection. Most clinicians will treat lesions for cure that are less than 3 to 4 cm in greatest diameter, that are limited to the bowel wall and preferably invading only the submucosa, and that are completely accessible to the treatment proctoscope. It is estimated that approximately, 3 to 10 percent of rectal carcinomas may be treated with endocavitary irradiation with the expectation of a good long-term outcome. The major factor restricting wider use of this treatment method is probably the limited availability of this equipment. The major problem with this technique is that the lesion cannot be staged because no histologic evaluation is performed.

Laser Vaporization.   Laser vaporization has not been used extensively in the United States or Europe for the primary treatment of early rectal cancers. The technique is usually applied when the patient is judged to be a very poor surgical candidate. A small Japanese series was presented in 1985 with good results.[502] The procedure may hold promise as a palliative option in certain selected elderly patients at high surgical risk.

Adjuvant Therapy

Of the approximately 45,000 carcinomas of the rectum diagnosed each year, about three fourths are amenable to surgical resection for cure. Unfortunately, close to one half of these patients subsequently die from metastatic disease. These rates have changed very little in the last few decades. Although aggressive surgery with complete excision and wide margins remains the single most important determinant of outcome, additional therapy to improve cure rates is desirable. Local recurrence is also a significant problem after surgical treatment, much more so than with colon cancers. This may be because of the limited radial margins attainable in the pelvis or because of a biologic difference in the disease.

Radiation Therapy

Primary External Beam Radiation Therapy

External beam radiation therapy has not proved to be an effective method of primary treatment. Even though rectal carcinomas are relatively radiosensitive, a high enough dose cannot be administered externally. Generally, treatment is limited to 50 to 60 gray because morbidity increases markedly beyond these dosages. Cummings and his associates at the Princess Margaret Hospital in Toronto reported the results of high-dose primary external beam radiation for rectal carcinoma in 123 patients. Surgery was performed for patients with residual tumor. The complication rate was fairly high, and cure was infrequent. An overall 5-year survival rate of only 21 percent was found. Patients with mobile lesions did better than those with fixed ones (38 versus 2 percent).[503] In collected series of external beam radiation—often supplemented with a local boost of brachytherapy—5-year survivals of 10 to 20 percent have been reported.[237,504-508] Endocavitary irradiation has been shown to be quite effective in the treatment of highly selected small carcinomas using doses of 120 to 160 gray (see Endocavitary Irradiation above). Trials of neutron beam radiation have not demonstrated any improvement but have been associated with marked increases in morbidity.

Radiation enteritis used to be a major limiting factor, making clinicians reluctant to use external beam therapy. However, with the development of multiple-field radiation techniques using high-voltage machines this complication has been reduced to less than 5 percent. By giving a portion of the radiation dose from the sides and the back as well as from the front, those areas where the beams cross receive the highest doses. Thus, much of the small bowel may be excluded from the treatment field. In addition, several techniques have been described to exclude the small bowel from the pelvis after surgery, further reducing the risk of complications.

Even though rectal carcinomas are generally sensitive to radiation, the tolerance of the surrounding structures limits the dosages used. The ureters, spinal cord, liver, lungs, and kidneys are particularly radiosensitive. Therefore, reasonable treatment with radiation therapy requires a balance between the therapeutic response and the undesirable side effects.[509]

Surgery and Radiation

It has recently become clear that there is a significant role for radiation therapy in the combined treatment of both primary and recurrent carcinoma of the rectum. Several prospectively randomized studies have shown a marked reduction in local recurrence when surgery was combined with radiation, although most do not show any improvement in overall survival. In a meta-analysis of evaluable studies from the English-language literature, improvement of up to 40 percent was seen with doses of 30 gray or more for patients with deeply invasive or node-positive carcinoma of the rectum.[510] It was estimated that to prevent local recurrence in 1 patient, 8 to 9 patients would have to be treated. It is reasonable to expect improvement only in local control with radiation since only the pelvis is treated. In addition, in the studies in which a statistically significant decrease in local recurrence was found after pelvic irradiation, the recurrence rates after surgery alone were unacceptably high. As has already been noted, Heald

and colleagues and Cawthorne and coworkers, achieved local recurrence rates with surgery alone which were much lower than those achieved with combined surgery and radiation.[76,98,99,429-431]

Postoperative Radiation Therapy

If radiation is used, there are several distinct advantages to delivering it after curative surgery. Surgery, which is clearly the most definitive treatment of the disease, is not delayed. Also, complete surgical and pathologic staging may be completed before therapy, allowing more accurate definition of treatment groups and, consequently, better results. In addition, accurate staging will stratify patients so that only those expected to derive significant benefit from radiation (Dukes B2 and C) will be treated. Last, operative exploration often helps to determine the limits of the treatment fields.

The disadvantages of waiting until after surgery for radiation include the theoretical considerations of decreased postoperative blood supply to the tumor bed, which may lead to a decreased biologic effect and larger numbers of viable tumor cells that could be shed during surgical manipulation and implant in the pelvis and abdomen. Practically, adhesions to and fixation of the small bowel and other structures may lead to a higher rate of complications with postoperative radiation.

Overall, postoperative radiation alone has produced a moderate decrease in the rate of local recurrence but has not had a significant effect on survival (Table 18-13).[514-516]

Table 18-13   Selected Studies of *Postoperative* Radiation Therapy (PRT) Versus Surgery Alone

Author/Year	Mean dose, gray	No. patients	Pelvic failure, %		Distant failure, %		5-yr survival, %	
			PRT	Surgery	PRT	Surgery	PRT	Surgery
GITSG[511] 1985	44	108	20	24	28	31	46	36
Balslev et al[512] 1986	50	90	17	35*				
Tepper et al[513]† 1987	45–50	165	19	29*			53	
Fisher et al NSABP[514] 1988	46	368	16	25*				
Schild et al[506]‡ 1989	50	139	22				59	

* Significant differences found.
† Stage B2–3 or C patients only. Median follow-up: 4.6 years. Compared with 142 historical control patients with surgery only. No difference in survival found.
‡ 47/139 patients had both postoperative radiation and chemotherapy. Mean follow-up 4.2 years. Patients with both radiation and chemotherapy had improved survival.

Preoperative Radiation Therapy

Preoperative radiotherapy has been proposed as a method of improving results in the treatment of rectal cancer. There are several theoretical advantages to the administration of ionizing radiation prior to surgery:

1. Large tumors may be reduced in size and radiation may increase their resectability rate.
2. The disease state may be downstaged by reducing or eliminating lymph node metastases.
3. The ability of tumor cells to metastasize or implant may be reduced before fresh tissue planes are opened and before manipulation of the tumor.
4. The biologic effects of radiation may be enhanced by an intact blood supply.
5. Injury to the small bowel may be lessened since the intestine has not descended into the pelvis and since it is not fixed by postoperative adhesions.
6. Postoperative complications will not delay therapy.

The most obvious disadvantages to preoperative radiation are that some patients (Dukes A and B1) are treated unnecessarily and that surgery is delayed. In addition, a change in the tumor size and extent may, in some authors' opinion, tempt the surgeon to do a less radical procedure, which may compromise the cure rate. The major problem in evaluating the effectiveness of preoperative radiation is that it may downstage lesions so that disease that may have originally been into the lymph nodes and labeled "C" may become a "B" lesion pathologically after treatment and be analyzed as such.[517] Thus, the benefits of preoperative radiation may be underestimated since our ability to stage disease preoperatively is limited.

Retrospective Studies.   In general, retrospective reviews of preoperative radiation therapy show that a significant reduction in local or pelvis failure may be realized (Table 18-14). Some studies support the notion that distant failure may also be improved along with survival. However, these studies must be interpreted with great caution because they tend to use historical controls for comparisons and the two groups may not be concurrent or analogous. Nevertheless, preoperative high-dose radiation has been shown to be safe and appears to markedly reduce local recurrence.[396,522]

Prospective Studies.   The results from a number of prospective randomized studies that compare preoperative radiation plus surgery with surgery alone support the contention that little additional morbidity is associated with preoperative therapy up to 60 gray. The single exception is an increased incidence of perineal wound breakdown. Overall, the majority of studies seem to support a decrease in tumor size and in the

Table 18-14   Selected Retrospective Studies of *Preoperative* Radiation Therapy (PRT) With Subsequent Surgery Versus Surgery Alone

Author/Year	Dosage, gray	No. patients	Pelvic failure, %		Distant failure, %		5-yr survival, %	
			PRT	Surgery	PRT	Surgery	PRT	Surgery
Friedmann et al[518] 1985	40–45	162	14	37			63	43a
Fortier et al[519] 1986	40–50	156	16	40			52	48
Reed et al[520] 1988	40–45	149	6d	18a,d	12	27a	68	52a
Mendenhall et al[521] 1988e	35–50	200	7.7	29a			66	38a

a Significant differences.

b 56/60 initially treated were resectable for cure at operation, versus 100 historical controls. No differences in survival were seen although the radiated patients had more advanced disease. Local control rates: 67% with 40 gray versus 91% with 50 gray.

c 40 radiated patients versus 109 patients undergoing surgery only. Improved survival was demonstrated; not seen in other studies. Severe complications occurred in 10% of patients receiving radiation.

d Isolated local recurrence.

e 65/74 initially treated were resected for cure at operation, versus 135 historical controls. Increasing from 35 gray to 40–50 gray rads improved local recurrence rates from 13% to 6% without an increase in postoperative complications.

Table 18-15   Prospective Studies of *Preoperative* Radiation Therapy (PRT) With Subsequent Surgery Versus Surgery Alone

Author/Year	Dosage, gray	No. patients	Pelvic failure, %		Distant failure, %		5-yr survival, %	
			PRT	Surgery	PRT	Surgery	PRT	Surgery
Kligerman et al[523] 1972	46	22	8	0	25	20		
Higgins et al[524] VASAG-I 1975	20–25	453	29	36	46	62	48	39
Kligerman[525] 1977	46	31	. . .	. . .	. . .	. . .	41	25
Leaming[526] 1980	20	538	11	17	22	15		
Stearns[527] 1980	20	790	. . .	. . .	. . .	. . .	57	58
Duncan[390] MRC 1984	5	552	40	42	47	50	. . .	. . .
Gerard et al[528] EORTC 1985	34	314	11	25	21	22	60	58
Gerard et al[379] EORTC 1988a	34	466	15	30	. . .	. . .	69	59
Reis Neto et al[529] 1989b	40	68	15	47	20	32	73	30
Dahl et al[522] 1991c	31	309	14	21	. . .	. . .	57	57

a 341 of 466 treated patients were resected for cure. Analysis included all patients who were randomized. Little or no survival benefit was found ($P = .08$), but there was significant improvement in the pelvic failure rate. One subgroup did show a survival benefit; those patients less than 55 years old had a 5-year survival of 80% after radiation and surgery versus 48% after surgery alone.
b Impressive tumor involution was seen with some shrinkage in all radiation patients. There seemed to be a downgrading of tumor grade and stage.
c 4.5% had no evidence of disease after preoperative radiation.

number of involved lymph nodes after preoperative radiation therapy. Nevertheless, little difference in overall survival has been found. Low-dose preoperative radiation (5–20 gray) appears to slightly reduce the number of involved lymph nodes but has little effect on local recurrence and no effect on survival. High-dose preoperative treatment (34.5–60 gray) including treatment of the superior hemorrhoidal lymphatic system improves local recurrence rates. This does not, however, seem to be accompanied by an improvement in survival in most studies (Table 18-15).[523] Again, the improvement is relative to local recurrence rates with surgery alone in excess of 30 to 40 percent.

There are few data comparing preoperative and postoperative radiation in a prospective randomized fashion. Pahlman and Glimelius[410] in a report from a randomized multicenter trial, compared patients resected for cure who were treated preoperatively with 25 gray over 5 to 7 days with operation within 1 week versus those who were treated postoperatively with 60 gray over 8 weeks. All 235 patients randomized to preoperative therapy were treated whereas only 115 of the 235 patients randomized to postoperative therapy were treated (49 percent). This was primarily because of pathologic staging, reserving radiation treatment for those patients with B2 and C lesions. The preoperative radiation was well tolerated, whereas only 9 patients underwent postoperative treatment without complications and 9 could not complete the therapy. Local recurrence was significantly lower in the preoperative radiation group (12 versus 21 percent); however, survival was not affected and the perineal wound infection rate was much higher (33 versus 18 percent).

It appears that short course preoperative radiation therapy followed immediately by surgery may be better tolerated than longer courses with delayed surgery and that preoperative radiation may be more effective at controlling local recurrence, even at lower dosages, probably because of better blood supply and undisturbed tissue planes that are not available for implantation. It is difficult to base conclusions regarding recurrence rates on studies such as Pahlman's,[410] since the entire group of preoperatively treated patients were compared with the Dukes B2 and C postoperatively treated patients. Inclusion of a number of A and B1 tumors in the preoperatively treated group could give a false impression of improved local control. Therefore, although it has been conclusively shown that pelvic radiation improves local control, the optimal timing for treatment is far from clear.

At this point it is believed that lesions limited to the submucosa or into but not through the muscularis with no lymphatic involvement are usually cured by surgery alone. Local recurrence rates may be much higher, however, with tumors that penetrate through the muscularis propria or have lymphatic spread. In these latter groups recurrence rates range from 30 to 50 percent. Radiation therapy may reduce this rate to 10 to 30 percent. Thus most patients are candidates for radiation therapy to reduce their risk of local recurrence. However, each surgeon needs to be cognizant of his or her own stage-stratified local recurrence rate to assess whether or not a significant advantage can be conferred by radiation.

Reduction of Unresectable Lesions

Preoperative radiation has been used to reduce locally unresectable lesions. Successes have been documented, allowing operations for cure. However, it is difficult to evaluate these reports clearly since the determination of resectability is a clinical one and likely varies considerably among surgeons, depending on their abilities and proclivities. The available literature suggests that full-dose preoperative radiation therapy may convert from 48 to 75 percent of patients to a "resectable" status. Still,

despite potentially curative resection with clear margins, local recurrence rates range from 16 to 55 percent, and 5-year survival is only 16 to 18 percent in most series.[530-532] Nevertheless, this remains a worthwhile approach since there are virtually no long-term survivors with incomplete resection or no treatment.

Sandwich Technique

Sandwich therapy is a combination of low-dose preoperative and full-dose postoperative radiation. This method has been proposed to offer the benefits of preoperative treatment while minimizing complications. In particular, it was hoped that the viability of the tumor cells would be reduced, avoiding local implantation or hematogenous spread at the time of surgery. In a small study of patients with B2 and C lesions surgery alone was compared with surgery plus preoperative, postoperative, or sandwich radiation.[533] Preoperative radiation seemed to reduce distant spread, while postoperative radiation improved local control. The sandwich technique appeared to improve both local and distant control, and this was associated with a significant improvement in survival (Table 18-16). Although few other studies of surgery and radiation without the addition of chemotherapy have documented a survival advantage, this approach bears further study, and a larger cohort is being developed.

Intraoperative radiation

Although intraoperative radiation was first described by Beck in 1909,[510] it was not extensively employed as a mode of adjuvant therapy until the 1980s. The clear advantage of this technique is that a relatively high dose of radiation may be administered directly to the tumor bed with precise boundaries, and adjacent tissues such as the small bowel and ureters may be excluded from the treatment field. Indeed, a given dose of radiation deliv-

Table 18-16 Treatment of Rectal Cancer With "Sandwich" Radiation Therapy

	No. patients	Local recurrence, %	Distant metastases, %	5-yr survival, %
Surgery only	88	26	57	34
Surgery + radiation				
50 gray preoperative	29	34	24	48
45 gray postoperative	26	11	50	29
Sandwich	31	7	13	78

From: Mohiuddin M, Derdel J, Marks G, Kramer S. Results of adjuvant radiation therapy in cancer of the rectum. Thomas Jefferson University Hospital experience. *Cancer.* 1985;55:350–353.[533]

ered intraoperatively is felt to be equivalent to two to three times the same dose given in standard fractions.[534] In addition, exclusion of dose-limiting structures allows larger doses to be administered. It is generally not practical to use this delivery method more than once per patient, so it is often combined with other techniques such as external beam radiation and brachytherapy.

Because of the equipment involved the technique of intraoperative radiation therapy is often demanding. Ideally, a dedicated operating room that houses a permanent electron accelerator will be available. When this is not the case, a room adjacent to the one housing the accelerator in the radiation therapy suite may be converted into an operating room. The patient must be anesthetized, the incision opened, and the treatment field exposed. A sterilized Lucite® applicator is selected to encompass the field and to exclude as much normal tissue as possible. The applicators differ in length, shape, and bevel of the distal end. If not in a dedicated operating room, the applicator must then be removed, and the patient is transported to the treatment room. The linear accelerator is moved into position over the patient, and the applicator is attached it to the head of the accelerator. Correct positioning is confirmed using a fiberoptic viewing system. Custom-shaped strips of lead shielding may be placed inside the treatment field to protect normal structures that cannot be moved from the site. A single boost of 15 to 20 gray may be given. The limits of the treatment field are marked with surgical clips prior to closure.[510,535]

Preoperative patient selection may be very difficult. Patients are candidates for curative treatment if the tumor is localized without evidence of spread beyond the regional lymph nodes, if the field is in a location accessible to the radiation beam with healthy tissue that may be displaced during treatment, and if the patient is a reasonable surgical candidate with a lesion that may not be controlled by surgery alone. These criteria may include patients with primary or recurrent lesions that are resected with incomplete or narrow margins.

Intraoperative radiation therapy is generally very well tolerated and has been associated with few complications. A rare late complication is a pain syndrome that may occasionally be associated with some sensory or motor deficit. This is thought to be due to a neuropathy caused by fibrosis. Ureteric obstruction may occur, but this is usually due to progression of the primary disease. Complications may be more frequent in patients with recurrent or unresectable disease.

Currently published results are limited to a few small series. O'Connell and colleagues[534] reported 85 percent local control in 20 highly selected patients. Sischy[509] treated patients with 45 to 50 gray of external beam radiation preoperatively, and then reevaluated them

after 4 weeks with CT. Intraoperative therapy was scheduled if the tumor appeared localized. With 3- to 5-year follow-up, survival rates of 50 percent for primary disease and 40 percent for recurrent disease were seen.

Tepper and co-workers from the Massachusetts General Hospital[536] described 40 patients with primary tumors who were treated preoperatively with 50.4 gray and went to surgery 4 to 6 weeks later. Intraoperatively a 10- to 20-gray boost was administered to the area of residual disease. Complete resections were performed in 29 patients, and they had only an 8 percent local failure rate after 3 years. Eleven patients with residual disease (5 gross, 6 microscopic) only had a 33 percent local failure rate after 3 years. Overall, 30 percent survived for 3 years.

Gunderson and associates at the Mayo Clinic reported 51 patients (15 primary and 36 recurrent tumors) treated preoperatively with 45 to 55 gray and with an additional 10 to 20 gray intraoperatively, depending on the volume of residual disease.[535] Some of these patients also received intravenous 5-fluorouracil (5-FU). At the time of report, 30 were alive and 22 (43 percent) were free of disease. Ten of 15 (67 percent) with primary disease were alive, 8 (53 percent) of whom had no evidence of disease after 10 to 64 months. Twenty of 36 patients (56 percent) with recurrent disease were alive, 14 (39 percent) of whom had no evidence of disease after 8 to 50 months. The 4-year actuarial survival rate was 53 percent with primary lesions and 23 percent for recurrences. After 1 year of follow-up local recurrence had developed in only 1 patient (2 percent) within the intraoperative treatment field and in 8 (18 percent) in the external beam field. All failures occurred in patients treated for recurrent cancer or in whom gross tumor had been left at the time of surgery. Expected failure rates in these situations would be at least 30 to 50 percent with standard external beam radiation and surgery.

These preliminary results are encouraging, but firm conclusions await larger studies. Still, because of its demands only a few specialized centers will employ this technique, and it is unlikely that this mode of therapy will be widely used in the near future.

Combination Chemoradiation

Radiation therapy appears to improve local control when added to surgery for the cure of rectal cancer. However, it has not been associated with any improvement in overall survival. This is not particularly surprising since radiation treatment only addresses the tumor bed and some of the lymphatic pathways. Some workers have suggested that radiation therapy may help to control distant spread by reducing further spread of local disease. However, it is likely that most distant disease progression is due to cells that metastasized prior to surgical therapy. Systemic chemotherapy attempts to address these distant deposits. These compounds may also act as sensitizing agents, improving the local results of radiation.[537]

A number of large, well-run trials have been completed recently and others are continuing.[511,514,536,538-540] Results to date were summarized by the National Cancer Institute at a Consensus Development Conference and updated in a Clinical Announcement on Adjuvant Therapy of Rectal Cancer, published in March 1991.[541,542] The panel felt that both postoperative radiation and chemotherapy are indicated for patients with TNM stage II and III disease because together they will reduce the risks of distant recurrence and local failure. Neither method alone was thought to be as effective as the combination of the two.

Most trials have used 5-FU as the standard chemotherapeutic agent, while some have added other drugs such as methyl-CCNU (semustine), vincristine, mitomycin-C, or methotrexate. Methyl-CCNU is only available as an investigational drug from the National Cancer Institute. With chronic administration, this drug has been associated with a 12-fold increased risk for secondary leukemia or preleukemia as well as with chronic renal toxicity.[543] The results from some studies have even suggested that methyl-CCNU is associated with a *poorer* outcome. Trials using methotrexate as part of the chemotherapeutic regimen have been discontinued because of the excessive morbidity and mortality related to treatment with this drug.[544]

At a Consensus Development Conference sponsored by the National Cancer Institute some guidelines for the use of adjuvant therapy by community practitioners were established. It was recommended that, unless enrolled in a specific adjuvant therapy trial, patients with stage II and III rectal cancer (extending beyond the submucosa or involving lymph nodes) should be treated with a sequential regimen of 5-FU and radiation therapy after curative resection of their tumor. It was also stated that community physicians should be encouraged to enroll their patients in ongoing clinical trials, since only large numbers of patients in these trials will give meaningful answers and thus improve the treatment of rectal cancer.[541,542]

The currently recommended treatment for patients with TNM stage III (Dukes B2, B3, and C) lesions not entered into ongoing trials is as follows (equivalent to the control arm of current Intergroup study INT 0114). Beginning 1 to 2 months postoperatively, 5-FU (500 mg/M²/day over 5 days) is given intravenously during weeks 1 and 5. Radiation therapy is begun during week 9, administering 45 gray over 6 weeks with a 5.4-gray boost in three fractions to the tumor bed. During the first and last weeks of radiation, 5-FU (500 mg/M²/day) is given for 3 days. During weeks 4 and 8 after completion of radiation, 5-FU (450 mg/M²/day) is given over 5 days. Adjustments in dosage and course should be made depending on toxicity and risk of small bowel injury.

If radiation therapy is contemplated, radioopaque clips placed during surgery to mark the borders of the tumor bed are helpful. Also, a sling to keep the small bowel out of the treatment field should be strongly considered.

Unfortunately, the recommendations of the N.C.I. Consensus panel were based on the results of a limited number of trials. Despite this limitation, the data were placed in such a light by the N.C.I. and the media so as to bind the hands of both investigators and clinitians. Because of this, other trials, which may have provided as good or better alternatives, or may have repudiated these early results, were prohibited. Many workers felt that the manner in which these data were disseminated through the lay media and not through peer-reviewed scientific meetings and journals was contrary to accepted scientific practice. This doctrine has made funding impossible for any trial that includes a surgery-alone arm. This does not take into account intersurgeon variability relative to technique and subsequent recurrence rates. Surgery alone may be a reasonable alternative for the treatment of rectal cancer if the patient clearly understands the potential benefits of adjuvant therapy and the significant risks and side effects of such treatment.

Chemotherapy and Immunotherapy

Although the combination of 5-FU and levamisole has been of significant benefit in patients with colon cancer, little is known about its effect in patients with rectal cancer.[545] 5-FU combined with leucovorin or levamisole may be a superior regimen for metastatic colorectal cancer versus 5-FU alone. Future research may concentrate on the use of immune modulators such as levamisole and leucovorin in combination with chemotherapeutic agents and radiation. Trials using these combinations as adjuvant therapy after surgery for rectal cancer are in progress.

Complications of Radiation Therapy

Radiation therapy is not a harmless treatment method. It is usually fairly well tolerated, but most patients will have some degree of symptomatic acute injury (60 to 75 percent). Although these early symptoms are usually self-limited, there may also be delayed complications in 5 to 20 percent of patients.[546]

Ionizing radiation delivers energy to the atoms in cells, causing electron excitation and chemical bond breakage. DNA molecules are particularly susceptible.

This damage results in cell death. Tissues that turn over rapidly are the most susceptible to this type of injury, and so the mucosa of the small bowel and rectum is at the highest risk for injury.

Tissue damage is generally divided into three phases. The first is the acute phase with depletion of the rapidly dividing cells of the mucosal crypts. This is usually seen in the first few days and weeks during and after treatment. The second or subacute phase involves a progressive obliterative arteritis with a fibroblastic response centered in the submucosa; this phase may last 1 to 2 years. The third phase is a chronic ischemia and fibrosis of the full bowel wall thickness, lasting for many years.

The tissue changes caused by radiation therapy occur to a greater or lesser degree in all patients receiving this treatment. The ability of the different tissues in the treatment field to withstand the effects of radiation differ markedly (Table 18-17). After the rectum, the terminal ileum is the organ most likely to be injured, with the sigmoid colon, cecum, vagina, and bladder also frequently involved. Most symptomatic patients will have several significant sites of injury.

The severity and extent of injury depend on several factors: the sensitivity and turnover rate of the tissues in the treatment field, the volume and distribution of tissue (increasing volume correlates with decreasing tolerance), and the mode of radiation delivery (total dosage, number of gray per fraction, number of fractions, and duration of treatment). There is a thin line between therapeutic and toxic dosages. Modification of these factors and the use of multiple radiation portals and patient positions have markedly reduced the incidence of postradiation complications. There are also a number of patient factors that predispose to greater injury.

Table 18-17   Radiation Therapy: Organ Tolerance Levels (gray)

Organ	TD 5/5*	TD 50/5†
Liver	35	45
Stomach	45	50
Small bowel	45	65
Colon	45	65
Rectum	55	80
Esophagus	60	75

* The dosage at which 5% of patients will sustain significant tissue injury.
† The dosage at which 50% of patients will sustain significant tissue injury.
From: Mohiudden M, Derdel J, Marks G, Kramer S. Results of adjuvant radiation therapy in cancer of the rectum. Thomas Jefferson University Hospital experience. *Cancer.* 1985;55:350–353.[533]

These include diabetes mellitus, hypertension, infection, concomitant chemotherapy, previous surgery with tissue fixation, and overlooking early symptoms of radiation enteritis, often masked by or treated with medications.

Symptoms

Early symptoms are usually self-limited and include nausea, abdominal cramps, tenesmus, and diarrhea. Rectal ulcerations and bleeding may also occur. Late complications include strictures; small bowel malabsorption; severe chronic diarrhea; fluid and electrolyte imbalances; malnutrition; fistulas to the small bowel, vagina, bladder, skin, or elsewhere; and chronic bleeding.

When evaluating these symptoms it is tempting to assume that the problem is limited. Unfortunately, the real extent of the process is generally much greater than that initially perceived. Bowel necrosis may be present with minimal signs or symptoms because of encasement of the viscera by fibrin which contains the process and limits the peritoneal response. This encasement also may decrease absorption of toxic products, reducing the incidence of early systemic signs. Therefore, a high index of suspicion should be maintained during the evaluation of these problems.

Radiation Proctitis

Radiation proctitis deserves special comment because it is common and often very difficult to treat. Though the ileal mucosa is more sensitive to radiation, the rectum is particularly likely to sustain injury because it is fixed in the pelvis. Radiation proctitis generally presents with tenesmus, crampy lower abdominal pains, mucous discharge, and bleeding. Patients may also complain of diarrhea and incontinence. Late sequelae include strictures and fistulas to the vagina or bladder. Proctoscopic examination reveals a loss of the normal vascular pattern, edema, friability, telangiectasias, mucosal ulcerations, and granularity. Evaluation should include a search for other sites of radiation injury. Manometric testing may reveal decreased rectal sensation, volume, and compliance, all indicative of wall fibrosis and rigidity.

Treatment of Radiation Injuries

Treatment is usually conservative. It involves dietary measures; oral administration of motility-slowing medications, bulking agents, and antispasmodics; steroid enemas; and belladonna and opium (B&O) suppositories. Many of the symptoms are mild and self-limiting. Bleeding may respond to these measures, but persistent or rapid bleeding may require operative intervention. Acute rectal bleeding occasionally is temporized by in-and-out rectal lavage with a cold, dilute epinephrine solution. Laser coagulation of telangiectasias has been quite successful in controlling this problem although repeated treatments are often necessary. Temporary or prolonged home total parenteral nutrition has a role in selected patients who are in poor condition and have debilitating symptoms such as a high-output fistula, malabsorption, or recalcitrant diarrhea.

Surgery is indicated for bowel necrosis, sepsis, or perforation. Chronic obstruction and uncontrolled hemorrhage are also reasons for urgent surgical intervention. Intractable symptoms, symptomatic fistulas, chronic bleeding, or an unwanted stoma may be relative indications. Throughout, the goals of preserving life and restoring function should be kept in mind. Procedures to consider in light of the patient's symptoms include proximal diversion with an ileostomy or colostomy, fistula closure, low anterior resection, coloanal anastomosis, abdominoperineal resection, or pelvic exenteration. Fortunately, these procedures are only rarely necessary. In the series from the Mayo clinic,[547] only 62 of 720 patients (8 percent) with radiation injuries of the rectum required surgical treatment. Morbidity was much higher after resection than after diversion, as it was in the Cleveland Clinic report.[548] The most common complications of surgery were anastomotic leakage, postoperative fistulas, and infections.

The colorectal surgeons at the Thomas Jefferson University in Philadelphia have adopted an aggressive surgical approach to the treatment of radiation injuries with fairly good results. In a review of their experience, indications for surgical treatment included perforation, bowel necrosis, obstruction, and fistulas; only one patient was operated on for severe hemorrhage.[546] Their management recommendations include avoiding operation when reasonably possible, optimizing preoperative nutrition, performing resections rather than bypass or simple fistula closure, and limiting adhesion lysis but doing as complete an exploration as possible, using meticulous surgical technique, and using nonradiated bowel for anastomoses. When performing surgery they recommend using ureteral catheters; recognizing early necrosis by the yellow-green coagulative color, edema, and liquid fibrin deposits; performing an adequate resection with a two-layered anastomosis; having a low threshold for creating a stoma; and assuming that the terminal ileum, cecum, and rectosigmoid are injured and that the hepatic flexure and descending colon are free of injury. Using these principles they have encountered much lower complication rates with surgery for radiation complications, mostly because of the emphasis on anastomosing the low rectum with its good blood supply to unirradiated upper descending or left transverse colon. In the majority of settings, however, diversion alone without resection is the most prudent course of therapy.[549]

Exclusion of the Small Bowel From the Pelvis

Radiation injury to the small bowel (radiation enteritis) typically occurs in at least 5 percent of patients being treated, but this rate may increase to 30 percent in some series and situations. Attempts have been made to reduce the incidence of small bowel radiation injury by excluding the small bowel from the pelvis. A variety of methods have been advanced including the use of omentum, muscle flaps, peritoneum, and silicone breast prostheses.[550-552] Absorbable mesh placed as a sling has been most successful, and is now the technique preferred by most clinicians.

The small bowel and, if necessary, the cecum and right colon are mobilized well above the sacral promontory and often to the level of the duodenum. Two large closed suction drains are placed in the pelvis. Beginning at the mid sacral promontory, a large sheet of polyglactin mesh (Vicryl, Ethicon, Somerville, NJ) is sutured in place using a running locked 2-0 polyglactin suture. Progressing in stages to the left and the right, the mesh is trimmed as necessary to keep it fairly flat and to minimize sagging into the pelvis. Careful attention must be given to avoid injury to the ureters and blood vessels. As progress is made laterally, it is best to angle up to the anterior abdominal wall to or just below the level of the umbilicus. Moving inferiorly to the pubis does not elevate the bowel sufficiently out of the radiation field. Too much elevation may, however, restrict the intraabdominal space enough to compromise respiratory excursions. When possible the omentum is brought down and sutured between the sling and the small bowel.[553,554]

Devereux and his colleagues accrued an early, large experience with this technique with laudatory results. They used polyglycolic acid mesh in 60 patients (42 rectal and 18 gynecological malignancies). Radiation therapy was begun within 3 weeks after surgery, and a mean of 55 gray of external beam radiation was administered. During the 28 months of follow-up there were no cases of radiation enteritis or mesh complications.[555,556]

Other studies have documented complications. Sener and associates noted one each of the following: pelvic abscess (drained percutaneously), wound dehiscence, and herniation of the small bowel between the pelvic sidewall and the mesh requiring small bowel resection. Two patients experienced late small bowel obstruction.[554] With the increasing use and proven efficacy of pelvic radiation, this technique is becoming more important and, in some centers, almost routine.

Postradiation Malignancies

Long after treatment of pelvic cancers by radiation, new anorectal malignancies may develop. This is thought to be a consequence of the radiation, but the actual incidence is unknown. The interval from treatment to the new tumor appears to be fairly long. In one study of 76 cases of colon or anorectal cancer developing after radiation treatment the mean interval was 15 years.[557] Of these lesions, 76 percent arose in patients treated for gynecologic malignancies, and one third were mucinous. Only 17 percent of patients had symptoms of radiation proctitis. The mean radiation doses given were not high. Five-year survival was 48 percent after treatment. Therefore, patients who have had radiation must be followed regularly not only to detect recurrence of the primary tumor but for surveillance for new cancers.

Photodynamic Therapy

Photodynamic therapy attempts to destroy tumor cells selectively, without disrupting normal tissue.[558] Although the concept of selective tissue concentration of certain compounds has been around since the turn of the century, it was not until the development of lasers and fiberoptic delivery systems that photodynamic therapy became clinically feasible.

The technique is based upon a photosensitizing agent that is concentrated in neoplastic tissue. When this agent is exposed to a certain wavelength of light, the compound is excited and interacts with molecular oxygen to create reactive singlet oxygen (O_2), the mediator of cytoxicity. This activated compound may also fluoresce when returning to ground state, permitting fluorescent detection of tumor cells. Hematoporphyrin derivative is the compound generally in use, although other, more purified substances are being developed. Hematoporphyrin derivative is concentrated in neoplastic tissue to a much greater degree than in most normal tissues, yet its concentration in liver, spleen, and kidney is consistently higher than that in tumor.

Hematoporphyrin derivative is prepared and kept in complete darkness until administered. It is administered by intravenous injection 48 to 72 hours before laser treatment.[559] The major risk is cutaneous photosensitivity which lasts for 4 to 6 weeks. During this period patients must avoid direct sunlight, although normal indoor activities may be pursued. Since hematoporphyrins are metabolized in the liver, they should be administered cautiously in patients with impaired liver function.

The extent of tissue destruction is related to the concentration of the sensitizing agent and the amount of energy delivered by the light source. Although hematoporphyrin derivative absorbs light maximally in the ultraviolet band (400 nm), red light (630 nm) is generally used because better tissue penetration may be achieved.[560] Under conditions that spare normal colonic tissue, tissue penetration is limited to about 5 mm.[561] Since most tumors are of some depth, repeated treatment or the use of interstitial optical fibers may be necessary. Combined treatment with chemotherapy or cytoreductive surgery may be helpful.

The first report of the clinical use of photodynamic therapy was from the Roswell Park Cancer Institute, where Dougherty treated dermatologic tumors.[562] Since then several thousand patients have been treated worldwide for a variety of tumors, mostly for palliation in uncontrolled trials.[164] Cutaneous tumors were an obvious place to start, and they continue to account for a large proportion of those treated. These include basal and squamous cell carcinoma, malignant melanoma, mycosis fungoides, Kaposi's sarcoma, and recurrent breast cancer on the chest wall. Other lesions treated include squamous cell carcinomas of the head and neck, gliomas of the central nervous system, melanomas and retinoblastomas of the eye, and transitional cell carcinoma of the bladder. Also, a number of esophageal, gastric, pulmonary, and vaginal tumors have been treated.[563-565]

Barr and associates treated 10 patients with colorectal carcinomas who were not thought to be surgical candidates. A flexible fiber was used via a colonoscope to treat up to four points of tumor per session. Two patients with small tumors had no evidence of disease at 20 and 28 months. There was one significant hemorrhage.[566] Patrice and co-workers in France described their initial experience with 54 patients with inoperable gastrointestinal carcinomas treated with endoscopic photodynamic therapy; 16 of these patients had rectosigmoid tumors. Follow-up was 13 months. Major complications occurred in 22 percent and included pain, skin photosensitization, perforation requiring surgery, and rectal stenosis complicated by death after dilatation. Treatment was judged to be successful in 50 percent of this diverse group, a partial response was seen in 32 percent, and no response was observed in 18 percent.[567]

Although this preliminary work is encouraging, much is left to do before photodynamic therapy becomes a common part of our armamentarium. Little work has been done in animal models, and questions remain about the optimum dosage of the sensitizing agents, the time between administration and treatment, the light intensity, and the exposure duration. There are also significant early and delayed complications including bleeding and perforation.[164] Because of the limited light penetration of tissues, superficial disease or treatment after debulking may be the most promising approaches.

Immunotherapy

The major problem with the nonsurgical treatment of cancer is targeting the neoplastic cells for destruction and sparing the normal tissue. This is particularly difficult since cancer cells develop from within the individual and are not easily recognized as "different." Radiolabeled antibodies for the localization of cancer were first created in 1948.[568] Their usefulness was limited because of their polyclonal source and their limited specificity. Since Kohler and Milstein first described the methods for producing monoclonal antibodies, a great deal of excitement has been generated.[569] Monoclonal antibodies may selectively identify antigens on tumor cells and thus have the potential for great specificity. Unfortunately, not all carcinomas elaborate the same antigens, and so the sensitivities of monoclonal antibody preparations are quite variable.

Monoclonal antibodies may be used for either diagnosis or treatment. When used for diagnosis, antibodies are "tagged" with an agent that may be imaged. Most tags used today are radioactive agents such as technetium, iodine compounds, or indium. These may then be viewed scintigraphically. Therapeutic approaches attempt to use these antibodies to guide chemotherapeutic compounds to the tumor, thereby increasing their concentration at the sites of disease with a relative reduction in the effects on normal tissues. This is especially attractive when attempting to eradicate occult foci of disease. Little practical work has yet been completed in the therapeutic arena, and so the following discussion focuses on imaging applications.

External imaging may be performed after the administration of monoclonal antibodies using standard scintigraphic equipment acquiring whole body images.[570] Beatty and colleagues studied 100 patients with known or suspected colorectal carcinomas who were given a murine monoclonal anti-CEA labeled with indium 111.[571] They found a sensitivity of 76 percent for primary tumors, 44 percent for hepatic metastases, and 78 percent for extraabdominal metastases. Of 46 patients thought to have spread limited to the liver by conventional preoperative imaging 17 (37 percent) had extrahepatic disease at exploration. Of these 17 cases, 9 were predicted by the preoperative scanning. The problem with this method is that the antibody used is extensively taken up by the liver so that lesions of the right and transverse colon may be obscured. Liver metastases may actually be seen as areas of relatively low uptake. Extraabdominal disease was much more reliably identified than intraabdominal disease. The false-positive rate was relatively high and the predictive value low. In this series, the findings did not alter management in any of the primary disease patients. If extrahepatic disease had been *reliably* found in patients explored for possible hepatic resection, operation could have been avoided. However, only 6 of 14 (43 percent) patients without preoperative evidence of extrahepatic intraabdominal disease were identified by a positive scan.

Radioimmunoguided Surgery (RIGS). The technique known as radioimmunoguided surgery (RIGS) is a particular application of monoclonal antibody imaging popularized by Martin at the Ohio State University. A radiolabeled monoclonal antibody is administered preoperatively.[572-574] During the surgical procedure a hand-held gamma detector (Neoprobe Corporation, Columbus, OH) is used to identify areas of increased activity which are presumed to be tumor deposits. A biopsy specimen may be taken from these areas for pathologic examination. If the findings are positive or suspicious, the resection may be extended to include these tissues. Any intraabdominal organ may be examined including the liver. The technique may be used as part of an initial exploration to assess completeness of resection or when attempting to identify recurrences such as during second-look surgery for an elevated CEA.

Early results have been encouraging with frequent identification of tumor sites that might have otherwise been missed. However, the specificities and sensitivities of the antibodies used continue to be a problem with significant false-negative and false-positive rates. Very early spread will not be detected since the lower limit of tumor size that may be detected is around 0.1 g. Also, the antibodies may be localized in areas of inflammation such as a duodenal ulcer or the uterus. Still, some small lesions may be found that are not detectable by any other methods.[575] Some disadvantages of the system include the possibility of anaphylactic reactions to the murine antibodies used and the time it takes for background levels to drop sufficiently after administration. This often takes 2 to 4 weeks, delaying surgery for this period. Multi-institutional cooperative studies are presently being conducted to evaluate the role of this interesting new application of monoclonal antibody technology. To make these techniques truly useful, the monoclonal antibodies must be made more specific and sensitive. Hybridoma technology may go a long way to meet these goals. It is unlikely that a single antibody will be effective in all patients. Rather, a unique antibody could be developed for each individual patient, based on the antigens expressed on that person's tumor. Such technology would make this method far more effective.

Treatment of Metastatic Disease

The hallmarks of malignancy are local invasion and distant spread (metastasis). Spread beyond the pelvis may occur through the lymphatic system or through the blood vessels. Lymphatic spread is usually the initial mode of extension and is indicated by examination of the regional lymph nodes after resectional surgery. Hematogenous spread is identified only when deposits of tumor are discovered in a noncontiguous location.

Metastases may be synchronous (found when treating the primary lesion) or metachronous (found after curative treatment of the primary). About one fourth of patients have unresectable local disease or distant spread at the time of their first diagnosis. The liver is the most common location of distant metastatic disease, followed by the lungs, bones, and other sites.[68,387,391,576-582]

Liver Metastases

Natural History

The liver is involved in 40 to 80 percent of patients dying of their disease.[583,584] Presumably, this is because of hematogenous spread of viable tumors cells through the portal circulation before or during surgery. Moreover, hepatic disease is the primary determinant of survival in cancer patients. At their primary operation 15 to 20 percent of patients have palpable liver metastases and at least 1 in 6 patients believed to have no hepatic disease by palpation will have occult lesions.[585-587] In patients whose disease progresses, the initial recurrence is isolated to the liver in 20 to 30 percent. Of these recurrences, 70 to 80 percent will manifest within 2 years.[384]

Symptoms due to hepatic metastases tend to be generalized; they include fever, fatigue, anorexia, loss of weight, and abdominal fullness. Specific symptoms including jaundice, ascites, and increasing abdominal girth are associated with advanced disease, and these lesions are usually not amenable to surgical intervention.

Longevity statistics for patients with liver metastases from colorectal carcinomas are based on historical controls. This is because, at present, it is unethical to randomize patients with apparently resectable disease to a no-treatment arm. Many retrospective reviews of unselected patients reveal mean survival rates of 6 to 9

months.[588-591] However, most of these patients were not candidates for curative resection. Since patients who present with symptoms are not likely to have resectable lesions, it is more reasonable to try to compare the results in treated patients with those in patients who did not receive treatment and who had limited asymptomatic disease: in other words, those who might have been candidates for surgical resection. Indeed, in this group, prolonged survival is found fairly often in untreated individuals.

Wagner and Adson reviewed 252 patients and found that the median survival times for those with unresected single or multiple lesions were 24 and 18 months, respectively. Patients with a solitary lesion that was not resected had a 20 percent 3-year survival rate.[592,593] However, there were no 5-year survivors. Scheele and coworkers reviewed 921 patients with unresectable disease and compared them with 62 patients with disease thought to be resectable but not treated.[594] Their median survivals were 6.9 and 14.2 months, respectively. Again, there were no 5-year survivors, and those patients who received incomplete resections survived only 13 months.

Finlay and McArdle have tried to estimate the growth rates of hepatic metastases by evaluation of serial CT scans.[586] Twenty-nine metastatic lesions were followed in 15 patients. Eleven of the lesions were "overt" and found at laparotomy; 18 were "occult" and seen only on postoperative CT scans. With overt and occult lesions, the mean doubling times were 155 ± 34 days and 86 ± 12 days ($P > 0.05$), the estimated ages of the metastases were 3.7 ± 0.9 and 2.3 ± 0.4 years, and the mean survivals of the patients were 10 ± 1.4 and 17 ± 1.8 months. All of these patients died within 3 years. It appeared that as the tumors increased in size, the growth rate diminished, presumably because of limiting factors such as nutrients, blood supply, and anatomy. Several reasons for the observed variability in growth rates were proposed: the metastases may not have arisen from a single cell but from clumps of cells of varying sizes, the lesions were probably part of a continuing metastatic process leading to metastases of different ages and growth rates, and very large tumor deposits would appear virtually to stop growing. Interestingly, the independently calculated overall lifespans for overt and occult lesions were quite similar at 52 and 47 months, respectively.

Detection

Accurate hepatic imaging is of critical importance and helps to make the diagnosis of hepatic metastases, to assess the extent of disease, to aid in the selection of patients for appropriate therapy, and to follow up the results of therapy. Preoperative CT scanning, ultrasonography, and arteriography have all been used but intraoperative ultrasonography, even more than palpation, has been clearly shown to be the most accurate method of identifying metastases.[595-597] Intraoperative ultrasound often detects lesions smaller than 1 to 2 cm that are deep in the hepatic parenchyma. Arterial portography with rapid sequence CT scanning may provide more information than any of the other preoperative methods studied, but its role and accuracy relative to these other studies are yet to be defined.[598]

Chemotherapy

Treatment of hepatic metastases with chemotherapy has been evolving for many years, and yet, though significant responses may be seen, survival has not been improved. Peripherally administered regimens, usually including 5- fluorouracil or FUDR alone or in combination with other agents, have achieved response rates of 15 to 45 percent.[599-602] Unfortunately, no improvements in survival have been seen, although toxicity and complications rise dramatically with combination regimens.

Hepatic artery ligation has been performed to reduce the blood flow to the tumor deposits. This seemed reasonable because these tumors, as opposed to normal liver parenchyma, derive a larger proportion of their blood supply from the arterial vessels than from the portal system. Although some palliation of symptoms may be seen, hepatic artery ligation has failed to prolong survival.[601,603]

Direct perfusion of the hepatic arterial supply may be performed after placement of a catheter in the hepatic artery with proximal ligation. Usually the catheter is introduced through the gastroduodenal artery. Hepatic arterial concentrations of the administered agents may be 5 to 10 times as much as when given peripherally, and hepatic extraction reduces systemic side effects including bone marrow toxicity. However, less systemic exposure means less systemic treatment, and so nonhepatic metastases are not affected. Hepatotoxicity is the limiting factor. Treatment may cause a chemical hepatitis, sclerosing cholangitis, cholecystitis, or gastritis in 50 to 75 percent of patients. In 70 to 90 percent of patients the CEA decreases, tumor diameter may decrease in 30 to 50 percent of patients, and approximately half experience alleviation of their symptoms. Nevertheless, the mean survival is only 16 to 18 months with patients dying of disseminated disease. For these reasons the technique has little merit.[603-607]

Regional delivery of cytotoxic agents to the tumor may be improved by using biodegradable starch or albumin microspheres. When given through a hepatic artery catheter, these microspheres cause a temporary blood flow statis that enhances regional uptake of simultaneously administered chemotherapeutic agents. This administration may also be combined with angiotensin II, which redistributes arterial blood flow toward the tumor. Although several trials of these techniques have demonstrated improved delivery of the agents and local tumor responses, no real survival benefit has been seen.[607-609]

Radiation

Irradiation of the liver has not been a useful therapy since the liver has little tolerance for the doses necessary to affect the disease.[610] Maximal tolerated doses are in the range of 25 to 35 gray, above which marked hepatotoxicity occurs. Webber attempted to combine low-dose radiation (25 gray) with FUDR infusion through the hepatic artery. Sixteen nonrandomized patients with less advanced disease were treated. A modest increase in survival was seen when compared with untreated patients (12 vs 6 mo), but whether this was attributable to the extent of their disease or to the treatment was not clear.[611]

Hyperthermia

Sporadic reports have been published of the use of hyperthermia to improve the effects of chemotherapy.[612] Hyperthermia may be induced by means of an electromagnetic coil to heat the region of the liver while giving infusional 5-fluorouracil or other agents. Storm and his colleagues at UCLA attempted to treat 36 patients with a variety of unresectable tumors.[613] Their initial problem was the inability to heat the liver adequately in many subjects. Success with their method was elusive, although some responses were seen.

Resection

Surgical resection of a portion of the liver is the preferred method of treatment of hepatic metastases. With selected patients and experienced surgeons, risks are fairly low and the results are good. Until recently, most surgeons assumed that if colorectal carcinoma had spread to the liver it was beyond surgical control and was a systemic disease. Because of the extremely poor results obtained with chemotherapy and other alternative approaches, an aggressive approach to surgical resection of the liver was taken by Adson at the Mayo Clinic, Fortner at the Memorial Sloan-Kettering Hospital in New York, Attiyeh at the Roosevelt Hospital in New York, and others. Over many years they have conclusively demonstrated that carefully selected patients have significant 5-year survival and cure rates, whereas untreated patients or those treated by any other means have virtually no chance of long-term survival.

Selection of patients to be considered for exploration and possible resection is critical. The recurrence or residual disease should be limited to the liver after complete extirpation of the primary lesion in a patient medically able to tolerate the surgery. Relative contraindications include more than four metastatic lesions, involvement of both major lobes, or involvement of the perihepatic lymph nodes or contiguous structures.[369,374,376,592,593,614-625]

It has been estimated that 20 to 30 percent of patients with hepatic metastases are candidates for resection.[369,614,623,624,626] In the United States 3000 to 5000 patients per year are projected to fulfill this criteria. Unfortunately, many fewer than that are evaluated for hepatic resection. In a survey of surgeons in England and Wales it appeared that fewer than one third of potentially operable patients actually underwent liver surgery.[608]

Preoperative evaluation includes examination and imaging studies to exclude other sites of disease, as well as to identify the extent and distribution of the hepatic deposits. These tests may include a chest x-ray; a CT scan of the pelvis, abdomen, and chest; ultrasonography and even, in some cases, hepatic angiography. Even with all of this information the resectability rate at the time of exploration may be less than 50 percent. Lefor, Hughes and colleagues reviewed 132 patients with apparently isolated liver metastases. During the preoperative evaluation, 25 were found to have intraabdominal spread. Surgical exploration was carried out in the remaining 107 patients, and at that time intraabdominal spread was identified in 28 (26 percent). In these authors' analysis, no factor was predictive, but intraabdominal spread tended to be associated with replacement of more than 25 percent of the liver parenchyma, symptoms, and a Dukes C (involved lymph nodes) primary lesion.[627]

The surgery performed does not appear to influence the outcome so long as all identified deposits are removed with at least a 1-cm margin.[369] Thus, wedge resections are as acceptable as formal lobectomies and each is appropriate with different distributions of disease and the associated hepatic anatomy.

Although the reported mortality has ranged from 1 to 12 percent, the trend is clearly towards a decrease and most centers with much experience are now recording mortality below 5 percent. Morbidity rates are 10 to 28 percent but also have been decreasing.[590]

Five-year survival averages 30 percent in most series (Table 18-18). Significant variation from this is proba-bly due to patient selection. Adson noted in his 1984 report that although the overall survival in his series at that time was 25 percent, some of these patients had extrahepatic disease and that when these were excluded the 5-year survival climbed to 46 percent.[593] The survival rates after hepatic resection begin to plateau at about 5 years, indicating that the course of the disease has been changed.[590] Adson feels that the risk of death in these patients is similar to that of the normal population.[626]

Most recurrences manifest within the first 12 months after hepatic resection.[590] Hughes and colleagues reported a 68 percent recurrence rate in 859 patients from their multi-institutional review. Only 10 percent of these recurrences were isolated to the liver; while 29 percent were extrahepatic only. Hughes thought that hepatic resection had altered the course of the disease in these patients.[634] Pulmonary recurrences were found in from 18 to 48 percent of patients, and the brain, abdominal cavity, pelvis, and bones were the site of most of the additional recurrent lesions.[634]

The factors that predict successful hepatic resection for cure vary somewhat from study to study, even though the long-term results in these studies are fairly similar. Factors that are strongly in favor of a good outcome include an absence of extrahepatic disease, fewer than four metastatic lesions, and tumor-free margins. Factors that are probably not significant are the latency or time from initial bowel resection to the detection of liver metastases, the size of the individual lesions, the patient's gender or age, the CEA level, and the site of the primary lesion (colon or rectum).[369,590,593,594,627,634] Factors that are of questionable value include the Dukes' stage of the primary tumor, the number of metastases fewer than 5, and whether the lesions are in one or both lobes.[369,595,630,634]

Occasionally, recurrence after hepatic resection is limited to the liver. This may be found when the CEA level rises or with a follow-up CT scan. Carefully selected patients may benefit from a second hepatic resection, especially if the relative proportion of liver removed initially was small.[625,635]

Surgery is the only curative alternative for patients with liver metastases from colorectal carcinoma. At this point, all other therapies are palliative at best, and none provides significant long-term survival. The survival rate after hepatic resection may rise as our ability to stage patients preoperatively and intraoperatively improves. The routine use of intraoperative hepatic ultrasonography may have a marked effect, helping to identify additional lesions that might have been missed and to preclude resection when the disease process is found to be too widespread for cure. Hepatic resection

Table 18-18   Hepatic Resection for Metastases From Colorectal Carcinomas: Operative Mortality and 5-year Survival

Author/Year	No. patients	Operative mortality, %	5-yr survival, %
Wilson, Adson[628] 1976	60	2	28
Foster[614] 1977	126	. . .	22
Morrow et al[629] 1982	38	10	27
Adson et al[593] 1984	141	2	25[a]
August et al[622] 1985	33	0	35
Cady and McDirmott[621] 1985	23	0	30
Butler et al[630b] 1986	62	10	34
Elkberg et al[623] 1986	72	. . .	16
Iwatsuki et al[631] 1986	60	0	45
Nordlinger et al[632] 1987	80	5	25
Attiyeh and Wichern[633] 1988	20	24	35
Hughes et al[634c] 1988	859	. . .	33
Fortner[624d] 1988	77	5	49
Fedorov and Shelygin[198] 1989	71	5	26
Scheele et al[594] 1990	183	5	31

a 46% in patients without extrahepatic disease.
b Recent operative mortality of 2%.
c Multi-institutional.
d Highly selected.

for colorectal carcinoma metastases is a good procedure in a selected group of patients.

Lung Metastases

In most series, the lungs are the second most common site of metastatic disease from a colorectal primary tumor. Portmortem studies reveal spread to the lungs in from 30 to 50 percent of patients dying of colorectal cancer.[636] Few reports differentiate between colonic and rectal primary sites. Approximately 10 percent of patients with colorectal cancer will have lung metastases detected during life, and 10 percent of these metastases will be isolated. Therefore, about 1 percent of all patients with colorectal cancer may have resectable disease.[580,636-638] The rate may be slightly higher for primary tumors of the rectum and left colon, perhaps because of the systemic vascular collaterals which bypass the liver.[639] A solitary pulmonary nodule in a patient with a history of colorectal cancer will represent a metastasis in about one half of cases and a primary lung neoplasm in the other half.[640]

CT scanning of the chest is the most accurate method of preoperative evaluation. Exploration is indicated if the primary lesion has been controlled, if the pulmonary disease is isolated, and if the patient is a reasonable operative risk.

The patient is explored through a median sternotomy. This approach is better tolerated than a thoracotomy and allows examination of both lungs.[580] Bilateral examination is quite important because there is a high incidence of unsuspected bilateral lesions.[369,641,642] Operative mortality is usually low (0–7 percent) and 5-year survival rates average 20 to 30 percent (Table 18-19). In comparison with hepatic lesions, pulmonary recurrences may occur as late as 7 years after lung resection.[580,648] Because of this prolonged recurrence period some of the good results reported may be a consequence of bias introduced by surgically reducing the volume of disease without really obtaining cure.[648]

The major prognostic factors are the presence of solitary metastatic lesions less than 3 cm in size and the tumor doubling time. Age, sex, type of surgery (wedge resection versus lobectomy or pneumonectomy), and the number of metastases resected do not appear to be significant factors.[648] Some authors think that a longer disease-free interval (the time from curative resection of the primary lesion until the diagnosis of recurrence) and the Dukes stage of the primary lesion are important factors.[646]

Thus, pulmonary resection for metastatic colorectal carcinoma may be applicable to as many as 1 percent of patients. These operations have a low mortality for selected patients, who will have a 20 to 30 percent overall survival after resection.

Metastases to Other Locations

Inguinal Lymph Nodes

Metastases to the inguinal lymph nodes are rare and are usually associated with disseminated disease. Graham and Hohn from the M.D. Anderson Hospital (Houston, TX) found 40 patients (1.2 percent) with inguinal lymph node involvement out of 3215 with colorectal cancers treated between 1949 and 1987.[649] Three groups were identified. The first group of 10 patients had unresectable primary lesions; 7 were treated with radiation therapy. Their median survival was 7 months. The second group, consisting of 22 patients, developed recurrent disease in both the inguinal nodes and other sites after a curative resection. Seven of these patients were treated with radiation, chemotherapy, or both. The median survival for this group of 22 patients was 9 months. The third group included 8 patients with apparently isolated inguinal node recurrence. Each underwent a superficial inguinal lymph node dissection and 2 had deep dissections as well. Their median survival was increased to 33 months. Only 2 of these patients were actually rendered disease free; one died of a myocardial infarction, and one was alive and well after 15 months of follow-up. Only one complication developed in these 40 patients, and this was treated with local wound care.

Patients with unresectable disease have limited survival, and their inguinal disease is not usually a major source of morbidity. These patients should be offered palliative treatment alone. Patients with multiple sites of recurrence are also generally treated palliatively. Patients with isolated disease may be offered inguinal lymph node dissection for cure. This may be combined with adjunctive therapy because of the high risk of subsequent local and systemic failure.

Ovarian Metastases

Metachronous metastases to the ovaries occur in 3 to 8 percent of women with colorectal cancer, most com-

Table 18-19 Survival After Resection of Pulmonary Metastases From Colorectal Carinoma

Author/Year	No. patients	5-yr survival, %
Cahan et al[640] 1974	31	30
Wilkins et al[643] 1978	34	27
McCormack and Attiyeh[580] 1979	35	22
Morrow et al[644] 1980	16	13
Mountain et al[645] 1984	28	28
Pihl et al[639] 1987	16	38
Brister et al[646] 1988	335	30
Scheele et al[647] 1989	45	44
Goya et al[648] 1989	62	42

monly after surgery for tumors located in the rectum and sigmoid.[650] The metastatic lesions are frequently bilateral and are confined to the ovaries in fewer than 7 percent of these women. Most women with ovarian involvement also have widespread disease and are not surgically treatable for cure. When limited disease is discovered, salpingo-oophorectomy is the only real treatment option and should be bilateral because of the high incidence of occult disease in the apparently uninvolved ovary. Mean survival after surgical treatment is 16 months, and cures are rarely achieved. Prognosis does not appear to be related to Dukes stage, menstrual status, or disease-free interval. Only the complete removal of all gross disease seems to influence the outcome.

Bone and Brain Metastases

Lesions in bone or the brain are evidence of widespread disease, and there is little curative treatment available. Of 765 patients with *disseminated* metastatic carcinoma of the colon and rectum treated at the Memorial Sloan-Kettering Cancer Center between 1960 and 1970, 53 (6.9 percent) had osseous lesions, 14 (1.8 percent) of whom had isolated deposits. The rates were higher in patients with rectal primaries (8.9 percent) than those with colonic primaries (5.1 percent). Several forms of palliative chemotherapy and radiation therapy are available for temporary symptomatic relief; radiation is particularly effective at pain relief. Survival after the diagnosis of osseous metastases averages 7 months. Headaches, visual changes, lethargy, and seizures are symptoms associated with brain metastases. Cerebral lesions are well imaged by CT and by MRI. Rarely, apparently isolated brain metastases may be resected.[651]

Follow-Up

The follow-up of patients treated for rectal carcinoma has two major goals.[652] The first is to detect recurrences early, if possible at a time when they are treatable. Unfortunately, the majority of recurrences found are at a stage when they are not treatable for cure.[653] The second goal is to identify new primary neoplasms early in their development, since these patients are at a significantly increased risk for metachronous polyps and carcinomas.

Close follow-up is important not only for the individual patient but also for the physician and other patients. It helps to document the morbidity and mortality as well as the local and distant recurrence rates for different methods of treatment. Accumulation of these data should help us assess and improve our approaches to these lesions.

Deaths due to colorectal carcinoma are related to the pattern of recurrence. Necropsy studies reveal that the vast majority of patient deaths are due to intraabdominal recurrence with liver failure and bowel and ureteral obstruction.[579,601] Generally, if a recurrence is symptomatic then it is likely to be advanced and not amenable to curative treatment.[371,654] Occasionally, small recurrences that may be treated are found on digital or sigmoidoscopic examination of the rectum.[655] Blind second-look operations have been abandoned because resectable disease is rarely found; usually either no disease or extensive, unresectable disease is present.[656-658] Close follow-up may improve detection of early lesions that are more amenable to curative treatment.[659-661]

Metachronous Neoplasms

A metachronous neoplasm is a primary carcinoma or adenoma that arises at a time subsequent to the diagnosis and surgical removal of an earlier carcinoma of the large bowel or rectum. All workers in this field agree that the incidence of new tumors in patients with a prior carcinoma far exceeds that found in the general population. However, to determine precisely what is a new lesion and what might have been missed at the time the index or primary lesion was treated is quite difficult. Some authors have arbitrarily stated that a lesion found after an interval of 6 months or 1, 2, or 3 years qualifies as a metachronous neoplasm. Studies in which clearance of the colon was initially obtained with a barium x-ray will probably have higher "metachronous" rates than ones in which all patients had a colonoscopy. This is simply because barium enema studies frequently miss small growths that are seen on colonoscopy. Also, the longer the follow-up period, the higher the rate will be.[662,663] Indeed, a third carcinoma will be discovered in some patients if they are followed long enough.[664]

Metachronous carcinomas have been reported to occur in from 1 to 4 percent of patients. This risk almost doubles if the cancer has been associated with other polyps. Metachronous polyps may be found in 35 to 75 percent of patients.[664] With close follow-up, these lesions should be discovered at an earlier stage than the typical cancer. Interestingly, the risk that these patients will die from a noncolorectal malignancy is just as high as their risk of getting a second intestinal cancer.

Malignancies that are common in colorectal cancer patients include breast, uterine, and kidney tumors.[665,666] Since women treated for a colorectal carcinoma have a higher than average risk of developing a gynecologic or breast malignancy, periodic Pap smears and regular breast examination should be a part of their follow-up. This is particularly important when there is a family history of malignancy. Survival rates after resection of a metachronous carcinoma are the same, stage for stage, as after treatment of an initial lesion.[664,667]

Detection of Recurrence

Close follow-up is aimed at detecting recurrent disease at a time when treatment for cure may be possible. Unfortunately, this will be true in only a small proportion of patients. Those with limited perineal or pelvic recurrence or those with resectable liver or lung metastases may be candidates. With early identification, significant salvage rates may be obtained in these groups of patients. In addition, metachronous tumors are sought.

Physical Examination

Palpation of the perineum together with transanal and transvaginal digital examination during the physical examination will detect many local recurrences. The inguinal regions and other sites should be examined for evidence of lymphatic spread.

Occult Blood Tests

Though useful for screening large groups with limited risks, tests for occult blood in the stool play no role in the follow-up of rectal cancer. In a series of 183 patients followed after a stapled anastomosis, occult blood tests were positive in only 18 percent of patients with recurrences, metachronous carcinomas, or polyps. All of these lesions were found by colonoscopy.[668]

Endoscopy

Rigid proctoscopy and anoscopy are the clearest and easiest methods for examining the remaining rectum and the anastomosis. Rigid examination of the rectum and anastomosis should be performed at each follow-up visit beginning at 3 months or earlier if indicated. No change in diet or preparation beyond a single enema is necessary and these examinations may be performed in the office.

Colonoscopy is the most accurate method of evaluating the remaining colon, but it is notoriously poor for examining the anal canal and low rectum. Examination of the colon is important not so much for the detection of local recurrences (which rarely cause early mucosal disruption[669]) but rather for the detection of metachronous neoplasms. Still, some recurrences will present with luminal manifestations and many of these may be detected at an earlier, possibly more resectable stage

by routine postoperative surveillance colonoscopy.[670,671] After perioperative clearance of the colon, periodic surveillance should be carried out for the remainder of the patient's life. Although there is general agreement that the first examination should be within 1 year after surgery, the optimal timing of subsequent examination is not clear.[45,375,672,673]

Liver Function Tests

Alterations in serum levels of alkaline phosphatase (AP), gamma-glutamyl transpeptidase (GGT), lactate dehydrogenase (LDH), leucine aminopeptidase (LAP), bilirubin and transaminases (SGOT, SGPT) are associated with progressive involvement of the liver by metastatic disease. However, a large volume of hepatic parenchyma must be replaced by tumor or the major bile ducts must become obstructed before these tests become significantly elevated.[371,671,674,675] Thus, changes in these tests are usually associated with advanced disease. In addition, it is unusual for these test results to rise before the CEA level rises (see below). Therefore, although they are frequently ordered, liver function tests are rarely an indicator of early recurrence.[652]

Barium Enema

Single-column barium enema studies are of little use. They provide little definition of the mucosa and will miss many new and recurrent lesions. Double-contrast barium studies are better at delineating mucosal detail but are still inferior to colonoscopy. They will overlook as many as 25 percent of early carcinomas and up to 56 percent of adenomas in asymptomatic patients.[668,676] They are used mainly in patients in whom complete colonoscopy cannot be performed for technical reasons or where colonoscopy is not available.[371]

Tumor Markers: CEA

Gold and Freedman were the first to identify an antigenic glycoprotein from malignant neoplasms.[677] This antigen seemed to arise from endodermally derived epithelium and was found in the embryonic and fetal gut, pancreas, and liver. Elevated serum and tissue levels of carcinoembryonic antigens (CEA) may be found in colorectal carcinomas, breast cancers, sarcomas, medullary thyroid cancers, biliary ductal tumors, carcinoma of the lung, gastric cancers, adenocarcinomas of the uterine cervix, and adenocarcinomas of the prostate. Although, determination of CEA levels is useful in the detection of tumor recurrence, the specificity and sensitivity of this test are not good enough to make it a useful screening tool.[678] Elevated levels may also be seen in benign diseases such as hepatobiliary disorders, pancreatitis, and inflammatory bowel diseases and also in cigarette smokers. In the case of colorectal carcinomas, elevated CEA levels are not detected preoperatively in all patients with known lesions, especially early ones. Although these levels tend to increase with more advanced disease, no direct inferences may be made from a single preoperative level.[679,680]

CEA levels are, at present, the single most effective noninvasive method of detecting tumor recurrence.[652,653,681] When these tests are performed regularly, relapses of colorectal cancer may often be detected months before any clinical signs appear.[680] Unfortunately, elevated levels will be found in fewer than 50 percent of patients with early or local recurrence, whereas about 75 percent of patients with disseminated disease will have this finding.[369,678] However, a rise in CEA level does not always mean recurrence. Transient elevations of CEA may occur in from 7 to 36 percent of patients in whom no recurrence is found. When CEA levels are used as part of a follow-up program, they must be performed serially, since the *trend* is of particular importance. Certain individuals may have a mildly elevated CEA level chronically because of smoking or other reasons. A rapid rise has been associated with the presence of liver metastases.[682,683] Asymptomatic recurrences found because of an elevated CEA value or trend are much more likely to be treatable for cure than those detected after symptoms begin.[684,685]

CEA-Directed Second-Look Surgery

A persistent elevation in CEA levels mandates a search for a site of recurrence. Often one will be found by means of physical examination, CT, MRI, chest x-rays, endoscopy, and bone scans. Whole body scintigraphic scans are now being evaluated for this purpose, as well. Occasionally, no recurrence is documented, yet the CEA continues to rise. Most of these patients will have intraabdominal or pelvic recurrence of their disease. Second-look laparotomy for an elevated CEA level will reveal recurrent disease in as many as 90 to 95 percent of these patients.[686] From 12 to 58 percent of patients with recurrent disease will have lesions that are resectable for cure.[686-689] Some authors suggest that more frequent determination of the CEA level, combined with aggressive evaluation of patients whose CEA levels are elevated, will increase this resectability rate and thereby improve survival rates.[369,690-692,658]

Martin and his colleagues at the Ohio State University have applied this approach particularly aggressively. Between 1971 and 1985, 146 asymptomatic patients underwent second-look operations because of a rising CEA level. Intraabdominal recurrences were found in 95 percent of these patients, and 58 percent

were resectable for cure. A CEA level of greater than 7.5 was thought to be indicative of recurrent tumor. Of the 45 patients operated upon between 1976 and 1979, 14 (31 percent) were living at the time of Martin's 1985 report.[686]

In 1989, Martin's group reported a series of 32 patients with metastatic colorectal carcinoma who underwent a second-look operation with the benefit of the RIGS (radioimmunoguided surgery) system. Preoperative evaluation with CT scanning detected only 41 percent of these recurrences, and this rate dropped to 27 percent when findings in the liver were excluded. The RIGS system was correct in detecting 81 percent of the intraabdominal recurrences, but only 41 percent of the liver lesions were identified. This low rate of detection was probably due to the very limited tissue penetration of the isotopes used. Six (18 percent) of these recurrences were detectable by RIGS only.[573,681]

Clearly, there is a role for second-look surgery in the management of recurrent carcinoma in the presence of an elevated CEA. The salvage rates, as noted, are quite variable, but this approach does yield some long-term survivors.[658,659,688,689]

Tumor Markers: Non-CEA

Other tumor markers have been found and examined, but none is as useful as CEA.[693-695] An elevated CA 19-9 level is found in only 30 percent of patients operated on for known residual or recurrent tumor. It tends to be highest in patients with liver disease and lowest with lung metastases or carcinomatosis. In one small study there was a suggestion that using both CEA and CA 19-9 may give some additional lead time, since an early phase of recurrence may be heralded by an elevation of one but not both.[696] When both had risen recurrence was always found, and it was often advanced. Fucini and his coworkers used CEA, CA 19-9, and TPC (tissue polypeptide antigen) prospectively to follow 52 patients who had been resected for cure[697]; 22 recurrences developed at a median of 47 months (12–72 mo). The sensitivities and specificities of CEA were 90 percent and 83 percent, of C 19-9 20 percent and 90 percent; and of TPA 60 percent and 50 percent. The predictive value of CEA determination was 69 percent.

Acute Phase Reactants

Acute phase reactant proteins (APRP), such as α_1-acid glycoprotein, α_1-antitrypsin, transferrin, haptoglobin, C-reactive protein, prealbumin, and retinol binding protein, are synthesized primarily in the liver in response to a variety of stimulants including malignancy. They may also be found in lymphatic and tumor cells. Although many of these substances may be elevated in the presence of malignancy, there is no evidence that their levels have prognostic significance or allow early detection.[674,698,699]

Chest X-ray

Chest x-rays are a routine part of the follow-up of patients who have had a rectal cancer. They are inexpensive, easy to obtain, and expose the patients to limited radiation. Unfortunately, they do not visualize a lesion until it is greater than 1 to 2 cm in size, and multiple, bilateral lesions may be present that are not seen but can be demonstrated on a CT scan.[371,669]

Computed Tomography

The accuracy of CT scanning in detecting locoregional recurrence varies markedly among studies, but it is clearly inadequate for detecting lymph node disease and small, early recurrences.[700,701] It may be of assistance in defining the extent of pelvic disease, but the scarring and fibrosis that typically occur after major resections are difficult to distinguish from true tumor.[702] A benign biopsy does not rule out recurrence.[703] A baseline examination obtained 6 to 8 weeks after surgery is useful to help differentiate scarring and altered anatomy from recurrence. Rapid injection of the contrast and thin (5-mm) slices may help to improve accuracy.

CT is still the most accurate method of imaging the liver, short of surgical exploration. Even so, lesions less than 1 to 2 cm in diameter will usually not be seen.[704,705] In a necropsy series, the mean diameter of liver metastases was found to be 1.4 cm, so many would have been missed on CT.[706] The major disadvantages of CT are its high cost, the radiation exposure to the patient, and the overuse of this technology in most medical centers. Many authors believe that an ultrasound examination is better initially. If it is unrevealing and there is a suspicion of recurrence, a CT scan may be performed subsequently. CT scanning of the chest is a very accurate method of defining metastases. Still, it is generally used after a suspicious chest x-ray or during evaluation of a patient with an elevated CEA level. Because of the high cost, limited access, and limited efficacy, routine CT scanning as part of a postoperative surveillance program is not practical.[652]

Ultrasonography

Ultrasonography is widely available at reasonable cost, is noninvasive, does not expose the patient to additional radiation, and is fairly sensitive. Liver metastases may be detected at a rate as high as 93 percent with greater sensitivity but less specificity than CT.[707] Thus, ultrasonography is a good choice as an initial examination

for the detection of recurrence, either on the basis of CEA elevation or abnormal liver function tests, or during routine screening in an aggressive follow-up program.[369]

A number of centers have used endorectal ultrasound extensively in the initial diagnosis and staging of rectal cancers (see Chapter 17). A few studies have attempted to evaluate its usefulness in the follow-up of patients who have had a low anterior resection with anastomosis. Women who have had an abdominoperineal resection may also be studied transvaginally. Romano and colleagues examined 42 patients and discovered a biopsy-confirmed local recurrence in 8.[708] There were 2 false-positive studies in this series. Beynon and associates followed 85 patients with physical examination, proctoscopy, and endorectal or endovaginal ultrasonography[709]; 22 local recurrences were found in 85 patients, 3 by endoluminal ultrasound alone. All were confirmed by biopsy, which was often ultrasound directed. As with CT scanning, it is best to perform a baseline examination within 3 months after surgery for later comparison. The pelvic anatomy changes markedly after surgical resection, with the uterus, tubes, and ovaries often taking up positions adjacent to the anastomosis. Suspected recurrences should be confirmed by biopsy.

Nuclear-Medicine Studies

Liver–spleen scanning has been all but abandoned for metastatic imaging because of its lack of specificity and sensitivity and because of the general availability of CT and ultrasonography. Magnetic resonance imaging (MRI) is in its infancy and so its ultimate role in the follow-up of rectal cancer is yet to be defined.[652] De-Lange and colleagues studied 11 patients with suspected recurrences.[710] Ten of twelve masses imaged were malignant and two were inflammatory on biopsy. No difference in signal intensity was discerned in their analysis. The major disadvantages of this technology are that it is expensive, and it is not yet generally available.[711]

Hepatic Arteriography

This study should not be used as a first-line diagnostic test because of its invasive nature, cost, and risk. It may be used selectively to define anatomy in patients who are candidates for elective hepatic resection.

Follow-Up Protocols

Although most workers believe that regular follow-up visits are important, no schedule or set of tests is accepted by all clinicians who treat patients with rectal carcinoma. Both the author and the editors use the following standard protocol for the continuing evaluation of patients treated curatively for rectal carcinoma. Adjuvant treatment programs have been discussed elsewhere in this chapter.

A CEA test is performed preoperatively and at the time of hospital discharge. Patients are seen 4 to 6 weeks after discharge for evaluation of bowel habits, diet, and the surgical wound. Patients with an ostomy are seen by the surgeon and the enterostomal therapist after 3 to 4 weeks when the stoma has lost its perioperative edema and refitting of the appliance is often necessary.

Beginning 3 months after surgery and continuing every 3 months until the 2-year anniversary of surgery is reached the patient is seen in the outpatient clinic for a brief history and physical examination. A proctoscopy or flexible sigmoidoscopy is performed and blood samples are drawn for a CBC and for CEA. After 2 to 3 years the interval between visits is lenghtened to 6 months. After 5 years visits become annual.

For the first 5 years, chest x-rays and endorectal or endovaginal and hepatic ultrasound are performed every 6 months if appropriate. If local recurrence is suspected or likely, for example, with close margins or a more advanced tumor, a CT scan of the pelvis is ordered 3 months after surgery and yearly thereafter. Colonoscopy is performed 1, 3, and 5 years after surgery and thereafter every 2 to 3 years so long as findings are negative. If polyps are found, the examination is repeated at least yearly until two consecutive studies are negative.

Local Recurrence

Local recurrences of rectal carcinoma occur in the pelvis. Theoretically these lesions arise from cells that either were not removed during the original excision or were shed during excision and implanted in the operative field. Solitary recurrences are more common after resection of rectal tumors than after resection of colonic tumors.[636,712,713]

Local recurrence rates increase as the level of the primary tumor in the rectum decreases.[235] They also increase with advancing Dukes stage (Table 18-20). Although recurrence is associated with a distal margin of less than 1 to 2 cm, increasing the margin beyond 2 cm has no effect.[90,366,725] The size of the primary tumor and the type of operation performed (abdominoperineal resection vs sphincter-saving procedure) also have no effect on recurrence rates.[69] In some studies, a higher local failure rate has been seen with less differentiated histology and with mucinous or colloid lesions, with ulcerating primaries, with venous or lymphatic invasion, and with less lymphatic stromal reaction.[684]

Many methods have been advanced to reduce the incidence of local recurrence including occluding the lumen with tapes, Turnbull's "no-touch" technique, luminal irrigation with various agents, and iodized sutures. All have little confirmed effectiveness. Complete mesorectal excision appears to significantly reduce the incidence of local recurrence, probably because lymphatic foci of residual tumor are removed.[99,366,429] Radiation therapy and radiation in combination with chemotherapy have also reduced the incidence of local recurrence in many studies.

Locally recurrent tumors may be divided into those that present with a perineal lesion, with an isolated anastomotic recurrence, with a pelvic mass, or with pelvic and distant disease. All but the last of these may be candidates for curative salvage.

Symptoms

Patients who have local recurrence may present without symptoms, and the neoplasm may be detected on routine follow-up examination. However, most recurrences are not detected until the patient becomes symptomatic. Unfortunately, by this time the lesion is often unresectable.[670] In one study, pain was the most common symptom and occurred initially in 30 percent of patients with recurrence.[584] Urinary or visceral symptoms accounted for 13 percent, altered bowel habits for 12 percent, and loss of weight for 11 percent. Other symptoms included weakness, bleeding per rectum, bloody mucous discharge, and tenesmus. Anemia and jaundice suggest extensive disease. Abdominal distention may be seen but is most common with recurrence of a colon carcinoma. Unrelenting pain beginning as a dull ache and progressing to a drilling sensation may imply sacral plexus or perineural invasion. This may progress to a cauda equina syndrome with an associated neurogenic bladder.[235]

Perineal Recurrence

Lesions may recur in the perineal closure scar after abdominoperineal resection and are found by physical examination. These recurrences may occasionally be isolated and cured by wide local excision.[235,726,727] A more radical method such as a combined transabdominal/perineal approach may improve results.[195] If the lesion cannot be removed entirely it is probably better to treat it palliatively with radiation than to perform an incomplete excision which will not heal and will leave a larger, infected, draining, and ulcerated wound. If such a wound occurs, before or after attempted excision, there may be a role for laser debulking.

Table 18-20   Review of Local Recurrence Rates

Author/Year	No. patients	Local recurrence Overall, %	By Dukes stage, % A	B	C
Patel et al[352] 1977	435	24	13	17	37
Hurst et al[714] 1982	34	32			
Vezeridis et al[715] 1982	49	2			
Localio et al[128] 1983	646		3	13	25
Anderberg et al[716] 1983	38	24			
Luke et al[717] 1983	44	23			
Ohman and Svenberg[718] 1983	21	10			
Fegiz et al[719] 1983	102	9			
Pheils et al[87] 1983	93	10			
Lasson et al[720] 1984	40	17			
Williams and Johnston[357] 1984	35	17			
Leff et al[721] 1985	70	11			
Rosen et al[722] 1985	76	21			
Kennedy et al[723] 1985	90	11			
McDermott et al[69] 1985	934	20	10	15	32
Heimann et al[90] 1986	320	16	0	14	24
Enker et al[184] 1986	412	28	14	30	41
Colombo et al[724] 1987	61	10			
Feil et al[684] 1988	90	20	7	17	40
Michelassi et al[186] **1988**	**154**	12		B1, 0; B2 9.6	21
Twomey et al[510] 1989	106	19			
Rubbini et al[725] 1990	183	24	2	25	39
McAnena et al[187] 1990	81	3			

Anastomotic Recurrence

True anastomotic recurrence is rare and is probably due to an inadequate distal margin with residual tumor or, theoretically, to free tumor cells implanting into the anastomosis at the time of the original resection.[728,729] The incidence has been reported to be in the range of 2 to 6 percent.[65,85,730-732] However, most "anastomotic recurrences" actually represent pelvic disease that has secondarily invaded the bowel and presents at or near the level of the anastomosis. It is more common after low anterior resection than after other colonic resections. Anastomotic recurrences may be detected at a treatable stage by digital examination, proctoscopy, and ultrasonography. The lesion is usually intramural and infiltrating; early in its course it may not cause mucosal changes. The treatment of choice is abdomino-perineal resection. Fewer than 50 percent of the few recurrences in this category are actually resectable for cure, and survival is somewhat less than 50 percent.[358,655,730,731,733,734]

Pelvic Recurrence

Most patients who present with pelvic recurrence beyond that discussed above are not candidates for curative resection,[180,195,358] but there are notable exceptions. Patients with locally aggressive recurrences that invade the urogenital organs anteriorly may be candidates for total or posterior pelvic exenteration. Those with invasion into the coccyx or sacrum may be able to undergo resection with the coccyx or a portion of the sacrum removed en bloc. These procedures are not to be undertaken lightly: they are associated with significant morbidity and most require a colostomy, an ileal conduit, or both. Prior to exploration, distant disease should be sought and the extent of the pelvic process should be defined to the extent possible. Preoperative consultations may include a medical oncologist, a radiation therapist, an enterostomal therapist, a urologist, and a social worker. Contraindications to major pelvic resections include sciatic pain, bilateral ureteral obstruction, lower extremity edema, aortic lymph node involvement, lateral/deep pelvic side wall invasion, adherence of multiple small bowel loops, and distant metastases.[195,735] These symptoms and findings indicate unresectable disease. There is little role for debulking procedures in the treatment of rectal cancer as they do not improve survival nor do they offer substantial palliation. When an incomplete resection is performed, intraoperative radiation may provide some control of the residual disease.

Patients who undergo complete resection may enjoy a prolonged disease-free period and significant palliation. The consequences of severe pelvic pain, tenesmus, and bleeding may be avoided because these patients tend to die of distant disease. In carefully selected patients, mortality is low although morbidity rates vary. Reports of patients undergoing apparently curative excision reveal 5-year survival rates of 8 to 34 percent.[195,577,659,736,737]

For larger recurrences in a pelvis that has not yet been maximally irradiated, radiation therapy may be added to resection. Beart and his coworkers at the Mayo Clinic treated 24 patients with isolated pelvic recurrences with 45 to 50 gray preoperatively using a multiple-field technique.[738] Even though repeated CT scans demonstrated localized disease, small amounts of tumor were left in the pelvis after surgery in all cases. An intraoperative radiation boost of 10 to 20 gray was administered during a separate surgical procedure. There were no treatment-related deaths and morbidity was minimal. With a mean follow-up of 20 months, 8 of 24 patients had died, 2 without evidence of recurrent disease; 13 of the 16 survivors remained disease-free during this limited period. Among the 8 patients who did develop recurrence, 3 patients had isolated local recurrence and 5 had disseminated disease. Therefore, this treatment regimen was locally effective in 85 percent of these patients, and prolonged survival was achieved in 67 percent. Still, this is a very small group with limited follow-up, and most patients with recurrence are not candidates for this type of approach.

En Bloc Sacral Excision

Resection of a portion of the sacrum may be performed en bloc with the recurrent tumor and adjacent viscera. If the bladder is uninvolved then sacrectomy up to the S-3 nerve roots may be performed without loss of bladder function. If the bladder is resected as well, then sacrectomy may be performed up to S-2 or even S-1. Excellent pain control is usually obtained after this procedure although the survival rates are poor. Pain is probably relieved because the tumor is removed but also because of surgically induced hypesthesia. Excision of the coccyx may be performed with little morbidity, excepting the rare patient who experiences persistent pain.

Only small groups of patients who have undergone this extensive procedure have been reported.[739,740] Takagi and colleagues reported 7 patients who underwent pelvic exenteration combined with sacral resection for locally recurrent rectal cancer.[741] Their two-phase procedure involves an abdominal exploration to assess resectability followed by a transsacral resection. If the anatomy appears appropriate and there is no evidence of distant disease, the aortoiliac vessels are dissected, ligating the hypogastric vessels which are removed with the specimen. The bladder is dissected anteriorly and laterally and the ileal conduit and colostomy are created. The abdomen is closed, and the patient is placed in the prone position. A wide perineal incision is made, and the gluteal muscles are dissected from the sacrum. The sacrotuberous and sacrospinous ligaments are severed while the sciatic nerves are carefully preserved. The sacrum is amputated at the lower end of the sacroiliac joints and the specimen is removed en bloc. The gluteal muscles are apposed, and the wound is closed over large drains.

In Takagi's 7 cases, the mean operating time was 8.8 hours, and between 2500 and 12,000 ml of blood were lost. The group thought that blood loss was lessened by completing the presacral venous plexus dissection from below, rather than from above. None of these 7 patients died in the perioperative period. Two complications were encountered: a perineal abscess in one patient and an intestinal fistula which required further surgery in another. All had relief of pain and were ambulatory. Three patients had died of their disease at 11, 16, and 17 months postoperatively, 2 were alive with disease at 26 and 32 months, and 2 had no evidence of disease at 3 and 22 months.

Palliative Treatment

Hippocrates said: "The physician should heal sometimes and alleviate suffering always."

The operability of rectal cancer varies widely among reports. These differences are probably related to the definition of operability and the patient populations seen. In some societies and ethnic groups late presentation is the rule, whereas in others closer surveillance and regular doctor visits make early detection possible.

When a patient is initially evaluated the ability of the surgeon to operate for cure depends on the local and distant extent of the tumor. In addition, the overall condition and desires of the patient must be considered. These issues are addressed in Chapter 17. If the tumor is judged incurable, palliative measures may be employed. When there is distant spread, resection of the primary tumor may still be in order to avoid the consequences of pelvic progression. If the patient's condition or the nature of the local disease does not allow resection, other measures may be used to ameliorate the local complications.

Unresected or recurrent rectal carcinoma will cause a number of significant local problems as it progresses: luminal obstruction, bleeding, copious discharge, local sepsis, perforation, fistulas, incontinence, and pain. The aims of palliative treatment are to improve and control these problems and to maintain a reasonable quality of life as long as possible.

Resections

Abdominoperineal resection or low anterior resection may be reasonable procedures to pursue in patients with metastatic disease. These procedures usually provide the best long-term control of the primary lesion, often avoiding any local problems at all. The vast majority of patients who have a formal resection will die of their distant disease. Of course, before a major resection is recommended, the benefits of local control must be weighed against the morbidity of the operation and, if necessary, a subsequent colostomy and the estimated longevity of the patient. If the local process is asymptomatic and the distant disease is such that very limited survival is anticipated, then there is little to be gained from surgery. If surgery is undertaken, much of the patient's remaining time may be consumed by the postoperative recovery.

However, if the patient is a good operative risk and the distant disease is not extensive, resection provides the best local palliation. Reports on this topic, though relying on retrospective data and selected patients, have also found that patients undergoing resection have twice the survival of those only having a colostomy.[742-745] The morbidity and mortality of these procedures appear to be little different from rates found in patients resected for cure, and many may be able to avoid a colostomy entirely.

Ostomy and Bypass

If the patient presents with obstruction, a proximal diverting colostomy may be used either as a prelude to subsequent resection or as the only palliative procedure because of extensive pelvic disease or poor medical condition. Yet, as early as 1947 Babcock[36] wrote that the permanent colostomy should be replaced by palliative resection whenever possible. A colostomy will ameliorate obstructive symptoms and may occasionally reduce bleeding and tenesmus in some patients. Pain, however, is not relieved. Such a colostomy should be either a loop or double-barreled type to allow venting of the distal limb above the lesion. An end sigmoid colostomy with a distal mucous fistula provides the best function; however, loop transverse colostomy is often the simplest procedure and is a good alternative for the patient who is in poor condition, has extensive disease, or has had high-dose radiation therapy.[746] Surprisingly, the postoperative mortality of a diverting colostomy is the same or higher than that of a palliative major resection. The survival of patients having a colostomy only approaches that of patients having no treatment at all (7–14 mo). Survival is roughly double this rate in patients having a palliative resection (14-27 mo).[742,743,745]

A loop of small bowel may become obstructed if entrapped in the pelvic process or when carcinomatosis develops. Bypassing an obstructing lesion is probably preferable to liberating it by cutting across the malignancy, since doing the latter may alter the progression of disease. A small-bowel ostomy may be necessary in patients with extensive carcinomatosis. These methods may provide several months of reasonable palliation; without intervention these patients die slowly and painfully of intestinal obstruction. A feeding jejunostomy or a decompressing gastrostomy may be useful if placed at the time of surgery. A hidden colostomy is another useful technique, although seldom indicated. If at the time of either primary or second-look laporotomy a resection is deemed unwise and a colostomy unnecessary, the probability of subsequent rectosigmoid obstruction should be estimated. If this probability is high, a loop of colon can be brought out superficial to the fascia but left deep to the skin. If obstruction subsequently occurs, a colostomy can be created in the office setting with local anesthesia.

Radiation Therapy

External beam radiation therapy has been the major mode of treatment of unresectable pelvic rectal carcinoma. Symptoms of pain, bloody discharge, and tenesmus may be alleviated in 60 to 80 percent of patients; however, survival is rarely affected and symptom control is of limited duration.[180,732,747-751] Pain due to neural or osseous invasion is particularly responsive. As noted above, a small proportion of these tumors will be rendered locally resectable.

Cummings and associates reported their results in 67 patients with unresectable rectal carcinoma. After greater than 40 gray, their actuarial survival was only 2 percent at 5 years, and only 9 percent had good local control.[752] Other authors have reported slightly better figures but all are fairly dismal.[505,732,753]

A combination of external beam radiation and either intracavitary radiation or brachytherapy may improve these results. Also, intraoperative radiation is useful in very selected cases. Chemotherapy alone or in combination with radiation or immunomodulating agents has not yet been particularly helpful in the treatment of these recurrences, although it may help to prolong the symptom-free period after radiation.[180,410,754]

Laser Therapy

Although lasers, in general, have had little impact on the curative treatment of colorectal neoplasms, their greatest contributions have been in the treatment of patients with obstruction and bleeding. As discussed above, recanalization may be performed in obstructed to allow preoperative bowel preparation prior to resection.[162] In the patient who is not a surgical candidate or has widespread local and/or distant metastases, lasers may be very effective in maintaining a patent lumen and avoiding a colostomy. The nd:YAG lasers have been used almost exclusively for this purpose because the beam may be administered through a flexible scope and has both vaporizing and coagulating properties. The tumor is treated retrograde whenever possible to reduce the risk of perforation. Initial patency may be established in as little as one session, but usually retreatment is necessary every 1 to 3 months.

Laser treatments may often be performed in an outpatient setting. Complications such as perforations, rectovaginal fistulas, bleeding, and strictures due to fibrosis do occur, and symptoms may not be adequately controlled in up to 10 percent of patients. Extensive series of patients with obstructing esophageal tumors have been published, but experience with colorectal lesions is more modest.[755,756] Different reports state that symptoms of bleeding, tenesmus, discharge, and obstruction may be adequately controlled in from 75 to 97 percent of patients.[757-770] Pelvic pain is not controlled by laser therapy and invasion into the sphincters is a relative contraindication to this form of therapy.[769,770]

Pain Control

Narcotic analgesics, given either orally or parenterally, are the major agents used for pain relief in progressive rectal cancer. These medications have many side effects including drowsiness, nausea, vomiting, and constipation. Eventually, the benefits decrease and, as higher dosages are needed, the individual is no longer able to function. Epidurally administered narcotics are used less frequently but may control pelvic pain.[771] A standard epidural catheter with intermittent injections may be used or the catheter may be connected to an implanted pump. Although transient nausea may occur, there are few other side effects at appropriate dosages. In a large unpublished series, quoted by Wexner and Brabbee (1986), 711 patients with intractable malignancies were treated by the Danish Epidural Opiate Study Group. Adequate pain relief was reported by 92 percent of the patients. Side effects were noted by 20 percent of patients and involved nausea, constipation, and urinary retention. Only 6 percent found it necessary to discontinue the therapy because of these symptoms.

Radiation therapy may provide dramatic pain relief.[746,772] Goligher notes that 75 percent of 117 patients treated for pain obtained long-lasting "good" or "fair" pain relief.[40] Ciatto and Pacini followed 108 patients treated with 35 to 55 gray of external beam radiation. Of these patients, 55 percent experienced adequate relief, but the pain was controlled for more than 12 months in fewer than 15 percent.[773] Resection remains the most effective method of long-lasting pain relief, but it is often not possible, as noted above.

Caudal or other nerve blocks may be used to relieve severe pelvic pain. The definitive procedure may be preceded by injection of the site with a local anesthetic to assess response. If good relief is obtained then a definitive ablation is performed using alcohol, phenol, or other agents. Some relief has been documented using epidural electrodes to stimulate electrical inhibition,[774] and intrathecal and intraventricular morphine have been tried.[775] Sacral rhizotomy and cordotomy may be used in selected cases.[776,777] In these patients, all other options have generally been exhausted.

References

1. John of Arderne; Power D'A, ed. *Treatises of Fistula-in-Ano and of Fistulae in Other Parts of the Body*. London: The Early English Test Society; 1910.

2. Wilson E. Local treatment of carcinoma of the rectum. *Dis Colon Rectum*. 1965;8:210–214.

3. Fain, S, Claman M, ed. *Surgery of Cancer of the Rectum*. Samuel Fain; 1982.

4. Lisfrank J. Mémoire sur l'excision de la partie inférieure du rectum devenue carcinomateuse [Observation on a cancerous condition of the rectum treated by excision. Translated in *Dis Colon Rectum*. 1983; 26:694–695.] *Rev Med Fr*. 1926;2:380.

5. Verneuil AA. *Etude sur la Extripation de l'Extremité Inferieure du Rectum* [Removal of the Lower Rectum]. Paris:1873. Quoted by Rankin FW. The technique of anterior resection of the rectosigmoid. *Surg Gynecol Obstet*. 1928;46:537–542.

6. Kraske P. Zur extirpation hochsitzender mastdarm-krebse [Extirpation of high carcinomas of the large bowel. Translated in *Dis Colon Rectum* 1984;27:499–503.] *Arch Klin Chir*. 1886;33:563.

7. Rehn L. Fortschritte in der technik der mastdarm-operatiomen. [Progress in the techniques of rectum operations.] *Arch Klin Chir*. 1900;61:1009.

8. Glenn F, McSherry CK. Carcinoma of the distal large bowel 32-year review of 1,026 cases. *Ann Surg*. 1960;163:838–849.

9. Hochenegg J. *Wien Klin Wochenschr*. 1888;1:254, 272, 290, 309, 324, 348.

10. Allingham W, Allingham HW. *The Diagnosis and Treatment of Diseases of the Rectum*. 7th ed. London: Bailliere; 1901.

11. Lockhart-Mummery JP. *Diseases of the Rectum*. 7th ed. London:Bailliere; 1907.

12. Lockhart-Mummery JP. Resection of the rectum for cancer. *Lancet*. 1920;1:20.

13. Lockhart-Mummery JP. Two hundred cases of cancer of the rectum treated by perineal excision. *Br J Surg*. 1926;14:110.

14. Mandl F. Uber den Mastdarmkrebs. *Dtsch Z Chir*. 1922;168:145.

15. Mandl F. Uber 1000 sakrale Mastdarmkrebsextirpa-tionen (Aus dem Hocheneggschen Material). *Dt Z Chir*. 1929;219:3.

16. Czerny (1833) quoted by Rankin FW, Bargen JA, Buie LA. *The Colon, Rectum and Anus*. Philadelphia: WB Saunders; 1932.

17. Bloodgood JC. Surgery of carcinoma of the upper portion of the rectum and sigmoid colon: combined sacral and abdominal operations. *Surg Gynecol Obstet*. 1906;3:284.

18. Miles WE. A method of performing abdominoper-ineal excision for carcinoma of the rectum and of the terminal portion of the pelvic colon. *Lancet*. 1908;2:1812.

19. Miles WE. *Cancer of the Rectum*. London:Harrison; 1926.

20. Dukes CE. The spread of cancer of the rectum. *Br J Surg*. 1930;17:643.

21. Coffey RC. The major procedure first in the two-stage operation for relief of cancer of the rectum. *Ann Surg*. 1915;61:446.

22. Jones DF, McKittrick LS. End results of operations for carcinoma of the rectum. *Ann Surg*. 1922; 76:386.

23. Choyce CC, Beattie JM, eds. *A System of Surgery*. 2nd ed. London:Cassell; 1923;vol 2:739.

24. Rankin FW: The technique of combined abdomino-perineal resection of the rectum. *Surg Gynecol Obstet*. 1929;49;193.

25. Lahey FH. Two-stage abdomino-perineal removal of cancer of the rectum. *Surg Gynecol Obstet*. 1930; 51:692.

26. Westhues H. Uber die Entstehung und Vermeidung des lokalen Rektumkarzinom-Rezidivs. *Arch Klin Chir*. 1930;161:582.

27. Gabriel WV. The end-results of perineal excision and of radium in the treatment of cancer of the rectum. *Br J Surg*. 1932;20;234.

28. Kirschner M. Das synchrone kombinierte Verfahren bei der Radikalbehandlung des Mastdarmkrebses. *Arch Klin Chir.* 1934;180:296.

29. Devine H. Excision of the rectum. *Br J Surg.* 1937;25:351.

30. Lloyd-Davies OV. Lithotomy-Trendelenburg position for resection of rectum and lower pelvic colon. *Lancet.* 1939;2:74.

31. Aleksandrov VB. University of Moscow (Russian). 1973. Thesis.

32. Hochenegg J. *J Wien Kiln Wochenschr.* 1895;1:287.

33. Dixon CF. Surgical removal of lesions occurring in the sigmoid and rectosigmoid. *Am J Surg.* 1939; 46:12–17.

34. Wangensteen OH. Primary resection (closed anastomosis) of rectal ampulla for malignancy with presevation of sphincteric function. *Surg Gynecol Obstet.* 1945;81:1.

35. Dixon CF. Anterior resection for malignant lesions of the upper part of the rectum and lower part of the sigmoid. *Ann Surg.* 1948;125:425.

36. Babcock WW. Radical single stage extirpation for cancer of the large bowel with retained functional anus. *Surg Gynecol Obstet.* 1947;1:1.

37. D'Allaines F. *Arch Fr Mal Appar Dig* 1948; 38:929.

38. Bacon HE. Pull-through procedure. What, when, why? *Dis Colon Rectum.* 1969;12:77.

39. Bacon HE. Present status of the pull-through sphincter-preserving procedure. *Cancer.* 1971; 28:196–203.

40. Goligher JC. *Surgery of the Anus, Rectum and Colon.* 4th ed. London:Balliere Tindall; 1984.

41. Saadia R, Schein M. Local treatment of carcinoma of the rectum. *Surg Gynecol Obstet.* 1988;166: 481–486.

42. Heald RJ, Bussey HJR. Clinical experiences at St. Mark's Hospital with multiple synchronous cancers of the colon and rectum. *Dis Colon Rectum.* 1975; 18:6–10.

43. Lasser A. Synchronous primary adenocarcinomas of the colon and rectum. *Dis Colon Rectum.* 1978; 21:20–22.

44. Welch JP. Multiple colorectal tumors: an appraisal of natural history and therapeutic options. *Am J Surg.* 1981;142:274–280.

45. Reilly JC, Russin LC, Theuerkauf FM Jr. Colonoscopy: its role in cancer of the colon and rectum. *Dis Colon Rectum.* 1982;25:532–538.

46. Langevin JM, Nivatvongs S. The true incidence of synchronous cancer of the large bowel: a prospective study. *Am J Surg.* 1984;147:330–333.

47. Thorson Ag, Christensen MA, David SJ. The role of colonoscopy in the assessment of patients with

colorectal cancer. *Dis Colon Rectum.* 1986;29: 306–311.

48. Askew A, Ward M, Cowen A. The influence of colonoscopy on the operative management of colorectal cancer. *Med J Aust.* 1986;145:254–255.

49. Shida H, Tamamoto T, Hiraiwa M, et al. Colorectal cancer and synchronous adenomatous or malignant polyps—factors influencing its incidence. *Gan No Rinsho.* 1984;33:929–935.

50. Carlsson G, Petrelli NJ, Herrera L, Nava H, Mittelman A. Endoscopic surveillance of patients following a curative resection for colorectal cancer. *J Surg Oncol.* 1988;38:80–82.

51. Adloff M, Arnaud JP, Bergamaschi R, Schloegel M. Synchronous carcinoma of the colon and rectum: prognostic and therapeutic implications. *Am J Surg.* 1989;157:299–302.

52. Barillari P, Ramacciato G, De Angelis R, et al. Effect of preoperative colonoscopy on the incidence of synchronous and metachronous neoplasms. *Acta Chir Scand.* 1990;156:163–166.

53. Wolff WI, Shinya H, Geffen A, Ozoktay S, DeBeer R. Comparison of colonoscopy and the contrast enema in five hundred patients with colorectal disease. *Am J Surg.* 1975;129:181–186.

54. Stearns MW, Deddish MR. Five year results of abdominal lymph node dissection for carcinoma of the rectum. *Dis Colon Rectum.* 1959;2:169–172.

55. Hojo K, Koyama Y, Moriya Y. Lymphatic spread and its prognostic value in patients with rectal cancer. *Am J Surg.* 1982;144:350–354.

56. Frigell A, Ottander M, Stenbeck H, Pahlman L. Quality of life of patients treated with abdominoperineal resection or anterior resection for rectal carcinoma. *Ann Chir Gynaecol.* 1990;79:26–30.

57. Lockhart-Mummery HE, Ritchie JK, Hawley PR. The results of surgical treatment for carcinoma of the rectum of St. Mark's Hospital from 1948–1972. *Br J Surg.* 1976;63:673–677.

58. Smart CR. Rectal cancer patterns of care. *Bull Am Coll Surg.* 1980;65:414–415.

59. McDermott FT, Hughes ES, Pihl EA, et al. Changing survival prospects in rectal carcinoma. A series of 1,306 patients managed by one surgeon. *Dis Colon Rectum.* 1986;29:798–803.

60. Black WA, Waugh JM. The intramural extension of carcinoma of the descending colon, sigmoid and rectosigmoid: a pathologic study. *Surg Gynecol Obstet.* 1948;87:457–464.

61. Grinnell RS. Distal intramural spread of carcinoma of the rectum and rectosigmoid. *Surg Gynecol Obstet.* 1954;99:421.

62. Madsen PM, Christiansen J. Distal intramural

spread of rectal carcinomas. *Dis Colon Rectum.* 1986;29:279–282.

63. Pollett WG, Nicholls RJ. The relationship between the extent of distal clearance and survival and local recurrence rates after curative anterior resection for carcinoma of the rectum. *Ann Surg.* 1983;198: 159–163.

64. Williams NS, Dixon MF, Johnston D. Reappraisal of the 5 centimetre rule of distal excision for carcinoma of the rectum: a study of distal intramural spread and of patients' survival. *Br J Surg.* 1983; 70:150–154.

65. Wilson SM, Beahrs OH. The curative treatment of carcinoma of the sigmoid, rectosigmoid, and rectum. *Ann Surg.* 1976;183:556–565.

66. Wolmark N, Fisher B. An analysis of survival and treatment failure following abdominoperineal and sphincter-saving resection in Dukes' B and C rectal carcinoma. A report of the NSABP clinical trials. National Surgical Adjuvant Breast and Bowel Project. *Ann Surg.* 1986;204:480–489.

67. Quer EA, Dahlin DC, Mayo CW. Retrograde intramural spread of carcinoma of the rectum and rectosigmoid: a microscopic study. *Surg Gynecol Obstet.* 1953;96:24–30.

68. Grinnell RS. Lymphatic metastasis and spread in carcinoma of the colon and rectum. *Ann Surg.* 1966;163:272–280.

69. McDermott FT, Hughes ES, Pihl E, Johnson WR, Price AB. Local recurrence after potentially curative resection for rectal cancer in a series of 1008 patients. *Br J Surg.* 1985;72:34–37.

70. Lazorthes F, Voigt JJ, Roques J, Chiotasso P, Chevreau P. Distal intramural spread of carcinoma of the rectum correlated with lymph nodal involvement. *Surg Gynecol Obstet.* 1990;170:45–48.

71. Villemin F, Huard P, Montagne M. Anatomical study of the lymphatics of the rectum and the anus for application in the surgical treatment of cancer. *Rev Chir.* 1925;63:39.

72. Jinnai. Quoted by: Goligher JC. *Surgery of the Anus, Rectum and Colon.* 4th ed. London: Balliere Tindall; 1984:774.

73. Bartholdson L, Hultborn A, Hulten L, Roos B, Rosencrantz M, Ahnen C. Lymph drainage from the upper and middle third of the rectum as demonstrated by Au. *Acta Radiol Ther.* 1977;16: 352–360.

74. Sauer I, Bacon HE. A new approach for excision of carcinoma of the lower portion of the rectum and anal canal. *Surg Gynecol Obstet.* 1952;95:229.

75. Dukes CE. The surgical pathology of rectal cancer. *Proc R Soc Med.* 1943;37:131.

76. Karanjia ND, Schache DJ, North WRS, Heald RJ. "Close Shave" in anterior resection. *Br J Surg.* 1990;77:510–512.

77. Waugh JM, Black MA, Gage RP. Three and 5-year survivals following combined abdominoperineal resection with sphincter preservation. *Ann Surg.* 1955; 142:752.

78. Deddish MR, Stearns MW Jr. Anterior resection for carcinoma of the rectum and rectosigmoid area. *Ann Surg.* 1961;154:961–966.

79. Gilbertsen VA. The results of the surgical treatment of cancer of the rectum. *Surg Gynecol Obstet.* 1962; 114:313.

80. Williams RD, Yurko AA, Kerr G, Zollinger RM. Comparison of anterior and abdominoperineal resections for low pelvic colon and rectal carcinoma. *Am J Surg.* 1966;111:114–119.

81. Palumbo LT, Sharpe WS. Anterior versus abdominoperineal resection for rectal and rectosigmoid carcinoma. *Am J Surg.* 1968;115:657.

82. Zollinger RM, Sheppard MH. Carcinoma of the rectum and the rectosigmoid. A review of 729 cases. *Arch Surg.* 1971;102:335–338.

83. Slanetz CA, Herter FP, Grinnell RS. Anterior resection versus abdominoperineal resection for cancer of the rectum and rectosigmoid. *Am J Surg.* 1972;123:110.

84. Stearns MS Jr. The choice among anterior resection, the pull through, and abdominoperineal resection of the rectum. *Cancer.* 1974;34:969.

85. Strauss RJ, Friedman M, Platt N, Wise L. Surgical treatment of rectal carcinoma: results of anterior resection vs. abdominoperineal resection at a community hospital. *Dis Colon Rectum.* 1978;21: 269–276.

86. Fick TE, Baeten CG, von Meyenfeldt MF, Obertop H. Recurrence and survival after abdominoperineal and low anterior resection for rectal cancer, without adjunctive therapy. *Eur J Surg Oncol.* 1990;16:105–108.

87. Pheils MT, Chapuis PH, Newland RC, Colquhoun K. Local recurrence following curative resection for carcinoma of the rectum. *Dis Colon Rectum.* 1983; 26:98–102.

88. Graf W, Pahlman L, Enblad P, Glimelius B. Anterior versus abdominoperineal resections in the management of mid-rectal tumours. *Acta Chir Scand.* 1990;156:231–235.

89. Amato A, Pescatori M, Butti A. Local recurrence following abdominoperineal excision and anterior resection for rectal carcinoma. *Dis Colon Rectum.* 1991;34:317–322.

90. Heimann TM, Szporn A, Bolnick K, Aufses AH

Jr. Local recurrence following surgical treatment of rectal cancer. Comparison of anterior and abdominoperineal resection. *Dis Colon Rectum.* 1986;29: 862–864.

91. Carlsson G, Petrelli NJ, Nava H, Herrera L, Mittelman A. The value of colonoscopic surveillance after curative resection for colorectal cancer or synchronous adenomatous polyps. *Arch Surg.* 1987; 122:1261–1263.

92. Neville R, Fielding LP, Amendola C. Local tumor recurrence after curative resection for rectal cancer. A ten-hospital review. *Dis Colon Rectum.* 1987; 30:12–17.

93. Athlin L, Bengtsson NO, Stenling R. Local recurrence and survival after radical resection of rectal carcinoma. *Acta Chir Scand.* 1988;154:225–229.

94. Christiansen J. Place of abdominoperineal excision in rectal cancer. *J R Soc Med.* 1988;81:143–145.

95. Fazio VW. The factors that make low colorectal anastomoses safe (symposium): sump suction and irrigation of the presacral space. *Dis Colon Rectum.* 1978;21:401–405.

96. Galandiuk S, Fazio VW. Postoperative irrigation-suction drainage after pelvic colonic surgery. A prospective randomized trial. *Dis Colon Rectum.* 1991;34:223–228.

97. Waits JO, Dozois RR, Kelly KA. Primary closure and continuous irrigation of the perineal wound after proctectomy. *Mayo Clin Proc.* 1982;57: 185–188.

98. Heald RJ, Husband EM, Ryall RD. The mesorectum in rectal cancer surgery—the clue to pelvic recurrence? *Br J Surg.* 1982;69:613–616.

99. Heald RJ, Ryall RD. Recurrence and survival after total mesorectal excision for rectal cancer. *Lancet.* 1986;1(8496):1476.

100. Beahrs OH. *An Atlas of the Surgical Techniques of Oliver H. Beahrs.* Philadelphia: WB Saunders; 1985.

101. Cajozzo M, Compagno G, DiTora P, Spallitta SI, Bazan P. Advantages and disadvantages of mechanical vs. manual anastomosis in colorectal surgery. A prospective study. *Acta Chir Scand.* 1990;156:167–169.

102. Fazio VW. Cancer of the rectum—sphincter-saving operation. Stapling techniques. *Surg Clin North Am.* 1988;68:1367–1382.

103. Baker JW. Low end-to-side rectosigmoidal anastomosis: description of technique. *Arch Surg.* 1950;67:143–157.

104. Khubchandani IT, Trimpi HD, Sheets JA. Low end-to-side rectoenteric anastomosis with single-layer wire. *Dis Colon Rectum.* 1975;18:308–310.

105. Beart RW Jr, Wolff BG. The use of staplers for anterior anastomoses. *World J Surg.* 1982;6: 525–530.

106. Feinberg Sm, Parker F, Cohen Z, et al. The double stapling technique for low anterior resection of rectal carcinoma. *Dis Colon Rectum.* 1986;29: 885–890.

107. Griffen FD, Knight CD Sr, Whitaker JM, Knight CD Jr. The double stapling technique for low anterior resection. Results, modifications, and observation. *Ann Surg.* 1989;211:745–751.

108. Varma JS, Chan AC, Li MK, Li AK. Low anterior resection of the rectum using a double stapling technique. *Br J Surg.* 1990;77:888–890.

109. Julian TB, Ravitch MM. Evaluation of the safety of end-to-end (EEA) stapling anastomoses across linear stapled closures. *Surg Clin North Am.* 1984;64:567–577.

110. Hilsabeck JR. The presacral space as a collector of fluid accumulations following rectal anastomosis: tolerance of rectal anastomosis to closed suction pelvic drainage. *Dis Colon Rectum.* 1982;25: 680–684.

111. Sehapayak S, McNatt M, Carter HG, Bailey W, Baldwin A Jr. Continuous sump-suction drainage of the pelvis after low anterior resection: a reappraisal. *Dis Colon Rectum.* 1973;16:485–489.

112. Gingold BS, Jagelman DG. The value of pelvic suction-irrigation in reducing morbidity of low anterior resection of the rectum: a ten-year experience. *Surgery.* 1982;91:384–398.

113. Broader JH, Masselink BA, Oates GD, Alexander-Williams J. Management of the pelvic space after proctectomy. *Br J Surg.* 1974;61:94–97.

114. Irvin TT, Goligher JC. A controlled clinical trial of three methods of perineal wound management following excision of the rectum. *Br J Surg.* 1975;62:287–291.

115. Terranova O, Sandei F, Rebuffat C, Maruotti R, Pezzuoli G. Management of the perineal wound after rectal excision for neoplastic disease: a controlled clinical trial. *Dis Colon Rectum.* 1979;22: 228–233.

116. Schrock TR, Deveney CW, Dunphy JE. Factors contributing to leakage of colonic anastomoses. *Ann Surg.* 1973;177:513–518.

117. Goligher JC, Graham NG, DeDombal FT. Anastomotic dehiscence after anterior resection of the rectum and sigmoid. *Br J Surg.* 1970;57:109–118.

118. Fielding LP, Stewart-Brown S, Hittinger R, Blesovsky L. Covering stoma for elective anterior resection of the rectum: an outmoded operation? *Am J Surg.* 1984;147:524–530.

119. Graffner H, Fredlund P, Olsson SA, Oscarson J, Peterson BG. Protective colostomy in low anterior

resection of the rectum using the EEA stapling instrument. A randomized study. *Dis Colon Rectum.* 1983;26:87–90.

120. Parks AG. Transanal technique in low rectal anastomosis. *Proc R Soc Med.* 1972;65:975–976.

121. Lazorthes F, Fages P, Chiotasso P, Lemozy J, Bloom E. Resection of the rectum with construction of a colonic reservoir and colo-anal anastomosis for carcinoma of the rectum. *Br J Surg.* 1986;73:136–138.

122. Parc R, Tiret E, Frileux P, Moszkowski E, Loygue J. Resection and colo-anal anastomosis with colonic reservoir for rectal carcinoma. *Br J Surg.* 1986;73:136–138.

123. Nicholls RJ, Lubowski DZ, Donaldson DR. Comparison of colonic reservoir and straight colo-anal reconstruction after rectal excision. *Br J Surg.* 1988;75:318–320.

124. Kocher T. Quoted by: Rankin FW, Bargen JA, Buie LA. *The Colon, Rectum and Anus.* Philadelphia:WB Saunders; 1932.

125. Kraske P. Ueber die Entstechung sek undarer Krebsqeschwure durch Impfung. *Zentralbl Chir.* 1984;11:801.

126. Turner CG. Conservative resection of the rectum by the lower route: the after results in seventeen cases. *Acta Chir Scand.* 1932;72:519–535.

127. Mason AY. Trans-sphincteric exposure for low rectal anastomosis. *Proc R Soc Med.* 1974;65:974.

128. Localio SA, Eng K, Coppa GF. Abdominosacral resection for midrectal cancer. A fifteen-year experience. *Ann Surg.* 1983;198:320–324.

129. Localio SA, Eng K. Abdominosacral resection. In: Beahrs OH, Higgins GA, Weinstein JJ, eds. *Colorectal Tumors.* Philadelphia:JB Lippincott; 1986: 185–190.

130. Marks G, Mohiuddin M, Borenstein BD. Preoperative radiation therapy and sphincter preservation by the combined abdomino-transsacral technique for selected rectal cancers. *Dis Colon Rectum.* 1985;28:565–571.

131. Murphy JB. Cholecysto-intestinal, gastrointestinal, entero-intestinal anastomosis and approximation without sutures. *Med Rec.* 1892;42:665–676.

132. Hardy TG Jr, Aguilar PS, Stewart WRC. Initial experience with a biofragmentable ring for sutureless bowel anastomosis. *Dis Colon Rectum.* 1987;30:55–61.

133. Hardy TG Jr, Stewart WRC, Aguilar PS. Biofragmentable ring for sutureless bowel anastomosis: early clinical experience. *Contemp Surg.* 1987; 31:39–44.

134. Maunsell HW. A new method of excising the two upper portions of the rectum and the lower segment of the sigmoid flexure of the colon. *Lancet.* 1892;2:474–476.

135. Weir RD. An improved method of treating high-seated tumors of the rectum. *JAMA.* 1901;37: 801–803.

136. Turnbull RB Jr, Cuthbertson JW. Abdominorectal pull-through resection for cancer and for Hirschsprung's disease. *Cleve Clin Q.* 1961;28:109–115.

137. Cutait DE, Figliolini FJ: A new method of colorectal anastomosis in abdominoperineal resection. *Dis Colon Rectum.* 1961;4:335–342.

138. Cutait DE, Cutait R, Ioshimoto M, Hypp'olito Da Silva J, Manzione A. Abdominoperineal endoanal pull-through resection. A comparative study between immediate and delayed colorectal anastomosis. *Dis Colon Rectum.* 1985;28:294–299.

139. Bear HD, MacIntyre J, Burns HJG, Jarrett F, Wilson RE. Colon and rectal carcinoma in the West of Scotland—symptoms, histologic characteristics, and outcome. *Am J Surg.* 1984;147: 441–446.

140. Phillips RKS, Hittinger R, Fry JS, Fielding LP. Malignant large bowel obstruction. *Br J Surg.* 1985;72:296–302.

141. Clark J, Hall AW, Moossa AR. Treatment of obstructing cancer of the colon and rectum. *Surg Gynecol Obstet.* 1975;141:541–544.

142. Dutton JW, Hreno A, Hampson LG: Mortality and prognosis of obstructing carcinoma of the large bowel. *Am J Surg.* 1976;131:36–41.

143. Goligher JC, Smiddy FG. The treatment of acute obstruction or perforation with carcinoma of the colon and rectum. *Br J Surg.* 1957;45:270–274.

144. Hughes ES. Mortality of acute large-bowel obstruction. *Br J Surg.* 1966;53:593–594.

145. Irwin TT, Greaney MG. The treatment of colonic cancer presenting with intestinal obstruction. *Br J Surg.* 1977;64:741–744.

146. Ohman U. Prognosis in patients with obstructing colorectal carcinoma. *Am J Surg.* 1982;143: 742–747.

147. Amsterdam E, Krispin M. Primary resection with colocolostomy for obstructing carcinoma of the left side of the colon. *Am J Surg.* 1985;150: 558–560.

148. Goldstein SD, Salvati EP, Rubin RJ, Eisenstat TE. Tube cecostomy with cecal extraperitonealization in the management of obstructing left sided carcinoma of the large intestine. *Surg Gynecol Obstet.* 1986;162:379–380.

149. Hoffman J, Jensen H-E. Tube cecostomy and staged resections for obstructing carcinoma of the left colon. *Dis Colon Rectum.* 1984;27:24–32.

150. Williams NS, Nasmyth DG, Jones D, Smith AH.

De-functioning stomas: a prospective controlled trial comparing loop ileostomy with loop transverse colostomy. *Br J Surg*. 1986;73:566–570.

151. Mirelman D, Corman ML, Veidenheimer MC, Coller JA. Colostomies—indications and contraindications: Lahey Clinic experience. 1963–1974. *Dis Colon Rectum*. 1978;21:172–176.

152. Mitchell WH, Kovalcik PJ, Cross GH. Complications of colostomy closure. *Dis Colon Rectum*. 1978;21:180–182.

153. Fielding LP, Stewart-Brown S, Blesovsky L. Large bowel obstruction caused by cancer: a prospective study. *Br Med J*. 1979;2:515–517.

154. Klatt GR, Martin WH, Gillespie JT. Subtotal colectomy with primary anastomosis without diversion in the treatment of obstructing carcinoma of the left colon. *Am J Surg*. 1981;141:557–558.

155. Brief DK, Brener BJ, Goldenkranz R. An argument for increased use of subtotal colectomy in the management of carcinoma of the colon. *Am Surg*. 1983;49:66–72.

156. Glass RL, Smith LE, Cochran RC. Subtotal colectomy for obstructing carcinoma of the left colon. *Am J Surg*. 1983;145:335–336.

157. Hughes ESR, McDermott FT, Polglase AL, Nottle P. Total and subtotal colectomy for colonic obstruction. *Dis Colon Rectum*. 1985;28:162–163.

158. White CM, Macfie J. Immediate colectomy and primary anastomosis for acute obstruction due to carcinoma of the left colon and rectum. *Dis Colon Rectum*. 1985;28:155–157.

159. Terry BG, Beart RW Jr. Emergency abdominal colectomy with primary anastomosis. *Dis Colon Rectum*. 1981;24:1–4.

160. Feng YS, Hsu H, Chen SS. One-stage operation for obstructing carcinomas of the left colon and rectum. *Dis Colon Rectum*. 1987;30:29–32.

161. Lelcuk S, Klausner JM, Merhav A. Endoscopic decompression of acute colonic obstruction. Avoiding staged surgery. *Ann Surg*. 1986;203:292–294.

162. Kiefhaber P, Kiefhaber K, Huber F. Preoperative neodymium-YAG laser treatment of obstructive colon cancer. *Endoscopy*. 1986;18:44–46.

163. Bown SG, Barr H, Matthewson K, et al. Endoscopic treatment of inoperable colorectal cancers with the Nd-YAG laser. *Br J Surg*. 1986;73:949–952.

164. Sankar MY, Joffe SN. Laser surgery in colonic and anorectal lesions. *Surg Clin North Am*. 1988;68(6):1447–1469.

165. Eckhauser ML, Imbembo AL, Mansour EG. The role of pre-resectional laser recanalization for obstructing carcinomas of the colon and rectum. *Surgery*. 1989;106:710–716.

166. Radcliffe AG, Dudley HA. Intraoperative antegrade irrigation of the large intestine. *Surg Gynecol Obstet*. 1983;156:721–723.

167. Koruth NM, Krukowski ZH, Younson GG, et al. Intra-operative colonic irrigation in the management of left-sided large bowel emergencies. *Br J Surg*. 1985;72:708–711.

168. Thomson WHF, Carter SStC. On-table lavage to achieve safe restorative rectal and emergency colonic resection without covering colostomy. *Br J Surg*. 1986;73:61–63.

169. Pollack AV, Palyforth MJ, Evans M. Peroperative lavage of the obstructed left colon to allow safe primary anastomosis. *Dis Colon Rectum*. 1987;30:171–173.

170. Morgan CN, Griffiths JD. High ligation of the inferior mesenteric artery during operations for carcinoma of the distal colon and rectum. *Surg Gynecol Obstet*. 1959;108:641.

171. Grinnell RS. Results in the treatment of carcinoma of the colon and rectum. *Surg Gynecol Obstet*. 1953;19:241.

172. Anet GW, Castro AF, Smith RS. Clinical study of ligation of the inferior mesenteric artery in left colon resection. *Surg Gynecol Obstet*. 1952;94:223–228.

173. Grinnell RS. Results of ligation of inferior mesenteric artery at the aorta in resections of carcinoma of the descending and sigmoid colon and rectum. *Surg Gynecol Obstet*. 1965;120:1031–1039.

174. Busuttil RW, Foglia R, Longmire WP Jr. Treatment of carcinoma of the sigmoid colon and upper rectum. A comparison of local segmental resection and left hemicolectomy. *Arch Surg*. 1977;112:920–923.

175. Pezim ME, Nicholls RJ. Survival after high or low ligation of the inferior mesenteric artery during curative surgery for rectal cancer. *Ann Surg*. 1984;200:729–733.

176. Surtees P, Ritchie JK, Phillips RKS. High versus low ligation of the inferior mesenteric artery in rectal cancer. *Br J Surg*. 1990;77:618–621.

177. Goligher JC. The adequacy of the marginal blood supply to the left colon after high ligation of the inferior mesenteric artery during excision of the rectum. *Br J Surg*. 1954;41:351.

178. Griffiths JD. Surgical anatomy of the blood supply of the distal colon. *Ann R Coll Surg Engl*. 1956;19:241.

179. Morgan CN. Quoted in: Griffiths JD. Surgical anatomy of the blood supply of the distal colon. *Ann R Coll Surg Engl*. 1956;19:241.

180. Stearns MW Jr. Diagnosis and management of recurrent pelvic malignancy following combined abdominoperineal resection. *Dis Colon Rectum.* 1980;23:359–361.

181. Koyama Y, Moriya Y, Hojo K. Effects of extended systematic lymphadenectomy for adenocarcinoma of the rectum—significant improvement of survival rate and decrease of local recurrence. *Jpn J Clin Oncol.* 1984;14:623–632.

182. Hojo K, Sawada T, Moriya Y. An analysis of survival and voiding, sexual function after wide iliopelvic lymphadenectomy in patients with carcinoma of the rectum, compared with conventional lymphadenectomy. *Dis Colon Rectum.* 1989;32:128–133.

183. Glass RE, Ritchie JK, Thompson HR, Mann CV. The results of surgical treatment of cancer of the rectum by radical resection and extended abdomino-iliac lymphadenectomy. *Br J Surg.* 1985;72:599–601.

184. Enker WE, Pilipshen SJ, Heilweil ML, et al. En bloc pelvic lymphadenectomy and sphincter preservation in the surgical management of rectal cancer. *Ann Surg.* 1986;203:426–433.

185. Kodaira S, Teramoto T. Extended radical operation of cancer of the rectum. *Gan No Rinsho.* 1986;32:1328–1332.

186. Michelassi F, Block GE, Vannucci L, Montag A, Chappell R. A 5- to 21-year follow-up and analysis of 250 patients with rectal adenocarcinoma. *Ann Surg.* 1988;208:379–389.

187. McAnena OH, Heald RJ, Lockhart-Mummery HE. Operative and functional results of total mesorectal excision with ultra-low anterior resection in the management of carcinoma of the lower one-third of the rectum. *Surg Gynecol Obstet.* 1990;170;517–521.

188. Boey J, Wong J, Ong GB. Pelvic exenteration for locally advanced colorectal carcinoma. *Ann Surg.* 1982;195:513–518.

189. Pittam MR, Thonton H, Ellis H. Survival after extended resection for locally advanced carcinomas of the colon and rectum. *Ann R Coll Surg Engl.* 1984;66:81–84.

190. Sugarbaker PH. Partial sacrectomy for en bloc excision of rectal cancer with posterior fixation. *Dis Colon Rectum.* 1982;25:708–711.

191. Davies GC, Ellis H. Radical surgery in locally advanced cancer of the large bowel. *Clin Oncol.* 1975;1:21–26.

192. Bonfanti G, Bozzetti F, Doci R, et al. Results of extended surgery for cancer of the rectum and sigmoid. *Br J Surg.* 1982;69:305–307.

193. Eldar S, Kemeny MM, Terz JJ. Extended resections for carcinoma of the colon and rectum. *Surg Gynecol Obstet.* 1985;161:319–322.

194. Hojo K, Koyama Y, Moriya Y. Radical surgery for advanced bowel cancer with the involvement to adjacent viscera or distant metastasis—combined resection of involved organs. *Gan No Rinsho.* 1984;30(9 suppl):1061–1066.

195. Cohen AM, Minsky BD. Aggressive surgical management of locally advanced primary and recurrent rectal cancer. Current status and future directions. *Dis Colon Rectum.* 1990;33:432–438.

196. Orkin BA, Dozois RR, Beart RW Jr, Patterson DE, Gunderson LL, Ilstrup DM. Extended resection for locally advanced primary adenocarcinoma of the rectum. *Dis Colon Rectum.* 1989;32:286–292.

197. Durdey P, Williams NS. The effect of malignant and inflammatory fixation of rectal carcinoma on prognosis after rectal excision. *Br J Surg.* 1984;71:787–790.

198. Fedorov VD, Shelygin YA. Treatment of patients with rectal cancer. *Dis Colon Rectum.* 1989;32:138–145.

199. Enker WE. Cancer of the rectum. In: Fazio VW, ed. *Current Therapy in Colon and Rectal Surgery.* Philadelphia:BC Decker; 1990:120–130.

200. Moriya Y, Hojo K, Sawada T. En bloc excision of lower ureter and internal iliac vessels for locally advanced upper rectal and rectosigmoid cancer. Use of ileal segment for ureteral repair. *Dis Colon Rectum.* 1988;31:872–877.

201. Ledesma EJ, Bruno S, Mittelman A. Total pelvic exenteration in colorectal disease: a 20-year experience. *Ann Surg.* 1981;194:701–703.

202. Wanebo HJ, Gaker DL, Whitehill R, Morgan RF, Constable WC. Pelvic recurrence of rectal cancer. Options for curative resection. *Ann Surg.* 1987;205:482–495.

203. Kraybill WG, Lopez MJ, Bricker EM. Total pelvic exenteration as a therapeutic option in advanced malignant disease of the pelvis. *Surg Gynecol Obstet.* 1988;166:259–263.

204. Williams LF Jr, Huddleston CB, Sawyers JL, Potts JR III, Sharp KW, McDougal SW. Is total pelvic exenteration reasonable primary treatment for rectal carcinoma? *Ann Surg.* 1988;207:670–678.

205. Touran T, Frost DB, O'Connell TX. Sacral resection. Operative technique and outcome. *Arch Surg.* 1990;125:911–913.

206. Block IR, Enquist IF. Lymphatic studies pertaining to local spread of carcinoma of the rectum in the female. *Surg Gynecol Obstet.* 1961;111:41.

207. Fazio VW, Pilipshen SJ. Techniques for the resection of colon cancer: an appraisal of the no-touch isolation technique. In: Beahrs OH, Higgins GA,

Weinstein JJ, eds. *Colorectal Tumors*. Philadelphia: JB Lippincott; 1986:159–169.

208. Quan SHG, Sehdev MK. Pelvic surgery concomitant with bowel resection for carcinoma. *Surg Clin North Am*. 1974;54:881–886.

209. Antoniades K, Spector HB, Hecksher RJ. Prophylactic oophorectomy in conjunction with large-bowel resection for cancer: report of two cases. *Dis Colon Rectum*. 1977;20:506–510.

210. Burt CA. Prophylactic oophorectomy with resection of the large bowel for cancer. *Am J Surg*. 1951;82:571.

211. Harcourt KF, Dennis DL. Laparotomy for ovarian tumors in unsuspected carcinoma of the colon. *Cancer*. 1968;21:1244–1246.

212. Knoepp LF, Ray JE, Overby I. Ovarian metastases from colorectal carcinoma. *Dis Colon Rectum*. 1973;16:305–311.

213. Leffel JM, Masson JC, Dockerty MB. Krukenberg's tumors: a survey of forty-four cases. *Ann Surg*. 1942;115:102.

214. Woodruff JD, Murthy YS, Bhaskar TN, Bordbar F, Tseng SS. Metastatic ovarian tumors. *Am J Obstet Gynecol*. 1970;107:202–209.

215. MacKeigan JM, Ferguson JA. Prophylactic oophorectomy and colorectal cancer in premenopausal patients. *Dis Colon Rectum*. 1979;22:401–405.

216. Graffner HOL, Alm POA, Oscarson JEA. Prophylactic oophorectomy in colorectal carcinoma. *Am J Surg*. 1983;146:233–235.

217. Blamey SL, McDermott FT, Pihl E, Hughes ESR. Resected ovarian recurrence from colorectal adenocarcinoma: a study of 13 cases. *Dis Colon Rectum*. 1981;24:272–275.

218. O'Brien PH, Neroton BB, Metcalf JS, Rittenbury MS. Oophorectomy in women with carcinoma of the colon and rectum. *Surg Gynecol Obstet*. 1981;153:827–830.

219. Cutait R, Lesser MC, Enker WE. Prophylactic oophorectomy in surgery for large bowel cancer. *Dis Colon Rectum*. 1983;26:6.

220. Birnkrant A, Sampson J, Sugarbaker PH. Ovarian metastases from colorectal cancer. *Dis Colon Rectum*. 1986;29:767–771.

221. Cole WH, Packard D, Southwick HW. Carcinoma of the colon with special reference to the prevention of recurrence. *JAMA*. 1954;155:1549.

222. Fisher ER, Turnbull RB. The cytologic demonstration and significance of tumor cells in the mesenteric venous bleed in patients with colorectal carcinomas. *Surg Gynecol Obstet*. 1955;100:102.

223. Griffiths JD, McKenna JA, Rowbotham HD, et al. Carcinoma of the colon and rectum: circulating malignant cells and five year survival. *Cancer*. 1973;31:226.

224. Barnes JP. Physiologic resection of the right colon. *Surg Gynecol Obstet*. 1952;94:722.

225. Turnbull RB, Kyle K, Watson FR, Spratt J. Cancer of the colon: the influence of the no-touch isolation technique on survival rates. *Ann Surg*. 1967;166:420–427.

226. Ackerman NB. Vascular influence on intestinal lymph flow and their relation to operation for carcinoma of the rectum. *Surg Gynecol Obstet*. 1973;137:801.

227. Wiggers T, Jeekel J, Arends JW, et al. No-touch isolation technique in colon cancer: a controlled prospective trial. *Br J Surg*. 1988;75:409–415.

228. Shafik A. A new concept of the anatomy of the anal sphincter mechanism and the physiology of defecation. Reversion to normal defecation after combined excision operation and end colostomy for rectal cancer. *Am J Surg*. 1986;151:278–284.

229. Williams NS, Hallan RI, Koeze TH, Watkins ES. Restoration of gastrointestinal continuity and continence after abdominoperineal excision of the rectum using an electrically stimulated neoanal sphincter. *Dis Colon Rectum*. 1990;33:561–565.

230. Cavina E, Seccia M, Evangelista G, et al. Perineal colostomy and electrostimulated gracilis "neosphincter" after abdominoperineal resection of the colon and anorectum: a surgical experience and follow-up study in 47 cases. *Int J Colorectal Dis*. 1990;5:6–11.

231. Spratt JS, Adcock RA, Muskovin M, Sherrill W, McKeown J. Clinical delivery system for intraperitoneal hyperthermic chemotherapy. *Cancer Res*. 1980;40:256–260.

232. Fujimoto S, Shrestha RD, Kokubun M, et al. Positive results of combined therapy of surgery and intraperitoneal hyperthermic perfusion for far-advanced gastric cancer. *Ann Surg*. 1990;212:592–596.

233. Fujimoto S, Shrestha RD, Kokubun M, et al. Clinical trial with surgery and intraperitoneal hyperthermic perfusion for peritoneal recurrence of gastrointestinal cancer. *Cancer*. 1989;64:154–160.

234. Fujimoto S, Takahashi M, Endoh F, et al. A clinical pilot study combining surgery with intraoperative pelvic hyperthermochemotherapy to prevent the local recurrence of rectal cancer. *Ann Surg*. 1991;213:43–47.

235. Davies RJ, Pilch YH. Diagnosis and management of local recurrences following primary resection of rectal carcinoma. *Surg Rounds*. August 1984;38–48.

236. Allee PE, Gunderson LL, Munzerrider JE. Postoperative radiation therapy for residual colorectal

carcinoma: ASTR Proceedings. *Int J Radiat Oncol Biol Phys.* 1981;7:1208.

237. Ghossein NA, Samala EC, Alpert S, et al. Elective postoperative radiotherapy after incomplete resection of colorectal cancer. *Dis Colon Rectum.* 1981; 24:252–256.

238. Schild SE, Martenson JA Jr, Gunderson LL, Dozois RR. Long-term survival and patterns of failure after postoperative radiation therapy for subtotally resected rectal adenocarcinoma. *Int J Radiat Oncol Biol Phys.* 1989;16:459–463.

239. Danjoux CE, Gelber RD, Catton GE, Klaassen DJ. Combination chemoradiotherapy for residual, recurrent, or inoperable carcinoma of the rectum: ECOG Study (EST 3276). *Int J Radiat Oncol Biol Phys.* 1985;11:765–771.

240. Morson BC. Histological criteria for local excision. *Br J Surg.* 1985;72 (suppl):S53–S54.

241. Hermanek P, Gall FP. Early (microinvasive) colorectal carcinoma: pathology, diagnosis and surgical treatment. *Int J Colorectal Dis.* 1986;1:79.

242. Mann CV. Techniques of local surgical excision for rectal carcinoma. *Br J Surg.* 1985;72(suppl): S57–S58.

243. Beynon J, McC Mortensen NJ, Foy DMA, Channer JL, Virjee J, Goddard P. Pre-operative assessment of local invasion in rectal cancer: digital examination, endoluminal sonography or computed tomography? *Br J Surg.* 1986;73:1015–1017.

244. Orrom WJ, Wong WD, Rothenberger DA, Jensen LL, Goldberg SM. Endorectal ultrasound in the preoperative staging of rectal tumors. A learning experience. *Dis Colon Rectum.* 1990;654–659.

245. Haggit RC, Glotzbach RE, Soffer EE, Wruble LD. Prognostic factors in colorectal carcinomas arising in adenomas: implications for lesions removed by endoscopic polypectomy. *Gastroenterology.* 1985;89:328–336.

246. Nivatvongs S, Rojanasakul A, Reiman HM, et al. The risk of lymph node metastasis in colorectal polyps with invasive adenocarcinoma. *Dis Colon Rectum.* 1991;34:323–328.

247. Morson BC, Whiteway JE, Jones EA, Macrae FA, Williams CB. Histopathology and prognosis of malignant colorectal polyps treated by endoscopic polypectomy. *Gut.* 1984;25:437–444.

248. Kipfmuller K, Buess G, Naruhn M, Junginger T. Training program for transanal endoscopic microsurgery. *Surg Endosc.* 1988;2:24–27.

249. Buess G, Kipfmuller K, Ibald R, et al. Clinical results of transanal endoscopic microsurgery. *Surg Endosc.* 1988;2:245–250.

250. Buess G, Theib R, Gunther M, Huttere F, Hepp M, Pichlmaier H. Endoscopic operative procedure for the removal of rectal polyps. *Coloproctology.* 1984;6:254–261.

251. Mason AY. Surgical access to the rectum: a transsphincteric exposure. *Proc R Soc Med.* 1970; 63(suppl):91–94.

252. Westbrook KC, Lang NP, Broadwater JR, Thompson BW. Posterior surgical approaches to the rectum. *Ann Surg.* 1982;195:677–685.

253. Stearns MW Jr, Sternberg SS, DeCosse JJ. Treatment alternatives: localized rectal cancer. *Cancer.* 1984;(suppl):2691–2694.

254. Eisenstat TE, Deak ST, Rubin RJ, Salvati EP, Greco RS. Five year survival in patients with carcinoma of the rectum treated by electrocoagulation. *Am J Surg.* 1982;143:127–132.

255. Strauss SF, Crawford RA, Strauss HA. Surgical diathermy of carcinoma of the rectum: its clinical end results. *JAMA.* 1935;104:1480.

256. Crile G Jr, Turnbull RB. The role of electrocoagulation in the treatment of carcinoma of the rectum. *Surg Gynecol Obstet.* 1972;135:391–396.

257. Madden JL, Kandalaft S. Electrocoagulation: a primary and preferred method of treatment for cancer of the rectum. *Ann Surg.* 1967;166:413–419.

258. Madden JL, Kandalaft SI. Long-term evaluation of electrocoagulation as a primary preferred method in the treatment of cancer of the rectum. In: Beahrs OH, Higgins GA, Weinstein JJ, eds. *Colorectal Tumors.* Philadelphia:JB Lippincott; 1986: 199–214.

259. Madden JL, Kandalaft S. Clinical evaluation of electrocoagulation in the treatment of cancer of the rectum. *Am J Surg.* 1971;122:347–352.

260. Hughes EP, Veidenheimer MC, Corman ML, Coller JA. Electrocoagulation of rectal cancer. *Dis Colon Rectum.* 1982;25:215–218.

261. Osborne DR, Higgins AF, Hobbs KE. Cryosurgery in the management of rectal tumours. *Br J Surg.* 1978;65:859–861.

262. Fritsch A, Seidl W, Walzel C. Palliative and adjunctive measures in rectal cancer. *World J Surg.* 1982;6:569–577.

263. Mlasowsky B, Bubey W, Jung D. Cryosurgery for palliation of rectal tumors. *J Exp Clin Cancer Res.* 1985;4:81–84.

264. Papillion J. Endocavitary irradiation of early rectal cancers for cure: a series of 123 cases. *Proc R Soc Med.* 1973;66:1179–1181.

265. Sischy B, Hinson EJ, Wilkinson DR. Definitive radiation therapy for selected cancers of the rectum. *Br J Surg.* 1988;75:901–903.

266. Kronlein RN. Quoted by: Glenn F, McSherry CK. Carcinoma of the distal large bowel: 32-year review of 1026 cases. *Ann Surg.* 1966;163:838.

267. Qinyao W, Weijin S, Youren S. New concepts in severe presacral hemorrhage during proctectomy. *Arch Surg.* 1985;120:1013–1020.

268. Zama N, Fazio VW, Jagelman DG, Lavery IC, Weakley FL, Church JM. Efficacy of pelvic packing in maintaining hemostasis after rectal excision for cancer. *Dis Colon Rectum.* 1988;31:923–928.

269. Nivatvongs S, Fang DT. The use of thumbtacks to stop massive presacral hemorrhage. *Dis Colon Rectum.* 1986;29:589–590.

270. Aso R, Yasutomi M. Urinary and sexual disturbances following radical surgery for rectal cancer, and pudendal nerve block as a countermeasure for urinary disturbance. *Am J Proctol.* 1974;25: 60–69.

271. Burgos FJ, Romero J, Fernandez E, Perales L, Tallada M. Risk factors for developing voiding dysfunction after abdominoperineal resection for adenocarcinoma of the rectum. *Dis Colon Rectum.* 1988;31:682–685.

272. Beahrs JR, Beahrs ON, Beahrs MM, Leary FJ. Urinary tract complications with rectal surgery. *Ann Surg.* 1978;187:542–548.

273. Aagaard J, Gerstenberg TC, Knudsen JJ. Urodynamic investigation predicts bladder dysfunction at an early stage after abdominoperineal resection of the rectum for cancer. *Surgery.* 1986;99:564–568.

274. Cass AS, Bubrick MP. Ureteral injuries in colonic surgery. *Urology.* 1981;18:359–364.

275. Leff EI, Groff W, Rubin RJ, Eisenstat TE, Salvati EP. Use of ureteral catheters in colonic and rectal surgery. *Dis Colon Rectum.* 1982;25:457–460.

276. Balslev I, Harling H. Sexual dysfunction following operation for carcinoma of the rectum. *Dis Colon Rectum.* 1983;26:785–788.

277. Danzi M, Ferulano GP, Abate S. Male sexual function after abdominoperineal resection for rectal cancer. *Dis Colon Rectum.* 1983;26:665–668.

278. Cirino E, Pepe G, Pepe F, Panella M, Rizza G, Cal'i V. Sexual complications after abdominoperineal resection. *Ital J Surg Sci.* 1987;17:315–318.

279. Walsh PC, Schlegel PN. Radical pelvic surgery with preservation of sexual function. *Ann Surg.* 1988;208:391–400.

280. Metcalf AM, Dozois RR, Kelly KA. Sexual function in women after proctocolectomy. *Ann Surg.* 1986;204:624–627.

281. Brotschi E, Noe JM, Silen W. Perineal hernias after proctectomy. *Am J Surg.* 1985;149:301–305.

282. Beck DE, Fazio VW, Jagelman DG. Postoperative perineal hernia. *Dis Colon Rectum.* 1987;30:21–24.

283. Baudot P, Keighley MR, Alexander-Williams J. Perineal wound healing after proctectomy for carcinoma and inflammatory disease. *Br J Surg.* 1980;67:275–276.

284. Tompkins RG, Warshaw AL. Improved management of the perineal wound after proctectomy. *Ann Surg.* 1985;202:760–765.

285. Page CP, Carlton PK Jr, Becker DW. Closure of the pelvic and perineal wounds after removal of the rectum and anus. *Dis Colon Rectum.* 1980;23:2–9.

286. Brough WA, Schofield PF. The value of the rectus abdominis myocutaneous flap in the treatment of complex perineal fistula. *Dis Colon Rectum.* 1991;34:148–150.

287. Bartholdsen L, Hulten L. Repair of persistent perineal sinuses by means of a pedicle of musculus gracilis. *Scand J Plast Reconstr Surg Hand Surg.* 1975;9:74–76.

288. Palmer JA, Vernon CP, Cummings BJ, Moffat FL. Gracilis myocutaneous flap for reconstructing perineal defects resulting from radiation and radical surgery. *Can J Surg.* 1983;26:510–512.

289. Taylor GI, Corlett RJ, Boyd JB. The versatile deep inferior epigastric (inferior rectus abdominis) flap. *Br J Plast Surg.* 1984;37:330–350.

290. Mann CV, Springall R. Use of a muscle graft for unhealed perineal sinus. *Br J Surg.* 1986;73: 1000–1001.

291. Young MR, Small JO, Leonard AG, McKelvey ST. Rectus abdominis muscle flap for persistent perineal sinus. *Br J Surg.* 1988;75:1228.

292. Baird WL, Hester TR, Nahai F. Management of perineal wounds following abdominoperineal resection with inferior gluteal flaps. *Arch Surg.* 1990;125:1486–1489.

293. Anthony JP, Mathes SJ. The recalcitrant wound after rectal extirpation. Applications of muscle flap closure. *Arch Surg.* 1990;125:1371–1376.

294. Goligher JC, Lee PW, Lintott DJ. Experience with the Russian model 249 suture gun for anastomosis of the rectum. *Surg Gynecol Obstet.* 1979;148:517–524.

295. Adloff M, Arnaud JP, Beehary S. Staples vs. sutured colorectal anastomosis. *Arch Surg.* 1980;115:1436–1438.

296. Bolton RA, Britton DC. Restorative surgery of the rectum with circumferential stapler. *Lancet.* 1980;1:850–851.

297. Smith LE. Anastomosis with EEA Stapler after anterior colonic resection. *Dis Colon Rectum.* 1981;24:236–246.

298. Beart RW Jr, Kelly KL. Randomized prospective

evaluation of the EEA stapler for colorectal anastomoses. *Am J Surg.* 1981;141:143–146.

299. Dorsey JS, Stone RM. Colorectal anastomosis with a surgical stapler. *Can J Surg.* 1981;24:555.

300. Heald RJ, Leicester RJ. The low stapled anastomosis. *Dis Colon Rectum.* 1981;24:437–444.

301. Detry RJ, Kestens PJ. Colorectal anastomoses with the EEA stapler. *World J Surg.* 1981;5:739–742.

302. Fazio VW, Jagelman DG, Lavery IC, McGonagle BA. Evaluation of the Proximate-ILS circular stapler. A prospective study. *Ann Surg.* 1985;201:108–114.

303. McGinn FP, Gartell PC, Clifford PC, Brunton FJ. Staples or sutures for low colorectal anastomoses: a prospective randomized trial. *Br J Surg.* 1985;72:603–605.

304. Antonsen HK, Fronborg O. Early complications after low anterior resection for rectal cancer using the EEA stapling device. A prospective trail. *Dis Colon Rectum.* 1987;30:579–583.

305. Belli L, Beati CA, Frangi M, Aseni P, Rondinara GF. Outcome of patients with rectal cancer treated by stapled anterior resection. *Br J Surg.* 1988;75:422–424.

306. West of Scotland and Highland Anastomosis Study Group. Suturing or stapling in gastrointestinal surgery: a prospective randomized study. *Br J Surg.* 1991;78:337–341.

307. Akwari OF, Kelly KL. Anterior resection for adenocarcinoma of the distal large bowel. *Am J Surg.* 1980;139:88–94.

308. Goligher JC, Lee PUG, Simpkins KC, Lintott DJ. A controlled comparison of one- and two-layer techniques of suture for high and low colorectal anastomoses. *Br J Surg.* 1977;64:609–614.

309. Ling L, Broome A, Ryden S. Low anterior resection using stapling instrument. *Acta Chir Scand.* 1979;145:487–489.

310. Dorricott NJ, Baddeley RM, Keighley MRB, Oates GD, Alexander-Williams J. Fifty rectal anastomoses with the EEA stapling instrument: clinical and radiological leak rates. *Gut.* 1980;21:A466.

311. Kirkegaard P, Christiansen J, Hjortrup A. Anterior resection for midrectal cancer with the EEA stapling instrument. *Am J Surg.* 1981;140:312–317.

312. Marti M, Fiala JM, Rohner A. EEA stapler in large bowel surgery. *World J Surg.* 1981;5:735–737.

313. Brennan SS, Pickford IR, Evans M, Pollock AV. Staples or sutures for colonic anastomoses? A controlled clinical trial. *Br J Surg.* In press.

314. Beard JD, Nicholson ML, Sayers RD, Lloyd D, Everson NW. Intraoperative air testing of colorectal anastomoses: a prospective, randomized trial. *Br J Surg.* 1990;77:1095–1097.

315. Fielding LP, Stewart-Brown S, Blesovsky L, Kearney G. Anastomotic integrity after operations for large bowel cancer: a multicentre study. *Br Med J.* 1980;281:911–914.

316. Metcalf AM, Dozois RR, Kelly KL, Beart RW Jr, Wolff BG. Ileal "J" pouch-anal anastomosis: clinical outcome. *Ann Surg.* 1985;202:735–739.

317. Everett WG, Friend PJ, Forty J. Comparison of stapling and hand-suture for left-sided large bowel anastomosis. *Br J Surg.* 1986;73:345–348.

318. Karanjia ND, Corder AP, Holdsworth PJ, Heald RJ. Risk of peritonitis and fatal septicaemia and the need to defunction the low anastomosis. *Br J Surg.* 1991;78:196–198.

319. Davies AH, Bartolo DCC, Richards AEM, Johnson CD, Mortensen MJM. Intraoperative air testing: an audit on rectal anastomosis. *Ann R Coll Surg Engl.* 1988;70:345–347.

320. Pritchard GA, Krouma FF, Stamatakis JD. Intraoperative testing of colorectal anastomosis can be misleading. *Br J Surg.* 1990;77:1105.

321. Chung RS, Hitch DC, Armstrong DN. The role of tissue ischemia in the pathogenesis of anastomotic stricture. *Surgery.* 1988;104:824–829.

322. Killingback M. Low anterior resection. *Aust N Z J Surg.* 1979;49:52–61.

323. Waxman BP, Ramsay AH. The effect of stapler diameter and proximal colostomy on narrowing at experimental circular stapled large bowel anastomoses. *Aust N Z J Surg.* 1986;56:797–801.

324. Pietropaolo V, Masoni L, Ferrara M, Montori A. Endoscopic dilation of colonic postoperative strictures. *Surg Endosc.* 1990;4:26–30.

325. Ross AH. Rectal stricture resection using the EEA autostapler. *Br J Surg.* 1980;67:281–282.

326. Hinton CP, Celestin LR. A new technique for excision of recurrent anastomotic strictures of the rectum. *Ann R Coll Surg Engl.* 1986;68:260–261.

327. Ovnat A, Peiser J, Avinoah E, Charuzi I. A new approach to rectal anastomotic stricture. *Dis Colon Rectum.* 1989;32:351–353.

328. Jao S, Beart RW, Wendorf LJ, Ilstrup DM. Irrigation management of sigmoid colostomy. *Arch Surg.* 1985;120:916–917.

329. Dlin B, Fisher H. Psychiatric aspects of colostomy and ileostomy. In: Howelis J, ed. *Modern Perspectives in the Psychiatric Aspects of Surgery.* New York:Brunner Mazel; 1976:321–341.

330. Gillies D. Body image changes following illness and injury. *J Enterostomal Ther.* 1984;11:186–189.

331. Birnbaum W, Ferrier P. Complication of abdominal colostomy. *Am J Surg*. 1952;83:64–67.

332. Bierman HJ, Tocker AM, Tocker LR. Statistical survey of problems in patients with colostomy or ileostomy. *Am J Surg*. 1956;112:7647–7650.

333. Burns FJ. Complications of colostomy. *Dis Colon Rectum*. 1970;13:448–450.

334. Hawley PR, Ritchie JK. Complications of ileostomy and colostomy following excisional surgery. *Clin Gastroenterol*. 1979;8:403–415.

335. Pearl RK, Prasad ML, Orsay CP, et al. Complications of intestinal stomas. *Contemp Surg*. 1984;24:17–23.

336. Stancanelli V, Ribichini P, Perrucci A, Montanari MC. Clinical and functional results of anterior resection in surgical treatment of rectal cancer. *Coloproctology*. 1990;12:280–282.

337. Williams JT, Slack WW. A prospective study of sexual function after major colorectal surgery. *Br J Surg*. 1980;67:772–774.

338. Batignani G, Monaci I, Ficari F, Tonelli F. What affects continence after anterior resection of the rectum? *Dis Colon Rectum*. 1991;34:329–335.

339. Catchpole BN. Motor pattern of the left colon before and after surgery for rectal cancer: possible implications in other disorders. *Gut*. 1988;29:624–630.

340. Pedersen IK, Christiansen J, Hint K, Jensen P, Olsen J, Mortensen PE. Anorectal function after low anterior resection for carcinoma. *Ann Surg*. 1986;204:133–135.

341. O'Connell PR, Horgan PG, Shinkwin C, Kirwan WO. The effect of low anterior resection on the anal sphincters. *Br J Surg*. 1988;75:604.

342. Horgan PG, O'Connell PR, Shinkwin CA, Kirwan WO. Effect of anterior resection on anal sphincter function. *Br J Surg*. 1989;76:783–786.

343. Iwai N, Hashimoto K, Yamane T, et al. Physiologic status of the anorectum following sphincter-saving resection for carcinoma of the rectum. *Dis Colon Rectum*. 1982;25:652–659.

344. Nakahara S, Itoh H, Mibu R, et al. Clinical and manometric evaluation of anorectal function following low anterior resection with low anastomotic line using an EEA stapler for rectal cancer. *Dis Colon Rectum*. 1988;31:762–766.

345. McDonald PS, Heald RJ. A survey of postoperative function after rectal anastomosis with circular stapling devices. *Br J Surg*. 1983;70:727–729.

346. Bussey HJ. The survival rate of patients with advanced rectal cancer. *Proc R Soc Med*. 1969;62:1221–1223.

347. Dukes CE. Cancer of the rectum: an analysis of 1000 cases. *J Pathol Bacteriol*. 1940;50:527.

348. Mayo CW, Fly OA. Analysis of five-year survival in carcinoma of the rectum and rectosigmoid. *Surg Gynecol Obstet*. 1956;103:94.

349. Gilbertsen VA. Adenocarcinoma of the rectum. A fifteen-year study with evaluation of the results of curative therapy. *Arch Surg*. 1960;80:135–143.

350. Lloyd-Davies OV. In: Maingot R, ed. *Abdominal Operations*. 5th ed. NY, New York:Appleton-Century-Crofts; 1969:1750–1751.

351. Whittaker M, Goligher JC. The prognosis after surgical treatment for carcinoma of the rectum. *Br J Surg*. 1976;63:384–388.

352. Patel SC, Tovee EB, Langer B. Twenty-five years of experience with radical surgical treatment of carcinoma of the extraperitoneal rectum. *Surgery*. 1977;82:460–465.

353. Corman ML, Veidenheimer MC, Coller JA. Colorectal carcinoma: a decade of experience at the Lahey Clinic. *Dis Colon Rectum*. 1979;22:477–479.

354. Enker WE, Laffer UT, Block GE. Enhanced survival of patients with colon and rectal cancer is based upon wide anatomic resection. *Ann Surg*. 1979;190:350–360.

355. Heberer G, Denecke H, Pratschke E, Teichmann R. Anterior and low anterior resection. *World J Surg*. 1982;6:517–524.

356. Rosen L, Veidenheimer MC, Coller JA, Corman ML. Mortality, morbidity, and patterns of recurrence after abdominoperineal resection for cancer of the rectum. *Dis Colon Rectum*. 1982;25:202–208.

357. Williams NG, Johnston D. Survival and recurrence after sphincter saving resection and abdominoperineal resection for carcinoma of the middle third of the rectum. *Br J Surg*. 1984;71:278–282.

358. Pilipshen AJ, Heilweil M, Quan SH, Sternberg SS, Enker WE. Patterns of pelvic recurrence following definitive resections of rectal cancer. *Cancer*. 1984;53:1354–1362.

359. Ohman U. Colorectal carcinoma. A survey of 1345 cases 1950–1984. *Acta Chir Scand*. 1985;151:675–679.

360. Isbister WH, Fraser J. Survival following resection for colorectal cancer. A New Zealand national study. *Dis Colon Rectum*. 1985;28:725–727.

361. Hojo K. Anastomotic recurrence after sphincter-saving resection for rectal cancer. Length of distal clearance of the bowel. *Dis Colon Rectum*. 1986;29:11–14.

362. Danzi M, Ferulano GP, Abate S, Dilillo S, Califano E. Survival and locations of recurrence

following abdomino-perineal resection for rectal cancer. *J Surg Oncol.* 1986;31:235–239.

363. Davis NE, Evans EB, Cohen JR, et al. Colorectal cancer: a large unselected Australian series. *Aust N Z J Surg.* 1987;57:153–159.

364. Kune GA, Kune S, Field B, et al. Survival in patients with large bowel cancer. A population-based investigation from the Melbourne colorectal cancer study. *Dis Colon Rectum.* 1990;33:938–946.

365. Dixon AR, Maxwell WA, Holmes J, Thornton T. Carcinoma of the rectum: a 10-year experience. *Br J Surg.* 1991;78:308–311.

366. Karanjia ND, Schache DJ, North WRS, Heald RJ. "Close shave" in anterior resection. *Br J Surg.* 1990;77:510–512.

367. Cass AW, Million RR, Pfaff WW. Patterns of recurrence following surgery alone for adenocarcinoma of the colon and rectum. *Cancer.* 1976;37:2861–2865.

368. Carlsson U, Lasson A, Ekelund G. Recurrence rates after curative surgery for rectal carcinoma, with special reference to their accuracy. *Dis Colon Rectum.* 1987;30:431–434.

369. Devesa JM, Morales V, Enriques JM, et al. Colorectal cancer. The bases for a comprehensive follow-up. *Dis Colon Rectum.* 1988;31:636–652.

370. Malcolm AW, Perencevich NP, Olson RM, Hanley JA, Chaffey JT, Wilson RE. Analysis of recurrence patterns following curative resection for carcinoma of the colon and rectum. *Surg Gynecol Obstet.* 1981;152:131–136.

371. Deveney KE, Way LW. Follow-up of patients with colorectal cancer. *Am J Surg.* 1984;48:717–722.

372. Phillips RK, Hittinger R, Blesovsky L, Fry JS, Fielding LP. Local recurrence following "curative" surgery for large bowel cancer,II: the rectum and sigmoid. *Br J Surg.* 1984;71:17–21.

373. Zhou XG, Yu BM, Shen YX. Surgical treatment of late results in 1226 cases of colorectal cancer. *Dis Colon Rectum.* 1983;26:250–256.

374. Butler J, Attiyeh FF, Daly JM. Hepatic resection for metastases of the colon and rectum. *Surg Gynecol Obstet.* 1986;162:109–113.

375. Nava HR, Pagana TJ. Postoperative surveillance of colorectal carcinoma. *Cancer.* 1982;49:1043–1047.

376. Coppa GF, Eng K, Ranson JH, Gouge TH, Localio A. Hepatic resection for metastatic colon and rectal cancer: an evaluation of preoperative and postoperative factors. *Ann Surg.* 1985;202:203–208.

377. Gilbert JM, Jeffrey I, Evans M, Kark AE. Sites of recurrent tumour after "curative" colorectal surgery: implications for adjuvant therapy. *Br J Surg.* 1984;71:203–205.

378. Veazey PR, McBride CM. Pelvic recurrence of cancer after abdominoperineal resection of the rectum. *South Med J.* 1979;72:1545–1547.

379. Gerard A, Buyse M, Nordlinger B, et al. Preoperative radiotherapy as adjuvant treatment in rectal cancer. Final results of a randomized study of the European Organization for Research and Treatment of Cancer (EORTC). *Ann Surg.* 1988;208:606–614.

380. Rao AR, Kagan AR, Chan PM, Gilbert HA, Nussbaum H, Hintz BL. Patterns of recurrence following curative resection alone for adenocarcinoma of the rectum and sigmoid colon. *Cancer.* 1981;48:1492–1495.

381. Dukes CE, Bussey HJ. The spread of rectal cancer and its effects on prognosis. *Br J Surg.* 1958;12:309–320.

382. Whittaker M, Goligher JC. The prognosis after surgical treatment for carcinoma of the rectum. *Br J Surg.* 1976;63:875–881.

383. Pihl E, Hughes ES, McDermott FT, Milne BJ, Korner JM, Price AB. Carcinoma of the rectum and rectosigmoid: cancer specific long-term survival. A series of 1061 cases treated by one surgeon: part 1. *Cancer.* 1980;45:2902–2907.

384. Fielding LP, Phillips RK, Fry JS, Hittinger R. Prediction of outcome after curative resection for large bowel cancer. *Lancet.* 1986;1:904–907.

385. Pahlman L, Glimelius B. Local recurrences after surgical treatment for rectal carcinoma. *Acta Chir Scand.* 1984;150:331–335.

386. Devereux DF, Dekers PJ. Contributions of pathologic margins and Dukes' stage to local recurrence in colorectal carcinoma. *Am J Surg.* 1985;149:323–326.

387. Eisenberg B, Decosse JJ, Harford F, Michalek J. Carcinoma of the colon and rectum: the natural history reviewed in 1704 patients. *Cancer.* 1982;49:1131–1134.

388. Hojo K, Koyama Y. Postoperative follow-up studies on cancer of the colon and rectum. *Am J Surg.* 1982;143:293–295.

389. Dukes CE. The classification of cancer of the rectum. *J Pathol Bacteriol.* 1932;35:323–332.

390. Duncan W. Adjuvant radiotherapy in rectal cancer: the MRC trials. *Br J Surg.* 1985;72(suppl):S59–S62.

391. Spratt JS Jr, Spjut HJ. Prevalence and prognosis of individual clinical and pathological variables associated with colorectal carcinoma. *Cancer.* 1967;10:1976–1985.

392. Syrjanenn KJ, Hjelt LH. Tumor-host relationships in colorectal carcinoma. *Dis Colon Rectum.* 1978;21:29–36.

393. Carlon CA, Fabris G, Arslan-Pagnini C, Pluchinotta AM, Chinelli E, Carniato S. Prognostic correlations of operable carcinoma of the rectum. *Dis Colon Rectum.* 1985;28:47–50.

394. Thynne GS, Moertel CG, Silvers A. Preoperative lymphocyte counts in peripheral blood in patients with colorectal neoplasms: a correlation with tumor type. Dukes' classification, site of primary tumor, and five-year survival rate in 1,000 patients. *Dis Colon Rectum.* 1979;22:221–222.

395. Jass JR, Love SB. Prognostic value of direct spread in Dukes' C cases of rectal cancer. *Dis Colon Rectum.* 1989;32:473–476.

396. Consensus Development Conference. *Clin Courier.* 1990;8(10):1–8.

397. Wolmark N, Wieand HS, Rockette HE, et al. The prognostic significance of tumor location and bowel obstruction in Dukes B and C colorectal cancer: findings from the NASBP clinical trials. *Ann Surg.* 1983;198:743–752.

398. Pescatori M, Maria G, Beltrani B, Mattana C. Site, emergency, and duration of symptoms in the prognosis of colorectal cancer. *Dis Colon Rectum.* 1982;25:33–40.

399. Steinberg SM, Barkin JS, Kaplan RS, Stablein DM. Prognostic indicators of colon tumors: the Gastrointestinal Tumor Study Group experience. *Cancer.* 1986;57:1866–1870.

400. Mzabi R, Himal HS, Demers R, MacLean LD. A multiparametric computer analysis of carcinoma of the colon. *Surg Gynecol Obstet.* 1976;143:959–964.

401. Gilbertson VA. The early diagnosis of adenocarcinoma of the large intestine: a report of 1884 cases including 5 year follow up survival data, results of surgery of the disease, and effect on survival prognosis of treatment earlier in the development of the disease. *Cancer.* 1971;27:143.

402. Sanfelippo PM, Beahrs OH. Factors in the prognosis of adenocarcinoma of the colon and rectum. *Arch Surg.* 1972;104:401.

403. Hertz REL, Deddish MR, Day E. Value of periodic examination in detecting cancer of the rectum and colon. *Post grad Med.* 1960;27:290.

404. Polisar L, Sim D, Francis A. Survival of colorectal cancer patients in relation to duration of symptoms and other prognostic factors. *Dis Colon Rectum.* 1981;24:364–369.

405. Chapuis PH, Dent OF, Fisher R, et al. A multivariate analysis of clinical and pathological variables in prognosis of resection of large bowel cancer. *Br J Surg.* 1985;72:698.

406. Ree PC, Marks JE, Moosa AR, Levin B, Platz CE. Rectal and rectosigmoid carcinoma: physician's prediction of local recurrence. *J Surg Res.* 1975;18:1–7.

407. Ranbarger KR, Johnston WD, Chang JC. Prognostic significance of surgical perforation of the rectum during abdominoperineal resection for rectal carcinoma. *Am J Surg.* 1982;143:186–188.

408. Slanetz CA Jr. The effect of inadvertent intraoperative perforation on survival and recurrence in colorectal cancer. *Dis Colon Rectum.* 1984;27:792–797.

409. Zirngibl H, Husemann B, Hermanek P. Intraoperative spillage of tumor cells in surgery for rectal cancer. *Dis Colon Rectum.* 1990;33:610–614.

410. Pahlman L, Glimelius B. Pre or postoperative radiotherapy in rectal and rectosigmoid carcinoma. Report from a randomized multicenter trial. *Ann Surg.* 1990;211:187–195.

411. Mayo WJ. Grafting and traumatic dissemination of carcinoma in the course of operations for malignant disease. *JAMA.* 1913;60:512–513.

412. Long RTL, Edward RH. Implantation metastasis as a cause of local recurrence in colorectal carcinoma. *Am J Surg.* 1989;157:194.

413. Umpleby HC, Williamson RCN. The efficacy of agents employed to prevent anastomotic recurrence in colorectal carcinoma. *Ann R Coll Surg Engl.* 1984;66:192.

414. Cohn I, Floyd CE, Atik M. Control of tumor implantation during operations on the colon. *Ann Surg.* 1963;157:825.

415. Kodner IJ, Shemesh EI, Fry RD, et al. Preoperative irradiation for rectal cancer. Improved local control and long-term survival. *Ann Surg.* 1989;209:194–199.

416. Sugarbaker PH. Carcinoma of the colon-prognosis and operative choice. *Curr Probl Surg.* 1981;28:756–801.

417. Blackshaw AJ, Bussey HJ, Morson BC. Neoplasms: pathology. In: Thomson JP, Nichols RS, Williams CB, eds. *Colorectal Disease.* London:William Heinemann; 1981:235–257.

418. Bentzen SM, Balslev I, Pedersen M, et al. A regression analysis of prognostic factors after resection of Dukes' B and C carcinoma of the rectum and rectosigmoid. Does post-operative radiotherapy change the prognosis? *Br J Cancer.* 1988;58:195–201.

419. Horn A, Dahl O, Morild I. The role of venous and neural invasion on survival in rectal adenocarcinoma. *Dis Colon Rectum.* 1990;33(7):598–601.

420. Khankhanian N, Maulight GM, Russel WO, Schimek M. Prognostic significance of vascular in-

vasion in colorectal cancer of Dukes B class. *Cancer.* 1977;39:1196–1200.

421. Talbot IC, Ritchie S, Leighton MH, Hughes AO, Bussey HJ, Morson BC. The clinical significance of invasion of veins by rectal cancer. *Br J Surg.* 1980;67:439–442.

422. Minsky BD, Mies C, Recht A, Tich TA, Chaffey JT. Resectable adenocarcinoma of the rectosigmoid and rectum: the influence of blood vessel invasion. *Cancer.* 1988;61:1417–1428.

423. Grinnell RS. The lymphatic and venous spread of carcinoma of the rectum. *Ann Surg.* 1942;116:200–215.

424. Sunderland DA. The significance of vein invasion by cancer of the rectum and sigmoid. *Cancer.* 1949;2:429–437.

425. Dukes CE, Bussey HJ. Venous spread in rectal cancer. *Proc R Soc Med.* 1941;34:571–581.

426. Seefeld PH, Bargen JA. The spread of carcinoma of the rectum, invasion of lymphatics, veins and nerves. *Ann Surg.* 1943;118:76–90.

427. Talbot IC, Ritchie S, Leighton MH, Hughes AO, Bussey HJ, Morson BC. Invasion of veins by carcinoma of rectum: method of detection, histological features and significance. *Histopathology.* 1981;5:141–163.

428. Talbot IC, Ritchie A, Leighton MH, Hughes AO, Bussey HJ, Morson BC. Spread of rectal cancer within veins. Histologic features and clinical significance. *Am J Surg.* 1981;141:15–17.

429. Cawthorn SJ, Parums DV, Gibbs NM, et al. Extent of mesorectal spread and involvement of lateral resection margin as prognostic factors after surgery for rectal cancer. Comment in: *Lancet.* 1990;5:335(8697):1067–1068. Comment in: *Lancet.* 1990;9:335(8702):1402-1403. *Lancet* 1990 May 5;334(8697):1055–1059.

430. Heald RJ. Rectal cancer: Anterior resection and local recurrence—a personal view. *Perspect Colorectal Surg.* 1988;1(2):1–26.

431. Breaching the mesorectum. *Lancet.* 1990;335:1067–1068. Editorial.

432. Taylor MC, Pounder D, Ali-Ridha W, Bodurtha A, MacMillin EC. Prognostic factors in colorectal carcinoma of young adults. *Can J Surg.* 1988;31:150–153.

433. Avni A, Fevcht M, Wagner MM. Juvenile versus adult colonic cancer: distinct different etiologic factors. *Dis Colon Rectum.* 1984;27:842.

434. Enblad G, Enblad P, Adami HO, Glimelius B, Krusemo U, Pahlman L. Relationship between age and survival in cancer of the colon and rectum with special reference to patients less than 40 years of age. *Br J Surg.* 1990;77:611–616.

435. Block GE, Enker WE. Survival after operations for rectal carcinoma in patients over 70 years of age. *Ann Surg.* 1971;174:521–529.

436. Irvin TT. Prognosis of colorectal cancer in the elderly. *Br J Surg.* 1988;75:419–421.

437. Morson PM, Carmen ML, Collar JA, Veidenheimer MC. Anterior resection for adenocarcinoma: Lahey Clinic experience for adenocarcinoma. *Am J Surg.* 1976;131:434–443.

438. Wolmark N, Cruz I, Redmond CE, et al. Tumor size and regional lymph node metastasis in colorectal cancer: a preliminary analysis from the NSABP clinical trials. *Cancer.* 1983;51:1315–1322.

439. Wolmark N, Fisher B, Wieand HS. The prognostic value of the modifications of the Dukes' C class of colorectal cancer. *Ann Surg.* 1986;203:115–122.

440. Stearns MW Jr, Deddish MR. The influence of size on prognosis of operable cancer of the rectum and distal sigmoid. *Cancer.* 1956;9:139.

441. Grinnell RS. The chance of cancer and lymphatic metastasis in small colon tumors discovered on x-ray examination. *Ann Surg.* 1964;159:132.

442. Phillips RK, Hittinger R, Blesovsky L, Fry JS, Fielding LP. Large bowel cancer: surgical pathology and its relationship to survival. *Br J Surg.* 1984;71:604–610.

443. Rankin RW, Olson PF. The hopeful prognosis in cases of carcinoma of the colon. *Surg Gynecol Obstet.* 1933;56:366.

444. Cohen AM, Wood WC, Gunderson LL, Shinnar M. Pathological studies in rectal cancer. *Cancer.* 1980;45:2965–2968.

445. Tribukait B, Hammarberg C, Rubio C. Ploidy and proliferation patterns in colo-rectal adenocarcinomas related to Dukes' classification and to histopathological differentiation. A flow-cytometric DNA study. *Acta Pathol Microbiol Immunol Scand (A).* 1983;91:89–95.

446. Forsslund G, Cedermark B, Ohman U, Erhardt K, Zetterberg A, Auer G. The significance of DNA distribution pattern in rectal carcinoma. *Dis Colon Rectum.* 1984;27:579–584.

447. Banner BF, Tomas-de la Vega JE, Roseman DL, Coon JS. Should flow cytometric DNA analyses precede definitive surgery for colon carcinoma? *Ann Surg.* 1986;202:740–744.

448. Scott NA, Rainwater LM, Wieand HS, et al. The relative prognostic value of flow cytometric DNA analysis and conventional clinicopathologic criteria in patients with operable rectal carcinoma. *Dis Colon Rectum.* 1987;30:513–520.

449. Moran K, Cooke T, Forster G, et al. Prognostic value of nucleolar organizer regions and ploidy

values in advanced colorectal cancer. *Br J Surg.* 1989;76:1152–1155.

450. Hood DL, Petras RE, Edinger M, Fazio V, Tubbs RR. Deoxyribonucleic acid ploidy and cell cycle analysis of colorectal carcinoma by flow cytometry. A prospective study of 137 cases using fresh whole cell suspensions. *Am J Clin Pathol.* 1990;93:615–620.

451. Armitage NC, Robins RA, Evans DF, Turner DR, Baldwin RW, Hardcastle JD. The influence of tumor cell DNA abnormalities on survival in colorectal cancer. *Br J Surg.* 1985;72:828–830.

452. Kokal WA, Duda RB, Azumi N, et al. Tumor DNA content in primary and metastatic colorectal carcinoma. *Arch Surg.* 1986;121:1434–1439.

453. Melamed MR, Enker JT, Banner P, Janov AJ, Kessler G, Darzynkiewicz Z. Flow cytometry of colorectal carcinoma with three-year follow-up. *Dis Colon Rectum.* 1986;29:184–186.

454. Bauer KD, Lincoln ST, Vera-Roman JM, et al. Prognostic implications of proliferative activity and DNA aneuploidy in colonic adenocarcinomas. *Lab Invest.* 1987;57:329–335.

455. Rognum TO, Thorud E, Lund E. Survival of large bowel carcinoma patients with different DNA ploidy. *Br J Cancer.* 1987;56(5):644–646.

456. Emdin SO, Sterling R, Roos G. Prognostic value of DNA content in colorectal carcinoma. A flow cytometric study with some methodologic aspects. *Cancer.* 1987;60(6):1282–1287.

457. Scott NA, Wieand HS, Moertel CG, Cha SS, Beart RW, Lieber MM. Colorectal cancer. Dukes' stage, tumor site, preoperative plasma CEA level, and patient prognosis related to tumor DNA ploidy pattern. *Arch Surg.* 1987;122:1375–1379.

458. Schutte B, Reynders MM, Wiggers T, et al. Retrospective analysis of the prognostic significance of DNA content and proliferative activity in large bowel carcinoma. *Cancer Res.* 1987;47:5494–5496.

459. Borkje B, Hostmark J, Skagen DW, Schrumpf E, Laerum OD. Flow cytometry of biopsy specimens from ulcerative colitis, colorectal adenomas, and carcinomas. *Scand J Gastroenterol.* 1987;22:1231–1237.

460. Bosquillon PG, Daver A, Page M, et al. Flow cytometric analysis of DNA abnormalities in colorectal carcinomas. *Bull Cancer (Paris).* 1989;76:291–300.

461. Fausel RE, Burleigh W, Kaminsky DB. DNA quantification in colorectal carcinoma using flow and image analysis cytometry. *Anal Quant Cytol Histol.* 1990;12:21–27.

462. Kouri M, Pyrhonen S, Mecklin JP, et al. The prognostic value of DNA-ploidy in colorectal carcinoma: a prospective study. *Br J Cancer.* 1990;62:976–981.

463. Yamaguchi A, Ishida T, Takegawa S, et al. Flow-cytometric analysis of colorectal cancer with hepatic metastases and its relationship to metastatic characteristics and prognosis. *Oncology.* 1990;47:478–482.

464. Schillaci A, Tirindelli DD, Ferri M, et al. Flow cytometric analysis in colorectal carcinoma: prognostic significance of cellular DNA content. *Int J Colorectal Dis.* 1990;5:223–227.

465. Crissman JD, Zarbo RJ, Ma CK, Visscher DW. Histopathologic parameters and DNA analysis in colorectal adenocarcinomas. *Pathol Annu.* 1989;24(pt 2):103–147.

466. Parks AG, Percy JP. Resection and sutured colo-anal anastomosis for rectal carcinoma. *Br J Surg.* 1982;69:301–304.

467. Hautefeuille P, Valleur P, Perniceni T, et al. Functional and oncological results after coloanal anastomosis for low rectal cancer. *Ann Surg.* 1988;207:61–64.

468. Rudd WW. The transanal anastomosis: a sphincter-saving operation with improved continence. *Dis Colon Rectum.* 1979;22:102–105.

469. Enker WE, Stearns MW Jr, Janov AJ. Perianal coloanal anastomosis following low anterior resection for rectal carcinoma. *Dis Colon Rectum.* 1985;28:576–581.

470. Vernava AM III, Robbins PL, Brabbee GW. Restorative resection: coloanal anastomosis for benign and malignant disease. *Dis Colon Rectum.* 1989;32:690–693.

471. Drake DB, Pemberton JH, Beart RW Jr, et al. Coloanal anastomosis in the management of benign and malignant rectal disease. *Ann Surg.* 1987;206:600–605.

472. Pappalardo G, Toccaceli S, Dionisio P, Castrini G, Ravo B. Preoperative and postoperative evaluation by manometric study of the anal sphincter after coloanal anastomosis for carcinoma. *Dis Colon Rectum.* 1988;31:119–122.

473. Morson BC, Bussey HJR, Samoorian S. Policy of local excision for early cancer of the colorectum. *Gut.* 1977;18:1045–1050.

474. Grigg M, McDermott FT, Pihl EA, Hughes ES. Curative local excision in the treatment of carcinoma of the rectum. *Dis Colon Rectum.* 1984;27:81–83.

475. Horn A, Halvorsen JF, Morild I. Transanal extirpation for early rectal cancer. *Dis Colon Rectum.* 1989;32:769–772.

476. Hagar TH, Gall FP, Hermanek P. Local excision of cancer of the rectum. *Dis Colon Rectum*. 1983;26:149–151.

477. Killingback MJ. Indications for local excision of rectal cancer. *Br J Surg*. 1985;72(suppl):S54–S56.

478. Cuthbertson AM, Simpson RL. Curative local excision of rectal adenocarcinoma. *Aust N Z J Surg*. 1986;56:229–231.

479. Biggers OR, Beart RW Jr, Ilstrup DM. Local excision of rectal cancer. *Dis Colon Rectum*. 1986;29:374–377.

480. DeCosse JJ, Wong RJ, Quan SH, Friedman NB, Sternberg SS. Conservative treatment of distal rectal cancer by local excision. *Cancer*. 1989; 63:219–223.

481. Ellis EM, Mendenhall WM, Bland KI, Copeland EM. Local excision and radiation therapy for early rectal cancer. *Am Surg*. 1988;54:217–220.

482. Despretz J, Otmezguine Y, Grimard L, Calitchi E, Julien M. Conservative management of tumors of the rectum by radiotherapy and local excision. *Dis Colon Rectum*. 1990;33:113–116.

483. Wilson SE, Gordon HE. Excision of rectal lesions by the Kraske approach. *Am J Surg*. 1969;118: 213–217.

484. Jorgensen SJ, Ottsen M. Posterior rectotomy for villous tumours of the rectum. *Acta Chir Scand*. 1975;141:680–682.

485. Richard CA, Clot PH, Cohen Solal JC. L'abord posterior du rectum: a propos de 40 cas. *Ann Chir*. 1980;34:281–283.

486. Allgower M, Durig M, Hochstetter AV, Huber A. The parasacral sphincter-splitting approach to the rectum. *World J Surg*. 1982;6:539–548.

487. Adloff M, Ollier JC, Arnaud JP, Py JM. L'abord posterieur du rectum: technique, indications, complications: a propos de 41 observations. *J Chir Paris*. 1983;120:205–210.

488. Thompson BW, Tucker WE. Trans-sphincteric approach to lesions of the rectum. *South Med J*. 1987;80:41–43.

489. Gall FP, Hermanek P. Cancer of the rectum—local excision. *Surg Clin North Am*. 1988;68: 1353–1365.

490. Lock MR, Cairns DW, Ritchie JK, Lockhart-Mummery HE. The treatment of early colorectal cancer by local excision. *Br J Surg*. 1978;65: 346–349.

491. Whiteway J, Nicholls RJ, Morson BC. The role of surgical local excision in the treatment of rectal cancer. *Br J Surg*. 1985;72:694–697.

492. Mentges B, Buess G. Personal communication, 1991.

493. Culp CE, Jackman RJ. Reappraisal of conservative management of certain selected cancers of the rectum. In: Najarian JS, Delaney JP, eds. *Surgery of the Gastrointestinal Tract*. New York:Intercontinental Medical; 1974:511–519.

494. van Slooten EA, Van Dobbenburg OA. Electrofulguration for rectal cancer. In: Welvaart K, ed. *Colorectal Cancer*. The Hague:Leiden University Press; 1980:175–180.

495. Hughes EP, Veidenheimer MC, Corman ML, Coller JA. Electrocoagulation of rectal cancer. *Dis Colon Rectum*. 1982;25:215–218.

496. Madden JL, Kandalaft SI. Electrocoagulation as a primary curative method in the treatment of carcinoma of the rectum. *Surg Gynecol Obstet*. 1983;157:164–179.

497. Hoekstra HJ, Verschueren RC, Oldhoff J, Van der Ploeg E. Palliative and curative electrocoagulation for rectal cancer. Experience and results. *Cancer*. 1985;55:210–213.

498. DeGraaf PW, Roussel JG, Gortzak E, Hart GA, Jongwan A, van Slooten EA. Early-stage rectal cancer: electrofulguration in comparison to abdominal extirpation or low-anterior resection. *J Surg Oncol*. 1985;19:123–128.

499. Salvati EP, Rubin RJ, Eisenstat TE, Siemons GO, Mangione JS. Electrocoagulation of selected carcinoma of the rectum. *Surg Gynecol Obstet*. 1988;166:393–396.

500. Papillon J. New prospects in the conservative treatment of rectal cancer. *Dis Colon Rectum*. 1984;27:695–700.

501. Lavery IC, Jones IT, Weakley FL, Saxton JP, Fazio VW, Jagelman DG. Definitive management of rectal cancer by contact (endocavitary) irradiation. *Dis Colon Rectum*. 1987;30:835–838.

502. Oguro Y, Tajiri H. Present status of laser medicine and laser endoscopic treatment of gastrointestinal cancers in Japan. Program of the Second International Nd:YAG Laser Conference; Munich, West Germany; 1985;323–328. Abstract.

503. Cummings BJ, Rider WA, Harwood AR, Keane TJ, Thomas GM. Radical external beam radiation therapy for adenocarcinoma of the rectum. *Dis Colon Rectum*. 1983;26:30–36.

504. Mendenhall WM, Million RR, Bland KI, Pfaff WW, Copeland EM. Preoperative radiation therapy for clinically resectable adenocarcinoma of the rectum. *Ann Surg*. 1985;202:215–222.

505. Rao AR, Kagan AR, Chan PYM, Gilbert HA, Nussbaum H. Effectiveness of local radiotherapy in colorectal carcinoma. *Cancer*. 1978;42: 1082–1086.

506. Schild SE, Martenson JA Jr, Gunderson LL, Dozois RR. Long-term survival and patterns of failure after postoperative radiation therapy for subtotally resected rectal adenocarcinoma. *Int J Radiat Oncol Biol Phys.* 1989;16:459–463.

507. Rominger CJ, Gelber RD, Gunderson LL, Conner N. Radiation therapy alone or in combination with chemotherapy in the treatment of residual or inoperable carcinoma of the rectum and rectosigmoid or pelvic recurrence following colorectal surgery. Radiation Therapy Oncology Group Study (76-16). *Am J Clin Oncol.* 1985;8:118–127.

508. Taylor RE, Kerr GR, Arnott SJ. External beam radiotherapy for rectal adenocarcinoma. *Br J Surg.* 1987;74:455–459.

509. Sischy B. Intraoperative electron beam radiation therapy with particular reference to the treatment of rectal carcinomas—primary and recurrent. *Dis Colon Rectum.* 1986;29:714–718.

510. Twomey P, Burchell M, Strawn D, Guernsey J. Local control in rectal cancer. A clinical review and meta-analysis. *Arch Surg.* 1989;124:1174–1178.

511. Gastrointestinal Tumor Study Group. Prolongation of the disease-free interval in surgically treated rectal carcinoma. *N Engl J Med.* 1985;312:1465–1472.

512. Balslev I, Pedersen M, Teglbjaerg PS, et al. Postoperative radiotherapy in Dukes' B and C carcinoma of the rectum and rectosigmoid. A randomized multicenter study. *Cancer.* 1986; 58:22–28.

513. Tepper JE, Cohen AM, Wood WC, Orlow EL, Hedberg SE. Postoperative radiation therapy of rectal cancer. *Int J Radiat Oncol Biol Phys.* 1987;13:5–10.

514. Fisher B, Wolmark N, Rockette H, et al. Postoperative adjuvant chemotherapy or radiation therapy for rectal cancer: results from NSABP protocol R-01. *J Natl Cancer Inst.* 1988;80:21–29.

515. Devereux DF, Eisenstate T, Zinkin L. The safe and effective use of postoperative radiation therapy in modified Astler Coller stage C3 rectal cancer. *Cancer.* 1989;63:2393–2396.

516. Treurniet-Donker AD, Van Putten WL, Wereldsma JC, et al. Postoperative radiation therapy for rectal cancer. An interim analysis of a prospective, randomized multicenter trial in The Netherlands. *Cancer.* 1991;67:2042–2048.

517. Roswit B, Higgins GA, Keehn RJ. Preoperative irradiation for carcinoma of the rectum and rectosigmoid colon: report of a National Veterans Administration randomized study. *Cancer.* 1975;35:1597–1602.

518. Friedmann P, Garb JL, Park WC, et al. Survival following moderate-dose preoperative radiation therapy for carcinoma of the rectum. *Cancer.* 1985;55:967–973.

519. Fortier GA, Constable WC, Meyers H, Wanebo HJ. Preoperative radiation therapy for rectal cancer. *Arch Surg.* 1986;121:1380–1385.

520. Reed WP, Garb JL, Park WC, Stark AJ, Chabot JR, Friedmann P. Long-term results and complications of preoperation radiation in the treatment of rectal cancer. *Surgery.* 1988;103:161–167.

521. Mendenhall WM, Bland KI, Pfaff WW, Million RR, Copeland EM III. Clinically resectable adenocarcinoma of the rectum treated with preoperative irradiation and surgery. *Dis Colon Rectum.* 1988;31:287–290.

522. Dahl O, Horn A, Morild I, et al. Low-dose preoperative radiation postpones recurrences in operable rectal cancer. Results of a randomized multicenter trial in western Norway. *Cancer.* 1990;66:2286–2294.

523. Kligerman MM, Urdaneta N, Knowlton A, Vidone R, Hartman PV, Vera R. Preoperative irradiation of rectosigmoid carcinoma including its regional lymph nodes. *Am J Roentgenol.* 1972;114: 498–503.

524. Higgins GA Jr, Conn JH, Jordan PH Jr, Humphrey EW, Roswit B, Keehn RJ. Veterans Administration Surgical Adjuvant Group. Preoperative radiotherapy for colorectal cancer. *Ann Surg.* 1975;181:624–631.

525. Kligerman MM. Radiotherapy and rectal cancer. *Cancer.* 1977;39:986–990.

526. Leaming R. Radiation therapy in the clinical management of neoplasms of the colon, rectum, and anus. In: Stearns MW Jr, ed. *Neoplasms of the Colon, Rectum and Anus.* New York:John Wiley & Sons; 1980:143–153.

527. Stearns MW. Pre- or postoperative radiation in resectable tumors. In: Welvaart K, Blumgart LH, Kreuning J, eds. *Colorectal Cancer.* The Hague:Leiden University Press; 1980:153–159.

528. Gerard A, Berrod J-L, Pene F, et al. Interim analysis of a phase III study on preoperative radiation therapy in resectable rectal carcinoma. *Cancer.* 1985;55:2373–2379.

529. Reis Neto JA, Quilici FA, Reis JA Jr. A comparison of nonoperative vs. preoperative radiotherapy in rectal carcinoma. A 10-year randomized trial. *Dis Colon Rectum.* 1989;32:702–710.

530. Dosporetz DE, Gunderson LL, Hedberg S, et al. Preoperative irradiation for unresectable rectal and rectosigmoid carcinomas. *Cancer.* 1983;52: 814–818.

531. Fortier GA, Korchak RJ, Jung AK, Constable

WC. Dose response to preoperative irradiation in rectal cancer: implications for local control and complications associated with sphincter sparing surgery and abdominoperineal resection. *Int J Radiat Oncol Biol Phys.* 1986;12:1559–1563.

532. Mendenhall WM, Million RR, Bland KI, Pfaff WW, Copeland EM III. Initially unresectable rectal adenocarcinoma treated with preoperative irradiation and surgery. *Ann Surg.* 1987;205:41–44.

533. Mohiuddin M, Derdel J, Marks G, Kramer S. Results of adjuvant radiation therapy in cancer of the rectum. Thomas Jefferson University Hospital experience. *Cancer.* 1985;55:350–353.

534. O'Connell MJ, Childs DS, Moertel CG, et al. A prospective controlled evaluation of combined pelvic radiotherapy and methanol extraction residue of BCG (MER) for locally unresectable or recurrent rectal carcinoma. *Int J Radiat Oncol Biol Phys.* 1982;8:1115–1119.

535. Gunderson LL, Martin JK, Beart RW. Intraoperative and external beam irradiation for locally advanced colorectal cancer. *Ann Surg.* 1988;207:52–60.

536. Tepper JE, Cohen AM, Wood WC, Hedberg SE, Orlow E. Intraoperative electron beam radiotherapy in the treatment of unresectable rectal carcinoma. *Arch Surg.* 1986;121:421–423.

537. Mayer B. Status of adjuvant therapy for colorectal cancer. *J Natl Cancer Inst.* 1989.

538. Danjoux CE, Gelber RD, Catton GE, Klaassen DJ. Combination chemo-radiotherapy for residual, recurrent or inoperable carcinoma of the rectum: E.C.O.G. Study (EST 3276). *Int J Radiat Oncol Biol Phys.* 1985;11:765–771.

539. Douglas HO Jr, Moertel CG, Mayer RJ, et al. Survival after postoperative combination treatment of rectal cancer. *N Engl J Med.* 1986;315:1294–1295. Letter.

540. Krook JE, Moertel CG, Gunderson LL, et al. Effective surgical adjuvant therapy for high-risk rectal carcinoma. *N Engl J Med.* 1991;324:709–715.

541. Consensus Development Conference. *Clin Courier.* 1990;8:1–8.

542. *National Cancer Institute Clinical Announcement on Adjuvant Therapy of Rectal Cancer.* March 14, 1991. US Dept of Health and Human Services, PHS, NIH, Bethesda, MD.

543. Boice JD Jr, Greene MH, Killen JY Jr, et al. Leukemia and preleukemia after adjuvant treatment of gastrointestinal cancer with semustine (methyl-CCNU). *N Engl J Med.* 1983;309:1079–1084.

544. Sparso BH, Von der Maase H, Kristensen D, et al. Complications following postoperative combined radiation and chemotherapy in adenocarcinoma of the rectum and rectosigmoid. A randomized trial that failed. *Cancer.* 1984;54:2363–2366.

545. Moertel CG, Fleming TR, Macdonald JS, et al. Levamisole and fluorouracil for adjuvant therapy of resected colon cancer. *N Engl J Med.* 1990;322:352–358.

546. Marks G, Mohiudden M. The surgical management of the radiation-injured bowel. *Surg Clin North Am.* 1983;63:81–96.

547. Jao SW, Beart RW Jr, Gunderson LL. Surgical treatment of radiation injuries of the colon and rectum. *Am J Surg.* 1986;151:272–277.

548. Anseline PF, Lavery IC, Fazio VW, Jagelman DG, Weakley FL. Radiation injury of the rectum: evaluation of surgical treatment. *Ann Surg.* 1981;194:716–724.

549. Jagelman DG, Rothenberger DA, Wexner SD. Irradiation injuries to the intestine. *Perspect Colorectal Surg.* 1990;3(2):275–296.

550. Russ JE, Smoron GL, Gagnon JD. Omental transposition flap in colorectal carcinoma: adjunctive use in prevention and treatment of radiation complications. *Int J Radiat Oncol Biol Phys.* 1984;10:55–62.

551. Bakare SC, Shafir M, McElhinney AJ. Exclusion of small bowel from pelvis for postoperative radiotherapy for rectal cancer. *J Surg Oncol.* 1987;35:55–58.

552. DeLuca FR, Ragins H. Construction of an omental envelope as a method of excluding the small intestine from the field of postoperative irradiation to the pelvis. *Surg Gynecol Obstet.* 1985;160:365–366.

553. Deutsch AA, Stern HS. Technique of insertion of pelvic Vicryl mesh sling to avoid postradiation enteritis. *Dis Colon Rectum.* 1989;32:628–630.

554. Sener SF, Imperto JP, Blum MD, et al. Technique and complications of reconstruction of the pelvic floor with polyglactin mesh. *Surg Gynecol Obstet.* 1989;168:475–480.

555. Devereux DF, Feldman MI, McIntosh TK, et al. Efficacy of polyglycolic acid mesh sling in keeping the small bowel in the upper abdomen after abdominal surgery: a 12-month study in baboons. *J Surg Oncol.* 1986;31:204–209.

556. Devereux DF, Chandler JJ, Eisenstat T, Zinkin L. Efficacy of an absorbable mesh in keeping the small bowel out of the human pelvis following surgery. *Dis Colon Rectum.* 1988;31:17–21.

557. Jao SW, Beart RW Jr, Reiman HM, Gunderson LL, Ilstrup DM. Colon and anorectal cancer after pelvic irradiation. *Dis Colon Rectum.* 1987;30:953–958.

558. DeLaney TF. Shedding light on localized solid tumors. *Contemp Oncol.* March/April 1991;14–25.

559. Brown SB, Vernon DI, Stribbling S. Fate of hematoporphoryn derivative after intravenous administration. *Photochem Photobiol.* 1990;51 (suppl):97s.

560. Moan J, Sommer S. Action spectra for hematoporphyrin derivative and Photofrin II with respect to sensitization of human cells in-vitro to photoinactivation. *Photochem Photobiol.* 1984;40:631.

561. Barr H, Bown SG, Krasner N, Boulos PB. Photodynamic therapy for colorectal disease. *Int J Colorectal Dis.* 1989;4:15–19.

562. Dougherty TJ. Photosensitization of malignant tumors. *Semin Surg Oncol.* 1986;2:24.

563. Cortese DA, Kinsey JH. Endoscopic management of lung cancer with hematoporphyrin derivative phototherapy. *Mayo Clin Proc.* 1982;57:543–547.

564. Dougherty JH, Kaufman JE, Goldfarb A. Photoradiation therapy for the treatment of malignant tumors. *Cancer Res.* 1978;38:2628–2633.

565. Forbes IJ, Cowled PA, Leong ASY, et al. Phototherapy of human tumors using hematoporphyrin derivative. *Med J Aust.* 1980;2:489–493.

566. Barr H, Krasner N, Boulos PB, Chatlani P, Bown SG. Photodynamic therapy for colorectal cancer: a quantitative pilot study. *Br J Surg.* 1990;77: 93–96.

567. Patrice T, Foultier MT, Yactayo S, et al. Endoscopic photodynamic therapy with hematoporphyrin derivative for primary treatment of gastrointestinal neoplasms in inoperable patients. *Dig Dis Sci.* 1990;35:545–552.

568. Pressman D, Keighley G. The zone of activity of antibodies as determined by the use of radioactive tracers: the zone of activity of nephrotoxic antikidney serum. *J Immunol.* 1948;59:141–146.

569. Kohler G, Milstein C. Continuous cultures of fused cells secreting antibody of predefines specificity. *Nature.* 1975;256:495–497.

570. Doerr RJ, Abdel-Nabi H, Merchant B. Indium III ZCE-025 immunoscintigraphy in occult recurrent colorectal cancer with elevated carcinoembryonic antigen level. *Arch Surg.* 1990;125:226–229.

571. Beatty JD, Hyams DM, Morton BA, et al. Impact of radiolabelled antibody imaging on management of colon cancer. *Am J Surg.* 1989;157:13–19.

572. Sickle-Santanello BJ, O'Dwyer PJ, Mojzisik C, et al. Radioimmunoguided surgery using the monoclonal antibody B73.2 in colorectal tumors. *Dis Colon Rectum.* 1987;30:761–764.

573. Sardi A, Workman M, Mojzisik C, Hinkle G, Nieroda C, Martin EW Jr. Intra-abdominal recurrence of colorectal cancer detected by radioimmunoguided surgery (RIGS system). *Arch Surg.* 1989;124:55–59.

574. Dawson PM, Blair SD, Begent RHJ, Kelly AMB, Boxer GM, Theodorou NA. The value of radioimmunoguided surgery in first and second look laparotomy for colorectal cancer. *Dis Colon Rectum.* 1991;34:217–222.

575. Moldofsky PJ, Sears HF, Mulhern CS Jr, et al. Detection of metastatic tumor in normal-sized retroperitoneal lymph nodes by monoclonal-antibody imaging. *N Engl J Med.* 1984;311:106–107.

576. Abrams HL, Spiro R, Goldstein N. Metastases in carcinoma: analysis of 1000 autopsied cases. *Cancer.* 1950;3:74–85.

577. Welch JP, Donaldson GA. Detection and treatment of recurrent cancer of the colon and rectum. *Am J Surg.* 1978;135:505–511.

578. Besbeas S, Stearns MW Jr. Osseous metastases from carcinomas of the colon and rectum. *Dis Colon Rectum.* 1978;21:266–268.

579. Welch JP, Donaldson GA. The clinical correlation of an autopsy study of recurrent colorectal cancer. *Ann Surg.* 1979;189:496–502.

580. McCormack PM, Attiyeh FF. Resected pulmonary metastases from colorectal cancer. *Dis Colon Rectum.* 1979;22:553–556.

581. Russell AH, Pelton J, Reheis CE, Wisbeck WM, Tong DY, Dawson LE. Adenocarcinoma of the colon: an autopsy study with implications for new therapeutic strategies. *Cancer.* 1985;56:1446–1451.

582. Willett CG, Tepper JE, Cohen AM, Orlow E, Welch CE. Failure patterns following curative resection of colonic carcinoma. *Ann Surg.* 1984;200:685–690.

583. Pestana C, Reitemeier RJ, Moertel CG, Judd ES, Dockerty MB. The natural history of carcinoma of the colon and rectum. *Am J Surg.* 1964;108:826.

584. Pihl E, Hughes ES, McDermott FT, Milne BJ, Price AB. Disease-free survival and recurrence after resection of colorectal carcinoma. *J Surg Oncol.* 1981;16:333–341.

585. Goligher JC. The operability of carcinoma of the rectum. *Br Med J.* 1941;2:393.

586. Finlay IG, McArdle CS. Occult hepatic metastases in colorectal carcinoma. *Br J Surg.* 1986;73: 732–735.

587. Palmer M, Petrelli NJ, Herrera L. No treatment option for liver metastases from colorectal adenocarcinoma. *Dis Colon Rectum.* 1989;32:698.

588. Jaffe BM, Donegan WL, Spratt JSJ. Factors influencing survival in patients with untreated hepatic metastases. *Surg Gynecol Obstet.* 1968;127:1–11.

589. Abrams MS, Lerner HJ. Survival of patients at Pennsylvania Hospital with hepatic metastases from carcinoma of the colon and rectum. *Dis Colon Rectum.* 1971;14:431.

590. Steele G, Ravikumar TS. Resection of hepatic me-

tastases from colorectal cancer. Biologic perspectives. *Ann Surg.* 1989;210:127–138.

591. Balslev I, Pedersen M, Teglbjaerg PS, et al. Prognosis in synchronous liver metastases from colorectal cancer. A multicenter study of patients with cancer of the rectum and rectosigmoid colon. *Ugeskr Laeger.* 1989;151:1045–1048.

592. Wagner JS, Adson MA, Van Heerden JA, Adson MH, Ilstrup DM. The natural history of hepatic metastases from colorectal cancer: a comparison with resective surgery. *Ann Surg.* 1984;199:502–508.

593. Adson MA, Van Heerden JA, Adson MH, Wagner JS, Ilstrup DM. Resection of hepatic metastases from colorectal cancer. *Arch Surg.* 1984;119:647–651.

594. Scheele J, Stangl R, Altendorf-Hofmann A. Hepatic metastases from colorectal carcinoma: impact of surgical resection on the natural history. *Br J Surg.* 1990;77:1241–1246.

595. Machi J, Isomoto H, Yamashita Y, Kurohiji T, Shirouzu K, Kakegawa T. Intraoperative ultrasonography in screening for liver metastases from colorectal cancer: comparative accuracy with traditional procedures. *Surgery.* 1987;101:678–684.

596. Russo A, Sparacino G, Plaja S, et al. Role of intraoperative ultrasound in the screening of liver metastases from colorectal carcinoma. *J Surg Oncol.* 1989;42:249–255.

597. Olsen AK. Intraoperative ultrasonography and the detection of liver metastases in patients with colorectal cancer. *Br J Surg.* 1990;77:998–999.

598. Yamaguchi A, Ishida T, Nishimura G, et al. Detection by CT during arterial photography of colorectal cancer metastases to liver. *Dis Colon Rectum.* 1991;34:37–40.

599. Grage TB, Vassilopoulos PP, Shingleton WW, et al. Results of a prospective randomized study of hepatic artery infusion with 5-fluorouracil versus intravenous 5-fluorouracil in patients with hepatic metastases from colorectal cancer: a Central Oncology Study Group study. *Surgery.* 1979;86:550–555.

600. Clark CG. Implantable vascular access devices in the treatment of colorectal liver metastases. *Br J Surg.* 1986;73:419–421.

601. Taylor I. Colorectal liver metastases: to treat or not to treat? *Br J Surg.* 1985;72:511–516.

602. Pernikoff BJ, Prats I, Fielding LP. Prevention of hepatic metastasis. *Perspect Colon Rectal Surg.* 1990;3:207–241.

603. Bengmark S, Fredlund P, Hafstrom LO, Vang J. Present experience with hepatic dearterialisation in liver neoplasms. *Prog Surg.* 1974;13:141–166.

604. Petrek JA, Minton JP. Treatment of hepatic me-

tastases by percutaneous hepatic arterial infusion. *Cancer.* 1979;43:2182–2188.

605. Larmi K, Karkola P, Klintrup HE, Heikkinen E. Treatment of patients with hepatic tumours and jaundice by ligation of the hepatic artery. *Arch Surg.* 1974;108:178–183.

606. Fujimoto S, Miyazaki M, Kitsukawa Y, Higuchi M, Okui K. Long-term survivors of colorectal cancer with unresectable hepatic metastases. *Dis Colon Rectum.* 1985;28:588–591.

607. Goldberg JA, Kerr DJ, Wilmott N, McKillop JH, McArdle CS. Regional chemotherapy for colorectal liver metastases: a phase II evaluation of targeted hepatic arterial 5-fluorouracil for colorectal liver metastases. *Br J Surg.* 1990;77:1238–1240.

608. Karanjia ND, Rees M, Schache D, Heald RJ. Hepatic resection for colorectal secondaries. *Br J Surg.* 1990;77:27–29.

609. Hunt TM, Flowerdew ADS, Birch SJ, Williams JD, Mullee MA, Taylor I. Prospective randomized controlled trial of hepatic arterial embolization or infusion chemotherapy with 5-fluorouracil and degradable starch microspheres for colorectal liver metastases. *Br J Surg.* 1990;77:779–782.

610. Taylor I. A critical review of the treatment of colorectal liver metastases. *Clin Oncol.* 1982;8:149–158.

611. Webber BM, Soderberg CH, Leone LA, Rege VB, Glickson AS. A combined treatment approach to management of hepatic metastases. *Cancer.* 1978;42:1087–1095.

612. Moffat FL, Falk RE, Calhoun K, et al. Effect of radiofrequency hyperthermia and chemotherapy on primary and secondary hepatic malignancies when used with metronidazole. *Surgery.* 1983;94:536–542.

613. Storm FK, Harrison WH, Elliott RS, Morton DL. Hyperthermic therapy for human neoplasms: thermal death time. *Cancer.* 1980;46:1849–1854.

614. Foster JH. Survival after liver resection for secondary tumours. *Am J Surg.* 1978;135:389–394.

615. Logan SE, Meier SJ, Ramming KP, Morton DL, Longmire WP Jr. Hepatic resection of metastatic colorectal carcinoma: a ten-year experience. *Arch Surg.* 1982;117:25–28.

616. Rapjal S, Dsmahapatra KS, Ledesma EJ, Mittelman A. Extensive resection of isolated metastasis from carcinoma of the colon and rectum. *Surg Gynecol Obstet.* 1982;155:813–816.

617. Iwatsuku S, Shaw BW Jr, Starzl TE. Experience with 150 liver resections. *Ann Surg.* 1983;197:247–259.

618. Kortz WJ, Meyers WC, Hanks JB, Schirmer BD, Jones RS. Hepatic resection of metastatic cancer. *Ann Surg.* 1984;199:182–186.

619. Fortner JC, Silva JS, Golbey RB, Cox EB, Maclean BJ. Multivariate analysis of a personal series of 247 consecutive patients with liver metastases from colorectal cancer, I: treatment by hepatic resection. *Ann Surg*. 1984;199:306–316.

620. Tomas-de la Vega JE, Donahue EJ, Doolas A, et al. A ten year experience with hepatic resection. *Surg Gynecol Obstet*. 1984;159:223–228.

621. Cady B, McDermott MV. Major hepatic resection for metachronous metastases from colon cancer. *Ann Surg*. 1985;201:204–209.

622. August DA, Sugarbaker PH, Ottow RT, Gianola FJ, Schneider PD. Hepatic resection of colorectal metastases: influence of clinical factors and adjuvant intraperitoneal 5-fluorouracil via Tenckhoff catheter on survival. *Ann Surg*. 1985;201:210–218.

623. Elkberg H, Tranberg K-G, Andersson R, et al. Determinants of survival in liver resection for colorectal secondaries. *Br J Surg*. 1986;73:727–731.

624. Fortner JG. Recurrence of colorectal cancer after hepatic resection. *Am J Surg*. 1988;155:378–382.

625. Griffith KD, Sugarbaker PH, Chang AE. Repeat hepatic resections for colorectal metastases. *Surgery*. 1990;107:101–104.

626. Adson MA. Resection of liver metastases—when is it worthwhile? *World J Surg*. 1987;11:511–520.

627. Lefor AT, Hughes KS, Shiloni E, et al. Intra-abdominal extrahepatic disease in patients with colorectal hepatic metastases. *Dis Colon Rectum*. 1988;31:100–103.

628. Wilson SM, Adson MA. A surgical treatment of hepatic metastasis from colorectal cancer. *Arch Surg*. 1976;113:551–557.

629. Morrow CE, Grage TB, Sutherland DE, Najarian JS. Hepatic resection for secondary neoplasms. *Surgery*. 1982;92:610–614.

630. Butler J, Attiyeh FF, Daly JM. Hepatic resection for metastases of the colon and rectum. *Surg Gynecol Obstet*. 1986;162:109–113.

631. Iwatsuki S, Esquivel CO, Gordon RD, Starzl TE. Liver resection for metastatic colorectal cancer. *Surgery*. 1986;100:804–810.

632. Nordlinger B, Quilichini MA, Parc R, Hannoun L, Dleva E, Hugent C. Surgical resection of liver metastases from colo-rectal cancers. *Int Surg*. 1987;72:70–72.

633. Attiyeh FF, Wichern WA Jr. Hepatic resection for primary and metastatic tumors. *Am J Surg*. 1988;156:368–373.

634. Hughes KS, Rosenstein RB, Songhorabodi S, et al. Resection of the liver for colorectal carcinoma metastases. A multi-institutional study of long-term survivors. *Dis Colon Rectum*. 1988;31:1–4.

635. Sardi A, Nieroda CA, Siddiqi MA, Minton JP, Martin EQ Jr. Carcinoembryonic antigen directed multiple surgical procedures for recurrent colon cancer confined to the liver. *Am J Surg*. 1990;56:255–259.

636. Welch JP, Donaldson GA. The clinical correlation of an autopsy study of recurrent colorectal cancer. *Ann Surg*. 1979;189:496–502.

637. Hughes ES, McConchie IH, McDermott FT, Johnson WR, Price AB. Resection of lung metastases in large bowel cancer. *Br J Surg*. 1982;69:410–412.

638. Wilking N, Petrelli NJ, Herrera L, Regal AM, Mittelman A. Surgical resection of pulmonary metastases from colorectal adenocarcinoma. *Dis Colon Rectum*. 1985;28:562–564.

639. Pihl E, Hughes ES, McDermott FT, Johnson WR, Katrivessis H. Lung recurrence after curative surgery for colorectal cancer. *Dis Colon Rectum*. 1987;30:417–419.

640. Cahan WG, Castro El B, Hajdu SI. The significance of a solitary lung shadow in patients with colon carcinoma. *Cancer*. 1974;33:414–421.

641. Johnson MR. Median sternotomy for resection of pulmonary metastases. *J Thorac Cardiovasc Surg*. 1983;85:516–522.

642. Regal AM, Reese P, Antkowiak J, Hart T, Takita H. Median sternotomy for metastatic lung lesions in 131 patients. *Cancer*. 1985;55:1334–1339.

643. Wilkins EJ Jr, Head JM, Burke JF. Pulmonary resection for metastatic neoplasms in the lung: experience at the Massachusetts General Hospital. *Am J Surg*. 1978;135:480–483.

644. Morrow CE, Vassilopoulos PP, Grage TB. Surgical resection for metastatic neoplasms of the lung: experience at the University of Minnesota hospitals. *Cancer*. 1981;45:2981–2985.

645. Mountain CF, McMurtrey MJ, Hermes KE. Surgery for pulmonary metastases: a 20 year experience. *Ann Thorac Surg*. 1984;38:323–340.

646. Brister SJ, deVarennes B, Gordon PH, Sheiner NM, Pym J. Contemporary operative management of pulmonary metastases of colorectal origin. *Dis Colon Rectum*. 1988;31:786.

647. Scheele J, Altendorf-Hofmann A, Stangle R, Groite H, Gall FP. Resection of lung metastases of colorectal cancer. Indications and indication limits. *Zentralbl Chir*. 1989;114:639–654.

648. Goya T, Miyazawa N, Kondo H, Tsuchiya R, Naruke T, Suemasu K. Surgical resection of pulmonary metastases from colorectal cancer. 10-year follow-up. *Cancer*. 1989;64:1418–1421.

649. Graham RA, Hohn DC. Management of inguinal lymph node metastases from adenocarcinoma of the rectum. *Dis Colon Rectum*. 1990;33:212–216.

650. Morrow M, Enker WE. Late ovarian metastases in carcinoma of the colon and rectum. *Arch Surg.* 1984;119:1385–1388.

651. Nakajima N, Ramadan H, Lapi N, et al. Rectal carcinoma with solitary metastasis: report of a case and review of the literature. *Dis Colon Rectum.* 1979;22:252.

652. Fantini GA, DeCosse JJ. Surveillance strategies after resection of carcinoma of the colon and rectum. *Surg Gynecol Obstet.* 1990;171:267–273.

653. Beart RW Jr, Metzger PP, O'Connell MJ, Schutt AJ. Postoperative screening of patients with carcinoma of the colon. *Dis Colon Rectum.* 1981;24:585–588.

654. Cochrane JP, Williams JT, Faber RC, Slack WW. Value of outpatient follow-up after curative surgery for carcinomas of the large bowel. *Br Med J.* 1980;280:593–595.

655. Vassilopoulos PP, Yoon JM, Ledesma EJ, Mittelman A. Treatment of recurrence of adenocarcinoma of the colon and rectum at the anastomotic site. *Surg Gynecol Obstet.* 1981;152:777–780.

656. Wangensteen OH, Lewis FJ, Tonnen LA. The "second look" in cancer surgery. *Lancet.* 1951;303–307.

657. Wanebo HJ, Gaker DL, Whitehill R, Morgan RF, Constable WC. Composite pelvic resection. *Arch Surg.* 1987;122:1401–1406.

658. Attiyeh FF, Stearns MW. Second-look laparotomy based on CEA elevations in colorectal cancer. *Cancer.* 1981;47:2119.

659. Schiessel R, Wunderlich M, Herbst F. Local recurrence of colorectal cancer: effect of early detection and aggressive surgery. *Br J Surg.* 1986;73:342–344.

660. Wenzl E, Wunderlich M, Herbest F, et al. Results of a rigorous follow-up system in colorectal cancer. *Int J Colorectal Dis.* 1988;3:176–180.

661. Adloff M, Arnaud JP, Ollier JC, Schloegel M. Can the prognosis of patients treated surgically in cancer of the rectum or colon be improved by follow-up? Prosopective study of 909 patients. *Chirurgie.* 1989;115:228–236.

662. Luchtefeld MA, Ross DS, Zander JD, Folse JR. Late development of metachronous colorectal cancer. *Dis Colon Rectum.* 1987;30:180–184.

663. Bulow S, Svendsen LB, Mellemgaard A. Metachronous colorectal carcinoma. *Br J Surg.* 1990;77:502–505.

664. Agrez MV, Ready R, Ilstrup D, Beart RW Jr. Metachronous colorectal malignancies. *Dis Colon Rectum.* 1982;25:569–574.

665. Morson B. Polyp-cancer sequence in the large bowel. *Proc R Soc Med.* 1974;67:451–457.

666. Weir JA. Colorectal cancer: metachronous and other associated neoplasms. *Dis Colon Rectum.* 1975;18:4–5.

667. Kiefer PJ, Thorson AG, Christensen MA. Metachronous colorectal cancer. Time interval to presentation of a metachronous cancer. *Dis Colon Rectum.* 1986;29:378–382.

668. Nava HR, Pagana TJ. Postoperative surveillance of colorectal carcinoma. *Cancer.* 1982;49:1043–1047.

669. Beart RW Jr, O'Connell MJ. Postoperative follow-up of patients with carcinoma of the colon. *Mayo Clin Proc.* 1983;58:361–363.

670. Buhler H, Seefeld U, Deyhle P, Buchmann P, Metzger U, Ammann R. Endoscopic follow-up after colorectal cancer surgery. Early detection of local recurrence? *Cancer.* 1984;54:791–793.

671. Barkin JS, Cohen ME, Flaxman M, et al. Value of a routine follow-up endoscopy program for the detection of recurrent colorectal carcinoma. *Am J Gastroenterol.* 1988;83:1355–1360.

672. Unger SW, Wanebo HJ. Colonoscopy: an essential monitoring technique after resection of colorectal cancer. *Am J Surg.* 1983;145:71–76.

673. Larson GM, Bond SJ, Shallcross C, Mullins R, Polk HC Jr. Colonoscopy after curative resection of colorectal cancer. *Arch Surg.* 1986;121:535–540.

674. Devesa J, Avedillo D, Morales V, Nunez-Puertas A. Automatic preoperative classification of carcinoma of the colon and rectum. *Surg Gynecol Obstet.* 1984;158:482–487.

675. Finan PJ, Marshall RJ, Cooper EH, Giles GR. Factors affecting survival in patients presenting with synchronous hepatic metastases from colorectal cancer: a clinical and computer analysis. *Br J Surg.* 1985;72:373–377.

676. de Roos A, Hermans J, Op den Orth JO. Polypoid lesions of the sigmoid colon: a comparison of single-contrast, double-contrast, and biphasic examinations. *Radiology.* 1984;151:597–599.

677. Gold P, Freedman SO. Demonstration of tumor specific antigens in human colonic carcinomata by immunological tolerance and absorption techniques. *J Exp Med.* 1965;121:439.

678. Moertel CG, Schutt AJ, Go VLW. Carcinoembryonic antigen for recurrent colorectal carcinoma: inadequacy for early detection. *JAMA.* 1978;239:1065.

679. Chapuis PH, Newland RC, Payne JE, MacPherson JG, Pheils MT. Perioperative carcinoembryonic antigen level and prognosis in colorectal cancer. *Med J Aust.* 1980;2:140–143.

680. Arnaud JP, Koehl C, Adloff M. Carcinoembryonic antigen (CEA) in diagnosis and prognosis of

colorectal carcinoma. *Dis Colon Rectum*. 1980;23: 141–144.

681. Sardi A, Agnone CM, Nieroda CA, et al. Radioimmunoguided surgery in recurrent colorectal cancer: the role of carcinoembryonic antigen, computerized tomography, and physical examination. *South Med J*. 1989;82:1235–1244.

682. Staab JH, Anderer FA, Brummendorf T, Stumpf E, Fisher R. Prognostic value of preoperative serum CEA levels compared with clinical staging, I: colorectal carcinoma. *Br J Cancer*. 1981;4: 652–662.

683. Lange MK, Martin EW Jr. Confronting recurrent colorectal cancer. *Contemp Gastroenterol*. 1991; 58–72.

684. Feil W, Wunderlich M, Kovats E, et al. Rectal cancer: factors influencing the development of local recurrence after radical anterior resection. *Int J Colorectal Dis*. 1988;3:195–200.

685. Behbehani AI, Al-Naqeeb N, Omar YT, et al. Serial determinations of serum CEA in monitoring management of patients with colorectal carcinoma. *Oncology*. 1990;47:303–307.

686. Martin EW Jr, Minton JP, Carey LC. CEA-directed second-look surgery in the asymptomatic patient after primary resection of colorectal carcinoma. *Ann Surg*. 1985;202:310–317.

687. Steele G Jr, Zamcheck N, Wilson R, et al. Results of CEA-initiated second-look surgery for recurrent colorectal cancer. *Am J Surg*. 1980;139: 544–548.

688. Wilking N, Petrelli NJ, Herrera L, Holyoke ED, Mittelman A. Abdominal exploration for suspected recurrent carcinoma of the colon and rectum based upon elevated carcinoembryonic antigen alone or in combination with other diagnostic methods. *Surg Gynecol Obstet*. 1986;162: 465–468.

689. Staab HJ, Anderer FA, Stumpf E, Hornung A, Fischer R, Kieninger G. Eighty-four second-look operations based on sequential carcinoembryonic antigen determinations and clinical investigations in patients with recurrent gastrointestinal cancer. *Am J Surg*. 1985;149:198–204.

690. Wanebo HJ, Stevens W. Surgical treatment of locally recurrent colorectal cancer. *Probl Gen Surg*. 1987;4:115–119.

691. Minton JP, Hoehn JL, Gerber DM, et al. Results of a 400-patient carcinoembryonic antigen second-look colorectal cancer study. *Cancer*. 1985;55: 1284–1290.

692. Martin EW Jr, Cooperman M, Carey LC, Minton JP. Sixty second-look procedures indicated primarily by rise in serial carcinoembryonic antigen. *J Surg Res*. 1980;28:389–394.

693. Holmgren J, ed. *Tumour Marker Antigens: Properties and Usefulness of Carcinoma Associated Antigens CEA, CA 19-9 and CA-50*. Lund: Studentlittertur; 1985.

694. Sugano K, Kodaira S, Teramoto T, Watanabe M, Mara A, Abe O. A new tumour marker defined by a monoclonal antibody, NCC-ST-439: its clinical usefulness for colorectal carcinoma. Presented at the Eleventh Biennial Congress of the International Society of University Colon and Rectal Surgeons; May 4–8 1986; Dallas, TX.

695. Armitage NC, Hardcastle JD. Neoplasms: screening and diagnosis. *Curr Opin Gastroenterol*. 1986; 2:16–21.

696. Delvillano BC, Zurawski VR Jr. The carbohydrate antigenic determinant 19-9 (CA 19-9): a monoclonal antibody defined tumour marker. *Immunodiagnostics*. 1983;269:82.

697. Fucini C, Tommasi SM, Rosi S, et al. Follow-up of colorectal cancer resected for cure. An experience with CEA, TPA, CA 19-9 analysis and second-look surgery. *Dis Colon Rectum*. 1987;30: 273–277.

698. Durdey P, Williams NS, Brown DA. Serum carcinoembryonic antigen and acute phase reactant proteins in the pre-operative detection of fixation of colorectal tumors. *Br J Surg*. 1984;71:881–884.

699. Durdey P, Cooper JC, Switala S, King RF, Williams NS. The role of peptidases in cancer of the rectum and sigmoid colon. *Br J Surg*. 1985;72: 378–381.

700. Mach JP, Vienny H, Jaeger P, et al. Long-term follow-up of colorectal carcinoma patients by repeated CEA radioimmunoassay. *Cancer*. 1979;49: 1043–1047.

701. Hodgman CG, MacCarty RL, Wolff BG, et al. Preoperative staging of rectal carcinoma by computed tomography and 0.15T magnetic resonance imaging: preliminary report. *Dis Colon Rectum*. 1986;29:446–450.

702. Kelvin FM, Korobkin M, Heaston DK, Grant JP, Akwari O. The pelvis after surgery for rectal carcinoma: serial CT observations with emphasis on nonneoplastic features. *Am J Radiol*. 1983;141: 959–964.

703. Lee JK, Stanley RJ, Sagel SS, Levitt RG, McLennan BL. CT appearance of the pelvis after abdomino-perineal resection for rectal carcinoma. *Radiology*. 1981;141:737–741.

704. Zaunbauer W, Haertel M, Fuchs WA. Computed tomography in carcinoma of the rectum. *Gastrointest Radiol*. 1981;6:79–84.

705. Havelaar IJ, Sugarbaker PH, Vermess M, Miller DL. Rate of growth of intraabdominal metastases from colorectal cancer. *Cancer*. 1984;54:163–171.

706. Schulz W, Hagen CH, Hort W. The distribution of liver metastases from colonic cancer: a quantitative post mortem study. *Virchows Arch [A]*. 1985;406:279–284.

707. Bartolozzi C, Ciatti S, Lucarelli E, Villari N, de Dominicis R. Ultrasound and computer tomography in the evaluation of focal liver disease. *Acta Radiol Diagn (Stockh)*. 1981;22:545–548.

708. Romano G, DeRosa P, Vallone G, Rotondo A, Grassi R, Santangelo ML. Intrarectal ultrasound and computed tomography in the pre- and postoperative assessment of patients with rectal carcinoma. *Br J Surg*. 1985;72(suppl):S117–S119.

709. Beynon J, Mortensen NJ, Foy DM, Channer JL, Rigby H, Virjee J. The detection and evaluation of locally recurrent rectal cancer with rectal endosonography. *Dis Colon Rectum*. 1989;32:509–512.

710. DeLange EE, Fechner RE, Wanebo HJ. Suspected recurrent rectosigmoid carcinoma after APR: MR imaging and histopathological findings. *Radiology*. 1990;170:323–328.

711. Johnson RJ, Jenkins JP, Isherwood I, James RD, Schofield PF. Quantitative magnetic resonance imaging in rectal cancer. *Br J Radiol*. 1987;60: 761–764.

712. Russell AH, Tong D, Dawson LE, Wisbeck W. Adenocarcinoma of the proximal colon: sites of initial dissemination and patterns of recurrence following surgery alone. *Cancer*. 1984;53:360–366.

713. Gunderson LL, Sosin H. Areas of failure found at reoperation (second or symptomatic look) following "curative surgery" for adenocarcinoma of the rectum: clinicopathologic correlation and implications for adjuvant therapy. *Cancer*. 1974;34: 1278–1292.

714. Hurst PA, Prout WG, Kelly JM, Bannister JJ, Walker RT. Local recurrence after low anterior resection using the staple gun. *Br J Surg*. 1982;69: 275–276.

715. Vezeridis M, Evans JT, Mittelman A, Ledesma EJ. EEA stapler in low anterior anastomosis. *Dis Colon Rectum*. 1982;25:364–367.

716. Anderberg B, Enblad P, Sjodahl R, Wetterfors J. The EEA-stapling device in anterior resection for carcinoma of the rectum. *Acta Chir Scand*. 1983; 149:99–103.

717. Luke M, Kirkegaard P, Lendorf A, Christiansen J. Pelvic recurrence rate after abdominoperineal resection and low anterior resection for rectal cancer before and after introduction of the stapling technique. *World J Surg*. 1983;7:616–619.

718. Ohman U, Svenberg T. EEA stapler for mid-rectum carcinoma. Review of recent literature and own initial experience. *Dis Colon Rectum*. 1983;26:775–784.

719. Fegiz G, Angelini L, Bezzi M. Rectal cancer: restorative surgery with the stapling device. *Int Surg*. 1983;68:13–18.

720. Lasson AL, Ekelund GR, Lindstrom CG. Recurrence risk after stapled anastomosis for rectal carcinoma. *Acta Chir Scand*. 1984;150:85–89.

721. Leff EI, Shaver JO, Hoexter B, et al. Anastomotic recurrences after low anterior resection. Stapled vs. hand-sewn. *Dis Colon Rectum*. 1985;28: 164–167.

722. Rosen CB, Beart RW Jr, Ilstrup DM. Local recurrence of rectal carcinoma after hand-sewn and stapled anastomoses. *Dis Colon Rectum*. 1985;28: 305–309.

723. Kennedy HL, Langevin JM, Goldberg SM, et al. Recurrence following stapled coloproctostomy for carcinomas of the mid portion of the rectum. *Surg Gynecol Obstet*. 1985;160:513–516.

724. Colombo PL, Foglieni CL, Morone C. Analysis of recurrence following curative low anterior resection and stapled anastomoses for carcinoma of the middle third and lower rectum. *Dis Colon Rectum*. 1987;30:457–464.

725. Rubbini M, Vettorello GF, Guerrera C, et al. A prospective study of local recurrence after resection and low stapled anastomosis in 183 patients with rectal cancer. *Dis Colon Rectum*. 1990;33: 117–121.

726. Polk HC Jr, Spratt JS Jr. The results of treatment of perineal recurrence of cancer of the rectum. *Cancer*. 1979;43:952–955.

727. Wilking N, Herrera L, Petrelli NJ, Mittelman A. Pelvic and perineal recurrences after abdominoperineal resection for adenocarcinoma of the rectum. *Am J Surg*. 1985;150:561–563.

728. Keynes WM. Implantation from the bowel lumen in cancer of the large intestine. *Ann Surg*. 1961; 153:357.

729. Southwick HW, Harradige WH, Cole WH. Recurrence at the suture line following resection for carcinoma of the colon: incidence following preventive measures. *Am J Surg*. 1962;103:86.

730. Andersen B, Clemmesen T, Sprechler M, Baden H. Anastomotic recurrences and five-year survival rate after low anterior resection for cure in 128 patients with rectal cancer. *Scand J Gastroenterol*. 1971;6:449–451.

731. Pihl E, Hughes ES, McDermott FT, Price AB. Recurrence of carcinoma of the colon and rectum at the anastomotic suture line. *Surg Gynecol Obstet*. 1981;153:495–496.

732. Pacini P, Cionini L, Pirtoli L, Clatto S, Tucci E, Sebaste L. Symptomatic recurrences of carcinoma of the rectum and sigmoid. *Dis Colon Rectum*. 1986;29:865–868.

733. Sannella NA. Abdominoperineal resection following anterior resection. *Cancer.* 1976;38:378–381.

734. Segall MM, Goldberg SM, Nivatvongs S, et al. Abdominoperineal resection for recurrent cancer following anterior resection. *Dis Colon Rectum.* 1981;24:80–84.

735. Ketcham AS. The management of recurrent rectal cancer. *Can J Surg.* 1985;28:422–424.

736. Vassilopoulos PP, Ledesma EJ, Yoon JM, Jung O, Mittelman A. Surgical treatment of metastatic colorectal adenocarcinoma. *Dis Colon Rectum.* 1981;24:265–271.

737. Benotti PN, Bothe A, Eyere RC, Cady B, McDermott MV, Steele G. Management of recurrent pelvic tumors. *Arch Surg.* 1987;122:457–460.

738. Beart RW Jr, Martin JK Jr, Gunderson LL. Management of recurrent rectal cancer. *Mayo Clin Proc.* 1986;61:448–450.

739. Sugarbaker PH, Corlew S. Influence of surgical techniques on survival in patients with colorectal cancer: a review. *Dis Colon Rectum.* 1982;25:545–557.

740. Pearlman NW, Stiegmann GV, Donohue RE. Extended resection of fixed rectal cancer. *Cancer.* 1989;63:2438–2441.

741. Takagi H, Morimoto T, Hara S, Suzuki R, Horio S. Seven cases of pelvic exenteration combined with sacral resection for locally recurrent rectal cancer. *J Surg Oncol.* 1986;32:184–188.

742. Donald EH, Welch CE, Nathanson J. One hundred untreated cancers of the rectum. *N Engl J Med.* 1936;214:451.

743. Lahey FH. Selection of operation and technique of abdominoperineal resection for carcinoma of the rectum. *Surg Clin North Am.* 1946;26:528.

744. Bordos DC, Baker RR, Cameron JL. An evaluation of palliative abdominoperineal resection for carcinoma of the rectum. *Surg Gynecol Obstet.* 1974;139:731–733.

745. Moran MR, Rothenberger DA, Lahr CJ, Buls JG, Goldberg SM. Palliation for rectal cancer. Resection? Anastomosis? *Arch Surg.* 1987;122:640–643.

746. Wexner SD, Brabbee GW. Treatment of locally recurrent rectal carcinoma: a multidisciplined approach. *Contemp Surg.* 1986;28:53–58.

747. Whiteley HW, Stearns MW, Leaming RH, Deddish MR. Radiation therapy in the palliative management of patients with recurrent cancer of the rectum and colon. *Surg Clin North Am.* 1969;49:381–387.

748. Kligerman MM. Radiation therapy for rectal carcinoma. *Semin Oncol.* 1976;3:407.

749. Boulware RJ, Caderao JB, Delclos L, Wharton JT, Peters LJ. Whole pelvis megavoltage irradiation with single dose of 1,000 rads to palliate advanced gynecologic cancers. *Int J Radiat Oncol Biol Phys.* 1979;5:333.

750. James RD, Johnson RJ, Eddleston B, Zheng GL, Jones JM. Prognostic factors in locally recurrent rectal carcinoma treated by radiotherapy. *Br J Surg.* 1983;70:469–472.

751. Dobrowsky W, Schmid AP. Radiotherapy of presacral recurrence following radical surgery for rectal carcinoma. *Dis Colon Rectum.* 1985;28:917–919.

752. Cummings BJ, Rider WA, Harwood AR, Keane TJ, Thomas GM. Radical external beam radiation therapy for adenocarcinoma of the rectum. *Dis Colon Rectum.* 1983;26:30–36.

753. Sischy B. The role of radiation therapy in the management of carcinoma of the rectum. *Contemp Surg.* 1987;30:13–26.

754. Taylor I. Neoplasms: radiotherapy, chemotherapy and immunotherapy. *Curr Opin Gastroenterol.* 1986;2:31–39.

755. Hunter JG, Bowers JH, Burt RW, et al. Lasers in endoscopic gastrointestinal surgery. *Am J Surg.* 1984;148:736–741.

756. Deschner WK, Fleischer DE. GI laser therapy: what's in store? *Contemp Gastroenterol.* May/June 1991:8–22.

757. Lambert R, Sabben G. Laser therapy for colorectal neoplasms. *Lasers Surg Med.* 1983;3:147.

758. Bowers J. Nd:YAG laser in malignant colorectal obstruction. In: Fleischer D, Jensen D, Bright-Asare P, eds. *Therapeutic Laser Endoscopy in Gastrointestinal Disease.* Boston: Martinus Nijhoff; 1983:139.

759. Kiefhaber P, Kiefhaber K, Haber F, et al. Endoscopic applications of Nd:YAG laser radiation in the gastrointestinal tract. In: Joffe SN, ed. *Nd:YAG Laser in Medicine and Surgery.* New York: Elsevier; 1983:5–14.

760. Groissier VW. YAG laser therapy of gastrointestinal tumors. *Gastrointest Endosc.* 1984;30:311–312.

761. Russin DJ, Kaplan SR, Goldberg RI, Barkin JS. Neodymium-TAG laser: a new palliative tool in the treatment of colorectal cancer. *Arch Surg.* 1986;121:1399–1403.

762. Mathus-Vliegen EM, Tytgat GN. Laser ablation and palliation in colorectal malignancy. Results of a multicenter inquiry. *Gastrointest Endosc.* 1986;32:393–396.

763. Escourrou J, Delvaux M, Frexinos J, et al. Treatment of rectal cancer with the neodymium-YAG laser. *Gastroenterol Clin Biol.* 1986;10:152–157.

764. Brunetaud JM, Maunoury V, Ducrotte P, Cochelard D, Cortot A, Paris JC. Palliative treat-

ment of rectosigmoid carcinoma by laser endoscopic photoablation. *Gastroenterology*. 1987;92: 663–668.

765. Barr H, Krasner N, Boulos PB, Chatlani P, Bown SG. Photodynamic therapy for colorectal cancer: a quantitative pilot study. *Br J Surg*. 1990;77(1): 93–96.

766. Low DE, Kozarek RA, Ball TJ, Patterson DJ, Hill LD. Colorectal neodymium-YAG photoablative therapy. Comparing applications and complications on both sides of the peritoneal reflection. *Arch Surg*. 1989;124:684–688.

767. Birnbaum PL, Mercer CD. Laser fulguration for palliation of rectal tumours. *Can J Surg*. 1990;33: 299–301.

768. Loizou LA, Grigg D, Boulos PB, Bown SG. Endoscopic Nd:YAG laser treatment of rectosigmoid cancer. *Gut*. 1990;31:812–816.

769. Mathus-Viegen EM, Tytgat GN. Nd:YAG laser photocoagulation in gastroenterology: its role in palliation of colorectal cancer. *Lasers Med Sci*. 1986;1:75–80.

770. Van Cutsem E, Boonen A, Geboes G, et al. Risk factors which determine long term outcome of neodymium-YAG laser palliation of colorectal carcinoma. *Int J Colorectal Dis*. 1989;4:9–11.

771. Coombs DW, Saunders RL, Gaylor MS, et al. Relief of continuous chronic pain by intraspinal narcotics infusion via an implanted reservoir. *JAMA*. 1983;250;2236–2239.

772. Gunderson LL, Cohen AM, Welch CE. Residual, inoperable or recurrent colorectal cancer: interaction of surgery and radiotherapy. *Am J Surg*. 1980;139:518–525.

773. Ciatto S, Pacini P. Radiation therapy of recurrences of carcinoma of the rectum and sigmoid after surgery. *Acta Radiol Oncol*. 1982;12:105–109.

774. Ray DR, Maurer DD. Electrical neurological stimulation systems: a review of contemporary methodology. *Surg Neurol*. 1975;4:82.

775. Onofrio BM, Yaksh TL, Arnold PG. Continuous low-dose intrathecal morphine administration in the treatment of chronic pain of malignant origin. *Mayo Clin Proc*. 1981;56:516.

776. Schwartz AG. High cervical cordotomy: techniques and results. *Clin Neurosurg*. 1962;8:282.

777. Leavens ME. Neurosurgical relief of pain in cancer patients. *Cancer Bull*. 1981;33:98.

CHAPTER 19

OTHER RECTAL NEOPLASMS

Frank J. Harford

Benign Rectal Neoplasms

Rectal polyps have the same morphologic and histologic characteristics as those found in other parts of the large bowel. They may be classified as neoplastic polyps, which include tubular adenomas, villous adenomas, and tubovillous adenomas, and nonneoplastic polyps, which include such entities as hyperplastic polyps, juvenile polyps, Peutz–Jeghers polyps, and inflammatory polyps (Table 19-1). The neoplastic polyps, as a group, may be referred to as adenomatous polyps.

Adenomatous Polyps

Tubular Adenoma

Tubular adenomas are composed of branching tubules lines by closely packed cells with reduced amounts of mucus. By definition all adenomatous polyps have dysplastic epithelium. This dysplasia ranges from mild to severe and varies from one area to another within the same polyp (Fig. 19-1A). Tubular adenomas may be sessile or pedunculated. When they are pedunculated, the stalk of the polyp is composed of normal mucosa and submucosa[1] (Fig. 19-1B).

Villous Adenoma

Villous adenomas consist of elongated papillae lined by epithelium which is similar to that found in the tubular adenoma. In a classic villous adenoma, the villi extend in an uninterrupted fashion from the muscularis mucosa to the surface of the polyp (Fig. 19-2A). Grossly they have a soft velvety consistency. Konoshi and Morson

Table 19-1 Rectal Neoplasms

BENIGN
Adenomatous polyps
   Tubular adenomas
   Villous adenomas
Hyperplastic polyps
Hamartomas
   Juvenile Polyps
   Peutz–Jeghers Polyps
Hemangiomas
Miscellaneous polyps

MALIGNANT
Adenocarcinomas (see Chapter 18)
Carcinoids
Lymphomas (see also Chapter 22)
Leiomyosarcomas
Melanomas (see Chapter 16)

require that 80 percent of the polyp have a villous configuration to classify it as a villous adenoma.[2] Frequently these polyps are sessile in character (Fig. 19-2B).

Tubovillous adenomas are polyps that contain both configurations. Konishi and Morson classify these lesions as those that contain from 20 to 80 percent villous components. When an adenomatous polyp is found on sigmoidoscopy, the incidence of synchronous neoplasms in the more proximal colon ranges between 30 and 60 percent. The finding of an adenoma in the rectum is an indication for colonoscopy regardless of the size or type of the rectal lesion.[3,4]

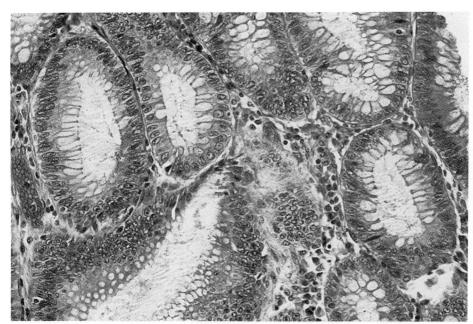

Figure 19-1. Tubular adenoma. (A) Histologic section demonstrating normal colonic glands on the right upper portion and adenamatous changes at the left lower portion and right side. Note crowded cells containing enlarged and hyperchromatic nuclei in the adenoma. (Hematoxylin and eosin, ×400). (Courtesy of Robert C. Petras, M.D., Cleveland, OH.) (B) Gross specimen demonstrating pedunculated polyp.

A

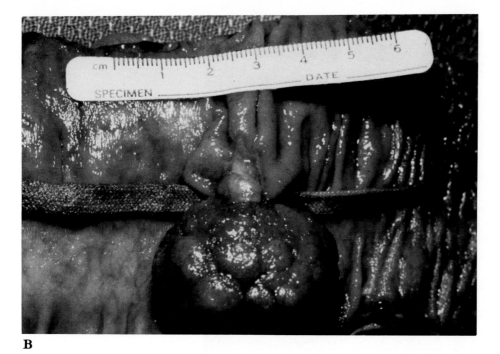

B

Carcinoma in Polyps

The incidence of carcinoma in polyps varies according to the histology of the polyp and its size. The incidence of carcinoma increases with increasing size of the polyp and the proportion of the polyp with a villous configuration (Tables 19-2 and 19-3).[5-8]

Invasive carcinoma is defined as that which invades the muscularis mucosa. If the malignant cells are confined to the mucosa or lamina propria, the lesion is termed carcinoma in situ. The importance of the muscularis mucosa is that the lymphatic vessels are found in the muscularis mucosa, but not above that level.[9] Thus lesions that are more superficial than the muscularis mucosa have no access to these lymphatics and have essentially no metastatic potential.

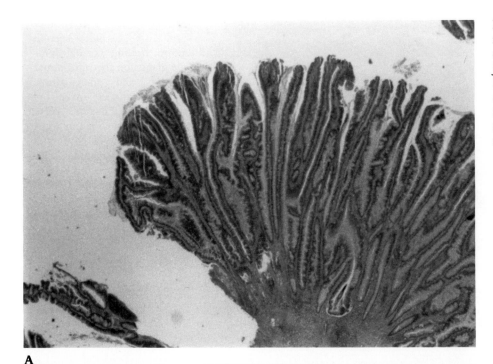

A

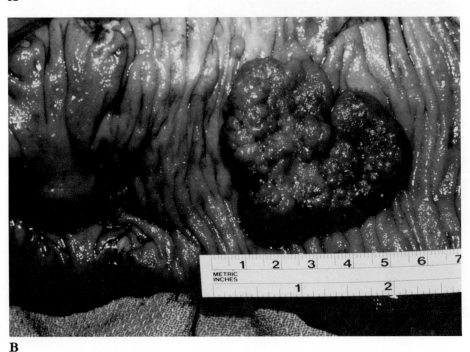

B

Figure 19-2. Villous adenoma. (A) Histologic section demonstrating fingerlike projections of mucosal epithelium. (Hematoxylin and eosin, ×15). (Courtesy of Scott Lee, M.D.) (B) Gross specimen demonstrating sessile polyp.

There is some controversy about whether the patient with an invasive carcinoma is adequately treated with polypectomy or should have a radical resection to remove potential regional lymphatic spread. There is a broad range of opinion in the literature regarding optimal management. There are those who favor radical surgical resection for all patients with invasive carcinoma, and others who favor a more selective policy.

Advocates of surgical resection for all polyps with invasive malignancy cite a study done by Colacchio and colleagues in which they demonstrated a 25 percent incidence of nodal metastases.[10] This study, however, is marred by the fact that not all the polyps in this series were removed endoscopically. Some were removed from resected specimens in the pathology laboratory. These polyps conceivably may not have been suitable

Table 19-2   Tubular Adenoma: Invasive Carcinoma, %

Author	<1 cm	1–2 cm	2–3 cm	>3 cm
Enterline et al[5]	1.1	15	60	100
Grinnel and Lane[6]	0.6	4.7	9.1	13.8
Day and Morson[7]	1	10.2	34*	

* All polyps > 2 cm.

for endoscopic polypectomy or would have had histologically positive margins if they were removed endoscopically rather than manually.

Wilcox and Beck, in a review of 39 studies, found the

incidence of nodal metastases to range between 1 and 7 percent.[11] Haggitt and colleagues have devised a staging system applicable to both pedunculated and sessile polyps in which the depth of malignant invasion can be depicted in an accurate and reproducible way (Fig. 19-3).[12] Level 1 carcinoma is limited to the head of the polyp. Level 2 carcinoma invades the neck of the adenoma. Level 3 invades the stalk, and Level 4 invades the submucosa below the polyp but does not extend into the muscularis propria. As can be seen in the illustration, any invasion into the submucosa in a sessile polyp is defined as level 4. Nivatvongs and co-workers at the Mayo Clinic reviewed 151 patients with colorectal polyps containing invasive carcinoma who were treated with resection.[13] In patients with sessile polyps, the

Table 19-3   Villous Adenoma: Invasive Carcinoma, %

Author	<1.0 cm	1–1.9 cm	2–2.9 cm	3–3.9 cm	4–6 cm
Enterline et al[5]	7.0	7.0	11.0	22	16
Grinnel and Lane[6]	12.5	26.7	21.4	436	37.2
Quan and Castro[8]	0	5	4	15.4	38.2
Day and Morson[7]	14	25.7	60.3*	0	0

* All polyps > 2 cm

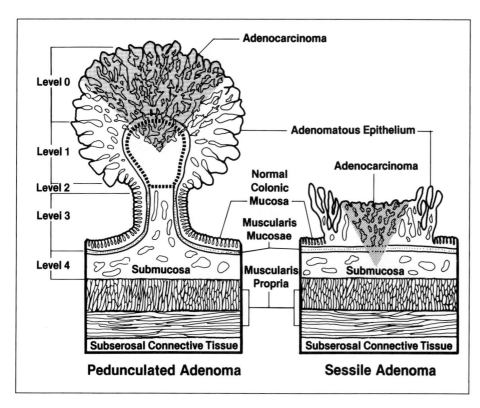

Figure 19-3. Polyp staging system. (*From*: Haggitt RC, Glotzbach RC, Soffer EE, et al. Prognostic factors in colorectal carcinomas arising in adenomas: implications for lesions removed by endoscopic polypectomy. *Gastroenterology*. 1985;89: 328–336.)

Table 19-4   Suggested Criteria for Colonic Resection

Sessile polyps removed piecemeal with level 4 invasion
Any polyp with invasion of the margin of resection
Any polyp with poorly differentiated carcinoma
Pedunculated polyp with level 4 invasion
Any polyp with invasion of submucosal lymphatic channels
Inability to achieve complete endoscopic resection with a tumor free margin

Modified from: Wexner SD. Management of the malignant polyp. *Semin Colon Rectal Surg.* 1991;2:22–27.

incidence of lymph node metastases was 10 percent. For pedunculated polyps, the overall incidence of lymph node metastases was 6 percent. However, there was no incidence of lymph node metastases when the depth of invasion was limited to the head, neck, and stalk of the polyp (levels 1, 2, and 3). When the depth of invasion reached to level 4 the risk of lymph node metastases was 27 percent.[12]

Wexner, in a review of the literature on malignant polyps, has suggested several criteria for colonic resection based on the available data (Table 19-4).[14] He emphasized the absolute necessity for clear communication between the endoscopist, the pathologist, and the surgeon to determine the most appropriate therapy for each individual. If the patient does not meet the criteria for surgical resection, endoscopy should be repeated at 3 and 6 months to observe the polypectomy site. If this can be identified, a biopsy should be taken to rule out local recurrence.

Treatment

Pedunculated and small sessile polyps can be easily treated endoscopically. Large sessile polyps must be treated surgically. Sessile polyps in the lower two thirds of the rectum can be excised or fulgurated transanally. The procedure is described in Figure 19-4. The technique includes submucosal injection of epinephrine in a 1:200,000 dilution. This enables the operator to resect the polyp in the submucosal plane and decreases bleeding. The mucosal defect may then be closed or may quite safely be left open. Completely circumferential lesions may be treated in this manner as well. There is no reason to do a proctectomy even for large circumferential tumors unless they harbor invasive malignancy. If a large circumferential lesion is removed, an attempt should be made to close the mucosa so as to avoid postoperative stricture. In circumferential lesions,

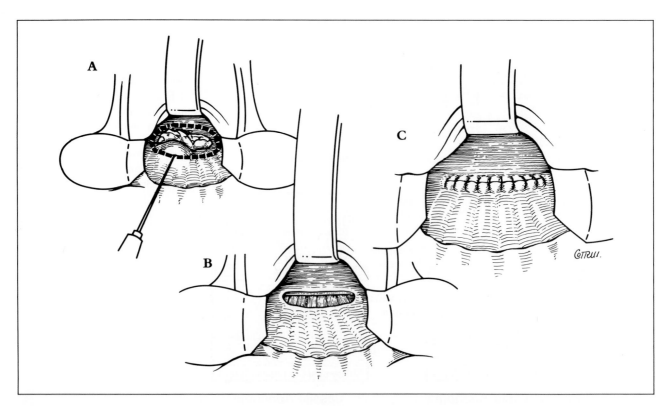

Figure 19-4.   Transanal excision. (A) Polyp excised. (B) Mucosal defect left open. (C) Mucosal defect closed.

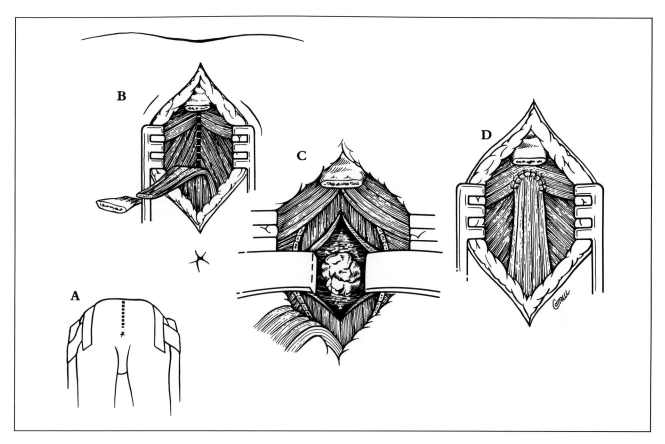

Figure 19-5.   Kraske approach. (A) Skin incision. (B) Anococcygeal ligament detached and coccyx excised. (C) Levator ani muscles incised and posterior rectum opened in midline exposing mass. (D) After excision of mass, divided layers and muscles are reapproximated.

this can be done by suturing the muscularis propria of the rectum in a manner similar to that described by Delorme for the treatment of rectal procidentia.[14] This shortens the rectum and permits primary suturing of the proximal and distal mucosa.[15]

If the lesion is more proximal, it may be approached by either the posterior Kraske approach (Fig. 19-5)[16] or the transsphincteric York–Mason technique (Fig. 19-6).[17] These techniques are discussed in more detail in Chapter 18.

If the diagnosis of invasive malignancy is established by biopsy, one can proceed to the definitive cancer operation without preliminary polypectomy. A negative biopsy, however, is not conclusive because the sampling error is great in these lesions. Therefore all polyps must be completely removed and carefully sectioned to exclude invasive carcinoma.

There has been some recent enthusiasm in the literature for laser ablation of these lesions.[18] There is some risk involved in laser ablation because the presence of invasive malignancy is not known unless the entire polyp is carefully examined microscopically.[19]

Hyperplastic Polyps

Hyperplastic polyps, sometimes referred to as meta-plastic polyps, are sessile growths that are usually slightly paler in color than the surrounding mucosa. Most are less than 5.0 mm in diameter; they can be single or multiple. Histologic examination reveals the crypts to be elongated. The upper parts of the crypts show papillary infoldings of normal-looking columnar, epithelial, and goblet cells. The lower parts of the crypts have epithelial cells with more basophilic cytoplasm and contain fewer goblet cells. The cells are crowded together and project into the lumen in folds or tufts. On cross section, this gives a characteristic stellate branching appearance of the glands (Fig. 19-7). These polyps are generally regarded as the result of a disorder of maturation of unknown origin. It should be noted that not all small sessile polyps seen in the rectum are hyperplastic. Biopsy is essential to identify the nature of the polyp accurately.[3] Although it was previously thought that there was no relationship between hyperplastic polyps and colonic adenomas, there has been some

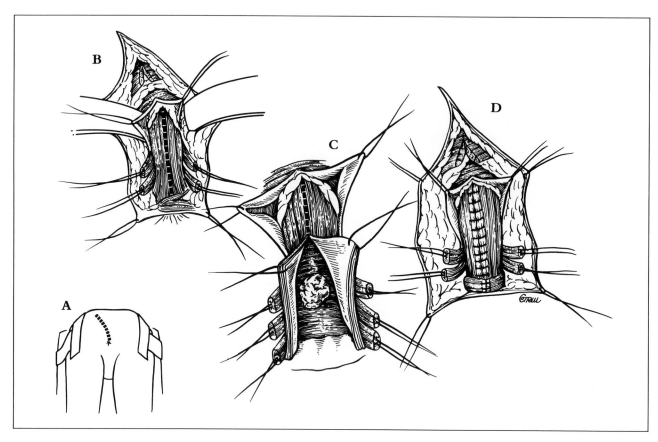

Figure 19-6.   York–Mason transsphincteric approach. (A) Skin incision. (B) Divided ends of external sphincter, puborectalis, and levator ani muscles. (C) Internal sphincter and rectal wall divided to expose mass. (D) After excision of mass, divided layers and muscles are reapproximated.

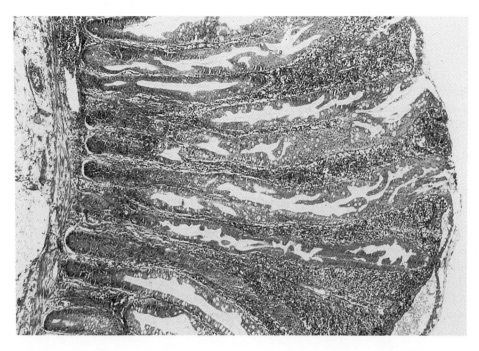

Figure 19-7.   Hyperplastic polyp with serrated configuration of glands. (Hematoxylin and eosin, ×400). (Courtesy of Robert C. Petras, M.D., Cleveland, OH.)

recent evidence that they too are indicators of more proximal adenomas and should prompt a complete colonoscopy.[20] Although this concept is not universally accepted, it is the policy of the editors to recommend colonoscopy to most patients in whom any rectosigmoid polyp is discovered.[21] This is done without preliminary sigmoidoscopic biopsy, since knowledge of the histopathology will not alter the decision-making process.

Juvenile Polyps

Juvenile polyps are usually spherical, smooth-surfaced polyps that often have a cherry red color. They can occur at any age but are the most commonly found polyp in the pediatric age group. They may be solitary or multiple and are most commonly found in the rectum.[22] They usually have a thin stalk and not uncommonly will spontaneously torque and autoamputate. Histologically, they are quite distinctive, consisting of normal columnar epithelial cells and goblet cells arranged in cystically dilated glands set in an abundant stroma (Fig. 19-8). The surface epithelium is often inflamed or ulcerated. These lesions are thought to be hamartomatous or inflammatory in nature and without any malignant potential. However, a juvenile polyposis syndrome has been described which does appear to be associated with an increased incidence of colorectal carcinoma.[23,24]

Peutz–Jeghers Polyps

These polyps are hamartomatous polyps that also have a very distinctive histologic appearance. Grossly, they can be either pedunculated or sessile and have a coarsely lobulated surface. Microscopically, they consist of elongated and branched glands lined by normal-appearing epithelial cells. The polyp is supported by a stroma of smooth muscle which is arranged in a treelike fashion (Fig. 19-9). The Peutz–Jeghers syndrome is a autosomal dominant inherited disease characterized by hamartomatous polyps of the gastrointestinal tract and mucocutaneous pigmentation. These polyps are predominantly located in the small bowel but are also found in the colon and rectum. These hamartomatous polyps are not generally regarded as being premalignant. However, several studies have found an excessive incidence of malignancy in patients with this syndrome. The malignancies were both intestinal and extraintestinal.[25,26] Spiegelman and colleagues, in a review of 72 patients with Peutz–Jeghers syndrome in the same St. Mark's Polyposis Registry, found malignant tumors in 22 percent of the patients.[26] All but 1 of these patients died of their tumors. There were 9 gastrointestinal tumors and 7 extraintestinal tumors. These authors recommended early and intensive surveillance as the chance of dying of cancer by the age of 57 in this series was 48 percent. If these patients do come to laparotomy, they should have intraoperative enteroscopy to ensure that the gastrointestinal tract is completely cleared of these tumors.[27]

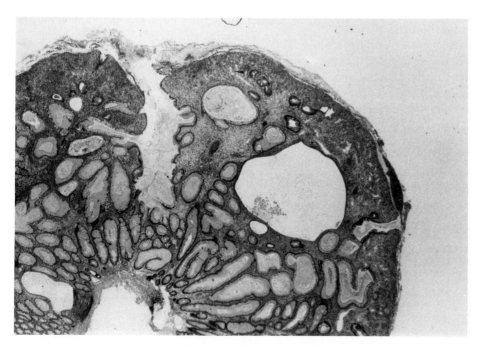

Figure 19-8. Juvenile polyp demonstrating surface ulceration covered by granulation tissue, cystically dilated glands filled with mucus, and inflamed and edematous stroma. (Hematoxylin and eosin, ×15). (Courtesy of Scott Lee, M.D., and Henry Cheu, M.D.)

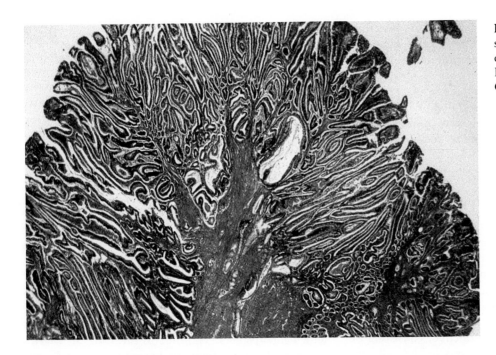

Figure 19-9. Peutz–Jeghers syndrome. (Hematoxylin and eosin, ×160). (Courtesy of Robert C. Petras, M.D., Cleveland, OH.)

Hemangiomas

A case of hemangioma of the rectum was first described by Philips in 1839.[28] Since that time, approximately 200 cases of hemangiomas of the large bowel have been reported.[29] The majority of these large-bowel lesions are located in the rectum or rectosigmoid.

Clinical Presentation

Patients with large-bowel hemangiomas usually present with a history of repeated episodes of hematochezia, often starting in childhood. Occasionally patients may have symptoms of tenesmus, urgency, or incomplete defecation. In the series of cases reported from St. Mark's Hospital, 80 percent of the patients had had at least one surgical procedure performed before the correct diagnosis was made.[30] Skin lesions may be seen in association with colorectal hemangiomas. Nader and Margolin found cutaneous lesions in half of the series of pediatric patients with large-bowel hemangiomas.[31] Those patients with associated skin lesions were likely to have multiple rather than solitary intestinal lesions. A familial tendency for gastrointestinal hemangiomas has also been noted. Cavernous hemangiomas may also be found occasionally in association with a Klippel–Trenaunay syndrome.[32]

Pathology

Hemangiomas can be classified as capillary, cavernous, or mixed. The large majority of large-bowel hemangiomas are cavernous. They are composed of networks of tiny capillary-like vascular structures. These vessels are closely packed together but have no true capsule. Cavernous hemangiomas are composed of large thin-walled vascular channels. These lesions may be discrete or diffuse and expansive or infiltrating. A variety of cavernous hemangiomas is called *multiple phlebectasia*. These are collections of small discrete cavernous lesions. A few hemangiomas have elements of both the capillary and the cavernous type of lesions. The expansive, infiltrating type of lesions may extend into adjacent structures such as the bladder or uterus, but they usually continue to be nourished by their own vascular supply and not that of the adjacent structure.[33]

Whether these lesions are truly neoplastic or are simply congenital vascular malformations remains the subject of some debate. There is, however, general agreement that they develop from embryonic sequestrations of mesodermal tissue. Capillary hemangiomas are considered to be a result of anomalous development in the first stage of mesodermal stem cell differentiation. Cavernous hemangiomas are aberrations in a later stage of development.[34]

Diagnosis

The diagnosis of rectal hemangioma can usually be made without difficulty on physical and proctoscopic examination. One should be alerted to the possibility of the diagnosis by a history of recurrent painless hematochezia, usually starting in childhood. Furthermore, any cutaneous hemangioma found on general physical examination should alert one's suspicions. A significant number of these patients are also anemic, although many patients are asymptomatic. Cavernous hemangiomas also may be associated with thrombocytopenia, defibrination, and depression of Factors V and VIII; this has been referred to as a Kasabach–Merritt syndrome.[35]

On digital examination, the tumor may be felt as a soft compressible mass that is poorly defined. The stool is often Hemoccult® positive. On proctoscopic examination, these lesions will be seen as wine- or plum-colored masses that collapse with insufflation or pressure from the proctoscope. The small cavernous hemangioma may present as a bluish discoloration on a polyp. Capillary hemangiomas often appear as cherry red spots on the mucosa. The rectal mucosa over the lesions may show chronic inflammatory changes both on gross examination and microscopically after superficial biopsy. This appearance, on occasion, will lead to a missed diagnosis.

If there is a fairly high suspicion that a cavernous hemangioma is present on digital and endoscopic examination, biopsy is ill advised. Total colonoscopy should be done to assess the extent of the lesion and the possibility of multiple lesions. Of the patients with intestinal hemangiomas, phlebolith clusters are noted on plain abdominal films in 50 percent. Mesenteric angiography will detect these lesions in two thirds of the cases, and some authors consider this study an essential part of the evaluation of a cavernous hemangioma because it defines the vascular supply of the lesion.[36] Computed tomography has recently been used in the evaluation of these lesions. It is useful when defining the limits of the lesion and detecting infiltration of local structures.[36] Magnetic resonance imaging (MRI) has also been used in the evaluation of these lesions.[37]

Treatment

Capillary hemangiomas or small cavernous hemangiomas may be treated endoscopically with electric snare cautery or local resection. Larger cavernous hemangiomas, however, do not lend themselves to local treatment. Several nonoperative remedies have been reported such as injection of sclerosing agents, radiotherapy, and cryosurgery, but surgical resection is clearly the therapy of choice in the medically fit patient.[29] Although abdominoperineal resection has been recommended[38] as treatment for rectal cavernous hemangiomas, recent successful applications of sphincter-sparing techniques have been reported.[39-41]

Miscellaneous Benign Tumors

Other rare lesions have been reported in the rectum including lymphangioma,[42] myoblastoma (granular cell tumor),[43] and neuroma,[44] as well as aggregations of ectopic tissue.[45] Lymphangiomas in the large bowel are usually small and can be treated endoscopically. However, there have been some cases in which the lesions were large and symptomatic and surgical resection was necessary. Ectopic tissue in the rectum usually presents as a small polyp or ulceration and is amenable to local treatment. The other lesions are usually small and discovered incidentally on examination.

Malignant Neoplasms

Carcinoids

Carcinoid tumors of the gastrointestinal tract may occur in the foregut, midgut, or hindgut. In most reported series of gastrointestinal carcinoids, the rectum is among the three most common sites along with the ileum and the appendix.[46-48]

Clinical Presentation

Most rectal carcinoids are asymptomatic and are found incidentally on screening examinations. The majority of these tumors are submucosal in location and are detected either by palpation or by proctoscopic examination. They usually appear as yellow submucosal nodules with an overlying intact mucosa. They are almost always solitary tumors, although multiple rectal carcinoids have been reported.[49,50] Several authors have found the anterior wall to be the most common location in the rectum. Some rectal carcinoids are polypoid, ulcerated, or even, in advanced cases, circumferential constricting lesions, but these are uncommon. Ulceration of the lesion is usually indicative of a more aggressive tumor.

Pathogenesis

These tumors are thought to arise from the entero-chromaffin cells in the crypts of Lieberkuhn which are first described by Kultschitzky in 1897. Gossett and Mason demonstrated that the granules of these Kultschitzky cells and those cells found in many carcinoid tumors had an affinity for silver[51]; for this reason, they are called carcinoids argentaffin tumors. Because of the similarity of the staining characteristics of these cells, it is generally accepted that carcinoid tumors arise from the Kultschitzky cell.

Pathology

Carcinoid tumors are composed of uniformly sized small polygonal, oval, or cuboid cells (Fig. 19-10) The

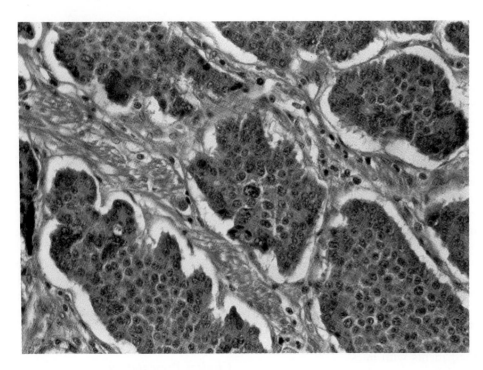

Figure 19-10. Carcinoid tumor of rectum. Note solid clumps and ribbons of uniform, pale cells. (Hematoxylin and eosin, ×1000.) (Courtesy of Robert C. Petras, M.D., Cleveland, OH.)

nuclei are very round and regular in size and mitotic figures are rare; multiple mitotic figures are usually associated with aggressive tumors. Conversely, the absence of mitoses does not argue for benign growth. Soga and Tazawa have characterized the morphology of these tumors and have divided them into five types: (1) tumors with nodular solid nests and peripheral invading cords, (2) tumors with a trabecular or ribbonlike structure, (3) tumors with an acinar or rosettelike structure, (4) tumors with structures of lesser or atypical differentiation, and (5) a mixed type of tumor with combinations of any of the four patterns.[52] Some authors have suggested that those tumors which are differentiated or have abundant mitotic figures should more properly be classified as neuroendocrine carcinomas.[53]

Histochemical Characteristics

Mason first described the staining of the granules in the cells of an appendiceal carcinoid with ammoniacal silver nitrate. This has been called the argentaffin reaction. Some tumors, however, will stain with silver salts only if a reducing agent is added. This reaction is termed agyrophilic. In earlier investigations, foregut carcinoids were usually found to be agyrophilic, midgut tumors were of the argentaffin type, and hindgut carcinoids generally did not stain with either method. Recent studies, however, using modified staining techniques,[54] have reported that some rectal carcinoids demonstrate a positive argentaffin reaction and a great many are agyrophilic.

Immunochemical stains used in the peroxidase method have been used to identify both general endocrine markers, and specific hormones. In a review of 84 carcinoids of the colon and rectum on file at the Armed Forces Institute of Technology, Federspiel and associates found that neuron-specific endolase was the most sensitive, being positive in 87 percent of the tumors.[55] The reactions, however, were often weak and usually diffuse. Fifty-eight percent of the tumors where chromogranin positive, and 50 percent showed diffuse reactivity to Leu-7. Serotonin and human pancreatic polypeptide was positive in 45 and 46 percent of the tumors respectively. These authors found a few tumors that stained for glucagon, somatostatin, ACTH, and gastrin. Prostatic acid phosphatase was present in 82 percent of the tumors and carcinoembryonic antigen (CEA) was present in 25 percent.

Treatment

Surgical treatment for rectal carcinoid is based on the findings of two studies of Peskin and Orloff published in 1959 and 1971, respectively.[56,57] They recommended that a tumor that is 2.0 cm or greater in size or that demonstrates invasion of the muscularis propria should be treated with radical resection, that is, low anterior resection or abdominoperineal resection. Tumors less than 2.0 cm in size and without muscularis propria invasion could be adequately treated with local transanal excision. This recommendation continues to be supported.[58] One recent review concluded that is the criteria for size and invasiveness were used to determine the need for a radical resection, only 6 percent of all tumors with nodal metastases would be inadequately treated.[59]

Despite generally widespread acceptance of the Peskin and Orloff guidelines, however, this recommendation has been recently challenged. Two series of patients have been reported in which all patients with rectal carcinoids with nodal metastases died of their tumor despite radical surgical resection.[60] The authors of these studies concluded that if the lesion can be completely resected with local excision, no benefit will be gained by a more radical procedure. This contrasted with the larger collected series from the National Cancer Institute in which a 5-year survival of 44 percent was reported for carcinoids of the rectum and rectosigmoid that had regional metastases.[47] One should keep in mind that often these carcinoid tumors are slow growing and a 5-year survival statistic may not accurately reflect the actual mortality from the disease.

Malignant Lymphoma

Malignant lymphoma of the rectum is rare; during a 27-year period at the Mayo Clinic only 61 cases of lymphoma with rectal involvement were noted.[61] In only 12 of these cases was the lymphoma confined to the rectum. In a 10-year period at Los Angeles County/USC Medical Center only 3 rectal lymphomas were noted.[62] During this same time period 233 rectal carcinomas were identified.

Clinical Presentation

There is little in the clinical presentation of rectal lymphoma to distinguish it from adenocarcinoma. It has been stated, however, that the triad of a large rectal tumor, a short clinical history, and a lack of emaciation might be suggestive of the diagnosis.[63]

Pathology

Most of these tumors are described as sessile or raised masses of variable dimensions. In the Mayo Clinic series, most of the tumors were described as nodular with overlying normal mucosa.[61] In 30 percent of those cases, the tumor had infiltrated through the mucosa and caused ulceration. Unlike adenocarcinomas, these lymphomatous ulcers were surrounded by folds or overlying mucosal edges. These thick rubbery folds appear to be caused by diffuse lymphocytic infiltration (Fig. 19-11). Sometimes, however, these lesions are indistinguishable from typical adenocarcinomas in their appearance. Polypoid lesions of the rectum may be seen in diffuse lymphomatous polyposis, a condition in which multiple polypoid lesions of malignant lymphoma are distributed throughout the gastrointestinal tract.[63,64]

Characterization of the histologic type of lymphoma is confusing because a plethora of classification systems are used to describe the paltry number of cases. Shepherd and associates, from St. Mark's Hospital, however, have analyzed 45 cases of colorectal lymphoma

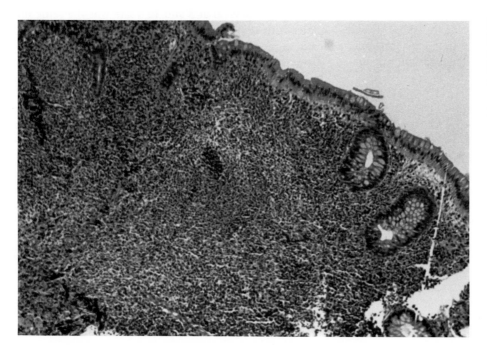

Figure 19-11. Non-Hodgkins lymphoma. The mucosa (lamina propria) is infiltrated by malignant lymphocytes. (Hematoxylin and eosin, ×75). (Courtesy of Scott Lee, M.D.)

morphologically and with immunohistochemistry and found that all tumors were of the B-cell phenotype.[65] Seven of the 45 patients had a history of ulcerative colitis, and other cases of lymphoma arising in ulcerative colitis have been reported.[66,67] There has been one case of rectal lymphoma arising in radiation-injured bowel.[68] Recently, there have been several reports of anorectal lymphoma in homosexual men, most of whom had proven AIDS.[69,70]

Treatment and Outcome

Patients in whom the rectal involvement is part of a more widespread lymphoma are not candidates for primary curative surgery. However, palliative procedures done for bleeding, obstruction, or perforation may be indicated. The available data indicate that patients with lymphoma confined to the rectum should be treated surgically if they are operative candidates.[61,71] Perry and associates reported that 8 of 10 patients with lymphoma confined to the rectum treated with radiotherapy, chemotherapy, or both died, whereas 5 of 9 patients treated by surgical resection survived.[72] Postoperative radiotherapy is usually recommended although there are too few cases to allow adequate study of the efficacy of this adjuvant therapy. There is some evidence that survival is enhanced in gastrointestinal lymphomas in general if surgical resection is followed by radiotherapy.[73]

Leiomyosarcoma

Leiomyoma and leiomyosarcoma are tumors which can arise in the rectum or the anus. Smooth muscle tumors of the rectum comprise 7 percent of those found throughout the gastrointestinal tract. Approximately half of the rectal tumors are benign and half are malignant. Leiomyosarcoma represents approximately 0.1 percent of all rectal malignancies.[74]

Clinical Presentation

The most frequent symptoms are rectal bleeding, constipation, rectal pain, and fullness or diarrhea.[75] The type and severity of symptoms are related to the location and size of the tumor. The great majority of these tumors can be felt on digital examination of the rectum.

Most of the tumors are firm in consistency. Ulceration of the rectal mucosa is found about 40 percent of the time.[76]

Pathology

There tumors may originate from the muscularis mucosa, the muscularis propria, or the smooth muscle in the arterial walls of the rectum. Microscopically, these tumors are composed of fusiform cells with eosinophilic cytoplasm and elongated nuclei. The degree of cellularity and pleomorphism is variable. Histologic distinctions between benign and malignant tumors are often difficult. The features that are more common to leiomyosarcoma are size $\geq$ 5.0 cm in diameter, mitosis $\geq$ 5 per 10 high-powered field, tumor cell necrosis, increased cellularity, and increased cellular atypia. Even tumors that do not fulfill any of these criteria for malignancy may prove to be malignant, however.[77] This aggressive behavior may be initially manifested by a recurrence or metastasis after excision. Hematogenous dissemination is much more common than is lymphatic spread.

Surgical Therapy and Outcome

Benign lesions are adequately treated by local excision. Diamante and Bacon noted an 80 percent recurrence in patients who were treated by local resection.[78] In a collected series, Khalifa and associates found that treatment of leiomyosarcoma by local excision was followed by a 67.5 percent recurrence. Although abdomino-perineal resection was associated with a 19.5 percent recurrence, survival at 5 and 10 years was the same for patients treated with local excision.[76] Quan and Berg have suggested that if the tumor is less than 2.0 cm. in diameter and of a low grade malignancy, local excision including a generous margin of normal tissue is sufficient therapy.[79] Experience at the Mayo Clinic prompted the recommendation of local excision for small lesions confined to the bowel wall and radical excision for larger or more extensive lesions.[75] Minsky and associates have reported the use of local resection with postoperative radiotherapy with good short-term results.[80] The 5- and 10-year survival in Khalifa's collected series is a 38.9 percent and 9.7 percent respectively.[76]

References

1. Robert LEV. *Adenomatous Polyps of the Colon*. New York:Springer-Verlag; 1990:7.
2. Konishi F, Morson B. Pathology of colorectal adenomas: a colonoscopic survey. *J Clin Pathol*. 1982;35:830–841.
3. Warden MJ, Patrelli NJ, Herrera L, Mittelman A.

The role of colonoscopy and flexible sigmoidoscopy in screening for colorectal carcinoma. *Dis Colon Rectum.* 1986;30:52–54.

4. Ryan ME, Norfleet RG, Kirchner JP, et al. The significance of diminutive colonic polyps found at flexible sigmoidoscopy. *Gastrointest Endosc.* 1989;35:85–89.

5. Enterline HT, Evans GW, Mercudo-Lugo R, et al. Malignant potential of adenomas of colon and rectum. *JAMA.* 1962;179:322.

6. Grinnell RS, Lane N. Benign and malignant adenomatous polyps and papillary adenomas of the colon and rectum: an analysis of 1856 tumors in 1335 patients. *Int Abstracts Surg.* 1958;106:519.

7. Day DW, Morson BC. The adenoma-carcinoma sequence. *Major Probl Pathol.* 1978;10:58–71.

8. Quan SHQ, Castro EB. Papillary adenomas (villous tumors): a review of 215 cases. *Dis Colon Rectum.* 1971;14:267.

9. Fenoglio CM, Kay GI, Lane N. Distribution of human colonic lymphatics in normal, hyperplastic, and adenomatous tissue. *Gastroenterology.* 1973;64:51–66.

10. Colacchio TA, Forde KA, Scantlebury VP. Endoscopic polypectomy: inadequate treatment for invasive colorectal carcinoma. *Ann Surg.* 1981;194:704–707.

11. Wilcox GM, Beck JR. Early invasive cancer in adenomatous colonic polyps ("malignant polyps"). Evaluation of the therapeutic options by decisive analysis. *Gastroenterology.* 1987;92:1159–1168.

12. Haggitt RC, Glotzbach RE, Soffer EE, et al. Prognostic factors in colorectal carcinomas arising in adenomas: implications for lesions removed by endoscopic polypectomy. *Gastroenterology.* 1985;89:328–336.

13. Nivatvongs S, Rojanasakul A, Reiman HM, et al. The risk of lymph node metastasis in colorectal polyps with invasive adenocarcinoma. *Dis Colon Rectum.* 1991;34:323–328.

14. Wexner SD. Management of the malignant polyp. *Semin Colon Rectal Surg.* 1991;2:22–27.

15. Parks AG, Stuart A. The management of villous tumors of the large bowel. *Br J Surg.* 1973;60:688.

16. Jorgensen SJ, Ottsen H. Posterior rectotomy for villous tumors of the rectum. *Acta Chir Scand.* 1975;141:680.

17. York-Mason A. Trans-sphincteric surgery of the rectum. *Prog Surg.* 1974;13:66–97.

18. Brunetaud JM, Mosquet L, Houcke M, et al. Villous adenomas of the rectum: results of endoscopic treatment with argon and Nd:YAG lasers. *Gastroenterology.* 1985;89:832–837.

19. Boyer T. Lasers and colon polyps. Technology and pathology: the courtship continues. *Gastroenterology.* 1986;90:2024–2025.

20. Blue MG, Sivak MV, Achkar E, et al. Hyperplastic polyps seen at sigmoidoscopy are markers for additional adenomas seen at colonoscopy. *Gastroenterology.* 1991;100:564–566.

21. Achkar E, Winawer SJ. A hyperplastic polyp is discovered on flexible sigmoidoscopy. Is a full colonoscopy indicated? *Am J Gastroenterol.* 1990;85:367–370.

22. Mazier WP, MacKeigan JM, Billingham RP, Dignan RD. Juvenile polyps of the colon and rectum. *Surg Gynecol Obstet.* 1982;154:829–832.

23. Veale AMO, McColl I, Bussey HJR, Morson BC. Juvenile polyposis coli. *J Med Genet.* 1966;3:5–16.

24. Gilinsky NH, Elliot MS, Price SK, et al. The nutritional consequences and neoplastic potential of juvenile polyposis coli. *Dis Colon Rectum.* 1986;29:417–420.

25. Giardiello FM, Welsh SB, Hamilton SR, et al. Increased risk of cancer in the Peutz–Jeghers syndrome. *N Engl J Med.* 1987;316:1511–1514.

26. Spiegelman AD, Murday V, Phillips RKS. Cancer and the Peutz–Jeghers syndrome. *Gut.* 1989;30:1588–1590.

27. Spiegelman AD, Thomson JPS, Phillips RKS. Towards decreasing the relaparotomy rate in the Peutz–Jeghers syndrome: the role of preoperative small bowel endoscopy. *Br J Surg.* 1990;77:301–302.

28. Philips B. Surgical cases. *London Med Gazette.* 1839;23:514–517.

29. Lyon DT, Mantia AG. Large bowel hemangiomas. *Dis Colon Rectum.* 1984;27:404–414.

30. Jeffrey PJ, Hawley PR, Parks AG. Colo-anal sleeve anastomosis in the treatment of diffuse cavernous hemangioma involving the rectum. *Br J Surg.* 1976;63:678–682.

31. Nader PR, Margolin F. Hemangioma causing gastrointestinal bleeding. *Am J Dis Child.* 1966;111:215–221.

32. Ghahremani GG, Kangarloo H, Volberg F, et al. Diffuse cavernous hemangioma of the colon in the Klippel–Trenaunay syndrome. *Radiology.* 1976;118:673–678.

33. Gentry RW, Docterty MB, Clagett OT. Vascular malformations and vascular tumors of the gastrointestinal tract. *Int Abstracts Surg.* 1949;88:281–323.

34. Bland RI, Abney HT, MacGregor AMC, et al. Hemangiomatosis of the colon and anorectum. *Am Surg.* 1974;40:626–635.

35. Rodriguez-Erdman F, Button L, Murray JE, Moroney WC. Kasabach–Merritt syndrome—coagulo-analytical observations. *Am J Sci.* 1971;261:9–15.

36. Aylward CA, Orangio GR, Lucas GW, Fazio VW. Diffuse cavernous hemangioma of the rectosigmoid—CT scan, a new diagnostic modality, and surgical management using sphincter-saving procedures: report of three cases. *Dis Colon Rectum.* 1988;31:797–802.

37. Lupetin AR. Diffuse cavernous hemangioma of the rectum: evaluation and MRI. *Gastrointest Radiol.* 1990;15:343–345.

38. Coppa GF, Eng K, Localio SA. Surgical management of diffuse cavernous hemangioma of the colon, rectum, and anus. *Surg Gynecol Obstet.* 1984;159:17–22.

39. Jeffrey PJ, Hawley PR, Parks AG. Colo-anal sleeve anastomosis in the treatment of diffuse cavernous haemangioma involving the rectum. *Br J Surg.* 1976;63:678–682.

40. Cunningham JA, Garcia V, Quispe G. Diffuse cavernous rectal hemangioma—sphincter-sparing approach to therapy. *Dis Colon Rectum.* 1989; 32:344–347.

41. Wang CH. Sphincter-saving procedure for treatment of diffuse cavernous hemangioma of the rectum and sigmoid colon. *Dis Colon Rectum.* 1985;28:604–607.

42. Kuramoto S, Sakai S, Tsuda K, et al. Lymphangioma of the large intestine: report of a case. *Dis Colon Rectum.* 1988;31:900–905.

43. Madiedo G, Komorowski RA, Jellani Dhar G. Granular cell tumor (myoblastoma) of the large intestine removed by colonoscopy. *Gastrointest Endosc.* 1980;26:108–109.

44. Attar B, Khurana D, Hlaing-Ray V, Levendoglu H. Mucosal neuroma of the rectosigmoid colon. *Gastrointest Endosc.* 1986;32:219–220.

45. Weitzner S. Ectopic salivary gland tissue in submucosa of rectum. *Dis Colon Rectum.* 1983; 26:814–817.

46. Hajdu SI, Winawer SJ, Laird Myers MP. Carcinoid tumors: a study of 204 cases. *Am J Clin Pathol.* 1974;61:521–528.

47. Godwin JD. Carcinoid tumors: an analysis of 2837 cases. *Cancer.* 1975;560–569.

48. Thompson GB, van Heeren JA, Martin JK, et al. Carcinoid tumors of the gastrointestinal tract: presentation, management, and prognosis. *Surgery.* 1985;98:1054–1062.

49. Scoma JA. Carcinoid tumors of the rectum. *Am J Surg.* 1978;135:708–709.

50. Kanter M, Lechago J. Multiple malignant rectal carcinoid tumors with immunocytochemical demonstration of multiple hormonal substances. *Cancer.* 1987;60:1782–1786.

51. Gosset A, Masson P. Tumeurs endocles de l'appendice. *Presse Med.* 1914;25:237–249.

52. Soga J, Tazawa K. Pathologic analysis of carcinoids: histologic reevaluation of 62 cases. *Cancer.* 1971;28:990–998.

53. Staren ED, Gould VE, Warren WH, et al. Neuroendocrine carcinomas of the colon and rectum: a clinicopathologic evaluation. *Surgery.* 1988;104: 1080–1089.

54. Smith DM, Haggitt RC. A comparative study of generic stains for carcinoid secretory granules. *Am J Surg Pathol.* 1983;7:61–68.

55. Federspiel BH, Burke AP, Sobin LH, Shekitka KM. Rectal and colonic carcinoids: a clinicopathologic study of 84 cases. *Cancer.* 1990;65:135–140.

56. Peskin GW, Orloff MJ. A clinical study of 25 patients with carcinoid tumors of the rectum. *Surg Gynecol Obstet.* 1959;100:673–682.

57. Orloff MJ. Carcinoid tumors of the rectum. *Cancer.* 1971;28:175–180.

58. Naunheim KS, Zeitels J, Kaplan EL, et al. Rectal carcinoid tumors—treatment and prognosis. *Surgery.* 1983;94:670–676.

59. Burke M, Shepherd N, Mann CV. Carcinoid tumours of the rectum and anus. *Br J Surg.* 1987;74:358–361.

60. Sauven P, Ridge JA, Quan SH, Sigurdson ER. Anorectal carcinoid tumors: is aggressive surgery warranted? *Ann Surg.* 1990;211:67–71.

61. Devine RM, Beart RW, Wolff BG. Malignant lymphoma of the rectum. *Dis Colon Rectum.* 1986; 29:821–824.

62. Vanden Heule B, Taylor CR, Terry R, Lukes RJ. Presentation of malignant lymphoma in the rectum. *Cancer.* 1982;49:2602–2607.

63. Ohri SK, Keane PF, Sackier JM, et al. Primary rectal lymphoma and malignant lymphomatous polyposis: two cases illustrating current methods in diagnosis and management. *Dis Colon Rectum.* 1989;32:1071–1074.

64. Fernandes BJ, Amato D, Goldfinger M. Diffuse lymphomatous polyposis of the gastrointestinal tract: a case report with immunohistochemical studies. *Gastroenterology.* 1985;88:1267–1270.

65. Shepherd NA, Hall PA, Coates PJ, Levison DA. Primary malignant lymphoma of the colon and rectum: a histopathological and immunohistochemical analysis of 45 cases with clinicopathological correlations. *Histopathology.* 1988;12:235–252.

66. Baker D, Chiprut RO, Rimer D, et al. Colonic lymphoma in ulcerative colitis. *J Clin Gastroenterol.* 1985;7(5):379–386.

67. Bartolo D, Goepel JR, Parsons MA. Rectal malig-

nant lymphoma in chronic ulcerative colitis. *Gut.* 1982;23:164–168.

68. Sibly TF, Keane RM, Lever JV, Southwood WFW. Rectal lymphoma in radiation injured bowel. *Br J Surg.* 1985;72:879–880.

69. Burkes RL, Meyer PR, Gill PS, et al. Rectal lymphoma in homosexual men. *Arch Intern Med.* 1986;146:913–915.

70. Lee MH, Waxman M, Gillooley JF. Primary malignant lymphoma of the anorectum in homosexual men. *Dis Colon Rectum.* 1986;29:413–416.

71. Richards MA. Lymphoma of the colon and rectum. *Postgrad Med J.* 1986;62:615–620.

72. Perry PM, Cross RM, Morson BC. Primary malignant lymphoma of the rectum (22 cases). *Proc Soc Med.* 1972;65:8.

73. Skudder PA, Schwartz SI. Primary lymphoma of the gastrointestinal tract. *Surg Gynecol Obstet.* 1985:160:5–8.

74. Anderson AP, Dockerty MB, Buie LA. Myomatous tumors of the rectum (leiomyomas and myosarcomas). *Surgery.* 1950;28:642–650.

75. Randleman CD, Wolff BG, Dozois RR, et al. Leiomyosarcoma of the rectum and anus: a series of 22 cases. *Int J Colorectal Dis.* 1989;4:91–96.

76. Khalifa AA, Bong WL, Rao VK, Williams MJ. Leiomyosarcoma of the rectum: report of a case and review of the literature. *Dis Colon Rectum.* 1986;29:427–432.

77. Serra J, Ruiz M, Lloveras B, et al. Surgical outlook regarding leiomyoma of the rectum: report of three cases. *Dis Colon Rectum.* 1989;32:884–887.

78. Diamante M, Bacon HE. Leiomyosarcoma of the rectum: report of a case. *Dis Colon Rectum.* 1967;10:347–351.

79. Quan SHQ, Berg JW. Leiomyoma and leiomyosarcoma of the rectum. *Dis Colon Rectum.* 1962;5:415–425.

80. Minsky BD, Cohen AM, Hajdu SI, Nori D. Sphincter preservation in rectal sarcoma. *Dis Colon Rectum.* 1990;33:319–322.

CHAPTER 20

PRESACRAL TUMORS IN ADULTS

Mark A. Christensen
and Garnet J. Blatchford

Presacral tumors represent an interesting, albeit rare, problem for the surgeon. Lesions in the area arise from a variety of tissues. A knowledge of these tumors is essential to providing appropriate treatment. Just as important is the ability to direct appropriate preoperative testing, avoiding pitfalls that can lead to serious morbidity and even death.

Incidence and Classification

Presacral tumors are rare. Whittaker and Pemberton[1] at the Mayo Clinic estimated the incidence to be 1 in 40,000 registrations. Using a system initially described by Lovelady and Dockerty,[2] these lesions can be classified as either congenital or neoplastic. Congenital lesions represent 40 percent and neoplastic lesions 60 percent. The neoplasms can be divided into three groups: (1) osseous, comprising 60 percent of the class; (2) neurogenic, 20 percent; and (3) all other lesions, also 20 percent (Table 20-1). The Mayo Clinic reported that 43 percent of presacral tumors were malignant.[3]

Not included in this classification are several other groups that could present as presacral masses. These include inflammatory masses, foreign material such as barium or oleogranuloma, and recurrent rectal cancer. Metastatic cancer from the prostate, bladder, ovary, or breast, and extrapelvic sarcomas have also been reported.[3]

Congenital Lesions

Congenital lesions are usually cystic but may contain some formed elements as well. Generally these fall into one of two groups: the developmental cysts and the meningoceles.

Developmental Cysts

The developmental cysts form the majority of the congenital lesions. These include, in order of frequency, mucus-secreting cysts, epidermoid cysts, teratomas, and teratocarcinomas. Classification of presacral cysts in the literature has been histologically confusing, so classification should be based on pathologic criteria.[3,4] Epidermoids and inclusion dermoids are simple cysts formed by nests of displaced ectoderm along the lines of embryonic fusion. Epidermoid cysts contain stratified squamous epithelium with keratohyaline granules. Inclusion dermoids are similar, but they also contain some skin appendages such as hair follicles, sweat glands, and sebaceous glands.[5] These can be confused with dermoid cysts of the teratoma variety such as an ovarian dermoid within a benign cystic teratoma. Many lesions described as dermoids in the literature are in fact epidermoid tumors. A teratoma has two or three germ cell layers and may contain cartilage, teeth, hair, brain, bone, or smooth muscle (Fig. 20-1). Middeldorpf[6] in 1885 described a mucus-secreting presacral tumor in a 1-year-old child. Since then many tumors in the area have been called Middeldorpf tumors. Strictly speaking, this term should refer only to teratomas.[7]

Mucus-secreting cysts containing columnar or cuboidal mucus-secreting epithelium are the most common developmental cysts. These may also contain squamous and transitional epithelium. Even though two germ layers are involved, the pathologic picture is different than it is for teratomas.[3] These have also been called "enterogenous cysts," "cystic hamartomas," "cystic teratomas," and "simple cysts." These thin-

Table 20-1   Classification of Presacral Masses Ranked by Relative Frequency Where Available

CONGENITAL LESIONS (40%)
1. Mucus-secreting cyst
2. Epidermoid cyst
3. Teratoma
4. Teratocarcinoma
   Adrenal rest tumor
   Duplication of the rectum
   Anterior sacral meningocele

NEOPLASTIC LESIONS (60%)
Osseous (60%)
1. Chordoma
2. Ewing's sarcoma
3. Giant cell tumor
   Osteogenic sarcoma
   Osteochondroma
   Aneurysmal bone cyst
   Chondrosarcoma
Neurogenic (20%)
1. Neurilemoma
2. Neurofibroma
3. Neurofibrosarcoma
   Ependymoma
   Ganglioneuroma
   Neuroblastoma
   Schwannoma
Miscellaneous (20%)
Fibrous, muscular, and adipose
   a. Fibroma and fibrosarcoma
   b. Leiomyoma and leiomyosarcoma
   c. Lipoma and liposarcoma
   d. Myelolipoma
Hematologic and lymphatic
   a. Lymphoma
   b. Lymphangioma and lymphangiosarcoma
   c. Plasmacytoma
   d. Hemangioma and hemangiosarcoma
   e. Leukemia
   f. Extramedullary hematopoiesis
Other
   a. Desmoid
   b. Endometrioma
   c. Histiocytoma
   d. Undifferentiated sarcoma

Modified from: Lovelady SB, Dockerty MB. Extragenital pelvic tumors in women. *Am J Obstet Gynecol.* 1949;58:215–234.

walled cysts are often multiloculated and contain clear mucoid material. Uhlig and Johnson[4] reported seven indeterminate cysts believed to be mucus-secreting cysts which became so inflamed that a microscopic diagnosis

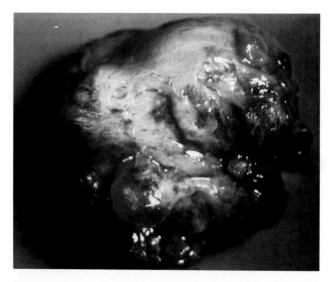

Figure 20-1.   Presacral teratoma containing cystic and solid areas.

was impossible. Most of these had been previously operated on. Excluding teratomas, malignancies in developmental cysts are rare, but have been reported in between 7 and 8.7 percent of epidermoid cysts, mucus-secreting cysts, and rectal duplications.[3,4]

Developmental cysts, except for teratomas, most often occur in adults. They occur in women up to 15 times more often than in men.[3] The size can range from 2 to 15 cm. The lesions can be asymptomatic and only diagnosed on routine examination. When symptoms are present they are often of a long duration (1–3.7 years),[3,4] in part because of a failure to establish the diagnosis. A history of recurrent perianal abscesses and multiple operations is not uncommon.[3]

A characteristic physical finding, in addition to the mass, is a postanal dimple—found in one third of these patients (Fig. 20-2). The opening is outside and posterior to the anus. The appearance is similar to a fistula in ano or pilonidal sinus, with which the lesion may be confused. Hair may be present in the tract.

Treatment of a benign cyst is by excision, which can usually be performed through a posterior approach. Large and high-lying lesions may require an anterior or a combined approach. Results are good when the lesion is completely removed, but with incomplete excision recurrence is likely. Aldridge and associates[8] described 12 cases of intramural dermoids with an internal opening. These are best removed transanally.

The great majority of sacrococcygeal teratomas occur in children; the incidence is 1 in 30,000 live births. In children the rate of malignancy increases with age up to 50 percent at 2 years. However, malignancy is less common after the second decade.[9] The rate of malignancy in adults ranges from 1 to 12.5 percent.[3,7,10]

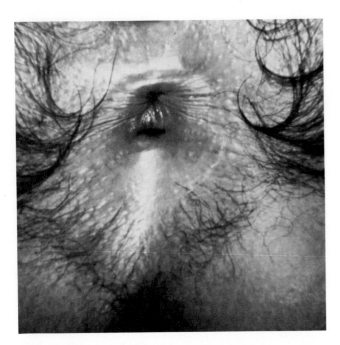

Figure 20-2. A typical postanal dimple. This lesion may be easily confused with a fistula in ano.

Teratocarcinoma is a very aggressive tumor. In addition to excision, radiation and chemotherapy with vincristine, actinomycin D, cyclophosphamide and doxorubicin may be required. CEA antigen, α-fetoprotein, and β-HCG levels may be monitored postoperatively to assess for recurrence.

Presacral teratomas and anterior sacral meningoceles can also be hereditary. The triad of hereditary sacral agenesis with a presacral mass and congenital anorectal stenosis was first described in 1981 by Currarino and coworkers.[11] More recently, O'Riordain and associates described a family with autosomal dominant inheritance of sacral agenesis.[12] Ten family members were affected; four had associated presacral teratomas and anterior sacral meningocele. Three of these lesions caused serious complications including bacterial meningitis, local recurrence of teratoma, and perianal sepsis. These authors stressed that early diagnosis and surgical excision of a presacral mass can prevent subsequent morbidity and death.

Anterior Sacral Meningocele

Anterior sacral meningocele is a congenital cystic structure containing cerebrospinal fluid (CSF). The outer portion is composed of the dural membrane and the inner surface of the arachnoid membrane. These membranes herniate through a defect in the anterior surface of the sacrum and are connected via a narrow neck to the dural sac.[13] Only rarely do these cysts contain neural elements; if they are present the lesion is a myelomeningocele. The size of the meningocele affects the development of the sacrum and coccyx, leaving a characteristic bony appearance.[14]

Anterior sacral meningoceles are detected more commonly in women than in men and usually present during adulthood when symptoms caused by the enlarging mass appear. Pressure is applied on adjacent organs causing urinary incontinence and retention, constipation, and backache. Pressure on the lesion from straining, coughing, or intercourse increases intracranial pressure and leads to headaches. Dystocia may occur.[14]

Digital rectal examination usually reveals a mass an-

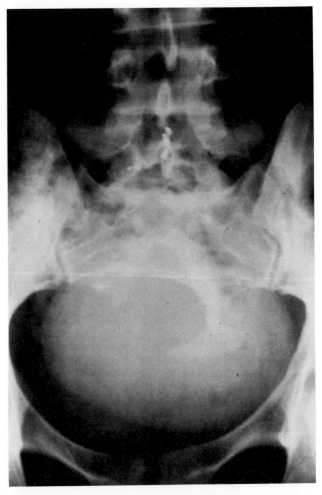

Figure 20-3. The "scimitar" sacrum. This characteristic radiographic finding is caused by pressure from the anterior sacral meningocele on the developing sacrum. (Courtesy of Charles D. Finae III, M.D. Minneapolis, MN.) (Reprinted with permission from Wexner SD, Jagelman DG. Pilonidal disease, presacral cysts, and pelvic and perianal pain. In: Zidema GD, Condon RE, eds. *Shackelford's Surgery of the Alimentary Tract*. 3rd ed. Philadelphia: WB Saunders; 1991:390–405.)

terior to the sacrum. The classic roentgenologic finding is the "scimitar" sacrum (Fig. 20-3). A portion of the sacrum and all the coccyx are absent, leaving a smooth, rounded bony edge next to normal bone. The concave border approximates the convex edge of an Arabian scimitar. Associated congenital anomalies such as duplication of the uterus and anal stenosis are common, as are pelvic tumors, usually teratomas or epidermoid cysts—rarely teratocarcinoma. These associated tumors should be sought out and removed. A CT scan with contrast, or preferably MRI, clearly defines the cyst, excludes associated lesions, and reveals the connection to the dural space. If the level of the tract is hard to discern, a myelogram may be indicated; lateral views can aid in revealing the level of the connection. A normal myelogram does not exclude the diagnosis because the opening can be so small that contrast takes a long time to enter the sac.[14] For this reason, delayed films are sometimes helpful.[7] These cysts must never be aspirated or drained. Meningitis has occurred after all routes of drainage, including transrectal, transvaginal, or even transabdominal aspiration performed during celiotomy. The consequent meningitis has caused deaths.

Both symptomatic and asymptomatic anterior sacral meningoceles should be resected to avoid infection[14] and to remove any adjacent congenital tumors. In women of childbearing age these lesions should be removed to prevent dystocia. The surgical procedure entails dividing the stalk of the meningocele, removing the cyst and any adjacent tumors, and tightly closing the neck of the sac. Low-lying anterior sacral meningoceles may be resected through a posterior approach whereas higher lesions require abdominal exposure. The operative technique is presented later.

Neoplastic Lesions

Osseous Tumors

Sacrococcygeal Chordoma

Chordomas can be located anywhere along the axial skeleton and are very rarely found in other locations. The frequency by location is sacrococcygeal 50 percent, sphenoccipital 35 percent, and vertebral 15 percent.[15]

A sacrococcygeal chordoma was first described by Henning in 1900. The Finnish Cancer Registry recorded an annual incidence in males and females of 0.3 and 0.18 per million population, respectively. For chordomas in the sacrococcygeal region the male:female ratio is 2:1.[15] Chordomas represent 1 to 4 percent of all bone tumors.[15] They have been reported at all ages, but over one half occur in persons aged 50 to 70.[16] The average age at the Mayo Clinic was 61 years and the average size

9 cm.[3] Sphenoccipital lesions are seen at a younger age because the tumor bulk produces symptoms earlier. Sacrococcygeal tumors, however, have a large area in which to expand prior to the onset of symptoms and hence are often diagnosed later in life.[17]

Chordomas are thought to arise from rests of the embryonic notochord. In the fourth through sixth weeks of development, the paraxial mesoderm encloses the notochord. In the sixth week, cartilage blocks appear around the notochord; these are the precursors of the vertebral bodies.[16] The notochord disappears except within the intervertebral disk where it expands to form the gelatinous center or nucleus pulposis. Theoretically, the notochord in the vertebral body does not completely degenerate and rests of this tissue persist and later degenerate into chordomas. Healey and Lane[17] note that it is enigmatic that these small rests of notochord can give rise to chordomas whereas chordomas do not occur in the normal nucleus pulposis.

Grossly, chordomas are lobulated, pseudoencapsulated, gelatinous masses. Their consistency is variable, with cystic areas of gelatinous material dispersed among firm areas of cartilaginous tissue. The lesions are malignant and tend to be locally aggressive growing along the path of least resistance. They often spread along the nerve roots in the sacral plexus. Although primary lesions do not usually infiltrate adjacent organs, reccurrent tumors have this tendency.

Histologically, abundant mucus production is noted. Near the center of the lobule, cords of cells appear to float in mucus.[16] Mucous droplets coalesce in single large vacuoles forming physaliferous cells which are characteristic of chordomas. Other elements seen include cartilage, fibrous tissue, giant cells, and inflammatory cells. The differential diagnosis includes mucinous adenocarcinoma, chondrosarcoma, chondroma, and myopapillary ependymoma.[18] Special stains and electron microscopy can be helpful in difficult cases.

Symptoms occur because of pressure caused by the tumor as it enlarges. Symptoms depend on the tumor location. Pain in the low back or pelvis is both the earliest and the most common symptom (Table 20-2). It may be a dull intermittent ache or severe and steady. Pain can also be felt in the buttocks, rectum, or perineum, or along the distribution of one or both sciatic nerves.[17] Standing may decrease the pain while sitting or straining, as for a bowel movement, may increase it. Low-lying tumors do not impinge on motor nerve roots, but higher tumors may. Difficulty in walking may be an early symptom.[17] Later, pressure on nerve roots can cause bladder and bowel dysfunction, hypoesthesia, anesthesia, or paralysis. A large tumor may compress the bowel causing constipation or problems emptying the rectum. Likewise, frequency, dysuria, and retention can occur if the bladder is affected.

Table 20-2   Reported Symptoms of Sacrococcygeal Chordoma in Order of Frequency in 222 Patients[15]

Symptoms	No. patients	%
Local pain	127	57
Constipation	49	22
Sciatica	37	17
Difficulty in urination and urinary retention	26	12
Difficulty in walking and leg weakness	20	9
Urinary incontinence	19	8
Fecal incontinence	15	7
Saddle anesthesia	15	7
Difficulty in defecation	10	4
Rectal bleeding	3	1

Chordomas are relentless slow-growing tumors. The Mayo Clinic[3] reported an overall 5-year survival of 75 percent in 30 patients. However, almost half the survivors were not disease free and 11 had one or more operations for recurrence. In 1975, Gray and associates[16] reported a 10-year survival of 16.4 percent, and in 1982 Cummings and colleagues[19] reported uncorrected 5- and 10-year survival rates of 62 percent and 28 percent, respectively. Most patients, however, had clinically detectable residual chordoma at the time of death or last contact.

Most patients die of local disease and distant metastases occur in 10 to 30 percent.[3,15] Although sacrococcygeal chordomas comprise 50 percent of all chordomas, they account for 73 percent of the metastases.[18] Metastases generally become apparent 1.5 to 3 years after diagnosis of the index lesion and are more likely if the primary tumor is anaplastic.[18] They occur through both hematogenous and lymphatic routes.[16] The most common sites of metastasis are, in order, lungs 58 percent, lymph nodes 33 percent, liver 22 percent, bones 17 percent, skin and others.[18] Despite these grim statistics, few patients die of metastatic disease and commonly it is asymptomatic.[15]

Giant Cell Tumors of the Sacrum

Giant cell tumor of bone is the second most common sacral tumor and is best treated by surgery.[20] Although curettage is the treatment most commonly used, it has a high recurrence rate. If total excision of the sacral lesion can be accomplished without major morbidity, this is the preferred approach. If major morbidity will occur, then an alternative approach is intralesional excision and packing with methyl methacrylate. The addition of methyl methacrylate to intralesional excision appears associated with a marked reduction in local recurrence compared to excision alone.[21]

Other osseous tumors occur infrequently and require individualized treatment.

Neurogenic Tumors

The neurogenic tumors are all uncommon. Of these, ependymomas are the most common tumors of glial origin, occurring in the region of the cauda equina. These may present in either the pre- or postsacral space. If presacral, their appearance is similar to that of the chordoma. The treatment is wide excision, but recurrence is common.[22]

Miscellaneous Tumors

A long list of diverse tumors have their origins in the hematopoietic system, the reticuloendothelial cell line, and soft tissues. These later tumors may arise from fibrous tissue, muscle, adipose tissue, or other cell lines. Treatment for each of these lesions must be individually selected.

Symptoms and Signs Associated with Presacral Tumors

One quarter of presacral tumors have no symptoms. They are found incidentally on routine physical examination or at childbirth. If symptoms are present, they average 6 to 12 months in duration at diagnosis.[3,15,23] Major reasons for the delay in diagnosis are the common symptom of nonspecific back pain with or without radiating leg pain, and the difficulty in obtaining and interpreting plain films of the sacrum.[24] The most common symptoms are pain, followed by change in bowel habits (often constipation), dysesthesia or weakness in the legs or perianal area, and urinary retention or incontinence. These later symptoms are significantly more common with malignant lesions. Benign lesions are more often associated with a postanal dimple, discharge of sebaceous material or hair protruding from a sinus, and dystocia. In addition, patients with benign lesions may have a history of recurrent perianal abscesses and may have had multiple perianal operations.

Pain is associated with 40 percent of benign lesions and with 60 to 80 percent of malignant ones.[3] It occurs most frequently in the sacrococcygeal area and less frequently in the buttocks, low back, anorectal area, or radiating into the lower extremities. Exacerbation of pain with sitting is common. Pain is present in all patients with osseous tumors and is common in patients with chordomas. Patients with low back and leg pain without an apparent cause should have a rectal examination and neurologic assessment of the sacral dermatomes and reflexes. Pain may also be associated with an infection in a congenital cyst.

Physical Examination

Presacral tumors are palpable in between 67 and 97 percent[3,24] of patients. Local tenderness may be elicited by pressure on the sacrum. Certain differentiating features among these tumors are worth noting. Developmental cysts are generally midline and are soft and nontender. In one third of congenital cysts there is a funnel-shaped postanal dimple. This dimple is located in the midline, posterior to the anus and caudal to the dentate line. It may or may not be connected with the sinus, and therefore can be confused with a pilonidal sinus or anal fistula.[4] Anterior sacral meningoceles feel similar, but an impulse may be felt when the patient coughs or strains. Also, pressure on the mass may cause a headache.[14] Chordomas are solid tumors adherent to the sacrum which often have attained a large size before being diagnosed. Neurofibromas are firm, smooth lesions which are felt high up and through the posterior rectal wall.[13] Osseous tumors may be solid or soft and giant cell tumors are very vascular and may pulsate.[21]

Proctoscopy confirms the extrarectal origin of the tumors. Small tumors are otherwise unremarkable while large tumors may narrow the lumen. A draining sinus may be seen in the posterior rectal wall if there is a communication from a cyst in the area.[25] This may result from an ill-advised transrectal biopsy of a congenital cyst.

Radiology

Plain Films

Plain x-rays of the sacrum are often obscured by overlying viscera containing gas, fecal material, or osseous structures—hence lesions are easily overlooked. The most common sacral neoplasm is due to metastatic disease. Benign sacral lesions are mostly osteoblastomas, giant cell tumors, and aneurysmal bone cysts. Marrow and metastatic lesions are found more frequently in the marrow-containing wings than the midline. The most common primary malignant neoplasm is the chordoma.[20] Chordomas produce a solitary presacral mass

containing calcific debris that displaces the rectum anteriorly; this finding is rare with other tumors.[23] Chordomas are more frequently in S-3, S-4, and S-5, whereas giant cell tumors, chondrosarcomas, and osteosarcomas are more common in the upper segments.[15] In sacrococcygeal chordoma, bony destruction is present in up to 78 percent of patients (Fig. 20-4). Osteosclerosis, osteolysis, or both may be seen, and a soft tissue mass is seen in 33 to 60 percent of patients.[15,26] Calcifications that represent tooth and bone fragments may be seen anterior to the sacrum in teratomas. Most patients with sacrococcygeal teratomas have no evidence of bony sacral involvement.[20]

Other abnormalities present on plain films include anterior displacement of the rectum which can be demonstrated with a barium enema.[24] Gas may be seen in the presacral area, suggesting a cyst with a communication to the rectum[25] or skin. The mass may resemble the soap-bubble appearance often seen with hemangiomas.[27] The scimitar sacrum, as previously de-

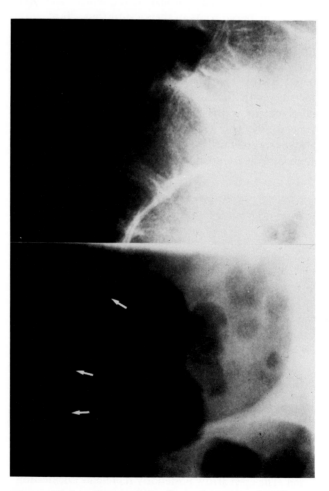

Figure 20-4. Presacral chordoma demonstrating disruption of the anterior sacral cortex on plain radiograph. Compare with MRI of the same tumor, Figure 20-8.

scribed, is the classic finding of an anterior meningomyelocele. Sacral deformities can also occur with developmental cysts.

Computed Tomography and Magnetic Resonance Imaging

CT, and now MRI, represent the best single examination to confirm the presence of a presacral tumor. It appears that each examination has its advantages. Both do a good job of measuring the size of the mass and defining its location. Likewise, both can demonstrate different tissue densities (Fig. 20-5). CT may offer superior definition of the spatial relationships between structures in the pelvis (Fig. 20-6). MRI shows bony involvement better. MRI, especially when used with contrast, is especially helpful when evaluating the spinal canal for extension of the tumor or drop lesions along the nerve roots (Fig. 20-7). It is helpful in distinguishing between sacral neoplasms of neural origin and those of bony origin. MRI also has the advantage of showing the anatomy in sagital and coronal planes, which can help in tracing the nerve roots in the sacrum (Fig. 20-8).

Evaluation of sacrococcygeal chordomas demonstrates an associated soft tissue mass in 90 percent (Fig. 20-9).[13] Levine and Batnitzky[28] and others[15] have noted a disproportionally large soft tissue mass associated with the tumor; this mass exceeds the bony involvement and is located anterior to the sacrum. In general, the soft tissue mass is of uniform density. However, one third[15] may contain one or more septated areas of low attenuation. Amorphous calcifications are

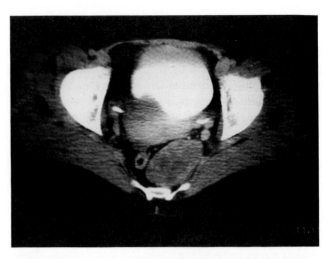

Figure 20-6. CT image of presacral ganglioneuroma. Large solid tumor anterior to the sacrum and displacing the rectum.

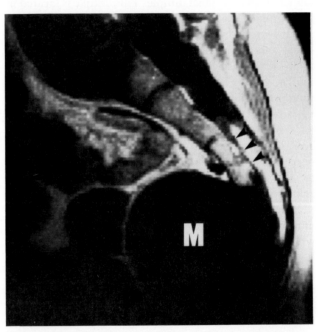

Figure 20-7. A T_2-weighted MRI clearly defines an anterior sacral meningocele. *Arrows* point out the dural defect and neck of the hernia sac. (From: Wetzel LH, Levin E. MR imaging of sacral and presacral lesions. *AJR.* 1990;154:771–775.)

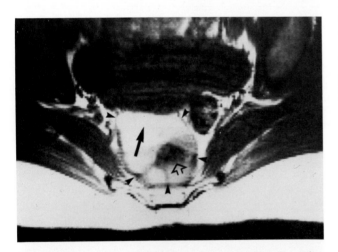

Figure 20-5. Axial MRI of a presacral teratoma. The mass is outlined by *arrowheads*. Large solid *arrow* shows high-intensity fat layering on lower-intensity fluid in the lesion. The open arrow posteriorly represents calcification. (From: Wetzel LH, Levin E. MR imaging of sacral and presacral lesions. *AJR.* 1990;154:771–775.)

found in 50 to 87 percent on CT, but only 44 percent on plain x-rays.[15]

In teratomas, both CT and MRI may reveal two or more tissue densities, suggesting the diagnosis. Ependymomas are better evaluated with MRI. Burchell presented an unusual case of a congenital cyst communicating with the rectum, that presented with

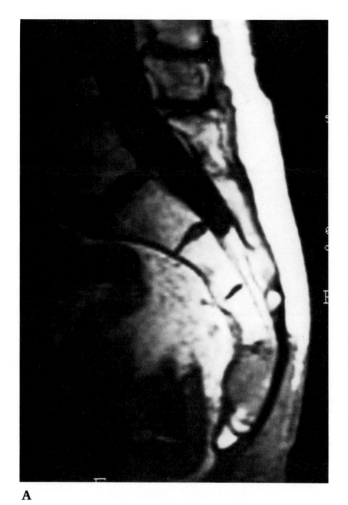

A

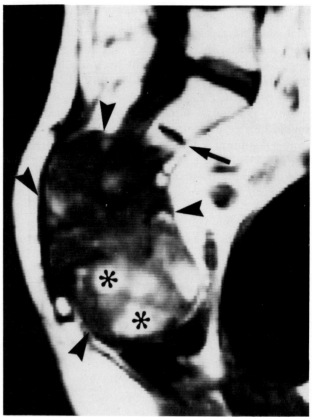

Figure 20-9. Large chordoma. Sagittal MR image showing extensive neoplasm (*arrows*) with obliteration of the sacral canal and pre- and postsacral extension. High intensity areas (*asterisks*) denote areas of hemorrhage in the tumor (From: Wetzel LH, Levin E. MR imaging of sacral and presacral lesions. *AJR.* 1990;154:771–775.)

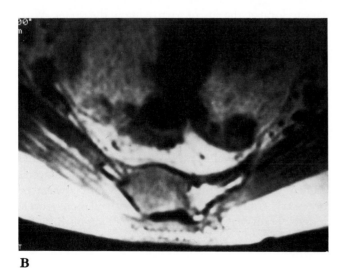

B

Figure 20-8.   A T$_2$-weighted MRI of a sacrococcygeal chordoma. Note the associated bony destruction. (A) Sagittal section. (B) Coronal view.

intermittent rectal drainage. When pelvic CT was used with contrast in the rectum a communication between the rectum and the cyst was seen.[25]

Bone Scans

Sacral tumors may be difficult to image with bone scintigraphy. The isotope may pool in the bladder and obscure a sacral lesion. Care should be taken to empty the bladder if this study is done, and to include lateral scans as well. Few large series have investigated the use of bone scans to evaluate chordomas, but Feldenzer and associates[24] reported 5 of 6 such examinations as positive. Smith and colleagues[15] reported that chordomas produce a pattern that can be helpful in the differential diagnosis: the main body of the tumor is "cold" and its peripheral margin is surrounded by a halo of increased activity. In general, CT or MRI can provide more information.

Ultrasonography

Transabdominal pelvic ultrasonography will display the size, position, and consistency of the pelvic lesion (Fig. 20-10). Simultaneously, the liver may be checked for metastatic disease and the kidneys for hydronephrosis. However, CT and MRI provide images of a higher quality. Transrectal ultrasound is also valuable.[29] It should be able to distinguish masses in the rectal wall from extramural lesions and cyctic from solid lesions (Fig. 20-11). In the case of primary lesions arising outside the rectum, transrectal ultrasonography may show whether the rectal wall is infiltrated and requires resection.

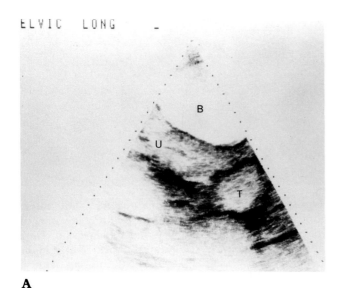

A

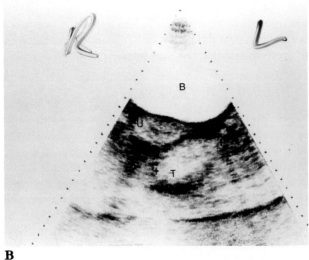

B

Figure 20-10.   Transabdominal pelvic ultrasonogram of presacral ganglioneuroma (see Fig. 20-6). (A) Longitudinal scan. (B) Transverse scan. T = tumor. B = bladder. U = uterus.

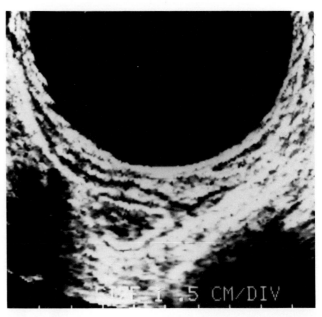

Figure 20-11.   Transrectal ultrasound of a presacral heterogeneous dermoid cyst. (Courtesy of WD Wong, M.D., St. Paul, MN.)

Sinography

This may be of use in an infected presacral cyst that connects to the skin.

Intravenous Pyelography

An intravenous pyelogram may not be necessary in small, circumscribed, low-lying lesions. If the initial CT or MRI suggests hydronephrosis, then an IVP is necessary to localize the site of narrowing in the ureter. With large and high-lying lesions it is of use in preoperative planning. It can show displacement of the bladder and obstruction or displacement of the ureters.

Myelography

Chordomas and ependymomas may extend into the spinal canal. Lesions in the proximal sacrum (S-1 and S-2) should be evaluated by a myelogram, as should even distal lesions if they are large. As experience is gained with MRI, myelography may not always be necessary. Conversely, with anterior sacral meningocele a myelogram may add information not supplied by the MRI.

Angiography

Before CT came into use, angiography was used to delineate presacral tumors. Pathologic circulation was not demonstrated and, despite subtraction techniques, abnormal vascularity was not seen.[15] Therefore it is not routinely used.

Surgical Technique

Surgical Indications

All presacral tumors should be removed even if the patient is asymptomatic. There are several reasons for this dictum. Cystic lesions may become infected either through a tract to the epithelial surface or after needle biopsy. Infection then makes the resection more difficult and prone to complications.[3] A high mortality is associated with untreated anterior sacral meningocele because of infection and secondary meningitis.[14,30] In women of childbearing age dystocia may occur. Finally, some lesions, namely teratoma or chordoma, may harbor the possibility of malignancy from the onset.

Biopsy

In the past, it has been accepted that presacral tumors should not be biopsied by needle or by an open technique. Biopsy has caused several undesirable complications. First, benign cysts have become infected, complicating their removal. Second, anterior meningoceles became infected and this proved highly lethal.[14] Third, with malignant lesions, there has been seeding of the biopsy tract with malignant cells. Therefore, taking a biopsy specimen through the rectum demands rectal resection even when the rectum might otherwise have been spared.

Currently available imaging methods are much better than earlier techniques in evaluating these lesions preoperatively. If a lesion is found to be cystic, biopsy is not necessary and in fact should be avoided. Solid tumors are more problematic. If the lesion clearly appears to be a chordoma, then a biopsy may not be necessary. If there is a question regarding its nature, then a biopsy may be appropriate and a perianal, parasacral, or direct posterior route should be selected. There appears to be no place for a transrectal biopsy which could infect the tumor and seed the otherwise uninvolved rectal wall, necessitating its removal.

Other tumors occurring presacrally are often treated preoperatively with chemotherapy, radiation, or both. Examples are osteogenic sarcoma and Ewing's sarcoma.[31] In these select instances, a preoperative biopsy may be beneficial. If a biopsy is performed, the tract should be removed at the time of a definitive operation. If the disease has already metastasized, then a biopsy may be performed to confirm the type of malignancy and to direct treatment.

Preoperative Preparation

If a major sacral resection is planned, the possibility of a colostomy and nerve dysfunction needs to be presented to the patient preoperatively. In all cases the preoperative evaluation should document the patient's sexual function and both urinary and fecal continence.[17]

Whether or not resection of the rectum is planned, both a mechanical and an antibiotic bowel preparation should be performed. It is advisable to prepare the bowel to minimize any contamination in case of an unplanned entry into the rectum. Perioperative prophylactic intravenous antibiotics are likewise appropriate.

The anus is left open in low-lying congenital lesions. Then if necessary, the surgeon or an assistant can double-glove and insert the index finger into the anus to put pressure on the mass, pushing it into the wound and facilitating its removal.[32] If pressure will not help and the anus is to be spared, it is temporarily closed with a suture to prevent contamination.[33] Visualization can be difficult at times and a fiberoptic headlight is helpful.

Some small lesions and all large or "high" lesions require a multidisciplinary team consisting of a colon and rectal surgeon, an orthopedic surgeon, and a neurosurgeon.

Operative Approach

The approach is dictated by the size and location of the lesion. The four approaches are pure abdominal, pure posterior, combined anteroposterior (either sequential or synchronous), and the rarely indicated transrectal approach. Sphincter-dividing approaches such as the York–Mason are rarely necessary because the lesions are usually well above the sphincter muscles and dividing them may lead to problems with continence. As a general rule, lesions that can be felt up to one half their entirety with the index finger on rectal examination can be approached posteriorly (Fig. 20-12). This would be approximately the S-4 level. If half or less of the tumor can be palpated, an abdominal approach is needed. This may have to be expanded to a combined approach if the sacrum or coccyx needs to be removed as well. An infected cyst that has ruptured into the rectum can be widely opened and curretted transanally; after the inflammation is resolved, it can be removed as a second-stage procedure.

The posterior approach is suitable for the majority of presacral cysts and teratomas. The patient is placed in the prone jackknife position with a firm roll elevating the hips and the buttocks spread and taped (Fig. 20-13).

Several different incisions have been used: a midline, a transverse, a paracoccygeal on the side of the tumor, or a "lazy S." The incision is carried down until the

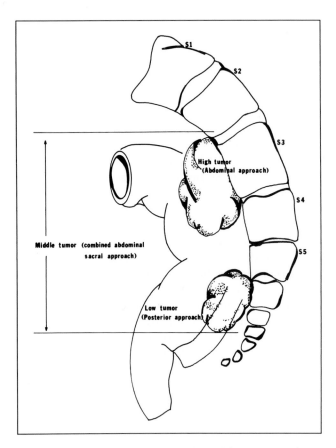

Figure 20-12. Location of high and low presacral tumors. Lesions that can be encompassed in at least one half of their height by transanal digital examination can generally be excised through a posterior approach. (Reprinted with permission from Wexner SD, Jagelman DG. Pilonidal disease, presacral cysts, and pelvic and perianal pain. In: Zidema GD, Condon RE, eds. *Shackelford's Surgery of the Alimentary Tract*. 3rd ed. Philadelphia: WB Saunders; 1991:390–405.)

sacrum, the coccyx, and the anococcygeal ligaments are identified. Self-retaining retractors help provide good exposure. Next, the fibrous attachments of the anococcygeal ligament and the pubococcygeus are freed from the coccyx. The coccyx is then disarticulated. This method provides good exposure with little or no residual morbidity.

It can be helpful to divide the anterior–superior attachments between the coccyx and the sacrum with electrocautery. The middle sacral artery lies just anterior to the midportion of this articulation and may at times retract and cause troublesome bleeding.

The foregoing procedure unroofs the lower part of the presacral space. At this time digital pressure exerted through the rectum can help elevate the lesion and improve exposure. Sharp and blunt dissection are used to free the lesion from adjacent structures. If a cyst is

present and adherent to the coccyx, it should be removed en bloc (Fig. 20-14), thereby possibily reducing the rate of recurrence.

If the rectum has been entered, it should be closed in two layers and the mucosa inverted. The anastomosis can be tested or a leak checked for by putting air in the rectum with the proctoscope, filling the wound with saline, and watching for bubbles. Careful hemostasis is obtained and a closed suction drain put in the space and brought out through a stab wound. The wound is irrigated and closed in layers.

McCarty and associates[34] outlined the classic approach for **low-lying sacrococcygeal chordomas**. The patient is placed in the prone position after a foley catheter has been inserted. The anus is temporarily closed with a suture. The entire area, including the sacrum, buttocks, and iliac crests, is prepared.

A midline incision is made beginning at the level of the iliac crests and ending just above the external anal sphincter. The lumbodorsal fascia and erector spinae are stripped from the sacrum. The gluteus muscles are retracted. If the tumor invades into the muscle, the involved portion of muscle should be resected en bloc with the specimen. The anococcygeal ligament is transected and the levator muscles are retracted. Careful blunt finger dissection is used to separate the rectum from the sacrum. Next the piriformis, sacrospinous,

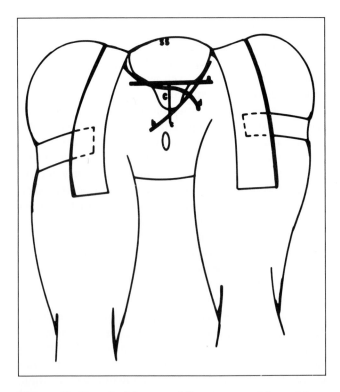

Figure 20-13. Incisions used for tumor excision with en bloc coccygectomy. (Reprinted with permission from *Shackelford's Surgery of the Alimentary Tract*, 390–405.)

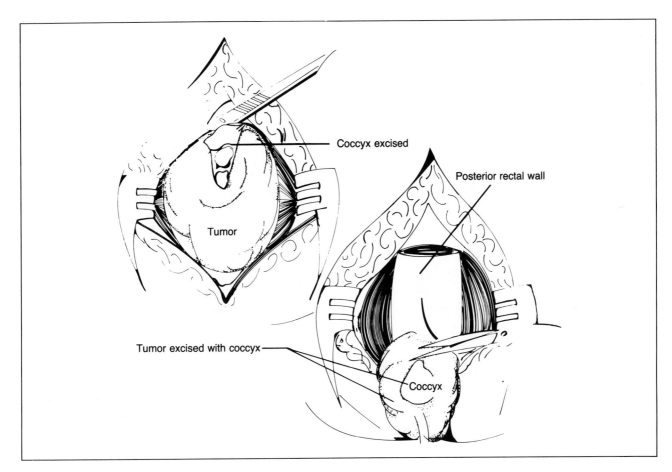

Figure 20-14.   Appropriate en bloc resection of a presacral cyst including the cyst and attached coccyx. (Reprinted with permission from *Shackelford's Surgery of the Alimentary Tract*, 390–405.)

and sacrotuberous ligaments and the coccygeus are divided close to the sacrum, thereby exposing the sciatic nerve. The pudendal nerve should also be identified and preserved. The index finger can be inserted in the sciatic notch and meet in the midline. This aids in separating the rectum from the sacrum and in defining the upper level of the lesion. A subperiosteal dissection posteriorly exposes the sacral laminae where the neuroforamina can be palpated anteriorly. A fine rongeurs is used to remove the fused sacral laminae at the line of resection.[35] Care is taken to identify and preserve the sacral roots. The dural sac of the cauda equina is suture ligated. The anterior cortex is then divided with an osteotome (Fig. 20-15). As the specimen is removed any residual attachments to the rectum are divided and hemostasis is obtained. The wound is closed in layers over a closed drainage system.

High sacral tumors that extend above the S-3 level require a combined anterior and posterior approach. The classic work of Stener and Gunterberg[33] describes this approach. Localio and associates[36], Huth and associates[37] and Michael and Decloed[38] have presented a combined abdominal transsacral approach and Kennedy and Mankin,[39] a posterolateral approach. The chief advantage of the latter two lies in their ability to provide neurovascular visualization during division of the sacrum and thereby ensure the correct direction for the osteotomy as the sacrum is divided.

The anterior–posterior approach includes a midline incision through which the abdomen is inspected to exclude metastatic disease. The presacral space is entered at the level of the sacral promontory and the rectum is mobilized to the upper margin of the tumor. Frequently, the tumor does not involve the rectum and the rectum can be separated from the tumor and preserved. En bloc rectal extirpation is indicated if the rectum is invaded by tumor or if a transrectal biopsy has been performed. In addition if the tumor is very large and displaces the rectum, thus precluding tumor excision with an adequate tissue margin, the rectum should be removed en bloc.

For **benign tumors**, efforts are generally made to preserve the first three sacral nerve roots bilaterally, although one S-3 root may be sacrificed with minimal

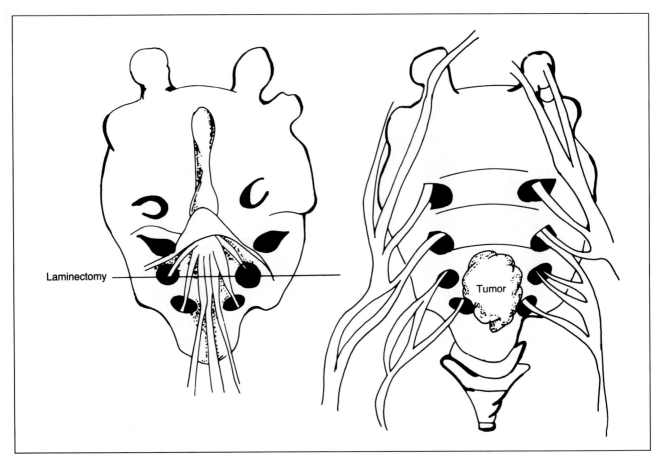

Figure 20-15.   The line of the sacral osteotomy above the tumor. The nerve roots exiting the foramen are preserved if not involved. (Reprinted with permission from Wexner SD, Jagelman DG. Pilonidal disease, presacral cysts, and pelvic and perianal pain. In: Zidema GD, Condon RE, eds. *Shackelford's Surgery of the Alimentary Tract.* 3rd ed. Philadelphia: WB Saunders; 1991:390–405.

impairment.[16] The loss of further nerve roots leads to neurologic deficits.[40] **Malignant lesions** that are potentially curable by resection may require the sacrifice of upper sacral nerves for complete removal of the lesion en bloc. If the S-3 roots are divided bilaterally, control of the anal sphincter is frequently lost. Many patients can cope with this by following a daily bowel-cleansing regimen.[31] However, a colostomy may be appropriate in selected patients.

Loss up to but not including S-1 has the following effects:

Denervation of the urinary bladder and uretheral sphincter: loss of bladder function necessitates self-catheterization or possibly a transurethral resection of the bladder neck; incontinence requires a urinary collecting system or diaper.

Genital function will be impaired with loss of sensation to the genitalia; other functions mediated through the sympathetic nerves may be preserved.

Anorectal incontinence follows but is usually not a problem so long as the stools are solid; daily evacuation is necessary and diapers may be required—a colostomy may be required if conservative measures fail.

A minor motor deficit in the lower extremities, manifested when climbing, can be compensated for in time by other muscle groups.

The loss of S-1 adds no major visceral effects so long as the adjacent sympathetics are spared in the dissection. If all the sacral nerves are sacrificed, acceptable leg function can be maintained.

The value of ligation of the internal iliac vessels and middle sacral vessels in treating chordoma is controversial. The vascular supply to this area usually does not come from the iliac vessels. Eilber[31] thinks that unless the tumor extends into these vessels, it is seldom necessary to ligate them. Dozios[41] suggests that blood loss is decreased during the perineal portion of the operation by ligation of the middle sacral vessels and the internal iliac vessels on the side containing the majority of the tumor. Sung and associates[42] recommend routine bilateral ligation of the internal iliac vessels. This is best achieved through the combined abdominosacral approach.

The rectum is mobilized laterally and then anteriorly at the level of the cul-de-sac. After this, the pelvic floor is reconstructed as much as possible, the midline incision is closed, and the stoma is matured. The patient is placed in the prone position and the posterior phase is completed as previously described. If the rectum is removed, the anus is included with the en bloc resection. The posterior wound is closed in layers again over a closed suction drainage system.

Division of the sacrum between S-1 and S-2, through the canals of the S-1 nerves, weakens the pelvis by 33 percent. When S-1 is divided above the canal the strength is decreased by 50 percent. Despite this, there is adequate strength for a normal load on the pelvis.[33] Stener and Gunterberg[33] found that if only the upper half of the body of S-1 remains, the pelvic girdle retains sufficient strength to permit standing immediately after

resection and collapse of the bony pelvis will not ensue. When full sacral resection has been performed, consideration is given to bone grafting or spinal instrumentation.[43] This procedure may be performed in stages.[17] In very advanced cases that still appear resectable, a hemipelvectomy in conjunction with a sacrectomy or full hemicorporectomy may be considered.[44] Figure 20-16 offers an algorithmic approach to the evaluation and management of presacral tumors in adults.

Radiation Therapy

Radiation therapy may play an important role in the treatment of some tumors such as Ewing's sarcoma. However, chordomas are radioresistant tumors and are rarely cured by partial tumor resection and conventional irradiation.[19] Nevertheless, it has been used to treat residual disease, local recurrences, and as primary therapy for large unresectable lesions.[17] High doses of 80 gray have been given, but Cummings and associates[19] found 40 to 55 gray of daily fractionated megavoltage equal in effectiveness to higher doses. Mean duration of symptomatic improvement after treatment

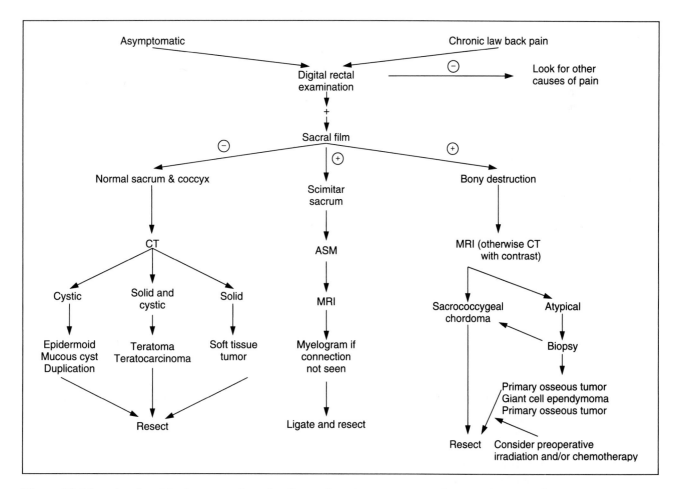

Figure 20-16. An algorithmic approach to the diagnosis and management of presacral cysts and tumors.

was 3.5 years.[19] Retreatment to a higher total dose can be given to patients developing a symptomatic recurrence. Limited success has been reported for preoperative irradiation,[39] proton therapy, and brachytherapy with I^{125}.

High grade malignant fibrohistiocytoma has been reported following radiotherapy for chordoma.[45]

Cryosurgery

Cryosurgery has a place as an adjunct to curative surgery and in palliation of chordomas.[46] Bone may be treated without resection, which may prove helpful in treating high sacral lesions. However, problems arise with skin and soft tissue necrosis, susceptibility of treated tissue to infection, and poor control over the extent of freezing.[47]

Repeat Resection

Resection for localized recurrence of chordoma definitely has a place because of the tumor's resistance to other forms of therapy and its indolent localized growth pattern. Postoperative irradiation may be advisable if it was not previously used.[48,49]

Chemotherapy

Chemotherapy has met with disappointing results for chordomas.[43]

References

1. Whittaker LD, Pemberton JD. Tumors ventral to the sacrum. *Ann Surg.* 1938;107:96–106.
2. Lovelady SB, Dockerty MB. Extragenital pelvic tumors in women. *Am J Obstet Gynecol.* 1949; 58:215–234.
3. Jao SW, Beart RW Jr, Spencer RJ, Reiman HM, Ilstrup DM. Retrorectal tumors: Mayo Clinic experience, 1960–1979. *Dis Colon Rectum.* 1984; 28:644–652.
4. Uhlig BE, Johnson RL. Presacral tumors and cysts in adults. *Dis Colon Rectum.* 1975;18:581–596.
5. Erich JB. Sebaceous, mucous, dermoid and epidermoid cysts. *Am J Surg.* 1940;50:672–677.
6. Middeldorpf K. Zur Kenntniss der angebornen Sacralgeschwulste. *Arch Pathol Anat Physiol.* 1885; 101:37–44.
7. Head HD, Gerstein JD, Muir RW. Presacral teratoma in the adult. *Am Surg.* 1975;240–247.
8. Aldridge MC, Boylston AW, Sim AJW. Dermoid cyst of the rectum. *Dis Colon Rectum.* 1983;26: 333–334.
9. Marcuse PM. Malignant presacral teratoma in an adult. *Cancer.* 1959;12:889–893.
10. Tolins SH, Cooper P. Presacral teratoma. *Am J Surg.* 1968;115:734–737.
11. Currarino G, Coln D, Votteler T. Triad of anorectal, sacral, and presacral anomalies. *Am J Radiol.* 1981;137:395–398.
12. O'Riordain DS, O'Connell PR, Kirwan WO. Hereditary sacral agenesis with presacral mass and anorectal stenosis: the Currarino triad. *Br J Surg.* 1991;78:536–538.
13. Kovalcik PJ, Burke JB. Anterior sacral meningocele and the scimitar sign. *Dis Colon Rectum.* 1988;31: 806–807.
14. Oren M, Lorber B, Lee SH, Truex RC Jr, Gennaro AR. Anterior sacral meningocele: report of five cases and review of the literature. *Dis Colon Rectum.* 1977;20:492–505.
15. Smith J, Ludwig RL, Marcove RC. Sacrococcygeal chordoma: clinicoradiological study of 60 patients. *Skeletal Radiol.* 1987;16:37–44.
16. Gray SW, Singhabhandhu B, Smith RA, Skandalakis JE. Sacrococcygeal chordoma: report of a case and review of the literature. *Surgery.* 1975; 78:573–582.
17. Healey JH, Lane JM. Chordoma: a critical review of diagnosis and treatment. *Orthop Clin North Am.* 1989;20:417–426.
18. Chambers PW, Schwinn CP. Chordoma: a clinicopathologic study of metastasis. *Am Soc Clin Pathol.* 1979;72:765–776.
19. Cummings BJ, Hodson DI, Bush RS. Chordoma: the results of megavoltage radiation therapy. *Int J Radiat Oncol Biol Phys.* 1983;9:633–642.
20. Wetzel LH, Levin E. MR imaging of sacral and presacral lesions. *AJR.* 1990;154:771–775.
21. Murray JA, Springfield DS. Giant cell tumor of bone. In: Evarts CM, ed. *Surgery of Musculoskeletal System.* 2nd ed. London: Churchill Livingstone; 1990:4822–4825.
22. Timmerman W, Bubrick MP. Presacral and postsacral extraspinal ependymoma: report of a case and review of the literature. *Dis Colon Rectum.* 1984; 27:114–119.
23. Cody HS, Marcove RC, Quan SH. Malignant retrorectal tumors: 28 years' experience at Memorial Sloan-Kettering Cancer Center. *Dis Colon Rectum.* 1981;24:501–506.
24. Feldenzer JA, McGauley JL, McGillicuddy JE. Sa-

cral and presacral tumors: problems in diagnosis and management. *Neurosurgery.* 1989;25:884–891.

25. Burchell MC. Radiologic impact on operative access to a retrorectal cyst. *Dis Colon Rectum.* 1987;30:396–397.

26. deBruine FT, Kroon HM. Spinal chordomas: radiologic features in 14 cases. *Am J Radiol.* 1988; 861–863.

27. Freir DT, Stanley JC, Thompson NW. Retrorectal tumors in adults. *Surg Gynecol Obstet.* 1971;132:681.

28. Levine E, Batnitzky S. Computed tomography of sacral and perisacral lesions. *Crit Rev Diagn Imaging.* 1984;21:307–374.

29. Rifkin MD, Marks GJ. Transrectal US as an adjunct in the diagnosis of rectal and extrarectal tumors. *Radiology.* 1985;157:499–502.

30. Amacher AL, Drake CG, McLachlin AD. Anterior sacral meningocele. *Surg Gynecol Obstet.* 1968; 126:986.

31. Eilber FR. Expert commentary. *Perspect Colon Rectal Surg.* 1990;3:252–253.

32. Spencer RJ, Jackman RJ. Surgical management of precoccygeal cysts. *Surg Gynecol Obstet.* 1962; 115:449.

33. Stener B, Gunterberg B. High amputation of the sacrum for extirpation of tumors: principles and technique. *Spine.* 1978;3:351–366.

34. MacCarty CS, Waugh JM, Mayo CW, et al. The surgical treatment of presacral tumors: a combined problem. *Proc Mayo Clin.* 1952;27:73.

35. Karakousis CP. Sacral resection with preservation of continence. *Surg Gynecol Obstet.* 1986;163: 271–273.

36. Localio SA, Eng K, Ranson JHC. Abdominosacral approach for retrorectal tumors. *Ann Surg.* 1980; 191:555–560.

37. Huth JF, Dawson EG, Eilber FR. Abdominosacral resection for malignant tumors of the sacrum. *Am J Surg.* 1984;148:157–161.

38. Michael LA, DeCloed TP. Synchronous abdominal and trans-sacral approach for excision of sacrococcygeal chordoma. *Acta Chir Belg.* 1989;316–319.

39. Kennedy CA, Mankin HJ. Sacral chordomas: surgical considerations. *Ortho Trans.* 1987;11(3):493.

40. Nakahara S, Itoh H, Mibu R, et al. Anorectal function after high sacrectomy with bilateral resection of S2–S5 nerves. *Dis Colon Rectum.* 1986;29: 271–274.

41. Dozois RR. Retrorectal tumors: spectrum of disease, diagnosis, and surgical management. *Perspect Colon Rectal Surg.* 1990;3:241–255.

42. Sung HW, Shu WP, Wang HM, et al. Surgical treatment of primary tumors of the sacrum. *Clin Orthop.* 1982;163:282.

43. Mindell ER. Chordoma. In: Evarts CM, ed. *Surgery of the musculoskeletal system.* 2nd ed. London: Churchill Livingstone; 1990;4946–4952.

44. Maroske D, Hupe K. Sacrococcygeal chordoma. Radical operation, a problem. *Chirurgie.* 1977; 48:118–122.

45. Halpeen J, Kopolovic J, Catane R. Malignant fibrous histiocytoma developing in irradiated sacral chordoma. *Cancer.* 1984;53:2661.

46. deVries J, Oldhoff J, Hadders HN. Cryosurgical treatment of sacrococcygeal chordoma. *Cancer.* 1986;58:2348–2354.

47. Wuismann P, Harle A, Matthiab HH, et al. Two-stage therapy in the treatment of sacral tumors. *Arch Orthop Trauma Surg.* 1989;108:255–260.

48. Rich TA, Schiller A, Suit HD, Mankin HJ. Clinical and pathologic review of 48 cases of chordoma. *Cancer.* 1985;56:182–187.

49. Ariel IM, Verdu C. Chordoma: an analysis of twenty cases treated over a 20 year span. *J Surg Oncol.* 1975;7:27.

CHAPTER 21

SEXUALLY TRANSMITTED AND INFECTIOUS DISEASES

Steven D. Wexner and
David E. Beck

During the past two decades, an explosive growth in the prevalence and variety of sexually transmitted diseases (STDs) and anorectal infections has occurred. This growth can be traced to increases in use of the anorectum for sexual gratification, promiscuity, and homosexuality. Anogenital, oroanal, and other anal-based erotic practices have increased; for example, an estimated 2 to 2.5 million British citizens regularly use the anorectum for sexual fulfillment.[1,2] Similarly, between 4 and 13 percent of the adult male population of the United States are predominantly homosexual or bisexual for at least a significant portion of their lives.[3] Promiscuity also plays a major role in the transmission of the vast majority of these diseases. It has been estimated that the average homosexual has about 1000 sexual partners during his lifetime,[4,5] and other studies suggest that a "moderately active" homosexual man will have sexual relations with 100 men per year.[6,7]

The frequent occurrence of STDs (estimated at over 12 million cases a year in the United States) and the gastrointestinal symptoms associated with these infections mandate a high index of suspicion to make an accurate diagnosis. Providers must remember that these patients commonly have more than one disease. Up to 55 percent of homosexual men with anorectal complaints have gonorrhea; 80 percent of the patients with syphilis are homosexuals. *Chlamydia* is found in 15 per-

cent of asymptomatic homosexual men, and up to one third of homosexuals have active anorectal herpes simplex virus. In addition, a host of parasites—bacterial, viral, and protozoan—are all rampant in the homosexual population. Although the term "gay bowel syndrome" has been used to include all STDs of the colon, rectum, and anus, this designation is somewhat of a misnomer because these STDs also can occur in women who practice anal intercourse.[8,9]

Finally, the global epidemic of the human immunodeficiency virus (HIV) and the resultant acquired immunodeficiency syndrome (AIDS) has produced a plethora of colorectal manifestations. Acute cytomegalovirus ileocolitis is the most common indication for emergency abdominal surgery in the homosexual AIDS population. Along with *Cryptosporidium* and *isospora*, the patient may present to the colorectal surgeon with bloody diarrhea and weight loss *before* the diagnosis of human immunodeficiency virus (HIV) disease. Other patients may present with colorectal Kaposi's sarcoma or anorectal lymphoma, and consequently will be found to have seropositivity for HIV. Moreover, in addition to these protean manifestations, one third of patients with AIDS consult the colorectal surgeon with either condylomata acuminata, anorectal sepsis, or proctitis before the diagnosis of HIV disease.

In view of the ever broadening geographic scope of STDs, it is of paramount importance that all colorectal providers have a working familiarity with each of these disorders. Tables 21-1 and 21-2 list the diseases covered in this chapter and include a summary of the presenting symptoms, physical findings, suggested diagnostic tests, and recommended treatment. Specific anorectal

The opinions expressed in this chapter are those of the authors and do not reflect the opinions of the United States Air Force or the Department of Defense.

Table 21-1   Sexually Transmitted and Infectious Organisms That Cause Anorectal Pathology

Organism	Symptoms	Anoscopy and proctoscopy	Laboratory test	Treatment*
BACTERIAL				
Gonorrhea	Rectal discharge	Proctitis, muco-purulent discharge	Thayer–Mayer culture of discharge	Ceftrlaxone 250 mg IM for 1 day and doxy-cycline 100 mg PO BID for 7 days
Syphillis	Rectal pain	Painful anal ulcer	Dark-field exam of fresh scrapings	Benzathine penicillin 2.4 million units IM
Chlamydia and lympho-granuloma venereum (LGV)	Tenesmus	Friable, often ulcerated rectal mucosa +/− rectal mass	Serologic antibody titer; biopsy for culture	Tetracycline 500 mg PO QID for 14 days (chlamydia) 21 days (LGV)
Hemophilus du-creyll (chancroid)	Perineal pain	Perianal abscess, ulcers	Culture	Erythromycin 500 mg PO BID for 7 days
Granuloma Inguinale	Perianal mass	Hard, shiny perianal masses	Biopsy of mass	Tetracycline 500 mg PO QID for 7 days
Hidradenitis suppurativa†	Pain, discharge from skin	Induration, scarring, discharge from sub-cutaneous tissue	Culture and biopsy	Complete surgical excision
VIRAL				
Mulluscum con-tageosum	Painless dermal lesions	Flattened round um-bilicated lesions	Excisional biopsy	Excision, cryotherapy
Human papillo-mavirus (HPV) (condylomata acuminata)	Pruritus, bleeding, discharge, pain	Perianal warts	Excisional biopsy with viral analysis	Destruction. See text.
Herpes simplex virus (HSV)	Anorectal pain, pruritus	Perianal erythema, vesicles, ulcers, dif-fusely inflamed, friable rectal mucosa	Cytologic exam of scrapings or viral culture of vesicular fluid	Symptomatic: acyclovir. See text.
Human immuno-deficiency virus (AIDS)‡	See text.‡	See text.‡	Western blot	AZT. See text.
Cytomegalovirus‡	Rectal bleeding	Multiple small white ulcers	Biopsy, viral culture, and antigen assay of ulcers	?DHPG (trials under-way)

* Many alternative regimes exist; some are described in the text.
† Discussed in Chapter 13.
‡ Discussed in Chapter 22.

disorders are covered first, followed by diseases that cause diarrhea as their major symptom. Anorectal abscesses, pilonidal infections, and AIDS are covered in other chapters. Infectious proctitides not discussed in this chapter are reviewed in Chapter 26. Medications and dosages are suggested, but clinicians are reminded to consult the full prescribing information before using any medication mentioned in this text.

Table 21-2   Sexually Transmitted and Infectious Organisms That Cause Diarrhea

Organism	Symptoms	Anoscopy and proctoscopy	Laboratory test	Treatment*
PARASITIC				
Entomeoba histolytica	Bloody diarrhea	Friable rectal mucosa; shallow ulcers with yellowish exudate and ring of erythema	Fresh stool exam (microscopy)	Metronidazole 750 mg PO TID for 10 days, then dilodohydroxyguinine 650 mg PO TID for 20 days
Giardia lamblia	Nausea, bloating, cramps, diarrhea	Normal sigmoidoscopy and anoscopy	Fresh stool exam (microscopy)	Metronidazole 250 mg PO TID for 7 days
Shigella	Abdominal cramps, fever, tenesmus, bloody diarrhea	Erythema, edema, grayish-white ulcerations of rectal mucosa	Culture stool	Trimethoprim-sulfamethoxazole (double strength) PO BID for 7 days
Campylobacter	Diarrhea, cramps, bloating	Erythema, edema, grayish-white ulcerations of rectal mucosa	Culture stool using selective media	Erythromycin 500 mg PO QID for 7 days
Cryptosporidia	Bloody, mucoid diarrhea, dehydration	Normal	Rectal biopsy (oocysts)	Hydration
Isospora	Vomiting, fever, abdominal pain	Normal	Acid-fast stain of stool; endoscopic biopsy	Trimethoprim-sulfamethoxazole (double strength) PO BID for 7 days
Mycobacterium avium-Intracellulare	Watery diarrhea	Normal	Acid-fast stain of stool; ileal biopsy	See text.

* Many alternative regimes exist; some are described in the text.

Specific Anorectal Disorders

Gonorrhea

Gonorrhea is a common STD caused by *Neisseria gonorrhoeae*, a gram-negative intracellular diplococcus that occurs in pairs or clusters and can infect the mucosal lining of all body orifices. The Centers for Disease Control estimated an incidence of 1.5 million cases in 1989 in the United States, and *N. gonorrhoeae* is probably the most common STD pathogen seen in homosexual men.[10] Up to 55 percent of homosexual men seen in screening clinics harbor gonorrhea.[11-14] The rectum is the only site infected in 40 to 50 percent of these patients, and the majority are asymptomatic.[10,15] Transmission, which is by anal intercourse, is followed by an incubation period of 5 to 7 days, after which a proctitis, cryptitis, or both ensue.[16] In women, gonorrhea can result from anal-receptive intercourse, but the vast majority of cases are caused by autoinoculation of vaginal gonorrhea into the lower rectum. Stansfield reported that only 6 percent of women have rectal gonorrhea in the absence of cervical or urethral involvement.[17]

Many patients with isolated gonorrheal proctitis are asymptomatic. If any symptoms do occur, they tend to include pruritus ani, bloody or mucoid rectal discharge, or tenesmus. In advanced cases, disseminated disease can occur. This includes perihepatitis, meningitis, endocarditis, pericarditis, and gonococcal arthritis. The latter manifestation is probably the most common of the disseminated group and tends to be a unilateral migratory purulent arthritis of large joints.

A mucopurulent discharge is the most suggestive diagnostic clue, especially when seen in combination with proctitis. This discharge appears as a thick, viscid, yellow exudate. Symptoms are nonspecific and include pruritus ani, tenesmus, and hematochezia[18] (Fig. 21-1).

Lubrication of the anoscope with anything other than water is not advisable since many lubricants and creams contain antibacterial agents. On endoscopic evaluation, the anal canal is classically uninvolved, while the rectum displays edema, friability, erythema, ulceration, and mucus. One classic finding is the ability to express mucopus from the anal crypts. This is best done by applying gentle external pressure while the anoscope is in place.

Diagnosis should be made by culture placed immediately on Thayer–Martin or Stuart's (anaerobic) medium. One can blindly swab the anal canal by inserting a pledget between 2.0 and 2.5 cm into the anal canal and then rotating it from side to side for several seconds. Swabbing the mucopus under direct anoscopic visualization, however, raises the positive yield on Gram's stain from 34 percent to 79 percent.[19-21] Rarely are the gram-negative intracellular diplococci seen, although positive identification facilitates immediate therapy. However, many nondiagnostic Gram stains are subsequently revealed to be false-negatives. For this reason, a high index of suspicion warrants empiric treatment pending final culture results. Conversely, positive identification of *N. gonorrhoeae* does not provide irrefutable proof of its responsibility for the patient's symptoms. Many homosexual male patients have coexistent STDs. *Neisseria meningitidis* may also be cultured from the rectum of homosexual male patients.[22]

Treatment must include screening for repeat gonorrheal infection in 3 months, as failure of initial treatment occurs in up to 35 percent of cases.[23] The traditionally preferred treatment is 4.8 million units of aqueous procaine penicillin G given intramuscularly plus 1 gram of probenecid given orally.[15] This regimen has two advantages: a low recurrence rate and the concomitant eradication of incubating syphilis.[24-26] However, there has been a tremendous rise in the prevalence of penicillinase-producing *Neisseria gonorrhoeae*.[27] These resistant strains are best treated with an alternative regimen: 250 mg ceftriaxone 250 mg given in a single intramuscular dose followed by 100 mg doxycycline given orally twice a day for 7 days is currently preferred.[28] Other authors prefer a single intramuscular dose of 2 g of spectinomycin hydrochloride, which has a 94.5 percent rate of success[18] or a single intramuscular dose of cefoxitin with 1 g of probenecid given orally.[29] The latter regimen has a slightly higher failure rate than the others. Additional treatment protocols are all multiple-dose regimens given over periods ranging from 3 to 10 days. They include trimethoprim–sulfamethoxazole, kanamycin, tetracycline, ampicillin, and ceftriaxone.[29,30]

As with other STDs, all sexual contacts must be treated to prevent recurrence. The importance of close follow-up examination with culture to assess disease eradication cannot be overemphasized. With careful follow-up and treatment of all sexual partners, a 95 percent cure rate is a reasonable expectation.

Syphilis

Primary anal syphilis is also largely a disease of homosexual men.[1,31,32] For example, 80 percent of cases of syphilis in central London clinics are in homosexual men.[33] Anal syphilis is caused by *Treponema pallidum*, a motile spirochete. The organism enters the anoderm or anal mucosa during anal-receptive intercourse; anal ulcers usually appear within 2 to 6 weeks after exposure but can occur up to 3 months later.[27,32] The initial lesion is a chancre at the anal margin or canal, which often causes exquisite pain and can therefore be mistaken for an anal fissure.[34] These lesions are usually raised, circular, and 1 to 2 cm in diameter. Inguinal adenopathy is typical and should assist in diagnosis. Ulcers may be eccentrically located, multiple, or irregular, and two ulcers may be opposite each other in a "mirror image" or "kissing" configuration (Fig. 21-2). Some chancres have been known to mimic polyps and lobulated masses.[27,35] If the chancre is of the painless variety, the patient may not seek medical advice, and the ulcer may heal in 3 to 4 weeks.[35] Proctitis in the absence of anogenital lesions has also been reported.[36] Rectal syphilis with inguinal adenopathy has been mistaken for lymphoma, as both diseases may present with rubbery inguinal lymphadenopathy and submucosal rectal irregularities.[37] Rectal syphilis, like lymphoma, is generally accompanied by tenesmus, mucoid discharge, and rectal pain.[38]

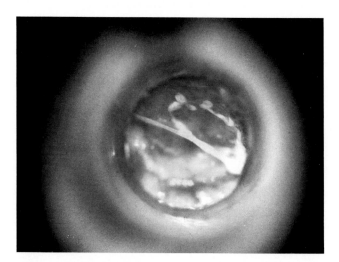

Figure 21-1.   The mucopurulent discharge of gonorrheal proctitis. (*From:* Wexner SD. Managing common anorectal sexually transmitted diseases. *Infect Surg.* 1990; June; 9–48.) (Photo courtesy of R. Copé, M.D., Paris, France.)

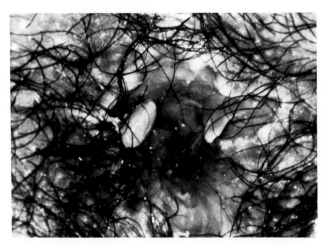

Figure 21-2. Atypical syphilitic chancre. (Courtesy of R. Cope, M.D., Paris, France.)

Because of the protean manifestations of syphilitic ulcers, any anal ulcer in a homosexual or bisexual man must be viewed with suspicion. Women with anal ulcers must be queried regarding anal-receptive intercourse. Early syphilis can be diagnosed by using anoscopy with dark-field examination of scrapings from the base of the chancre, and also by serology; early lesions should be teeming with spirochetes.[15] When viewed with dark-field microscopy, the treponemes appear as corkscrew-shaped, motile, fluorescent yellow-green organisms. In untreated primary syphilis, the Venereal Disease Research Laboratory (VDRL) assay is reactive in about 75 percent of cases. In early latent syphilis, reactivity occurs in about 95 percent of cases, and in the secondary stage 100 percent should react. The fluorescent treponemal antibody (FTA) absorption test usually becomes positive about 4 to 6 weeks after the initial infection.[27] Thus, the VDRL is usually reactive after the FTA. Some laboratories use the rapid plasma reagin (RPR) test, which is also positive after the FTA. The RPR test can be automated, making it useful in mass screening. Currently the FTA and dark-field microscopy constitute the initial diagnostic maneuvers. Because of these prolonged serologic latencies, clinically suspicious lesions should be treated pending laboratory confirmation.

The second stage of anal syphilis will appear in untreated patients 6 to 8 weeks after the chancre has healed (Fig. 21-3). It may present as a condyloma latum, a pale-brown or pink flat verrucous lesion with numerous spirochetes, or as a mucocutaneous rash.[16] The patient will often have an accompanying fever, malaise, lymphadenopathy, and arthropathy. The condyloma latum is a large perianal mass composed of many raised, moist, smooth warts. These warts tend to secrete mucus and consequently are associated with pruritus ani and a

foul odor. The secondary lesion and the primary chancre may coexist. The differential diagnosis includes condyloma acuminatum, but the latter wart is more desiccated and keratinized than is the condyloma latum. All three serologic tests for syphilis will invariably be positive in high titers during secondary syphilis.[32] Although exceedingly rare in western countries at this time, a tertiary stage (tabes dorsalis) can occur; it produces anal sphincter paralysis and severe perianal pain. Syphilitic rectal gumma are exceedingly rare and may be confused with malignant growths.[34]

The initial treatment of patients with syphilis is a single dose of 2.4 million units of benzathine penicillin G given in one intramuscular injection. Patients with long-standing disease may require this dose repeated at weekly intervals for 3 weeks. Penicillin-allergic patients can be effectively treated with 500 mg tetracycline or 500 mg erythromycin given orally four times a day for 15 to 30 days.[32] All sexual contacts of patients with primary, secondary, or early tertiary syphilis should be prophylactically treated. Adequate disease eradication includes treatment of all partners with whom sexual activity occurred during the preceding 12 months. Patients and contacts must abstain from all sexual contacts until proved noninfective by low titers. Patients who have had syphilis for greater than 1 year or have symptoms of neural involvement require a cerebral spinal fluid (CSF) examination. If the CSF is involved, additional therapy is indicated. Follow-up testing with the VDRL or RPR should be undertaken at 3-month intervals for 1 year.

Lymphogranuloma Venereum and Other Chlamydiae

Chlamydiae, small intracellular organisms, related to bacteria, have been implicated in a number of clinical

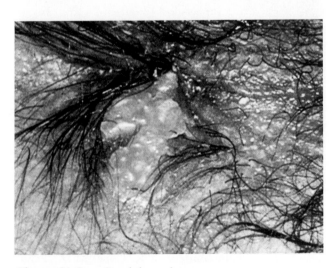

Figure 21-3. Condyloma latum.

syndromes including cervicitis, nongonococcal urethritis, and proctitis. Symptoms are related to inflammation of the infected mucosa. Chlamydial infection is currently the most common STD in the United States and is becoming a more frequent cause of proctitis in both men and women who practice anal-receptive intercourse.[39-41] Chlamydial proctitis may coexist with other rectal STDs, especially gonorrhea. Chlamydial rectal infections are currently found in up to 15 percent of asymptomatic homosexual men.[42] Both anal-receptive intercourse and oral-anal intercourse have been implicated as causative behaviors. Of the 15 known immunotypes of *Chlamydia trachomatis*, serotypes D through K are responsible for proctitis and serotypes L_1, L_2, and L_3 are responsible for lymphogranuloma venereum (LGV). Symptoms of rectal infection generally include fever, malaise, anorexia, headache, joint pain, tenesmus, rectal pain, and a mucoid or bloody rectal discharge. The LGV serovars tend to cause painful anal or perianal ulcers (Fig. 21-4); rectovaginal fistulae can occur. Inguinal adenopathy is associated with both serovars D through K and with L_1 through L_3 perianal infections. The nodes may fuse into a large indurated mass with erythema of the overlying skin producing a clinical picture similar to syphilis. Chronic inflammation of the lymph nodes may result in lymphedema.

Sigmoidoscopic findings generally include severe nonspecific granular proctitis with mucosal erythema, friability, and ulceration (Fig. 21-5). Late findings may include an intraluminal stricture or mass, although this is more common in women. Biopsy of the rectal mucosa will reveal findings consistent with infectious proctitis; these microscopic features include crypt abscesses, infectious granulomata, and giant cells.[42,43] Because *Chlamydia* is an obligate intracellular pathogen,

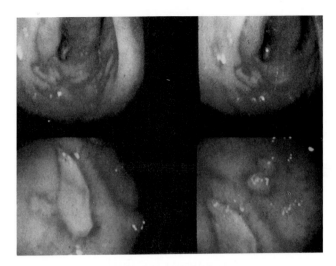

Figure 21-5.   Rectal chlamydial ulcer.

rectal culture is usually unrewarding, and the complement fixation test may not be positive.[44] The microimmunofluorescent antibody titer is the most sensitive serotyping test and is becoming more readily available.[45] However, the test is not yet universally available, and many clinicians prefer to culture a biopsy of the inflamed rectal mucosa. The biopsy for culture is best obtained under direct visualization and transported in sucrose phosphate medium on ice for immediate tissue culture inoculation. Antichlamydial antibody titers, as determined by the complement fixation test, are 1:80 or greater.[27] Titer elevation generally occurs 1 month or more after infection. However, low-level antibody response should not form the cornerstone of diagnostic reliability. Either microimmunofluorescent or tissue culture testing must be positive for confirmation.

C. trachomatis infections generally respond to either oral tetracycline or erythromycin, 500 mg four times a day. Alternatively, 100 mg oral doxycycline given twice a day for a 6-month course has been suggested.[46] With the exception of Vibramycin®, the duration of antibiotic administration is from 7 to 14 days for non-LGV and 21 days for LGV-strain infections.[47]

Residual rectal strictures have been reported as a late complication of these infections.[34] The strictures may be from single or multiple and may have short segments of long ones that can extend from 3 cm above the anal verge to the splenic flexure. Other more common causes of stricture, such as inflammatory bowel disease and ischemia, must be excluded. Asymptomatic strictures require no treatment; the treatment of symptomatic strictures should first include a 3-week course of erythromycin, tetracycline, or doxycycline. If this does not relieve symptoms, sphincter-saving excisional surgery may be the only curative alternative.

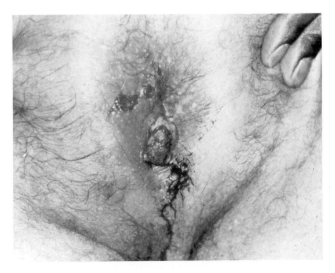

Figure 21-4.   Perianal LGV ulcer. (Courtesy of T. H. Dailey, M.D., New York, NY.)

Chancroid

Chancroid is caused by *Hemophilus ducreyi*, a small gram-negative, nonmotile, non-spore-forming aerobic bacillus. The infection is characterized by adenopathy, multiple perineal abscesses, and ulcers.[48] The diagnosis is confirmed by culture. Treatment is accomplished with 600 mg erythromycin given orally twice a day for 7 days *or* 1 trimethoprim/sulfamethoxazole tablet given orally twice a day for 7 days. Antibiotic susceptibility of this organism varies. If clinical improvement does not occur after the initial course of therapy, a different antibiotic should be tried. Resolution of the adenopathy will lag behind resolution of the ulcers.[49]

Granuloma Inguinale

Granuloma inguinale is caused by *Calymmatobacterium granulomatis*, a gram-negative bacillus. It produces chronic granulomatous infections that present as hard, shiny masses in the perineal area. The diagnosis is confirmed by biopsy. Treatment is 500 mg tetracycline given orally four times a day for 7 days or 500 to 1000 mg streptomycin given intramuscularly twice a day.[49]

Herpes Simplex Virus

Herpes simplex (HSV) is a DNA virus that is endemic in the United States. Two serotypes cause anorectal problems: type 1 is usually associated with oral lesions and type 2 is associated with genital infections. Most cases of herpetic proctitis are caused by herpes simplex (also known as herpes hominis) virus type 2 (HSV-2) and are acquired by direct inoculation during anal-receptive intercourse.[50] The type 1 infection accounts for approximately 10 percent of anal infections, and type 2 for almost all of the rest; the zoster-varicella variety is occasionally encountered. Herpes simplex virus has been found on rectal cultures in 6 to 30 percent of homosexual patients with rectal symptomatology, and in one third of these cases it is associated with other pathogenic organisms.[51-53]

Serologic tests have revealed that more than 95 percent of homosexual male patients may have been infected with HSV-2.[54] The Centers for Disease Control (CDC) recently revised the diagnostic criteria for AIDS to include chronic mucocutaneous HSV infection.[55] Ulcerative perianal HSV-2 (among other varieties) present for at least 1 month in a patient with no other identifiable cause of immunodeficiency or who has laboratory-evidenced HIV infection is diagnostic of AIDS.

The HSV causes symptoms more commonly than most other anorectal infections, generally beginning 4 to 21 days after anal-receptive intercourse.[32] Ninety-five percent of patients have anorectal pain or burning,

exacerbated by enemas, intercourse, and bowel movements.[53,56] Pruritus ani affects approximately 50 to 85 percent of patients.[57] Other findings include mucoid or bloody bowel movements, tenesmus, psychogenic constipation, and less commonly the systemic manifestations of fever, chills, and malaise.[53] Bilateral tender inguinal lymphadenopathy is reported occasionally.[16]

Some patients present with the constellation of urinary dysfunction, sacral paresthesias, impotence, and pain in the lower abdomen, thighs, and buttocks.[32] Occasionally, the bulbocavernous reflex is absent. This syndrome is secondary to the lumbosacral radiculopathy caused by the HSV and is found in up to 50 percent of HSV-infected men.[58] The symptoms of the radiculopathy and a deep-seated severe pelvic pain often outlast the active clinical infection.[59] The disease is highly contagious from the first appearance of the vesicles until perianal reepithelialization is complete. Rarely, HSV is transmitted even after complete healing.

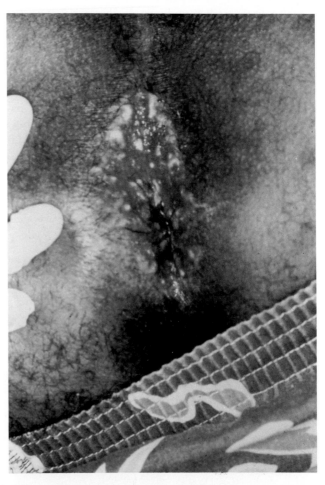

Figure 21-6.   Perianal herpes simplex virus. The vesicles have already encrusted and coalesced. (*From:* Wexner SD. AIDS: what the colorectal surgeon needs to know. *Perspect Colorectal Surg.* 1989; 2(2): 19–55.)

During the acute phase, the anorectum usually is exquisitely tender, and an accurate examination may be impossible without typical anesthesia. Acute lesions range from small (1–2 mm) vesicles with red areolae, to larger ruptured vesicles, to aphthous coalesced ulcers (Fig. 21-6). These lesions are usually painful, contain clear fluid, and occur on the perianal skin, in the anal canal, or less frequently in the rectum. Shallow perianal ulcers may coalesce and extend to the sacrococygeal area in a butterfly distribution. The differential diagnosis includes herpes zoster. The zoster ulcers, however, occur along a dermatomal distribution, as shown in Figure 21-7.

The sigmoidoscopic findings of HSV proctitis typically include friable mucosa, diffuse ulcerations, and occasional intact vesicles and pustules (Fig. 21-8). These changes are almost always limited to the distal 10 cm of the rectum. Ulcerations in the anal canal may become secondarily infected, and appear as grayish crypts with erythematous borders. Crusting of the lesions is followed by healing in approximately 2 weeks. A chronic relapsing course is common, with recurrence rates of 40 percent.[60] In some patients, an inciting factor such as trauma or exposure to sunlight may be related to the recurrence. Lesions usually recur in the same dermatome distribution as did the initial infection. Sacral paresthesias and severe perianal and buttock pain often precede the recurrence of vesicles by several days. Cytologic scrapings or biopsies taken from the bed of an ulcer will reveal the typical intranuclear inclusion bodies or multinucleated giant cells (Fig. 21-9) diagnostic of the virus.[50] Crypt abscesses and lamina propria neutrophils occur in about one half of all specimens. Although

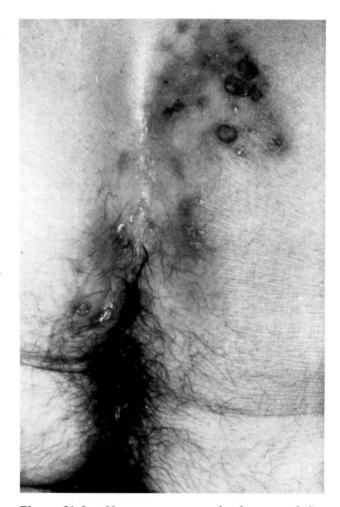

Figure 21-8. Herpes zoster; note the dermatomal distribution.

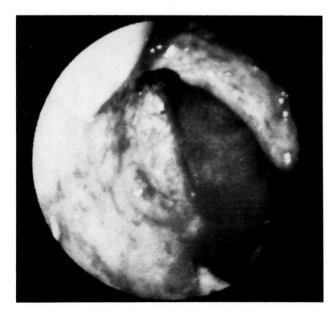

Figure 21-7. Herpes proctitis.

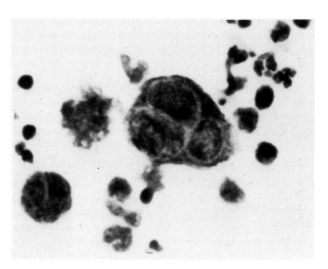

Figure 21-9. Microscopic identification of multinucleate giant cells from the cytologic scraping of a perianal ulcer. (*From:* Wexner SD. AIDS: what the colorectal surgeon needs to know. *Perspect Colorectal Surg.* 1989; 2(2) 19–55.)

routine stains are usually sufficient to identify typical cytologic alterations, intranuclear inclusion bodies can be selectively stained with anti-HSV-2 antiserum using special techniques. Viral culture and direct immunofluorescent staining of the vesicular fluid are also diagnostic.[61]

Treatment of HSV has traditionally been symptomatic, with sitz baths, lidocaine ointment, cool compresses, and oral analgesics.[56] Hygiene is important to prevent a bacterial superinfection. Recently, however, acyclovir has produced improvement in the acute setting, although it does not eradicate the HSV or cure the disease.[52,62] Acyclovir, administered orally and topically, has been effective in lengthening the asymptomatic period, promoting healing of lesions, and shortening the period of viral shedding.[63-65] Administered orally, acyclovir may suppress the frequency of recurrence, provided the drug is taken for life.[66]

Rompalo and associates[67] enrolled 29 homosexual men with first-episode rectal HSV-2 in a double-blind prospective trial of oral acyclovir (400 mg 5 times daily) and placebo. In 80 percent of those who received acyclovir as compared with only 25 percent of placebo recipients, viral shedding ceased within 3 days of the start of therapy. The median durations of viral excretion from the herpetic lesions and of the presence of the lesions themselves were significantly shorter in the acyclovir group. This latter group also reported a more rapid resolution of rectal pain, discharge, and other subjective symptoms of proctitis. Whitley and associates[68] reported very similar results as did Mertz and associates.[69]

Topical acyclovir is less effective than is either oral or intravenous therapy.[70] Treatment should be continued until all mucocutaneous surfaces have completely re-epithelialized. Most patients with perianal herpes infections can be effectively treated with 200 to 400 mg acyclovir given orally five times each day for 10 days. In addition, topical acyclovir ointment can be used five times daily. Patients with severe perianal infections or with herpes proctitis may benefit from intravenous acyclovir at a dosage of 5 mg/kg every 8 hours for 5 to 7 days. Since many patients with AIDS suffer from frequent recurrences, suppressive therapy is possible; the dosage is generally 200 mg or 400 mg given orally between two and five times daily. AIDS patients with HSV perianal ulcerations that are resistant to acyclovir may be candidates for either foscarnet or vidarabine, two newer compounds.[71-73]

Stamm and associates[74] and Holmberg and associates[75] have independently reported a statistically significant association between HSV-2 infection and subsequent HIV infection. The HSV-2 must be recognized not only as an ulcerative pathogen but as a harbinger of HIV infection. All patients with anorectal herpes infections should be counseled regarding HIV testing.

Molluscum Contagiosum

The disease known as molluscum contagiosum is caused by a virus of the pox group and is transmitted by direct body contact. After an incubation period of 3 to 6 weeks, the patient develops painless 3-mm flattened round umbilicated lesions. Although the disease is benign and self-limiting, treatment is used both to prevent spread and for cosmetic purposes. Treatment options include local destruction with phenol, surgical removal, and cryotherapy.[49] Cryotherapy is probably the most commonly used.

Condylomata Acuminata

Condylomata acumulata (anal and perianal warts) are the most common sexually transmitted disease seen by the colorectal surgeon.[76] The CDC reported a 500 percent increase in the incidence of condylomata between 1966 and 1981.[77] Condylomata acuminata are epithelialized raised wartlike lesions that can arise alone or more often in groups. The lesions can range in size from a few millimeters to a cauliflower-like Buschke–Lowenstein type lesion (Figs. 21-10 and 21-11). Anal condylomata may occur in combination with genital (penile or vaginal) condylomata. They may occur on the perianal skin, or in the anal canal. In nonimmunocompromised patients they do not extend cephalad to the dentate line. The usual mode of transmission is by anal-insertive intercourse, although autoinnoculation from genital warts may occur. The condylomata may be asymptomatic or may cause pruritus ani or a mass. They rarely bleed and pain should not be a presenting symptom.

The human papillomavirus (HPV) is responsible for condylomata acuminata. Over 40 subtypes of HPV have been isolated in association with a wide range of lesions from the common digital wart to intraepithelial cervical neoplasia.[78] Although HPV subtypes 6, 11, 16, and 18 have been recovered from perianal condylomata, type 6 is the most common.[79] Types 16 or 18 behave more aggressively and are more frequently associated with dysplasia and malignant transformation than are types 6 and 11.[80] Scholefield and colleagues used magnification colposcopy, and HPV typing to determine the incidence of the HPV virus in perianal tissue that was not condylomatous on gross inspection.[81] Palmer and coworkers reported similar findings.[82] The significance of the potential premalignant type of HPV in perianal condylomata cannot be overemphasized. The condylomata may undergo malignant transformation and develop into either carcinoma in situ or invasive carcinoma. Nash and colleagues reported 20 cases of histologically atypical and mucosal lesions, ranging from atypical condylomata to carcinoma in situ[83]: 92 percent of the patients were male and 75 percent of these were known homosexuals. Croxson and associates reported 7 homosexual men in whom condylomata revealed carcinoma in situ.[84] Other authors have observed that homosexual men are at increased risk for the development of invasive anal carcinoma.[85–87] Gail and associates have used immunohistochemical techniques to implicate HPV in anal squamous cell carcinoma in homosexual men.[88]

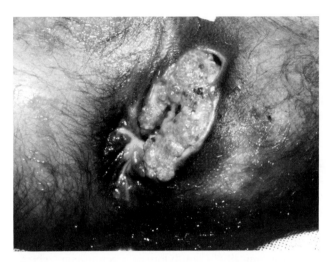

Figure 21-11. Florid condylomata acuminata with carcinoma in situ. (*From:* Wexner SD, Smithy WB, Milson JW, Dailey TH. The surgical management of anorectal diseases in AIDS and pre-AIDS patients. *Dis Colon Rectum.* 1986, 29:719–723.)

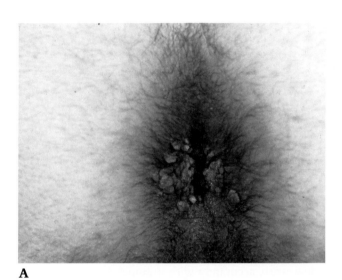

A

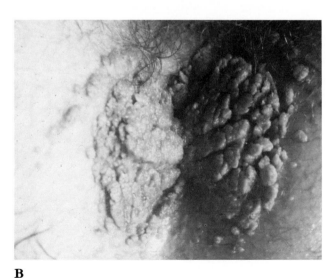

B

Figure 21-10. (A) Condylomata acuminata. (B) Extensive condylomata acuminata.

Prevalence

Although perianal condylomata can be seen in women and in heterosexual men, the typical patient is a sexually active homosexual or bisexual male. Forty to 70 percent of homosexual men have condylomata,[89] and 90 percent of patients with anal condylomata report the practice of anal-receptive intercourse.[90] Associated genital condylomata are common in 80 percent of women (on the external genitalia, vagina, or cervix) and in 16 percent of men (on the penis).[90] Urethral warts have also been reported, and warts may occur in the anal canal. Symptoms are related to the lesions' location: patients without visible anogenital warts may be asymptomatic. As many as 50 percent to 75 percent of asymptomatic homosexual men harbor anal canal condylomata,[91,92] leading to important epidemiologic implications. Sohn and Robilotti reported that the condylomata were confined to the perianal area in only 6 percent of symptomatic homosexual males, whereas both perianal and intraanal lesions were noted in 84 percent.[91] Furthermore 10 percent of the symptomatic patients had only intraanal condylomata. This highlights the importance of anoscopy performed with adequate sphincter relaxation, good direct lighting, and possible colposcopy, acetic acid staining, or loupe magnification.[82,93]

Evaluation

Symptoms include pruritus ani, bleeding, discharge, persistent perianal wetness, and pain.[70] Very few patients complain of a lump or mass. The lesions can be single, pinkish-white, cauliflower-like pinheads (see Fig. 21-10) or may form many multiple large clusters that appear as a confluent sheet that may obliterate the anus from view (see Figure 21-11). This latter pattern is typically seen in the AIDS patient.[94] The differential diagnosis of these lesions includes condylomata latum, molluscum contagiosum, and hypertrophied anal papillae. Condylomata latum (secondary syphilitic sores) are smoother, flatter, and moister than condylomata and demonstrate spirochetes on dark-field examination. The lesions of molluscum contagiosum are small, raised, centrally umbilicated, and pinkish-white, whereas hypertrophied anal papillae are usually not as friable as are condylomata.

Microscopically, condylomata acuminata show marked acanthosis of the epidermis with hyperplasia of the prickle cels, parakeratosis, and an underlying chronic inflammatory cell infiltration.[95] Vacuolization of the upper prickle layer (koilocytosis) may also be present and orthokeratosis is often seen.

Successful therapy requires accurate diagnosis and eradication of all warts. Therefore, all patients should undergo anoscopy, proctosigmoidoscopy, and either a vaginal or penile examination. In addition, other coexisting alimentary or sexually transmitted pathogens (as described in this chapter) should be identified and treated.

Many types of therapy have been used to manage anal condylomata, as outlined in Table 21-3. Evaluation of each method has been complicated by occasional spontaneous regression of the warts, uncertainty about whether the warts identified after treatment are true recurrences or reinfection, and the lack of prospective controlled clinical trials. Results of therapy have varied, with reported recurrence rates ranging from 10 to 75 percent. The method used to eliminate the warts, appears to be less important than limiting the damage to the surrounding normal skin. Each method has advantages and disadvantages which are presented below.

Specific Therapy

Excision. Condylomata can be excised either in the office with local anesthesia or in the outpatient operating room with a regional block. Excision allows precise removal of the condylomata and complete histopathologic microscopic examination. This is especially important considering the rising incidence of malignant transformation of condylomata.[86]

The excisional technique used by the authors involves giving the patient two disposable phosphate enemas 30 to 60 minutes prior to the procedure. The patient is assisted to the prone-jacknife position with the buttocks taped apart. A headlight provides excellent

Table 21-3   Some of the More Commonly Used Treatment Options for Condylomata Acuminata

EXCISIONAL

DESTRUCTIVE
Podophyllin
Bichlorocetic acid (BCCA)
Electrocautery
Cryotherapy
Laser
    Carbon dioxide
    Contact ND: YAG

IMMUNOTHERAPY
Interferon injection
    Intramuscular
    Intralesional

CHEMOTHERAPY
5-Fluororacil
Bleomycin
Other

illumination of the anus and perianal region and is indispensable in the identification of smaller condylomata.[76] A solution of 0.5% lidocaine with 0.25% bupivicaine and 1:200,000 epinephrine is used to obtain a perianal field block as described in Chapter 5. If regional or general anesthesia is administered, a 1:200,000 epinephrine solution is still used because it reduces blood loss and elevates and separates the warts (Fig. 21-12), thereby improving the operator's ability to excise individual warts accurately with minimal damage to inter-

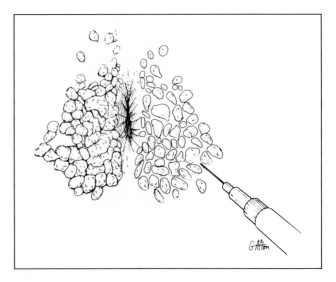

Figure 21-12. Epinephrine solution injected subdermally elevates and separates warts (*right*).

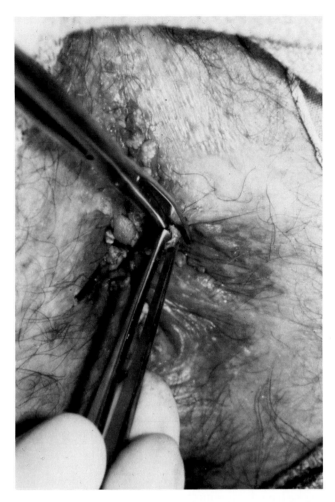

Figure 21-13.   Excision of individual warts with fine scissors.

vening skin. Prior to wart excision, anoscopy and proctoscopy should be undertaken if these examinations have not been previously accomplished. The warts are then individually excised with a fine iris or fistula scissors (Fig. 21-13). Preservation of anoderm (Fig. 21-14) and especially anal canal mucosa is of paramount importance to minimize perioperative discomfort, complications, and healing time. In the vast majority of patients all the condylomata can be excised in a single session with postoperative bleeding as the most frequent complication (2 to 3 percent).[96] Electrocautery applied to the base of each wart helps prevent early postoperative bleeding, although delayed bleeding after the eschar sloughs is still possible. The rate of recurrence is less than 10 percent.[97]

Podophyllin.   Podophyllin is the resin of podophyllum, an agent that is cytoxic to condylomata and very irritating to normal skin. It is generally applied in either liquid paraffin or tincture of benzoin, the latter adhering best to the warts. Although concentrations from 5% to 50% have been used, a 25% suspension is readily available and seems optimal. The mixture is carefully applied directly to the condylomata, ensuring that the intervening normal skin bridges are not treated. A sharpened wooden dowel is a good vehicle of delivery. After application, talcum powder is applied to the skin. Six to eight hours later the patient should thoroughly wash the entire area to prevent skin damage.

Because of autoinnoculation, repeated treatments are often required. Furthermore, because podophyllin is toxic to skin or mucosa, it cannot be applied to anal canal warts. Local complications include skin necrosis, fistula in ano, dermatitis, and anal stenosis. In addition, large doses may cause systemic effects including hepatic, renal, gastrointestinal, respiratory, and neurologic problems.[98,99] Particularly disturbing is the fact that podophyllin causes histologic changes in the treated warts that are difficult to distinguish from carcinoma in situ.[95] These histologic changes, including dispersion of

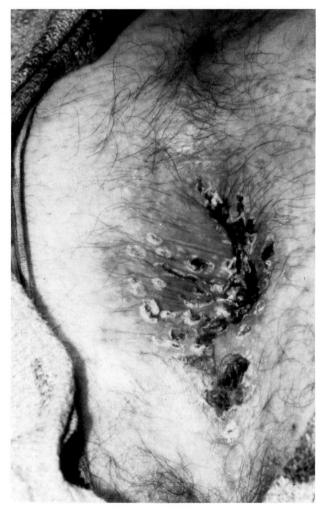

Figure 21-14.   Warts have been excised and the base electrocauterized with preservation of anoderm.

chromatin, paranuclear vacuolization, and nuclear changes, reverse within 4 weeks of the last podophyllin application.[100] Several treatments are often required to eradicate all warty tissue. Jensen reported a prospective radomized trial in which 25% podophyllin application was compared with surgical excision in 60 patients with first-episode condylomata.[101] The podophyllin was applied weekly for up to 6 weeks. Although the warts resolved in 77 percent of patients treated with podophyllin, the warts had recurred at 12 months in 65 percent. This compared to 93 percent resolution and 29 percent recurrence after surgical excision. Thus excision produced more rapid initial clearance and a lower incidence of recurrence than did podophyllin.

Bichloroacetic Acid.   Bichloroacetic acid (BCAA) can be applied to warts in a similar way as podophyllin. The major differences are that BCAA can be applied to anal canal warts, does not have systemic toxicity, and does not cause histologic changes that mimic carcinoma in situ. The recurrence rate is approximately 25 percent after a mean of 5 treatments and up to 13 treatments are necessary to achieve resolution of the condylomata.[102] Treatments can be performed at weekly intervals.

Electrocoagulation.   Electrocoagulation requires the use of local or regional anesthesia. The aim is to produce a white coagulum, which is the equivalent of a superficial second-degree burn. The procedure is best effected with a high current setting. Patients are prepared and positioned as described for excision. The cautery tip is placed near, but not into, the wart and a spark gap is created.[95] A white coagulum is produced which can then be wiped away. If any black eschar appears, a deep second- or third-degree burn has been created. The danger of such a burn is a major drawback of this procedure, especially in the anal canal. Electrocoagulation may also cause intense pain and sphincter spasm, both during and after the procedure. For this reason a general anesthetic may be necessary when a large volume of condylomata are present. Furthermore, an ample quantity of oral analgesics should be given to the patient on discharge home. Obviously anal stenosis is a potential complication. Recurrence rates range from 10 to 25 percent.

Cryotherapy.   Advocates of cryotherapy report that anesthesia is unnecessary, but this has not been the overall experience. The procedure is inexact because the depth of destruction cannot be accurately gauged intraoperatively. Typically, cryotherapy creates wide, deep wounds that are associated with delayed painful tissue sloughing. Moreover, a foul-smelling discharge accompanies the sloughing ulcer. A cotton-tipped applicator, however, may be used to carefully treat individual warts. Since storage of the liquid nitrogen is cumbersome and the compound itself has a limited storage life, cryotherapy has little if any value.[103]

Laser Therapy.   A laser can also be used to destroy warts. Although advocates claim that this method is followed by less pain and fewer recurrences than other therapies, randomized studies have not yet confirmed this view. Billingham and Lewis treated 38 patients with extensive warts with a carbon dioxide laser on the right and electrocautery on the left half of the anus.[104] The patients were blinded as to which half was treated with which modality. Use of the laser was accompanied by more pain and by a more rapid recurrence of condylomata. An additional risk of using the laser is the problem of aerosalized active viral particles in the laser plume (smoke). Viable viral particles have been recovered from this plume,[105,106] and cases of medical providers developing condylomata in their respiratory tracts after using a laser to treat condylomata have been reported.[107] To reduce this possibility, special filter masks and devices to evacuate the smoke are recommended any time a laser is used.[108] Transmission of viral particles appears to be less of a problem with the smoke from electrocautery, which consists of larger particles.[106] Finally, the laser is vastly more expensive than cautery and requires special training by both the physician and the ancillary staff. For these reasons and the lack of proven effectiveness many colorectal surgeons have been reluctant to adopt the laser.

During any operative or therapeutic procedures, several condylomata should biopsied for pathologic review. This confirms the clinical diagnosis and excludes the presence of an invasive squamous cell cancer (Buschke–Lowenstein tumor) which may mimic condylomata.

Nonsurgical Therapy

Immunotherapy.   A method of immunotherapy has been described by Abcarian and associates.[90,109] At least 5 grams of condylomata are used to prepare an autologous vaccine. Six weekly intramuscular injections of 0.5 ml of the vaccine are undertaken. No adverse sequelae of the injections were reported. Eighty-four percent of the 200 patients treated by Abcarian experienced disappearance of the warts and all remained free of disease during the 46-month follow-up. An additional 11 percent had significant reductions in the volume of condylomata which permitted complete eradication after a single session of local excision. Only 5 percent of patients did not benefit from the vaccine and half of those responded to a second course of immunotherapy. Others subsequently reported similar results.[110] Immunotherapy, therefore, may be the treatment of choice in patients with extensive, persistent, or recurrent warts.

Interferon.   Several studies have reported the use of an injection of interferon-α 2b, either intramuscularly or intralesionally. Schonfeld and coworkers treated 22 patients in a double-blind trial with either 2 million units of intramuscular interferon or placebo.[111] Complete remission was reported in 82 percent of the interferon group and 18 percent of the placebo group. Gall and associates, using 5 million units of intralesional interferon daily for 1 month, noted complete response in 69 percent of patients and partial response in 25 percent.[112] Eron and colleagues used 1 million units intralesionally thrice weekly for 3 weeks.[113] One week after the conclusion of therapy there was a 62 percent decrease in the area of the warts, compared to a 1 percent increase in the placebo group. Twelve weeks later the interferon group still had a 40 percent reduction whereas the placebo group then had a 46 percent increase. Friedman-Kien and associates reported a double-blind randomized trial in which 62 percent of interferon patients had complete elimination or improvement of warts compared to only 21 percent of placebo-treated patients.[114] The side effects of interferon include fever, chills, myalgia, headache, fatigue, and leukopenia.

Management in the HIV-Seropositive Patient.   A recent clinical problem of increasing importance has been the management of condylomata in HIV-positive patients. The authors' experience includes over 119 (18 percent) of our HIV-positive patients with anal condylomata.[115] The demographics and risk factors of these patients were similar to those for the HIV-positive patients without condylomata, and 60 percent of the condylomata patients had at least one other sexually transmitted disease. This patient group was obtained from mandatory screening of U.S. military personnel.

Anal condylomata or anogenital warts in HIV-positive patients are managed in the following manner: Observation is recommended for asymptomatic patients or patients with late stage disease (Walter Reed class 3–4 or CDC III or IV). Symptomatic patients with warts limited to the anal margin are treated with one or two applications of podophyllin (5% in benzoin) or BCAA. Patients with anal canal lesions are offered excision, fulguration, or both with either general or regional anesthesia.

Of the 23 percent of HIV-positive condylomata patients who underwent excision and fulguration under a general or regional anesthetic, all had biopsy-proven condylomata acuminata. There were no significant perioperative complications and wounds healed in all patients. In follow-up averaging more than 1 year, the recurrence rate for condylomata in the treated patients was 26 percent after local treatment with podophyllin and 4 percent after fulguration and excision. Although these HIV-positive condylomata patients were a select group, similar results can be expected in early stage HIV-positive patients.

Condylomata Acuminata: A Preferred Clinical Approach

All patients with condylomata are at high risk for recurrence, regardless of the therapeutic method employed. All sexual partners should be screened, and treated patients should be examined monthly for at least 3 months after disappearance of all warts. The authors' preference, based on the data presented herein, is either to excise multiple condylomata and to cauterize the bases for hemostasis and additional tissue destruction, or to fulgurate the warts using electrocautery. Excision permits histologic examination and is well tolerated by the patient. Excised warts are grouped into quadrants, labeled as such, and separately delivered to the pathologist. Should carcinoma in situ be discovered, the quadrant in question can be biopsied, obviating the need for a complete perianal reevaluation.

If an invasive carcinoma is identified it is managed as described in Chapter 16. Isolated innocuous warts and limited recurrences are treated in the office with BCAA or podophyllin. This is true whether the patient's HIV status is seropositive, seronegative, or unknown. Recurrent condylomata and refractory cases are treated in the operating room with an anesthetic to ensure adequate sphincter relaxation. This permits the identification and elimination of all warty tissue. If this technique fails to eradicate all condylomata, immunotherapy should be considered. Regardless of the therapy employed, patients are instructed to abstain from sexual activity until protracted resolution has been documented. Monthly office visits are imperative.

Human Immunodeficiency Virus

The human immunodeficiency virus (HIV) and the resultant acquired immune deficiency syndrome (AIDs) are covered in Chapter 22.

Infectious Diarrheal Disorders

There are many parasitic infestations, previously considered rare in an urban setting, that are now seen with impressive regularity in the homosexual and bisexual male populations.[116] These diseases include amebiasis, giardiasis, and infections with *Enterobius vermicularis* and other helminths.[27,117-120]

Amebiasis

Entamoeba histolyica is a protozoan which commonly infects humans. It is the most common cause of parasitic colitis seen by surgeons in the United States and is endemic in several parts of the world. Transmission is related to sanitation measures or sexual activity. Recently, 40 percent of all cases of amebiasis in the United States occurred in New York City, and 80 percent of these were in men in Manhattan.[121] The prevalence rate for infection with *E. histolytica* among homosexual and bisexual men ranges from 20 to 32 percent, and between 26 and 70 percent of the homosexual population with diarrhea is found to harbor one or more protozoan organisms in the stool.[121-123] Amebic cysts may be ingested in contaminated food or drink, but in the homosexual and bisexual populations transmission usually occurs through oroanal intercourse with an infected partner. The evaluation and treatment of amebiasis is discussed in Chapter 26.

Giardiasis

Giardia lamblia are intestinal flagellates which inhabit the upper small intestine and biliary tract of infected individuals. This protozoan is also transmitted through oroanal intercourse with an infected partner. The incidence of giardiasis is probably between 4 percent and 18 percent in the homosexual population.[119] It is the only infectious protozoan organism that has a significant correlation with symptomatic enteritis.[119] Although these organisms do not infect the lower gastrointestinal tract, they may produce mild to severe cramps, bloating, anorexia, and weight loss accompanied by malabsorption syndromes with frequent foul, greasy, loose stools. Anoscopic and sigmoidoscopic findings are usually normal but may reveal diffuse ulcerations.[27] The diagnosis is made by identification of characteristic trophozoites in a fresh stool specimen, in the scrapings from an ulcer base, or in jejunal biopsies. Three to five stool specimens should be collected at least 2 days apart, and as for *E. hitolytica* they must be examined within 1 hour of collection. Barium and mineral oil may give false-negative test results.[7] If a diagnosis cannot be made after three attempts at identification of the parasite in the patient's stool, a duodenal aspirate or small bowel biopsy may be required. The recommended therapy is 50 mg metronidazole given by mouth three times daily for 7 days. Quinacrine, tinidazole, furazolidone, and paramomycin are other useful agents in the treatment of giardiasis.[124]

Shigella Infection

Forty percent of asymptomatic homosexual men harbor at least one enteric pathogen, and *Shigella* is virtually endemic.[119] The first reports of *Shigella flexneri* as an infection common in homosexuals who lived in major U.S. cities were published in 1974.[125-128] The true incidence of *S. flexneri* in the homosexual population is unknown; however, 30 to 50 percent to cases of shigellosis in New York City, San Francisco, and Seattle are in this group.[125,128,129] Sexual transmission is by direct or indirect fecal–oral contamination, which is a highly efficient mode of spread because infection can be caused by as few as 10 organisms.[27] The evaluation and management of shigellosis is discussed in Chapter 26.

Campylobacter Infection

Campylobacter jejuni has recently been recognized as a common cause of enterocolitis or infectious diarrhea. It can be transmitted by ingestion of infected milk or meat. Although no proof of sexual transmission exists, *Campylobacter jejuni*, *Campylobacter fetus*, and *Campylobacter intestinalis* are seen in homosexual men more frequently than in matched heterosexual controls.[27] *Campylobacter* has been cultured in 3 percent of asymptomatic homosexual men and in 6 percent of those with gastrointestinal symptoms.[117] The evaluation and management of campylobacter is discussed in Chapter 26.

Cryptosporidiosis

Cryptosporidial colitis induces a self-limited infection in nonimmunocompromised patients; however, in patients with AIDS, it produces a life-threatening colitis.[130] Cryptosporidial enterocolitis has been reported in 3 to 4 percent of patients with AIDS.[131] A profuse, often bloody mucoid diarrhea is caused from the tiny protozoans that inhabit the microvilli; electrolyte imbalance, dehydration, and prostration ensue.[132] Diarrhea in excess of 5 to 10 liters per day has been seen.[133] The diagnosis can be established from histopathologic examination of rectal biopsy specimens, which may demonstrate the characteristic oocysts. Alternatively, the organisms may be seen on either routine or modified acid-fast (Kinyoun) stain. Very thin tissue sections and proper fixation are necessary to identify these minuscule protozoans.

The treatment of cryptosporidiosis is largely supportive, with rehydration and nutritional support being the basis of therapy. Although a wide variety of antiparasitic agents have been employed, none has yielded impressive results. Since cryptosporidiosis is not commonly seen in non–HIV-infected homosexuals, its presence should alert the physician to the need for HIV testing.

Isosporiasis

Isospora belli, an opportunistic protozoan, has as much lower prevalence than does *Cryptosporidium* in patients with AIDS. The estimated incidence is less than 0.2 percent in patients with AIDS in the United States.[131] *I. belli* causes symptoms similar those caused by *Cryptosporidium*: diarrhea, vomiting, fever, and abdominal pain. As a rule, however, the quantity of diarrhea tends to be less with Isosporiasis and consequently patients tend to present with less weight loss and malnutrition.

As with cryptosporidiosis, the diagnosis of *Isopora* enterocolitis may be made by using a modified acid-fast stain on a fresh stool specimen. Alternatively, endoscopic biopsy followed by histopathologic tissue examination may reveal the organism. In distinct contrast to cryptosporidiosis, isosporiasis responds promptly to antiprotozoal therapy. Both clinical and microbiologic proof of organism eradication is usually achieved within 7 days of initiation of trimethoprim and sulfamethoxazole therapy.[134] Since the relapse rate is high, prophylaxis with a nightly dose of double-strength trimethoprim and sulfamethoxazole is suggested.[131] Furazolidone is an alternative pharmacologic agent against *Isospora belli*.

Mycobacterium Avium-intracellulare Infection

Mycobacterium avium-intracellulare is another opportunistic microbial infection often seen in patients with AIDS. Some patients remain asymptomatic carriers, whereas others develop profuse watery diarrhea, with dehydration, malabsorption, and severe abdominal pain. If suspicion of *M. avium-intracellulare* infection exists, stool should be sent for acid-fast stains. If acid-fast staining of stool is nondiagnostic, an ileal colonoscopic biopsy should be the next step. The characteristic hisopathologic finding is macrophages filled with acid-fast mycobacteria.[135] Biopsies may also show blunted villi shortened and widened by an infiltrate of histiocytes. These findings resemble those seen with Whipple's disease and account for the severe and often seen malabsorption.[136] Granuloma formation is rare because of the lack of cell-mediated immunity in these individuals.

Small-intestinal involvement is often associated with markedly enlarged mesenteric lymph nodes; in one report, a 10-cm abdominal mass was actually a clump of *M. avium-intracellulare* infected nodes.[137] Other authors have reported a small-bowel obstruction that presented as an extensive *M. avium-intracellulare* infection of the terminal ileum.[138] Radiologic findings of ileal narrowing and ulceration may suggest Crohn's disease preoperatively.[139]

The colon may be involved by *M. avium-intracellulare*, but this is usually less obvious. A normal-appearing routine colonic biopsy stain may reveal acid-fast bacilli in scattered subepithelial macrophages. Because of *M. avium-intracellulare*, as well as *Cryptosporidium* and *Isospora*, all colonic biopsies in patients with AIDS should be assessed with acid-fast stains. Tests with acid-fast stains should also be performed in all patients with AIDS who have perianal suppuration, as *M. avium-intracellulare* perianal abscesses have been noted.

Rosengart and Coppa analyzed 14 patients with AIDS who had abdominal mycobacterial infections.[140] Sites of extrapulmonary involvement included the ileocecal region, the psoas muscle, the liver, and the peritoneum. The patients with ileocecal *M. avium-intracellulare* presented with abdominal pain and a normal white blood cell count. Interestingly, the purified protein derivative test (PPD) was usually negative because many patients with AIDS were anergic. Therefore, as with many diseases in patients with AIDS, a high index of suspicion must exist because laboratory tests are often unreliable.

The treatment for intestinal *M. avium-intracellulare* infection is discouraging. These organisms are nearly always resistant to standard antituberculosis agents, and newer agents such as clofazimine and ansamycin have not yet demonstrated clinical utility. The complications of abdominal *M. avium-intracellulare* infections, which usually require operation, include obstruction in 30 percent, fistulas in 2 to 20 percent, perforation in 5 percent, and bleeding in 20 percent of patients.[141] Surgery is more likely to be necessary in those patients who present with abdominal pain than in those who present with other symptoms.[140] Surgical judgment must be based on the patient's history, the physical examination, and an abdominal CT scan, as culture confirmation may take up to 6 weeks. The 1-year survival has been reported to be as high as 66 percent and is largely contingent on the presence or absence of opportunistic infections.[141]

The increase in incidence and variety of STD and infectious diseases can be expected to increase. Regardless of the STD encountered, treatment will fail unless all sexual contacts are adequately screened and tested. Patients must also refrain from sexual activity until they and all of their partners are rendered free of disease. Knowledge of common diseases, the almost uniform presence of multiple diseases, and a high index of suspicion are essential if the provider is to make the correct diagnoses and provide appropriate treatments.

References

1. Felman YM, Morrison JM. Examining the homosexual male for sexually transmitted diseases. *JAMA*. 1977;238:2046–2047.

2. Wilcox RR. The rectum as viewed by the venereologist. *Br J Venereal Dis*. 1981;57:1–6.

3. Kinsey AC, Pomeroy WB, Martin LE. Sexual behaviour in the human male. Philadelphia: WB Saunders; 1948:650–651.

4. Kinsey AC, Pomeroy WB, Martin LE. Sexual behaviour in the human male. Philadelphia: WB Saunders; 1948:610.

5. Darrow WW, Barrett D, Jay K, et al. The gay report on sexually transmitted diseases. *Am J Public Health*. 1981;71:1004–1011.

6. Gebhard PH. The exposure factor. The venereal disease crisis. In: *Report of International Venereal Disease Symposium*. St. Louis: Pfizer Laboratories;1978.

7. William DC. The sexual transmission of parasitic infections in gay men. *J Homosex*. 1980;5:291–294.

8. Kazal HL, Sohn N, Carrasco JI, et al. The gay bowel syndrome clinicopathologic correlation in 260 cases. *Am Clin Lab Sci*. 1976;6:184–192.

9. Weller IV. The gay bowel. *Gut*. 1985;26:869–875.

10. Judson FN, Penley KA, Robinson ME, et al. Prevalence and site pathogen studies of *Neisseria meningitides* and *Neisseria gonorrhea* in homosexual men. *Am J Epidemiol*. 1980;112:836–843.

11. Dritz SK. Medical aspects of homosexuality. *N Engl J Med*. 1980;302:463–464.

12. Janda WM, Bonhoff M, Morgello JA, et al. Prevalence and site pathogen studies of *Neisseria meningitides* and *Nisseria gonorrhea* in homosexual men. *JAMA*. 1980;244:2060–2064.

13. Ostrow DG, Shaskey D, Steffen, et al. Epidemiology of gonorrhea infections in gay men. *J Homosex*. 1980;5:285–289.

14. Pariser H, Marino AF. Gonorrhea—frequently unrecognized reservoirs. *South Med J*. 1970;63:198–201.

15. Baker RW, Peppercorn MA. Gastrointestinal ailments of homosexual men. *Medicine*. 1982;61:390–405.

16. Buls JB. Sexually transmitted diseases of the anorectum. In: Goldberg SM, Nivatvongs S, Gordon PH, eds. *Essentials of Anorectal Surgery*. Philadelphia: JB Lippincott; 1980:150–152.

17. Stansfield VA. Diagnosis and management of anorectal gonorrhea in women. *Br J Venereal Dis*. 1980;56:319–321.

18. Fluker JL, Deherogada P, Flatt DJ, et al. Rectal gonorrhea in male homosexuals: presentations and therapy. *Br J Venereal Dis*. 1980;56:397–399.

19. Deherogada P. Diagnosis of rectal gonorrhea by blind anorectal swabs taken via proctoscope. *Br J Venereal Dis*. 1977;53:311–313.

20. Danielsson D, Johannisson G. Culture diagnosis of gonorrhea: a comparison of the yield with selective and non-selective gonococcal culture media inoculated in the clinic after transport of specimens. *Acta Derm Venereol (Stockh)*. 1973;53:75–80.

21. Daniel DC, Felman YM, Riccardi NB. The utility of anoscopy in the rapid diagnosis of symptomatic anorectal gonorrhea in men. *Sex Transm Dis*. 1981;8:16–17.

22. Janda WM, Bohnhoff M, Morello JA, Lerner SA. Prevalence and site—pathogen studies of *Neisseria meningitides* and *N. gonorrhoeae* in homosexual men. *JAMA*. 1980;244:2060–2064.

23. Klein EF, Fisher LS, Chow AD, Guz LB. Anorectal gonococcal infection: a clinical review. *Ann Intern Med*. 1977;86:340–346.

24. Fluker JL. A 10-year study of homosexually transmitted infection. *Br J Venereal Dis*. 1976;52:155–160.

25. Lebedeff DR, Hochman EB. Rectal gonorrhea in men: diagnosis and treatment. *Ann Intern Med*. 1980;92:463–466.

26. Schroeter AL, Turner RH, Lucas JB, et al. Therapy for incubating syphilis: effectiveness of gonorrheal treatment. *JAMA*. 1971;218:711–717.

27. Knapp JS, Zenilman JM, Thompson SE. Gonorrhea. In: Morse SA, Moreland AA, Thompson SE, eds. *Sexually Transmitted Diseasese*. Philadelphia: JB Lippincott; 1990:512–522.

28. Schwarcz SK, Zenilman JM, Schnell D, et al. National surveillance of antimicrobial resistance in *Neisseria gonorrhoeae*. *JAMA*. 1990;264:1413–1417.

29. Rompalo AM, Stamm WE. Anorectal and enteric infections in homosexual men. *West J Med*. 1985;142:647–652.

30. Stamm WE, Guinan ME, Johnson C, et al. Effect of treatment regiments for *Neisseria gonorrhea* on simultaneous infection with *Chlamydia trachomatis*. *N Engl J Med*. 1984;310;545–549.

31. Venereal aspects of gastroenterology—Medical Staff Conference. University of California at San Francisco. *West J Med*. 1979;130:236–246.

32. Catterall RD. Sexually transmitted diseases of the anus and rectum. *Clin Gastroenterol*. 1975;4:659–669.

33. British cooperative clinical group. Homosexuality and venereal diseases in the United Kingdom: A second study. *Br J Venereal Dis*. 1980;56:6–11.

34. Goligher JC. Sexually transmitted diseases. In:

Diseases of the Anus, Rectum, and Colon. 5th ed. London: Balliere Tindall; 1985:1033–1045.

35. Venereal diseases of the anal canal and rectum. In: Hughes E, Cuthbertson AM, Killingback MK, eds. *Colorectal Surgery.* New York: Churchill Livingstone; 1983:203–208.

36. Akdamarr K, Martin RJ, Ichinase H. Syphilitic proctitis. *Dig Dis.* 1977;22:701–704.

37. Drusin LM, Singer C, Valenti AJ, Armstrong D. Infectious syphilis mimicking neoplastic disease. *Arch Intern Med.* 1977;137:156–160.

38. Faris MR, Perry JJ, Westermeier TG, Redmond J III. Rectal syphilis mimicking histiocytic lymphoma. *Am J Clin Pathol.* 1983;80:719–721.

39. Holmes K. The chlamydia epidemic. *JAMA.* 1981;245:1718–1723.

40. McCormack WM, Mardh P. Fifth International Symposium on Chlamydial Infections. *Sex Transm Dis.* 1982;9:216–232.

41. McMillan A, Sommerville RG, McKee PMK. Chlamydial infections in homosexual men: frequency of isolation of *Chlamydia trachomatis* from the urethra, anorectum, and pharynx. *Br J Venereal Dis.* 1981;57:47–49.

42. Quinn TC, Goodell SE, Mkrtichian EE, et al. *Chlamydia trachomatis* proctitis. *N Engl J Med.* 1981;305:195–200.

43. Levine JS, Smith PD, Brugge WR. Chronic proctitis in male homosexuals due to lymphogranuloma vereum. *Gastroenterology.* 1980;79:563–565.

44. Goodell SE, Quinn TC, Mkrtichian EE, et al. The infectious etiology and histopathology of proctitis and enteritis in homosexual men. *Gastroenterology.* 1981;80:1159. Abstract.

45. Wang SP, Grayston JT, Alexander ER, Holmes KK. A simplified microimmunofluorescent test with trachoma–lymphogranuloma venereum (*Chlamydia trachomatis*) antigen for use as a screening test for antibody. *J Clin Microbiol.* 1975;1:250–255.

46. Rodier B, Catalan F, Harboun A. Severe proctitis due to chlamydia of serotype D. *Coloproctology.* 1987;9:341–344.

47. Hansfield HH. Sexually transmitted disease. *Hosp Pract.* 1982;17:99–116.

48. Beck DE. Sexually transmitted and infectious diseases. In: *Patient Care in Colorectal Surgery.* Little, Brown; 1991:267–278.

49. Baker DA. *Clinical Management of Sexually Transmitted Diseases.* Vol. 2: *Treatment and Management of STDs.* Charlotte, NC: Burroughs Welcome; 1989.

50. Goodell SE, Quinn TC, Mktrichian EE, et al. Herpes simplex virus proctitis in homosexual men: clinical, sigmoidoscopic and histopathologic features. *N Engl J Med.* 1983;308:868–871.

51. Goldmeier D. Proctitis and herpes simplex virus in homosexual men. *Br J Venereal Dis.* 1980;56:111–114.

52. Quinn TC, Corey L, Chaffee RG, et al. The etiology of anorectal infections in homosexual men. *Am J Med.* 1981;71:395–406.

53. Goodell SE, Quinn TC, Mkritchian EE, et al. Herpes simplex virus: an important cause of acute proctitis in homosexual men. *Gastroenterology.* 1981;80:1159. Abstract.

54. Nerurkar L, Goedert J, Wallen W, et al. Study of antiviral antibodies in sera of homosexual men. *Federation Proceedings.* 1983;42:6109.

55. Revision of the CDC surveillance case definition for acquired immunodeficiency syndrome. *MMWR.* 1987;36(suppl):1–15s.

56. Jacobs E. Anal infections caused by herpes simplex virus. *Dis Colon Rectum.* 1976;19:151–157.

57. Wexner SD, Dailey TH. Pruritus ani: diagnosis and management. *J Skin Dis.* 1986;7:5–9.

58. Samarasinghe PL, Oates JK, MacLennan IPB. Herpetic proctitis and sacral radiculomyelopathy—a hazard for homosexual men. *Br Med J.* 1979;2:365–366.

59. Baringer JR. Recovery of herpes simplex virus from human sacral ganglions. *N Engl J Med.* 1974;291:828–830.

60. Goldmeier D. Herpetic proctitis and sacral radiculomyelopathy in homosexual men. *Br Med J.* 1979;2:549.

61. Rotterdam H, Sommers SC. Alimentary tract biopsy lesions in the acquired immune deficiency syndrome. *Pathology.* 1985;17:181–192.

62. Corey L. The diagnosis and treatment of genital herpes. *JAMA.* 1982;248:1041–1049.

63. Bryson YJ, Dillon M, Lovett M, et al. Treatment of first episodes of genital herpes simplex virus infection with oral acyclovir: a randomized controlled trial in normal subjects. *N Engl J Med.* 1983;308:916–921.

64. Reichman RC, Badger GJ, Merttz GJ, et al. Treatment of recurrent genital herpes simplex infections with oral acyclovir. *JAMA.* 1984;251:2103–2107.

65. Douglas JM, Critchlow C, Benedetti J, et al. A double-blind study of oral acyclovir for suppression of recurrences of genital herpes simplex virus infection. *N Engl J Med.* 1984;310:155–156.

66. Straus SE, Takiff HE, Seidlin M, et al. Suppression of frequently recurring genital herpes: a placebo-controlled double-blind trial of oral acyclovir. *N Engl J Med.* 1984;310:1545–1550.

67. Rompalo AM, Mertz GJ, Davis LG, et al. Oral acyclovir for treatment of first-episode herpes simplex virus proctitis. *JAMA.* 1988;259:2879–2881.

68. Whitley RJ, Levin M, Barton N, et al. Infections

caused by herpes simplex virus in the immunocompromised host: natural history and topical acyclovir therapy. *J Infect Dis.* 1984;150:323–329.

69. Mertz GJ, Jones CC, Mils J, et al. Long-term acyclovir suppression of frequently recurring genital herpes simplex virus infection. *JAMA.* 1988; 260:201–206.

70. Wexner SD. Sexually transmitted diseases of the colon, rectum, and anus. The challenge of the nineties. *Dis Colon Rectum.* 1990;33:1048–1062.

71. Erlich KS, Mills J, Chatis P, et al. Acyclovir-resistant herpes simplex virus infections in patients with the acquired immunodeficiency syndrome. *N Engl J Med.* 1989;320:293–296.

72. Chatis PA, Miller GH, Schrager LE, Crumpacker CS. Successful treatment with Foscarnet of an acyclovir-resistant mucocutaneous infection with herpes simplex virus in a patient with acquired immunodeficiency syndrome. *N Engl J Med.* 1989;320:297–300.

73. Wexner SD. Treatment of AIDS patients with herpes simplex virus infections resistant to acyclovir. *Colon and Rectal Surgery Outlook.* 1989;2:1–2.

74. Stamm WE, Handsfield H, Rompalo AM, et al. The association between genital ulcer disease and acquisition of HIV infection in homosexual men. *JAMA.* 1988;260:1429–1433.

75. Holmberg SD, Stewart JA, Gerber AR, et al. Prior herpes simplex virus type 2 infection as a risk factor for HIV infection. *JAMA.* 1988; 259:1048–1050.

76. Wexner SD. Managing common anorectal sexually transmitted diseases. *Infect Surg.* 1990 (June); 9–48.

77. Condylomata acuminatum—United States, 1966–1981: current trends. *MMWR.* 1983;32: 306–308.

78. Brescia RJ, Jenson B, Lancaster WD, et al. The role of human papilloma virus in the pathogenesis and histologic classification of precancerous lesions of the cervix. *Hum Pathol.* 1986;17:555–559.

79. Gissmann L, Schwarz E. Persistence and expression of human papillomavirus DNA in genital cancer. Papillomavirus. *Clin Found Symp.* 1986;120:90–97.

80. Syrjanen SM, Von Krough G, Syrjanen KJ. Detection of human papillomavirus DNA in anogenital condylomata in men using in-situ DNA hybridisation applied to paraffin secretions. *Genitour in Med.* 1987;63:32–39.

81. Scholefield JH, Sonnex C, Talbot IC, et al. Anal and cervical intraepithelial neoplasia: possible parallel. *Lancet.* 1989;2:765–769.

82. Palmer JG, Scholefield JH, Coates PJ, et al. Anal cancer and human papillomaviruses. *Dis Colon Rectum.* 1989;32:1016–1022.

83. Nash G, Allen W, Nash S. Atypical lesions of the anal mucosa in homosexual men. *JAMA.* 1986; 256:873–876.

84. Croxson T, Chabon AB, Rorat E, Barash IM. Intraepithelial carcinoma of the anus in homosexual men. *Dis Colon Rectum.* 1984;27:325–330.

85. Cooper HS, Patchefsky AS, Markus G. Cloacogenic carcinoma of the anorectum in homosexual men: an observation of four cases. *Dis Colon Rectum.* 1979;22:557–558.

86. Wexner SD, Milsom JW, Dailey TH. The demographics of anal cancers are changing: identification of a high-risk population. *Dis Colon Rectum.* 1987;30:942–946.

87. Peters RK, Mack TM. Patterns of anal carcinoma by gender and marital status in Los Angeles county. *Br J Cancer.* 1983;48:629–636.

88. Gall AA, Meyer PR, Taylor CR. Papillomavirus antigens in anorectal condylomata and carcinoma in homosexual men. *JAMA.* 1987;257:337–340.

89. Car G, William DC. Anal warts in a population of gay men in New York City. *Sex Transm Dis.* 1977;4:56–57.

90. Abcarian H, Sharon N. The effectiveness of immunotherapy in the treatment of anal condylomata acuminatum. *J Surg Res.* 1977:22;231–236.

91. Sohn N, Robilotti JG. The gay bowel syndrome, a review of colonic and rectal conditions in 200 male homosexuals. *Am J Gastroenterol.* 1977;67: 478–483.

92. Schlappner OLA, Shaffer FA. Anorectal condylomata acuminata: a missed part of the condylomata spectrum. *Can Med Assoc J.* 1978;118:172–173.

93. Bailey HR. Personal communication.

94. Wexner SD, Smithy WB, Milson JW, Dailey TH. The surgical management of anorectal diseases in AIDS and pre-AIDs patients. *Dis Colon Rectum.* 1986;29:719–723.

95. Connors RC, Ackerman AB. Histologic pseudomalignancies of the skin. *Arch Dermatol.* 1976;112:1767–1780.

96. Thompson JPS, Grace PH. The treatment of perianal and anal condylomata: a new operative technique. *Proc R Soc Med.* 1978;71:180–185.

97. Gollock JM, Slatford K, Hunter JM Scissor excision of anorectal warts. *Br J Venereol Dis.* 1982; 58:400–401.

98. Moher LM, Maurer SA. Podophyllum toxicity: case report and literature review. *J Fam Pract.* 1979;9:237–234.

99. Montadil DH, Giambrone JP, Courey NG, Taefi P. Podophyllin poisoning associated with the

treatment of condyloma acuminatum: a case report. *Am J Obstet Gynecol.* 1974;119:1130–1131.

100. Prasad ML, Abcarian H. Malignant potential of perianal condyloma acuminatum. *Dis Colon Rectum.* 1980;23:191–197.

101. Jensen SL. Comparison of podophyllin application with simple surgical excision in clearance and recurrence of perianal condyloma acuminata. *Lancet.* 1985:1146–1148.

102. Swerdlow DB, Salvait EP. Condylomata acuminatum. *Dis Colon Rectum.* 1971;14:226–229.

103. Corman ML. *Colon and Rectal Surgery.* 2nd ed. Philadelphia: JB Lippincott; 1989.

104. Billingham RP, Lewis FG. Laser versus electrical cautery in the treatment of condylomata acuminata of the anus. *Surg Gynecol Obstet.* 1982;155: 865–867.

105. Garden JM, O'Banion KO, Sheintz LS, et al. Papillomavirus in vapor of carbon dioxide laser-treated verrucae. *JAMA.* 1988;259:1199–2102.

106. Sawchuk WS, Weber PJ, Lowy DR, Dzubow LM. Infectious papillomavirus in the vapor of warts treated with carbon dioxide laser or electrocoagulation: detection and protection. *J Am Acad Dermatol.* 1989;21:41–49.

107. Volen D. Intact viruses in CO_2 laser plumes spur safety concern. *Clin Laser Monthly.* 1987;5:101–103.

108. Sawchuk WS. Infectious potential of aerosolized particles. *Arch Dermatol.* 1989;125:1689–1692.

109. Abcarian H, Sharon N. Long term effectiveness of the immunotherapy of anal condylomata. *Dis Colon Rectum.* 1982;25:648–651.

110. Eftaiha MS, Amshel AL, Shonberg IL, Batshon B. Giant and recurrent condyloma acuminatum: appraisal of immunotherapy. *Dis Colon Rectum.* 1982;25:136–138.

111. Schonfeld A, Schattner A, Crespi M, et al. Intramuscular human interferon-B injections in treatment of condylomata acuminata. *Lancet.* 1984;1:1038–1041.

112. Gall SA, Hughes CE, Whisnant J, Weck P. Therapy of resistant condylomata with lymphoblastoid interferon. *J Cell Biochem.* 1985;(supl 9 C): 91–92.

113. Eron LJ, Judson F, Tucker S, et al. Interferon therapy for condyloma acuminata. *N Engl J Med.* 1986;315:1059–1064.

114. Friedman-Kien AE, Eron LJ, Conant M, et al. Natural interferon alpha for treatment of condylomata acuminata. *JAMA.* 1988;259:533–538.

115. Beck DE, Jaso RG, Zajac RA. Surgical management of anal condylomata in the HIV-positive patient. *Dis Colon Rectum.* 1990;33:180–183.

116. Most M. Manhattan: "A tropical isle?" *Am J Trop Med Hyg.* 1968;17:33.

117. Burnham WR, Reeve RS, Finch RG. *Entamoeba histolytica* infection in male homosexuals. *Gut.* 1980;21:1097–1099.

118. Dritz SK, Ainsworth TE, Back A. Patterns of sexually transmitted enteric diseases in a city. *Lancet.* 1977;2:3–4.

119. Quinn TC, Stamm WE, Goodell SE, et al. The polymicrobial origin of intestinal infections in homosexual men. *N Engl J Med.* 1983;309: 576–582.

120. McMillan A. Thread worms in homosexual males. *Br Med J.* 1978;1:367.

121. Pomerantz BM, Marr JS, Goldman WD. Amebiasis in New York City 1958–1978: identification of the male homosexual high risk population. *Bull N Y Acad Med.* 1980; 56:232–244.

122. William DC, Shukhoff HB, Felman YM, et al. High rates of enteric protozoal infections in selected homosexual men attending a venereal disease clinic. *Sex Transm Dis.* 1978;5:155.

123. Phillips SC, Mildvan D, William DC, et al. Sexual transmission of enteric protozoa and helminths in a venereal disease clinic population. *N Engl J Med.* 1981;305:603–606.

124. Peppercorn MA. Enteric infections in homosexual men with AIDS. *Contemp Gastroenterol.* 1989;2: 23–32.

125. Allason-Jones E, Mindel A. Sex and the bowel. *Int J Colorectal Dis.* 1987;2:32–37.

126. Dritz SK, Back AF. *Shigella* enteritis venereally transmitted. *N Engl J Med.* 1974;291:1194.

127. Drusin LM, Genvert G, Topf-Olstein B, Levy-Zomeck E. Shigellosis: another sexually transmitted disease? *Br J Venereal Dis.* 1976;52:348–350.

128. Bader M, Pederson AHB, Williams R, et al. Venereal transmission of shigellosis in Seattle–King County. *Sex Transm Dis.* 1977;4:89–91.

129. William DC, Felman YM, Marr JS, et al. Sexually transmitted enteric pathogens in male homosexual populations. *N Y State J Med.* 1977;77:2050–2052.

130. Quinn TC. Gastrointestinal manifestations of AIDs. *Pract Gastroenterol.* 1985;9:23–34.

131. Soave R. Cryptosporidiasis and isosporiasis in patients with AIDS. *Infect Dis Clin North Am.* 1988; 2;485–493.

132. Currant WL, Reese NC, Ernst JV, et al. Human cryptosporidiosis in immunocompetent and imuunodeficient persons: studies of an outbreak and experimental transmission. *N Engl J Med.* 1985; 305:1252–1257.

133. Rodgers VD, Kagnoff MF. Gastrointestinal manifestations of the acquired immunodeficiency syndrome. *West J Med.* 1987;146:57–67.

134. DeHovitz JA, Pape JW, Boncy M, et al. Clinical manifestations and therapy of *Isospora belli* infec-

tion in patients with acquired immunodeficiency syndrome. *N Engl J Med.* 1986;315:87–90.

135. Cello JP. Gastrointestinal manifestations of AIDS. *Infect Dis Clin North Am.* 1988;2:387–396.

136. Santangelo WC, Krejs GT. Gastrointestinal manifestations of the acquired immunodificiency syndrome. *American Journal of the Medical Sciences.* 1986;292:328–334.

137. Walsman J, Rotterdam H, Neidt GN, et al. Biopsy pathology of acquired immune deficiency syndrome. *Pathology.* 1985;17:181–182.

138. Schneebaum CW, Novick DM, Chabin AB, et al. Terminal ileitis associated with mycobacterium avium intracellulare infection in a homosexual man with the acquired immune deficiency syndrome. *Gastroenterology.* 1987;92:1127–1130.

139. Wexner SD. AIDS: What the colorectal surgeon needs to know. *Colon Rectal Surg.* 1989;2:19–54.

140. Rosengart TK, Coppa GF. Abdominal mycobacterial infections in immunocompromised patients. *Am J Surg.* 1990;159:125–131.

141. Haddad FS, Ghossain A, Sawaya E, Nelson AR. Abdominal tuberculosis. *Dis Colon Rectum.* 1987; 30:724–735.

CHAPTER 22

ACQUIRED IMMUNODEFICIENCY SYNDROME

Steven D. Wexner and
David E. Beck

The human immunodeficiency virus (HIV) is a retro-virus that infects and can progressively destroy the population of helper-inducer lymphoctyes. These helper cells play a key role in the human immunologic system and are known as either OKT4, CD4, or T4 lymphocytes (synonymous labels referring to the cells' surface epitopes).[1] The HIV may also infect monocytes, macrophages, and other cells.[2] It is self-evident that compromising the OKT4, monocyte, and macrophage populations can have a disastrous effect on the patient's immune system as demonstrated by the plethora of HIV manifestations. These maladies range from subclinical laboratory abnormalities to the full-blown spectrum of the acquired immune deficiency syndrome (AIDS).

This chapter briefly reviews the current experience with AIDS as it applies to the colorectal surgeon. It also includes information about etiology, diagnosis, and treatment. Additional knowledge of appropriate infection control measures and a systematic approach for evaluation and management are presented to help the surgeon care for AIDS patients.

Epidemiology

As of January 1992, more than 205,000 cases of AIDS had been diagnosed in the United States.[3] In addition an estimated 1 million to 2 million people in the United States are believed to be infected with AIDS.[4] It is expected that at least 25 and 35 percent of those infected with HIV will develop AIDS within 2 years of becoming infected.[4,5]

Currently, the single most common risk factor for infection with HIV or for the subsequent development of AIDS in the United States is homosexuality.[6] Male AIDS patients outnumber female AIDS patients by a ratio of 10:1 and on questioning 75 percent of these males report homosexual of bisexual activity.[3] The mode of transmission also weighs heavily upon the subsequent manifestations of the disease, because the homosexual and bisexual male populations tend to present with a different spectrum of disorders than do those HIV-infected persons who are heterosexual intravenous drug abusers, or hemophiliacs.[7]

A study by Wexner and coworkers found that 15 percent of patients with AIDS or what were formerly known as AIDS-related complex (ARC) and pre-AIDS presented with anorectal pathology *prior to* the diagnosis of AIDS.[8] In addition, 116 of 340 AIDS, ARC, and pre-AIDS patients (34 percent) manifested some form of anorectal disease during their illness. The single most common manifestations was perianal sepsis, observed in 58 percent of the patients studied. Other commonly noted diseases included perianal condylomata acuminata, Kaposi's sarcoma (KS), cytomegalovirus, carcinoma in situ, lymphoma, tuberculous proctitis, perianal histoplasmosis, invasive cancer, and nonhealing anal ulcers. Perianal herpes simplex virus (HSV) infections were notably absent from this series, because only patients who underwent anorectal surgery were reported on. Edwards and coworkers reviewed 160

* *Modified from*: Beck DE, Wexner SD. AIDS and the colorectal surgeon. Part II: anorectal disease. *Postgraduate Advances in Colorectal Surgery*. 1990;2(7):1–14.

The views expressed in this chapter are those of the authors and do not necessarily represent the opinions of the United States Air Force or the Department of Defense.

seropositive patients; 33 percent had anorectal symptomatology.[9] More recently Beck and associates and other authors have reported similar findings.[10-14] In Britain the incidence of anorectal disease is about 14-fold more common in HIV-positive male homosexuals than in the age and sex-matched general population.[15]

In stark contrast to the findings in all of the above cited series, anorectal STDs in heterosexual intravenous drug abusers (IVDAs) with AIDS are exceedingly rare.[16] Wolkomir and associates compared the results of anorectal surgery between 14 heterosexual IVDAs and 6 homosexual AIDS patients. In the IVDA group one third of the wounds had failed to heal at 1-month follow-up. In the AIDS group, none of the wounds healed at 1-month follow-up. Although the rate of wound healing appeared higher in the IVDAs, the authors attributed this to a small sample size with few associated anorectal infectious diseases. They concluded that both homosexual and IVDA groups of AIDS patients experience prolonged wound healing and high short-term postoperative mortality after minor anorectal surgery.

Diagnosis and Staging

After a latency period of variable length, often up to two years, the HIV produces diminished immunologic function, which culminates as AIDS.[17] Exposure and infection with HIV can be documented by the methods described by Greco and Simms and by Wexner.[18,19] As a brief review, an enzyme-linked immunoassay (ELISA) against HIV antibody serves as the primary screening test. If a positive result is obtained, the test is repeated and confirmed by the Western blot technique.[19] This combination of tests is 99 percent sensitive and specific.[18] The reported interval between viral exposure and the development of antibodies ranges from 6 weeks to 3 years.

The natural history of HIV infection continues to be elucidated. Acute infection may be associated with a short viral-like illness (3 to 14 days). An asymptomatic carrier phase follows, and finally the patient demonstrates symptoms of diminished immunologic function. The true duration of each phase and the rate or certainty of disease progression have yet to be determined.

In 1986, the Centers for Disease Control (CDC) described a four-group classification system for HIV disease and AIDS (Table 22-1).[20] In this system, group I patients have acute infection symptoms, group II are asymptomatic, group III have persistent generalized lymphadenopathy, and group IV have AIDS-related diseases (constitutional diseases, neurologic diseases, secondary infections, secondary cancers, and other conditions).

The Walter Reed classification system uses both clinical and laboratory findings to group patients for prognostic purposes (Table 22-2).[21] The Walter Reed classification relies heavily on the CD4 T-helper cell count; the premise is that the CD4 T-cell is the principal

Table 22-1   Centers for Disease Control (CDC) Classification System

Group	Description
I	Acute infection
II	Asymptomatic infection
III	Persistent generalized lymphadenopathy
IV	Other disease
Subgroup A	Constitutional disease
Subgroup B	Neurologic disease
Subgroup C	Secondary infectious diseases
Category C-1	Specified secondary infectious diseases listed in the CDC surveillance definition for AIDS*
Category C-2	Other specified secondary infectious diseases
Subgroup D	Secondary cancers, including those within the CDC surveillance definition for AIDS*
Subgroup E	Other conditions

* See Table 22-3 for the CDC surveillance definition for AIDS.

Adapted from: Centers for Disease Control. Classification system for human T-lymphotropic virus type III/lymphadenopathy–associated virus infections. *MMWR.* 1986;35:334–339.

Table 22-2   Walter Reed Staging Classification (Adults)

Stage (WR)	HTLV III AB/Virus	Chronic lymphadenopathy	T-Helper cells/mm	Delayed cutaneous hypersensitivity	Thrush	Opportunistic infections
0	−	−	> 400	Normal	−	−
1	+	−	> 400	Normal	−	−
2	+	+/−	> 400	Normal	−	−
3	+	+/−	< 400	Normal	−	−
4	+	+/−	< 400	Partial	−	−
5	+	+/−	< 400	Complete	+	−
6	+	+/−	< 400	Partial/complete	+/−	+

Adapted from: Redfield RR, Wright DC, Tramont EC. The Walter Reed classification for HTLV-III/LAV infection. *N Engl J Med.* 1986:314;131–132.

target cell of the HIV virus and therefore the number of these cells per cubic millimeter is a major prognosticator.

The essential feature of both classification systems is that early stage patients (WR 1 and 2 and CDC I and II) have minimal alterations of their immune systems. Patients with more advanced disease stages have signficant immunologic dysfunction which results in accelerated morbidity and mortality. Although the Walter Reed classification may provide a better prognostic index, it requires extensive laboratory investigations.

Infection Control

Because HIV is transmitted sexually, by contaminated needles, by infected body fluids, and perhaps by tissue, infection control measures are very important. The CDC, American Hospital Association (AHA), and American Academy of Orthopaedic Surgeons (AAOS) have all recommended "universal precautions" for routine patient contact and additional protective measures for invasive procedures.[22-24]

Universal precautions demand protecting the examiner's skin and mucous membranes from body fluids (eg, blood, vaginal secretions, saliva, tears). The potential for exposure determines the measures the examiner should use. Appropriate protective attire for performing invasive procedures includes gloves (double or triple), goggles, a mask, and a gown. If the patient is known to be HIV-positive, many surgeons will wear an additional waterproof apron under the gown. To reduce the chance of inadvertant needle punctures only experienced personnel should participate in the operation and extra care is required in handling all sharp objects.

Most patients seen in the office require only a proc-toscopic or anoscopic examination for an adequate evaluation to be made; for added safety, the use of disposable instruments is preferred. Traditional sterilization measures can be safely employed if nondisposable instruments are used. Recommendations for handling endoscopic instruments include the use of universal precautions both during and after the procedure.[25] Endoscopists and their assistants should wear gloves and protective garments. After use, instruments must be thoroughly cleaned with detergent both internally and externally to remove all blood, secretions, and debris. Subsequently, instruments should be completely immersed for at least 10 minutes in 2 percent activated glutaraldehyde (Cidex, Surgikos, Inc., Arlington, TX) to inactivate bacteria and viruses. Each instrument should then be rinsed and flushed. Nonimmersible instruments should be cold gas sterilized with ethylene oxide. Biopsy forceps and other accessory equipment must undergo similar disinfection. If large numbers of HIV-positive patients are treated, some institutions designate endoscopic instruments and equipment to be used only on these patients. In addition, it may be preferable to perform invasive procedures on HIV-infected patients at the end of the day. This scheduling maneuver facilitates thorough disinfection and overnight air drying of the room before it is used again.

Patient Evaluation

An adequate history is essential to an appreciation of a patient's potential risk factors for HIV infection or AIDS. This history includes questions about sexual preference, intravenous drug usage, and exposure to blood products or to HIV-positive individuals. Table 22-3 lists high-risk sexual practices related to HIV infec-

Table 22-3 Sexual Practices Associated With Increased Risk of Infection With HIV

HIGHEST RISK FACTORS*
Contact with infected semen or blood
Receptive anal intercourse (especially with ejaculation)
Receptive vaginal intercourse (especially with ejaculation)
Fellatio involving contact with semen

MODERATE/SIGNIFICANT RISK FACTORS*
Insertive anal intercourse
Insertive vaginal intercourse
Brachloproctic eroticism
Use of enemas/rectal douches
Use of sexual devices
Oral–anal contact
Fellatio without contact with semen

LESSER RISK FACTORS†
Contact with urine
Mutual masturbation with ejaculation on partner
"Deep" kissing
Cunnilingus

* Based on current epidemiologic evidence.
† Based on weaker evidence and/or presumed risk.
Adapted from: Glasel M. High risk sexual practices in the transmission of AIDS. In: DeVita VT Jr, Hellman S, Rosenberg SA, eds. *AIDS. Etiology, Diagnosis, Treatment and Presentation.* 2nd ed. Philadelphia: JB Lippincott; 1988:355–367.

tion and AIDS. Patients suspected of exposure to HIV should be encouraged to undergo testing for antibodies to HIV. The patient must be made to understand that a surgeon's lack of knowledge about the patient's HIV status may preclude selecting appropriate invasive therapeutic procedures.

Specific queries must seek out chronic productive cough, pruritic dermatitis, or a history of lymphoadenopathy, oropharyngeal candidiasis, or chronic and progressive herpes simplex or herpes zoster infections. Any of these problems allows a provisional clinical surveillance definition of AIDS to be made.[26] In addition, loss of more than 10 percent of preailment weight, or fever or diarrhea of unknown etiology lasting for at least 1 month, warrant evaluation of the patient's HIV status.[19]

The basic physical examination is identical to that performed on all other patients. In addition, extra attention is directed toward the various lymph node groups and the skin. Specifically, the physician is seeking to exclude lymphadenopathy and Kaposi's sarcoma.

Routine laboratory evaluations should include a complete blood count, a biochemical profile, and serologic tests for common sexually transmitted diseases (syphilis and *Chlamydia trachomatis*)[27] In HIV-

positive patients with gastrointestinal symptoms, it is essential to evaluate the patient's stool for pathogens by cultures or special stains, and to evaluate for ova and parasites. Specifically, the modified Kinyoun stain is useful for detecting cryptosporidiosis and isosporiasis (see Chapter 21). India ink or acid-fast stains are best for identifying *Mycobactrium avium-intracellulare.*[28]

The diseases identified in HIV patients can be grouped into three categories: First, certain diseases are associated with HIV infections. Second, common proctologic and colonic conditions routinely discovered in the general population may be seen in HIV-positive patients. Third, diseases associated with high-risk groups such as homosexual males and intravenous drug users can also be seen. These latter diseases, however,

Table 22-4 Commonly Seen Colorectal Manifestations of AIDS

PROCTOCOLITIDES
Viral
    Cytomegalovirus (CMV)
    Herpes simplex virus (HSV)
    Human immunodeficiency virus (HIV)
Fungal and protozoan
    Cryptosporidiosis
    Isosporosis
    Candidiasis
    Histoplasmosis
Bacterial
    Mycobacterium avium-intracellulare (MAI)
HIV wasting syndrome
    Amebiasis
    Salmonellosis
    Shigellosis

COLORECTAL TUMORS
Histoplasmoma
    Non-B-cell immunoblastic
    Burkitt's
    Reticulosarcoma
    Other
Lymphoma
Kaposi's sarcoma

ANAL AND PERIANAL PATHOLOGY
Malignant
    Condylomata with carcinoma
    Cloacogenic cancer
    Lymphoma
    Kaposi's sarcoma (KS)
Benign
    Condylomata
    Histoplasmoma

are not pathognomic of or seen exclusively in HIV-positive patients and include *Chlamydia trachomatis*, hepatitis B, condylomata acuminata, lymphogranuloma venereum, syphillis, gonorrhea, and herpes simplex. Many of the common colorectal manifestations of AIDS are listed in Table 22-4.

Beck and associates reported their experience with 677 HIV-positive patients who were evaluated from 1986 to 1988.[10] The patients ranged in age from 19 to 70 years (mean = 25 yr). Ninety-five percent were male, 52 percent were white, 41 percent were black, and 7 percent were other races, primarily Hispanic. Only 10 percent reported homosexual activity and only 2 percent admitted to intravenous drug abuse (the accuracy of these etiologic factors is questionable because of the military status of these patients). According to the Walter Reed classification system, at initial presentation 54 percent of patients were stage 1, 24 percent were stage 2, 10 percent were stage 3, 3 percent were stage 4, 6 percent were stage 5, and 3 percent were stage 6.

Evaluation revealed common nonsexually related anorectal conditions in 7 per cent of these patients. In contrast to this small number of nonsexually related problems, more than 60 percent of the patients had at least one sexually transmitted disease (Table 22-5). Positive serologies for *Chlamydia* (58 percent) and hepatitis (35 percent) were the most common conditions, followed by anal condylomata (18 percent). Combining patients with nonsexually related anorectal diseases (such as fissures and hemorrhoids) and those with anal condylomata, 24 percent had treatable anorectal conditions.

This patient population is distinctive for several reasons: First, the age, sex, and race characteristics reflect active duty military forces (children, females, and elderly are underrepresented). Second, the population had

been medically prescreened (candidates with underlying chronic illnesses such as diabetes and hypertension were not selected for active duty service). Third, and most important in comparing these patients with other groups, most of these patients were asymptomatic and were identified by mandatory mass screening.

Specific Anorectal Disorders

Opportunistic Infections and Anal Ulcerations

Cytomegalovirus

Cytomegalovirus (CMV) is the most common infectious organism in AIDS patients; more than 90 percent of AIDS patients develop an active CMV infection.[11,14] CMV can cause inflammation, hemorrhage, ulceration, or perforation in the gastrointestinal (GI) tract. Ileocolitis secondary to CMV is the most common intestinal manifestation of AIDS.[14,29] Symptomatic CMV proctitis occurs in at least 10 percent of AIDS patients. The patient may present with tenesmus, diarrhea, and weight loss or, less commonly, with melena or hematochezia. The diagnosis of CMV proctitis can be confirmed by endoscopy or biopsy. Endoscopic findings range from submucosal hemorrhage and erythematous patches with or without punctate ulcers to multiple wide, deep ulcers (Fig. 22-1). Microscopic evaluation of

Table 22-5 Sexually Related Diseases in HIV-positive Patients

Condition	No. patients (%)
Chlamydia trachomatis	391 (58)
Hepatitis B serology	234 (35)
Condylomata acuminata	119 (18)
Lymphogranuloma venereum	100 (15)
RPR/FTA	100 (15)
Herpes simplex (I, II)	92 (60)
1036 conditions in 407 patients (60%)*	

* Several patients had more than one disease.
RPR/FTA = rapid plasma reagin/fluorescent treponeonal antibody.

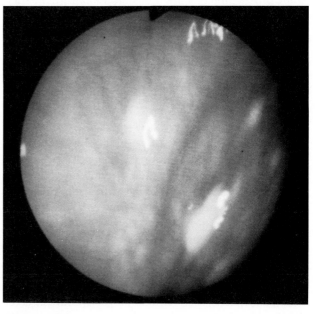

Figure 22-1. Rectal cytomegalic ulcerations. (*From:* Wexner SD, Smithy WB, Trillo C, Hopkins, BS, Dailey TH. Emergency colectomy for cytomegalovirus ileocolitis in patients with the acquired immune deficiency syndrome. *Dis Colon Rectum.* 1988;31:755–761.)

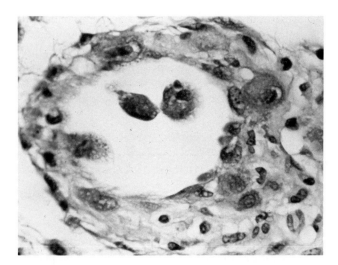

Figure 22-2. Intranuclear inclusion bodies representative of cytomegalovirus infection. (*From:* Wexner SD, Smithy WB, Trillo C, Hopkins BS, Dailey TH. Emergency colectomy for cytomegalavirus ileocolitis in patients with the acquired immune deficiency syndrome. *Dis Colon Rectum.* 1988;31:755–761.)

biopsied tissue demonstrates vasculitis; neutrophilic infiltration; large basophilic, intranuclear cytomegalic viral inclusions; and, less often, granular cytoplasmic inclusions[30] (Fig. 22-2). Viral culture of the biopsy specimen may also reveal CMV, although this test is less specific for active infection. Barium enema findings include diffuse mucosal aphthous ulceration, granularity, skip lesions, thumbprinting, and linear ulceration.[31] Because these findings are nonspecific, the most common misdiagnoses are Crohn's disease, mucosal ulcerative colitis, and ischemic colitis.[30,31]

CMV proctocolitis often requires surgery because of multifocal bleeding or perforation.[14,32] Surgery for CMV complications accounts for 64 to 100 percent of emergent laparotomies in AIDS patients. It is not surprising that these high risk operations are accompanied by a 71 percent 30-day mortality.[14]

If surgery is necessary, the procedure of choice is a total abdominal colectomy and end-ileostomy. Medical treatment of less severe cases of CMV proctocolitis includes intravenous ganciclovir.[28] Clinical improvement has been reported in 85 percent of patients, although cure does not occur.[29]

In addition to colonic ulcerations, CMV is also associated with anal ulcers (Fig. 22-3). Horn and Hood examined five consecutive skin biopsy specimens taken from perianal ulcers on immunosuppressed patients.[33] Each specimen was formalin fixed and in addition to routine microscopy was evaluated with anti-CMV immunoperoxidase. All five ulcers had demonstrable

CMV although in none of the cases was the virus successfully cultured. Treatment of these ulcers is often frustrating and unrewarding. Moreover gangiclovir can be administered only in the intravenous form. This usually requires placement of an indwelling intravenous catheter. Moreover, lifelong maintenance therapy is usually necessary.[29] Neutropenia is the chief toxicity noted in approximately 40 percent of patients.[29] Other toxicities include thrombocytopenia, central nervous system aberrations, and GI disturbances. Thus the physician must weigh lifelong dependency upon intravenous administration of a toxic substance against perianal ulcer symptoms. If ganciclovir is chosen, the entire course of therapy should be orchestrated and supervised by an infectious disease specialist.

Herpes Simplex Virus

Although herpes simplex proctitis and herpes simplex perianal lesions are not seen exclusively in AIDS pa-

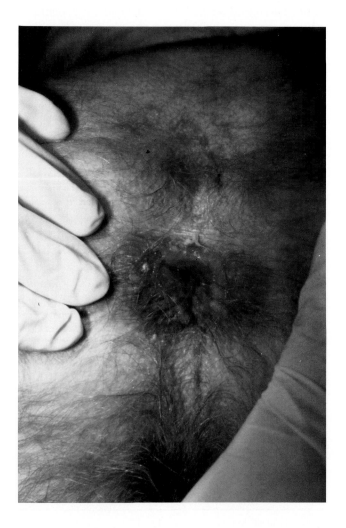

tients, they occur frequently in this group.[34,35] Serologic tests revealed that more than 95 percent of homosexual men with AIDS have been previously infected with HSV-2.[36] Chronic mucocutaneous HSV infection suggests immunoincompetence, and the CDC has recently revised the diagnostic criteria for AIDS to include this condition.[37] Thus, ulcerative HSV infection, including perianal HSV-2, present for 1 month or longer in a patient in whom no other cause of underlying immunodeficiency exists and one who has laboratory evidence of HIV infection, is diagnostic of AIDS.

Herpes simplex virus (HSV) is the most frequent cause of nongonococcal proctitis in sexually active homosexual men,[38,39] and HSV causes symptoms more often than do most other anorectal infections. Symptoms, patient evaluation, and treatment of HSV are discussed in Chapter 21. This information is applicable to the HIV-positive patient with clinically active HSV. In addition, many AIDS patients suffer from frequent HSV recurrences. They can be managed with suppressive acyclovir therapy in dosage ranges from 200 mg three times a day to 400 mg four times daily; GI side effects will generally limit the dosage. Acyclovir resistance has been reported.[40] Alternative treatment regimens include foscarnet (insodium phosphonoformate) and vidarabine.

Infectious Diarrheas

Infectious diarrheas are also common in HIV patients (50 to 80 percent of patients during their illnesses).[41] The evaluation and treatment of these conditions are covered in Chapters 21 and 26.

Idiopathic Anal Ulceration

Idiopathic anal ulcers in HIV-seropositive homosexual and bisexual males are a particularly challenging problem. The ulcers may be due to a plethora of benign and malignant causes. Two initial facets of diagnosis are imperative prior to embarkation upon therapeutic interventions. First, the ulcer must be distinguished from a fissure. Benign anal fissures should be either in the posterior or anterior midline. They should be accompanied by a "garden variety" skin tag and should be visible upon buttock retraction. This picture is in sharp contradistinction to that of the HIV-related ulcer. The latter entity is similar to a Crohn's anal fissure, as the ulcers are eccentric or multiple, often deep or cavitating, and show little or no signs of healing (Fig. 22-4). In addition, the accompanying "skin tags" are not ubiquitous and if present they are often edematous and bluish-purple in hue. The major difference between a Crohn's anal ulcer and an HIV anal ulcer is that the

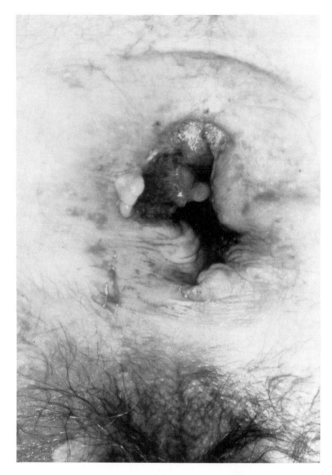

Figure 22-4.   An HIV-associated anal ulcer. (*From:* Wexner SD. AIDS: what the colorectal surgeon needs to know. *Perspect Colorectal Surg.* 1989;2(2):19–55.)

Crohn's type is associated with anal stenosis whereas the HIV type is usually accompanied by anal sphincter hypotonia. Wastell has suggested the term "gay anus syndrome" to describe the clinical picture of a homosexual male with a moist anus (due to mucous leakage, sphincter hypotonia, or both), skin tags, and condylomata.[42] Gottesman has described these skin tags as "bridging."[43]

The second initial facet of diagnosis is to exclude treatable benign and malignant ulcer etiologies. Table 22-6 lists causes of anal ulceration; these conditions are discussed in Chapters 21 and 26. Some of those etiologies, such as HIV ulcers, are seen only in HIV seropositive patients. Other etiologies, however, may be seen in HIV seronegative patients of either sex.

Initial examination includes ulcer biopsy. This can be done in the office or another outpatient setting. If the patient is cooperative and preferably thin, the buttocks can be taped apart to limit the potential for needle stick injury. The contralateral hand should *not* assist in but-

Table 22-6   Causes of HIV-Associated Anal Ulceration

MALIGNANT
Anal carcinoma
Kaposi's sarcoma
Perianal and anal lymphoma
Condyloma-in-situ ("malignant" condylomata)

TRAUMATIC
Insertive
   Penile
   Foreign body
   Fist
   Other
Iatrogenic
   Nonhealing surgical site
Fissure

INFECTIOUS
Viral
   Herpes simplex (HSV)
   Herpes zoster (HZV)
   Cytomegalovirus (CMV)
   Human immunodeficiency (HIV)
   Human papilloma (HPV)
Fungal
   Cryptococcus neoformans
   Mycobacterium avium-intracellulare (MAI)
   Histoplasma capsulatum
Bacterial
   Nisseria gonorrheae
   Chlamydia trachomatis
   Chancroid
Other
   Treponema pallidum

tock retraction, nor should the hand of any assistant be placed on the field. A 30-gauge, 3/8-inch long needle is used to slowly administer a mixture of 0.5% lidocaine, 0.25% bipuvacaine, and 1:200,000 units of epinephrine. The anal examination is usually facilitated by the baseline sphincter hypotonia that many male homosexual HIV-seropositive patients with anal ulcers exhibit. If the patient is unable to tolerate infiltration with a local anesthetic or if he is in severe pain, an examination under anesthesia is warranted.

If the ulcers are perianal, 3- to 5-mm punch biopsies are taken from the center and edges of the ulcer. If the ulcer is in the distal anal canal or at the anal verge, the edges are excised and the base curetted. Ulcers located proximal to the dentate line are biopsied only in the operating room after administration of a regional or general anesthetic. This limits the opportunity for needle-stick injury and enhances visualization.

Biopsies are obtained for routine hematoxylin and eosin histopathologic examination, for viral culture, for acid-fast stain, and for RNA-HIV probes. The initial pathogens being sought are CMV, HSV, mycobacterium avium-intracellulare (MAI), and HIV. In addition, a dark-field examination can also be performed to exclude syphilis. If the ulcer is chronic, periodic acid-Schiff staining should also be undertaken to exclude *Cryptococcus neoformans*.[44] In addition, a VDRL blood test should be requested if suspicion of syphilis exists. If any adjacent vesicles are present, fluid should be obtained and sent for viral culture because this appearance is typical for HSV. Occult sepsis must be excluded wherein the ulcer represents the visible portion of a deep excavating cavity. These lesions can be quite impressive in magnitude, involving the anal sphincters, the ischiorectal fossae, or even the supralevator space.[42]

A few practical aspects relative to anorectal biopsies in HIV-positive patients are worth noting:

1. Blunt-tipped electrocautery or scissors are the only instruments used to cut tissue; scalpels are not permitted on the field.
2. Vesicle fluid has the highest yield for the diagnosis by viral culture of HSV.
3. A viral culture should be obtained with a plastic- or metal-shafted cotton-tipped swab and sent immediately in special viral transport medium; the standard wooden-tipped swabs may inactivate the viruses.
4. Rigid proctoscopy should be performed to assess the rectal mucosa for synchronous lesions.
5. Some tissue should always be placed aside in normal saline; this can then be used for MAI culture and sensitivity, for acid-fast staining for an RNA-HIV probe assay, for HPV typing, or for other more esoteric assays.

If the patient has a history of HSV or if the lesions are suggestive of this infection, empiric topical 5% acylovir ointment therapy may be commenced. The initial therapeutic trial consists of applications five times daily for 1 to 2 weeks. Local application of 5% lidocaine jelly may also be helpful for pain relief. Oral acyclovir, 400 mg five times daily, can be started with the anticipation of symptomatic relief within a few days.[43] Failure of oral and topical acylovir therapy mandates the use of intravenous acylovir. Suppressive oral therapy of 200 mg to 400 mg three times a day should be considered in all patients after resolution of the initial lesion.[45]

Despite a multitude of laboratory evaluations, the etiology of some ulcers remains elusive. They may be due to the HIV itself, as viral particles can be identified using RNA probes.[43,46] Gottesman has reported initial success with the injection of depomedrol, 1 to 2 ml of 80 mg/ml, into the ulcer base.[43] In some cases, however, the only method of ameliorating the excruciating pain of these idiopathic ulcers is by complete fecal diversion.[8,43]

After exclusion of all possible STDs, anal manometry is performed. If sphincter hypertension exists, if the patient does not have chronic diarrhea, and if the patient is asymptomatic from HIV disease (WR stage 1–3 or CDC I), a limited sphincterotomy can be performed with the anticipation of symptomatic improvement.

Current understanding of perianal ulcerations and fissure in the HIV-positive patient has increased exponentially since 1986. New drugs, such as diDeoxycytidine (dDI) and diDeoxycytosine (dDC) and others have improved the prognosis for these patients. "Cautiously aggressive" surgery can sometimes be beneficial rather than detrimental to these patients.[47]

Anal Malignancies

Kaposi's Sarcoma

Kaposi's sarcoma is the most common malignant tumor in AIDS patients.[48] It is a malignant tumor of endothelial origin that was traditionally an indolent cutaneous sarcoma found almost exclusively in elderly males from Mediterranean Europe. In this latter group of patients, the gastrointestinal tract was the most common extracutaneous location, although GI lesions were seldom seen. This experience contrasts sharply with AIDS population, in whom disseminated lesions have been identified in 50 percent of those with Kaposi's sarcoma of the skin and in between 25 percent and 77 percent of all patients.[49-51] Traditional Kaposi's sarcoma is associated with a 10:1 to 15:1 male:female ratio and an elderly population (83 percent over 40 years of age). In stark comparison, the AIDS-associated type occurs during the third or fourth decades of life with a male:female ratio of 50:1.[52-54] Forty-three percent of homosexual and bisexual male AIDS patients have Kaposi's sarcoma.[55] It is of interest that the rates of colorectal lesions are markedly lower in heterosexual AIDS patients. Cytomegalovirus has been recovered from Kaposi's sarcomas and may play a permissive role for clinical expression of this malignancy.[56]

Clinically, the disease in homosexual and bisexual AIDS patients tends to be widespread, with frequent involvement of mucosal surfaces, visceral organs, lymph nodes, and skin.[57,58] Kaposi's sarcoma has been reported from the mouth to the anus and is more common in the upper GI tract than in the colon. Most patients are completely asymptomatic, although bleed-

ing, obstruction, perforation, and mesenteric cyst formation have all been reported.[59]

The endoscopic appearance of Kaposi's sarcoma is quite characteristic, with raised, round, sessile red nodules ranging from several millimeters to several centimeters in diameter (Fig. 22-5). Larger lesions often have a soft central umbilication. The edges of the lesions are quite smooth and invariably symmetric. The deep red or purplish color is due to the highly vascular nature of the lesion and the chronic extravasation of erythrocytes resulting in hemosiderin deposition (Fig. 22-6). Occasionally patients develop a macular variety, rather than the traditional nodular type. These macules often resemble submucosal ecchymoses or granulation tissue.

Diagnosis is made by proctosigmoidoscopy and biopsy. Because of the submucosal nature of the lesion, histopathologic confirmation is often impossible.[60] One study reported only 23 percent success in histopathologic diagnosis.[51] Despite the tumor's vascular appearance, excessive bleeding has not been problematic, even after biopsy with an 8-mm proctoscopic biopsy

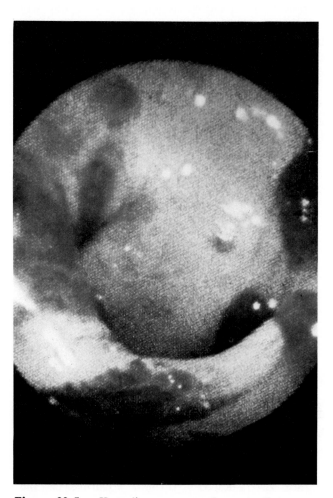

Figure 22-5.   Kaposi's sarcoma, endoscopic view.

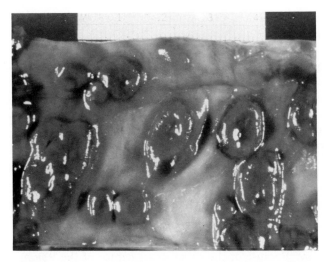

Figure 22-6. Kaposi's sarcoma, gross lesion. (*From*: Wexner SD. Cytomegalovirus ileocolitis and Kaposi's sarcoma in AIDS. In: Fazio VW, ed. *Current Therapy in Colon and Rectal Surgery*. Toronto: BC Decker; 1990:217–221.)

forceps.[50,51,61] A superficial biopsy (<3 to 4 mm) will almost certainly be unrewarding.[50] Two patients have been reported in whom the only abnormality that led to diagnosis was posterior rectal wall thickening seen on CT scanning.[62]

In the classic nodular variety, histopathologic studies show spindle-shaped cels with central hemorrhage, vascular slits, and extravasated erythrocytes (Fig. 22-7).[63] Inflammatory cells are generally absent, but hemosiderin-laden macrophages and nuclear and cytologic atypia are seen instead. The thin endothelial cells lining the abnormally shaped vascular spaces stain for Factor VIII using indirect immunoperoxidase techniques. This

points to an endothelial cell origin for Kaposi's sarcoma.[64]

Diagnosis is most useful as a prognosticator, since no effective medical treatment is available at present. Chemotherapy with single and combined agents, irradiation, and interferon have all been relatively disappointing.[65-67] Zidovudine is currently under investigation for the treatment of Kaposi's sarcoma.[68] The mean duration of response to most chemotherapeutic regimens is only between 2 and 8 months.[50] Except in cases of pulmonary involvement, which has a rapid and universally fatal outcome, Kaposi's sarcoma is rarely the immediate cause of death.[50,68] As with AIDS in general, patients most often die of coexisting opportunistic infections. In fact, patients with Kaposi's sarcoma who do not have an opportunistic infection have an 80 percent 28-month survival, whereas those with Kaposi's sarcoma and opportunistic infection have only a 20 percent 28-month survival.[64]

Friedman, Wright, and Altman[51] found a significantly death rate at 12, 18, and 24 months in AIDS patients with GI lesions as compared with those who had only cutaneous Kaposi's sarcoma. At 24 months, 89 percent of the GI group had died compared with only 12 percent of the cutaneous group. Interestingly, they also found that GI involvement increased with the number of cutaneous lesions: 33 percent of patients with 10 or fewer cutaneous lesions had GI lesions as compared with 80 percent of those with 11 or more skin lesions.

Surgical resection should be contemplated only to control massive exsanguination, perforation, or obstruction in an AIDS patient who might otherwise be expected to have a reasonably long life expectancy. Surgical results, however, have generally been disappointing.

A recent report on 8 homosexual male patients with Kaposi's sarcoma of the rectum noted a mean age of 34 years with an age range of 24 to 39 years.[69] Common presenting symptoms were proctalgia in 62 percent, hematochezia in 50 percent, and diarrhea in 50 percent. Associated anorectal conditions were condylomata acuminata in 75 percent, rectal HSV in 25 percent, CMV in 13 percent, and fistulae in 13 percent. Five patients (62 percent) had disseminated lesions and 3 (36 percent) had disease limited to the rectum. Three patients were treated with radiation or chemotherapy. Five patients received no specific treatment. Three patients from each group were alive 1 month to 5 years after diagnosis. The authors concluded that aggressive surgical treatment of anorectal Kaposi's sarcoma is not indicated. Surgical excision should be limited to biopsy for diagnosis. These authors also reconfirmed that neither chemotherapy, radiotherapy, nor immunotherapy is of proven

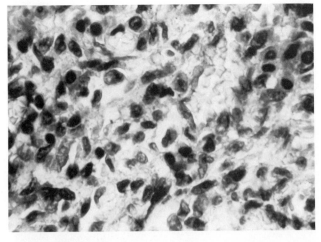

Figure 22-7. Kaposi's sarcoma. (Hematoxylin and eosin, × 250.)

benefit. There may, however, be some value to palliative radiation for local control of painful lesions.

Lymphoma

HIV patients have an increased incidence of malignant lymphomas.[70,71] Although Hodgkin's lymphoma of the rectum has been reported in this population, the overwhelming majority of cases of intestinal lymphomas are of the non-Hodgkin's variety.[72,73] Seventy percent of these are of B-cell origin and most are high grade.[74] Lymphoma in AIDS patients is frequently extranodular and highly aggressive. These high grade B-cell lymphomas may be related to Epstein–Barr viral infection and usually present as advanced extralymphatic disease.

Within the GI tract, the rectum is the second most common site, exceeded in incidence only by the stomach. Identification of an anorectal lymphoma is generally difficult, because in most cases these lesions are extraluminal. Although discrete non-Hodgkin's rectal lymphoma is occasionally seen, the typical presentation is a diffuse, deep-seated form.[75] Most patients are brought to the operating room wth perirectal abscess as the preoperative diagnosis.[76,77] All that may be noticed on initial consultation is erythema, or perhaps some induration in the perianal region or within the pelvis that can be felt on rectal examination. However, larger ulcerative lesions may be present (Figs. 22-8A and B). In addition, because the majority of homosexual patients, especially those with AIDS, have shotty inguinal adenopathy, this sign is of little value. Therefore, in a high-risk patient with symptoms of tenesmus, fever, and perirectal pain, examination under anesthesia is often warranted. Treatment consists of a broad assortment of aggressive multimodal chemotherapeutic regimens. Results of chemotherapy have been poorer than in non-AIDS patients because of a lack of bone marrow reserve and frequent opportunistic infections. Median survival in these patients is generally less than 12 months.[76,78]

Anal Carcinoma

Anal carcinoma in situ has been described with increasing frequency in homosexual men with condylomata acuminata.[79,80] Nash and colleagues reported 20 cases of histologically atypical anal mucosal lesions ranging from atypical condylomata to Bowen's disease.[81] Of these patients 92 percent were male, and more than 75 percent of the males were known homosexuals. The most common site of atypia was at the junction of the anal transitional zone with the rectal mucosa. Croxson and associates reported 7 homosexual men in whom condylomata acuminata revealed carcinoma in situ.[82]

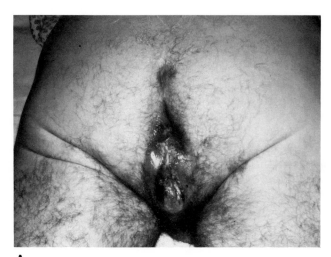
A

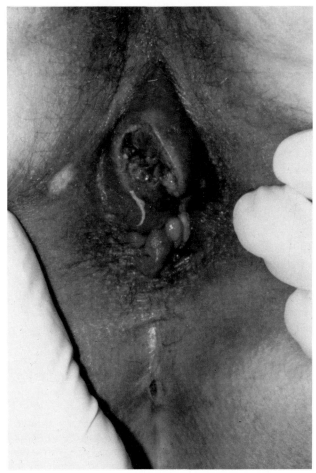
B

Figure 22-8.   (A) and (B) Perianal lymphoma. (Figure A *from*: Wexner SD. AIDS: what the colorectal surgeon needs to know. *Perspect Colorectal Surg.* 1989;2(2):19–55.)

Cooper and other authors have also noted an increased incidence of cloacogenic, squamous, and in situ carcinomas in homosexual and bisexual men, and especially in AIDS patients.[42,83-86]

Recent epidemiologic studies have shown significantly more anal cancers in single than in married men.[86-89] The authors of these studies suggest that anal cancer may follow habitual anal-receptive intercourse. The transition from condylomata acuminata to carcinoma in situ may well be analogous to the transition seen in the cervix from papilloma virus to carcinoma.[90,91] Another epidemiologic study found the anal carcinoma risk in homosexual and bisexual men to be 25- to 50-fold higher than the equivalent risk in heterosexual men.[84] All of these data are related to the almost universal finding of human papillomavirus (HPV) in anorectal carcinomas in homosexual men.[80]

Scholefield and coworkers prospectively evaluated 82 patients with anal HPV infection and found that 23 had anal intraepithelial neoplasia.[92] The prevalence of anal intraepithelial neoplasia in men with HPV infection was significantly higher among homosexuals than it was among heterosexuals (17 of 28 vs 1 of 26). In a similar study, Palmer and colleagues further supported the association between HPV and squamous cell anal cancer.[93] After DNA analysis, the authors found that HPV 16 was present in 23 of 41 (56 percent) anal cancers. In addition, HPV 18 DNA was found in another 5 percent. No detectable HPV 6 or 11 DNA was noted in any of the cancers. Nonmalignant anorectal epithelium did not contain any HPV. This investigation supports the concept of HPV as a cofactor or initiator in malignant transformation in anal lesions. Additional experience in patients with chronic epithelial infection supports the oncogenic potential of HPV. The high incidence of condylomata acuminata in HIV patients, and their associated immunosuppression, suggests a potential for developing epidermoid anal cancers.

Careful evaluation and biopsy of any anal lesions will lead to early diagnosis. As with other malignancies already described, the selection of therapy should be based on the patient's immunologic and health status. The standard and currently accepted regimen of combined chemotherapy and radiation therapy is probably appropriate treatment for squamous cell cancer in the asymptomatic HIV-seropositive patient.[94]

Patients with more advanced disease, however, have a poor prognosis and may not tolerate either chemotherapy or radiation therapy.

Treatment

Because of the preselected population of asymptomatic, mandatorily screened HIV-positive military recruits,

the study by Beck and colleagues[10] stands in stark contrast to those described elsewhere.[8,95] Wexner and coworkers reviewed 73 anorectal procedures performed on 51 patients with symptomatic AIDS.[8] Fifteen percent of these patients presented with anorectal disease prior to the diagnosis of AIDS and half were dead within 7.4 months of presentation. As in the study by Beck and colleagues,[10] the majority of patients had multiple sexually transmitted anorectal disease either active or past.[8] A total of 118 sexually transmitted diseases were diagnosed in 39 patients. These included hepatitis B, HSV, herpes zoster virus, condylomata acuminata, gonorrhea, syphillis, and giardiasis.

The majority of procedures performed in this study were minor and elective, such as fistulotomies, transrectal biopsies, or incision and drainage of small abscesses. Despite the relatively limited intervention undertaken, the wounds of only 6 of the 51 patients (12 percent) healed uneventfully within 1 month of surgery, and 17 patients (34 percent) required longer than 6 months to heal. Furthermore, all 10 of the AIDS patients who underwent sphincterotomy were rendered at least partially incontinent.

The studies by Beck and colleagues and by Wexner and coworkers illustrate the importance of asking *every* patient with "suspicious" anorectal disease about sexual preferences. A history of homosexual or bisexual behavior or of anorectal or enteric STD should prompt HIV testing. Failure to do so augurs a poor outcome. In many regions, however, HIV testing can be performed only after informed consent and can be refused by the patient. This underlines the importance of the surgeon's own assessment of risk factors.[92]

In retrospect, many nonhealing "fissures" treated by sphincterotomy may have been HIV ulcers.[8,96] Carr and associates retrospectively reviewed the outcome of anorectal surgery in 34 homosexual men.[95] Within this series were 8 HIV-negative patients, 4 asymptomatic HIV-positive patients, 12 symptomatic HIV-patients, and 10 in whom the HIV status was unknown. Surgery consisted of abscess drainage or fistulotomy in 19 patients, treatment of fissure in 15 patients, excision of tags or hemorrhoids in 8 patients, and other procedures in 2 patients. Several patients underwent more than one procedure. Irrespective of the type of surgery performed, healing occurred within 6 weeks of surgery in all HIV-negative and asymptomatic HIV-positive patients. However, the wounds of 8 of 9 symptomatic HIV-positive patients failed to heal.

Moenning and colleagues retrospectively reviewed a series of 52 HIV-positive and AIDS patients with anorectal disorders.[97] Of these patients, 16 underwent anorectal surgery with a morbidity of 62 percent, a mortality of 6 percent, and a recurrence rate of 56 percent. Patients with advanced-stage disease had significant rates of morbidity and mortality, and the results of operative therapy were dismal. Again, these data confirm those cited above and reflect the consequences of surgical intervention in the face of markedly altered immunologic function.[8,10,94–98]

In view of these data, the authors are hesitant to perform aggressive surgical procedures on late-stage patients (WR stage 4–6, CDC stages III and IV). However, conservative proctologic procedures in early-stage patients can be performed with reasonable results. Following the guidelines of conservatism in advanced HIV disease and "cautiously aggressive" surgery in early-stage HIV disease, Beck and coworkers reported their results[99]: 119 HIV-positive patients had anal condylomata. On presentation, the patients with condylomata were similar to the overall HIV-positive group for age, sex, race, etiologic risk factors, and Walter Reed classification. Evaluation revealed that in addition to the condylomata, 60 percent of the patients had at least one other sexually transmitted disease, including hepatitis B in 55 percent of patients, HSV (type 2) in 42 percent, chlamydia in 36 percent, and syphilis in 13 percent.

Anal condylomata were managed in the following manner: Sixty-one patients who were asymptomatic or had late Walter Reed stage (3–6) disease were observed. Thirty-one symptomatic patients with condylomata limited to the anal margin were treated with one or two applications of 5% podophyllin in benzoin. Twenty-seven patients with anal canal condylomata underwent excision and fulguration under general or regional anesthesia. During the operative procedure, several of the condylomata from each patient, were biopsied for pathologic review and all were confirmed to be condylomata acuminata. There were no significant perioperative complications, and all patients' wounds healed.

Follow-up of the condylomata patients ranged from 4 to 26 months (mean = 12 mo). The recurrence rate for condylomata in the treated patients was 26 percent after local treatment with podophyllin and 4 percent after fulguration and excision. Progression of Walter Reed staging at follow-up occurred in 29 percent of patients, and 29 HIV-positive patients died during follow-up. The low recurrence rate and absence of significant complications after fulguration in early-stage patients, supports its use in symptomatic patients with extensive lesions.

Asymptomatic HIV-seropositive patients can be expected to have good results with few complications following limited anorectal procedures. The safest way to proceed with therapy might be after T4 cell counts are made. Moenning and colleagues evaluated the T4 counts in 39 HIV-positive and AIDS patients with anorectal disease (personal communication). Of these patients, 2 had T4 counts ≤200 and 16 had T4 counts >200. The <200 group had a 65 percent morbidity rate whereas the >200 group had only a 7 percent morbidity rate.

Jaso and associates have suggested that in early-stage HIV-positive patients the presence of anorectal disease appears to be a marker for more rapid disease progression.[100] Thus benign anorectal disease must be viewed with suspicion, evualated with thorough attention to HIV status, and treated only after complete knowledge of HIV disease status. Although well-intentioned surgical intervention may bring transient symptomatic relief to the advanced-stage AIDS patient, the long-term sequelae of such action may be disastrous.[101] Similarly, withholding appropriate intervention from an early-stage asymptomatic HIV-positive individual may be unnecessary.[102]

Several surgical tips are worth emphasizing.

1. Scalpels and needles are not permitted on the field; electrocautery is used for all incisions, dissection, and hemostasis.
2. Two or three pairs of gloves and eye protection are worn by all personnel.
3. On those rare occassions when suturing is required the instruments are *never* manually passed. Instead, the nurse places the loaded needle-holder on a tray from which it is retrieved by the surgeon. The same procedure is reversed when the suturing is completed. Only the person using the needle is permitted to put hands in the operating field. An instrument, rather than the contralateral hand is used to retrieve the needle.
4. All patients receive broad spectrum antibiotics preoperatively and for 1 week postoperatively. In addition, all patients are maintained on Zidovudine®, diDeoxycytidine (ODC), diDeoxyinosine (dDI), or another reverse transcriptase inhibitor.
5. *All* patients, regardless of the thoroughness of preoperative investigation and disease staging, are alerted to the possibilities of nonhealing wounds and fecal incontinence.

Conclusions

The management of HIV-positive patients continues to challenge surgeons. The epidemologic and treatment information presented in this chapter should update the practitioner. Until a vaccine or definitive treatment for the viral infection becomes available, increasing numbers of patients will require care. As progress is made in treating the infectious complications associated with diminished immunity, additional and unusual malignancies may become apparent in these patients. Their management will be challenging and will require a multidisciplinary approach.

References

1. Popovic M, Sargadharan MG, Read E, et al. Detection, isolation, and continuous production or cytopathic retrovirus (HTLV-III) from patients with AIDS and pre-AIDS. *Science.* 1984; 225:497–500.

2. Gartner S, Markovits P, Markovitz DM, et al. The role of mononuclear phagocytes in HTLV-III/LAV infection. *Science.* 1986;233:215–220.

3. Centers for Disease Control. HIV/AIDS surveillance report. January 1992:1–22.

4. Curran JW, Jaffe WH, Hardy AM, et al. Epidemiology of HIV infection and AIDS in the United States. *Science.* 1988;239:610–618.

5. Coolfont report: A public health service plan for prevention and control of AIDS and AIDS virus. *Public Health Serv Rep.* 1986;101:341–348.

6. Lui KJ, Darrow WW, Rutherford GW III. A model-based estimate of the mean incubation period for AIDS in homosexual men. *Science.* 1988;240:1333–1335.

7. DeVita VT Jr, Hellman S, Rosenberg SA, eds. *AIDS. Etiology, Diagnosis, Treatment and Presentation.* 2nd ed. Philadelphia: JB Lippincott; 1988.

8. Wexner SD, Smithy WB, Milsom JW, Dailey TH. The surgical management of anorectal diseases in AIDS and pre-AIDS patients. *Dis Colon Rectum* 1986;29:719–723.

9. Edwards P, Wodak A, Cooper DA, Thompson IL, Penny R. The gastrointestinal manifestation of AIDS. Aust *N Z/J Med.* 1990;20:141–148.

10. Beck DE, Jaso RG, Zajac RA. Proctologic management of the HIV (+) patient. *South Med J.* 1990;83:898–892.

11. Wexner SD. Cytomegalovirus ileocolitis and Kaposi's sarcoma in AIDS. In: Fazio VW, ed. *Current Therapy in Colon and Rectal Surgery.* Toronto: BC Decker; 1990:217–221.

12. Kaplan LD. AIDS-associated lymphomas. *Infect Dis Clin North Am.* 1988;2:525–532.

13. Croxson T, Chabon AB, Rorat E, Barash IM. Intraepithelial carcinoma of the anus in homosexual men. *Dis Colon Rectum.* 1984;27:325–330.

14. Wexner SD, Smithy WB, Trillo C, Hopkins BS, Dailey TH. Emergency colectomy for cytomegalovirus ileocolitis in patients with the acquired immune deficiency syndrome. *Dis Colon Rectum.* 1988;31:755–761.

15. Allen-Mersh TG, Gottesman LG, Miles AJG, et al. The management of anorectal diseases in HIV-positive patients. *Int J Colorectal Dis.* 1990;5:61–72.

16. Wolkomir AF, Barone JE, Hardy HW III, Cottone FJ. Abdominal and anorectal surgery and the acquired immune deficiency syndrome in heterosexual intravenous drug users. *Dis Colon Rectum.* 1990;33:267–270.

17. Ranki A, Valle S-L, Krohn M, Antonen J, et al. Long latency precedes overt seroconversion in sexually transmitted human-immunodeficiency-virus infection. *Lancet.* 1987;2:589–593.

18. Greco TP, Simms MF. Acquired immune deficiency syndrome and the surgeon. *Postgrad Adv Colorectal Surg.* 1988;1(3):1–20.

19. Wexner SD. Epidemiology of human immunodeficiency virus (HIV) transmission relative to the anorectal manifestations of AIDS. In: Gottesman L, Mersh TA, eds. Anorectal disease in AIDS. London: Edward Arnold; 1991; 14–27.

20. Centers for Disease Control: Classification system for human T-lymphotropic virus type III/lymphadenopathy–associated virus infections. *MMWR.* 1986;35:334–339.

21. Redfield RR, Wright DC, Tramont EC. The Walter Reed classification for HTLV-III/LAV infection. *N Engl J Med.* 1986:314;131–132.

22. Fleming DO. Hazard control of infectious agents. *Occup Med.* 1987;2:499–510.

23. The Task Force on AIDS. *Recommendations for the Prevention of Human Immunodeficiency Virus (HIV) Transmission in the Practice of Orthopaedic Surgery.* Chicago, IL: American Academy of Orthopaedic Surgeons; 1989.

24. Lifson AR, Rutherford GW, Jaffe HW. The natural history of human immunodeficiency virus infection. *J Infect Dis.* 1988:158; 1360–1367.

25. Valenzuela JE. AIDS and gastrointestinal diseases. *Pract Gastrointest.* 1990:2;11–15.

26. Colebunder R, Mann JM, Francis H, et al. Evaluation of a clinical case—definition of acquired immunodeficiency syndrome in Africa. *Lancet.* 1987;1:492.

27. Wexner SD. Sexually transmitted diseases: the challenge of the nineties. *Dis Colon Rectum.* 1990;33(12):1048–1062.

28. Wexner SD. AIDS: what the colorectal surgeon

needs to know. *Perspect Colorectal Surg.* 1990; 2(2):19–54.

29. Drew WL, Buhles W, Erlich KS. Herpesvirus infections (cytomegalovirus, herpes simplex virus, varicella-zoster virus). *Infect Dis Clin North Am.* 1988:2;495–509.

30. Frager DH, Frager JD, Wolf EL, et al. Cytomegalovirus colitis in acquired immunodeficiency syndrome: radiology spectrum. *Gastrointest Radiol.* 1986;11:241–246.

31. Culpepper-Morgan JA, Kotler DP, Scholes JV, et al. Evaluation of diagnostic criteria for mucosal cytomegalic inclusion disease in the acquired immune deficiency syndrome. *Am J Gastroenterol.* 1978;82:1264–1270.

32. Wexner SD. Infectional resection in AIDS patients. In: Rothenberger DA, Nyhus L, eds. *Problems in General Surgery.* Philadelphia: JB Lippincott. In press.

33. Horn TD, Hood AF. Cytomegalovirus is predictably present in perineal ulcers from immunosuppressed patients. *Arch Dermatol.* 1990; 126:642–644.

34. Allason-Jones E, Mindel A. Sex and the bowel. *Int J Colorectal Dis.* 1987:2:32–37.

35. Wexner SD. Managing common anorectal sexually transmitted diseases. *Infect Surg.* 1990; 9(6):9–48.

36. Nerurkar L, Goedert J, Wallen W, et al. Study of antiviral antibodies in sera of homosexual men. *Federation Proceedings* 1983:42:6109.

37. Revision of the CDC surveillance case definition for acquired immunodeficiency syndrome. *MMWR.* 1987;36(suppl):1s–15s.

38. Goodell SE, Quinn TC, Mktrichian EE, et al. Herpes simplex virus proctitis in homosexual men: clinical sigmoidoscopic, and histopathologic features. *N Engl J Med.* 1983:308:868–871.

39. Siegal FP, Lopez C, Hammer GS, et al. Severe acquired immunodeficiency in male homosexuals manifested by chronic perianal ulcerative herpes simplex lesions. *N Engl J Med.* 1981;305: 1439–1444.

40. Wexner SD. Treatment of AIDS patients with herpes simplex virus infections resistant to acyclovir. *Colon Rectal Surg Outlook.* 1989; 2(8):1–2.

41. Antony MA, Brandt LJ, Klein KS, Nernstein LH. Infectious diarrhea in patients with AIDS. *Dig Dis Sci.* 1988:33;1141–1146.

42. Wastell C. AIDS and the surgeon: an update. In: *Surgery.* Oxford: Oxford University Press; 1989;69:9–10. Medicine International Series.

43. Gottesman L. Treatment of anorectal ulcers in the HIV-positive patient. *Perspect Colorectal Surg.* 1991;4(1):19–30.

44. Van Calck M, Motte S, Rickaert F, Serruys E, Adler M, Wybran J. Cryptococcal anal ulceration in a patient with AIDS. *Am J Gastroenterol.* 1988; 83:1306–1308.

45. Milson JW. Anal disease in the immunocompromised patient. *Semin in Colon and Rectal Surgery.* 1990;1(4):241–246.

46. Kotter DP, Wilson CS, Haroutiounian G, Fox CH. Detection of human immunodeficiency virus-1 by 35s-RNA in situ hybridization in solitary esophageal ulcers in two patients with the acquired immune deficiency syndrome. *Am J Gastroenterol.* 1989;84:313–317.

47. Wexner SD. Anal surgery in the HIV-positive patient. *J R Soc Med.* 1991;84(4):191–192.

48. Mitsuyasu RT. Kaposi's sarcoma in the acquired immunodeficiency syndrome. *Infect Dis Clin North Am.* 1988:2;511–523.

49. Gottlieb MS, Croopman JE, Weinstein WM, et al. The acquired immunodeficiency syndrome. *Ann Intern Med.* 1983;99:208–220.

50. Mitsuvasu RT. Kaposi's sarcoma in the acquired immunodeficiency syndrome. *Infect Dis Clin North Am.* 1988;2:511–523.

51. Friedman SL, Wright TL, Altman DF. Gastrointestinal Kaposi's sarcoma in patients with acquired immunodificiency syndrome. *Gastroenterology.* 1985;89:102–106.

52. Reynolds WS, Windelmann RK, Soule EH. Kaposi's sarcoma: clinicopathologic study with particular reference to its relationship to the reticuloendothelial system. *Medicine.* 1965;44: 419–443.

53. Rothman S. Remarks on sex, age, and racial distribution of Kaposi's sarcoma and on possible pathogenic factors. *Acta Int Cancer.* 1962; 18:326–329.

54. Cox FH, Helwig EB. Kaposi's sarcoma. *Cancer.* 1959;12:289–298.

55. Steis RG, Longo DL. Clinical, biologic, and therapeutic aspects of malignancies associated with the acquired immunodeficiency syndrome: part 1. *Ann Allergy.* 1988;60:310–323.

56. Daul CB, DeShazo RD. Acquired immunodeficiency syndrome: an update and interpretation. *Ann Allergy.* 1983;51:351–361.

57. Friedman-Klen AE, Laubenstein LJ, Rubenstein P, et al. Disseminated Kaposi's sarcoma in homosexual men. *Ann Intern Med.* 1982;86:693–700.

58. Hymes KB, Greene JB, Marcus A, et al. Kaposi's sarcoma in homosexual men—a report of eight cases. *Lancet.* 1981;2:598–600.

59. Macho JR. Gastrointestinal surgery in the AIDS patient. *Gastroenterol Clin North Am.* 1988: 17:563–571.

60. Cone LA, Wodard DR, Potts BE, et al. An update on the acquired immunodeficiency syndrome (AIDS). *Dis Colon Rectum.* 1986:29;60–64.

61. Walsman J, Rotterdam H, Niedt GN, et al. AIDS: an overview of the pathology. *Pathol Res Pract.* 1987;182:729–754.

62. Jeffrey RB, Nyberg DA, Bottles K, et al. Abdominal CT in acquired immunodeficiency syndrome. *AJR.* 1986;146:7–13.

63. Francis ND, Parkin JM, Weber J, et al. Kaposi's sarcoma in acquired immune deficiency syndrome (AIDS). *J Clin Pathol.* 1986;39:469–474.

64. Krigel RL, Friedman-Kien AE. Kaposi's sarcoma in AIDS: diagnosis and treatment. In: DeVita VT, Hellman S, Rosenberg SA, eds. *AIDS: Etiology, Diagnosis, Treatment, and Prevention.* 2nd ed. Philadelphia: JB Lippincott; 1988:245–261.

65. Krown SE, Real FX, Cumingham-Rundles S, et al. Preliminary observations on the effect of recombinant leukocyte-A interferon in homosexual men with Kaposi's sarcoma. *N Engl J. Med.* 1983;308:1071–1076.

66. Real FX, Oettgen HF, Krown SE. Kaposi's sarcoma and the acquired immunodeficiency syndrome: treatment with high and low doses of recombinant leukocyte A interferon. *J Clin Oncol.* 1986;4:544–551.

67. Gelman EP, Lango D, Lane HC, et al. Combination chemotherapy of disseminated Kaposi's sarcoma in patients with the acquired immune deficiency syndrome. *Am J Med.* 1987;82:11–18.

68. Meduri GV, Stover DE, Lee M, et al. Pulmonary Kaposi's sarcoma in the acquired immmonodeficiency syndrome. Clinical, radiologic, and pathologic manifestations. *Am J Med.* 1985;81:11–18.

69. Lorenz P, Wilson W, Leigh B, Schecter WP. Kaposi's sarcoma of the rectum in patients with the acquired immunodeficiency syndrome. *Am J Surg.* 1990;160:681–683.

70. Zwigler JL. Non-Hodgkin's lymphoma in 90 homosexual men: relationship to generalized lymphadenopathy and acquired immunodeficiency syndrome. *N Engl J Med.* 1984:311:565–571.

71. Lowenthal DA, Safai B, Koziner B. Malignant neoplasia in AIDS. *Infect Surg.* July 1987:413–420.

72. Coonley CJ, Strauss DJ, Filippa D. Hodgkin's disease presenting with rectal symptoms. *Cancer Invest.* 1984:2:279–284.

73. Joachim HL, Cooper ML, Hellman GC. Lymphoma in men at high risk for acquired immune deficiency syndrome. *Cancer.* 1985:56:2831–2842.

74. Kaplan LD. AIDS-associated lymphomas. *Infect Dis Clin North Am.* 1988:2:525–532.

75. Morrison JG, Scharfenberg JC, Timmcke AE. Perianal lymphoma as a manifestation of the acquired immunodeficiency syndrome. Report of a case. *Dis Colon Rectum.* 1989;32:521–523.

76. Kaplan LD, Abrams DI, Feigal E, et al. AIDS-associated non-Hodgkin's lymphoma in San Francisco. *JAMA.* 1989;261:719–724.

77. Burkes R, Meyer PR, Parkash SG, et al. Rectal lymphoma in homosexual men. *Arch Intern Med.* 1986:146:913–915.

78. Levin AM. Reactive and neoplastic lymphoproliferative disorders and other miscellaneous cancers associated with HIV infection. In: DeVita VT, Hellman S, Rosenberg SA, eds. *AIDS: Etiology, Diagnosis, Treatment, and Prevention.* 2nd ed. Philadelphia: JB Lippincott; 1988:263–275.

79. Lee SH, McGregor DH, Kuziez MN. Malignant transformation of perianal condyloma acuminatum. A case report with review of the literature. *Dis Colon Rectum.* 1981:24:462–467.

80. Gal AA, Meyer PR, Taylor CR. Papillomavirus antigens in anorectal condyloma and carcinoma in homosexual men. *JAMA.* 1987:257:337–340.

81. Nash G, Allen W, Nash S. Atypical lesions of the anal mucosa in homosexual men. *JAMA.* 1986:256:873–876.

82. Croxson T, Chabon AB, Rorat E, et al. Intraepithelial carcinoma of the anus in homosexual men. *Dis Colon Rectum.* 1984;27:325–330.

83. Cooper HS, Patchefsky AS, Marks G. Cloacogenic carcinoma of the anorectum in homosexual men. An observation of four cases. *Dis Colon Rectum.* 1979:22:557–558.

84. Daling JR, Weiss NS, Klopfenstein LL, et al. Correlates of homosexual behavior and the incidence of anal cancer. *JAMA.* 1982:247:1988–1990.

85. Wexner SD, Milsom JW, Daily TH. The demographics of anal cancers are changing: identification of a high risk populaton. *Dis Colon Rectum.* 1987:30:942–946.

86. Creasman C, Haas PA, Fox TA, Balazs M. Malignant transformation of anorectal giant condyloma (Buschke-Lowenstein tumor). *Dis Colon Rectum.* 1989:532:481–487.

87. Austin DF. Etiological clues from descriptive epidemiology squamous carcinoma of the rectum or anus. In: Henderson BF, ed. *Third Symposium on Epidemiology and Cancer Registries in the Pacific Basin.* Bethesda, MD: National Cancer Institute; 1982:89–90. Monograph 62.

88. Peters RK, Mack TM. Patterns of anal carcinoma by gender and marital status in Los Angeles County. *Br J Cancer.* 1983;48:629–636.

89. Peters RK, Mack TM, Berstein L. Parallels in the epidemiology of selected anogenital carcinomas. *J Clin Natl Cancer Inst.* 1984:72:609–615.

90. Syrjanen KJ. Human papilloma virus (HPV) infections of the female genital tract and their associations with intraepithelial neoplasia and squamous cell carcinoma. In: Sommers SC, Rosen PP, Fechner RE, eds. *Pathology Annual.* Norwalk, CN: Appleton Century Crofts; 1986:53–89.

91. Bescia RJ, Jenson B, Lancaster WD, et al. The role of human papilloma virus in the pathogenesis and histologic classification of precancerous lesions of the cervix. *Hum Pathol.* 1986:17:555–559.

92. Scholefield JM, Sonnex C, Talbot I, et al. Anal and cervical intraepithelial neoplasia: possible parallel. *Lancet.* 1989;1:765–769.

93. Palmer JG, Scholefield JM, Coates PJ, et al. Anal cancer and human papillomaviruses. *Dis Colon Rectum.* 1989:2:1016–1022.

94. Scholfield JH, Northover JMA, Carr ND. Male homosexuality HIV infection and colorectal surgery. *Br J Surg.* 1990;77:493–496.

95. Carr ND, Mercey D, Slack WW. Non-condylomatous perianal disease in homosexual men. *Br J Surg.* 1989;76:1064–1066.

96. Safavi A, Gottesman C, Dailey T. Anorectal surgery in the HIV (+) patients. Presented at annual meeting of the American Society of Colon and Rectal Surgeons; April 29–May 4, 1990; St. Louis, MO.

97. Moenning S, Simonton C, Huber P, Nightengale S, Odom C, Kaplan E. Presentation and treatment of anorectal disorders in the HIV +/AIDS patient. Presented at the annual meeting of the American Society of Colon and Rectal Surgeons. April 29–May 4, 1990; St. Louis, MO.

98. Buchmann P, Christen D, Rudlinger R. HIV positivity and its importance on proctologic treatment. Presented at the Tripartite Meeting of the American Society of Colon and Rectal Surgeons, the section of Coloproctology of the Royal Society of Medicine of England and the Section of Colon and Rectal Surgery of the Royal Australian College of Surgeons; June 19–24, 1989; Birmingham, England.

99. Beck DE, Jaso RG, Zajac RA. Surgical management of anal condylomata in the HIV-positive patient. *Dis Colon Rectum.* 1990:33:12–15.

100. Jaso RG, Zajac RA, Beck DE. Human immunodeficiency virus progression associated with anorectal disease. (Personal communication, January 1992.)

101. Buchmann P, Seefeld V. Rubber band ligation of a pile can be disasterous in HIV positive patient. *Int J Colorectal Dis.* 1989;4:57–58.

102. Schmitt SL, Wexner SD, Reiter W, et al. Is aggressive management of perianal ulcers in HIV-positive patients justifiable? Presented at the annual meeting of The American Society of Colon and Rectal Surgeons; June 7-12, 1992; San Francisco, CA.

CHAPTER 23

ANORECTAL TRAUMA AND NECROTIZING INFECTIONS

Jorge E. Marcet and
Lester Gottesman

Anorectal trauma, although infrequent in its occurrence, continues to challenge surgeons. The principles of its management evolved from military experience and have been successfully applied to civilian rectal trauma. Early recognition with prompt and appropriate surgical treatment can decrease the high morbidity and mortality associated with these injuries.

Etiology

Trauma to the rectum and anus may occur from a variety of causes (Table 23-1). The rectum is afforded a fair degree of protection from injury by its anatomic location within the bony pelvis. Consequently, in the multiple-trauma patient, the rectum is injured less frequently than other organs are. Conversely, if the trauma is severe enough to injure the rectum, the injury will commonly involve other organs.

Gunshot wounds to the lower abdomen or pelvis are the most common cause of penetrating trauma to the rectum.[1] A missile may cause injury by direct penetration of the rectal wall, by blast effect, or by penetration from fragmented bone.[2] Stab wounds to the lower abdomen or buttocks caused by long sharp objects may also penetrate the rectum.

Blunt trauma, such as that seen in a motor vehicle accident, rarely causes rectal injury. Rectal prolapse[3] and rectosigmoid tears with transanal evisceration[4] have been attributed to blunt trauma; however, most significant rectal injuries are associated with pelvic fractures, which may result in perforation or laceration by fractured bone edges.[5]

Rectal impalement is an even more unusual form of rectal injury. The typical mechanism of injury is a jump or a fall onto an impaling object, such as a fence or rake.

Table 23-1   Etiology of Anorectal Trauma

BLUNT
Motor vehicle accident
Fall
Other

PENETRATING
Transabdominal
  Projectile
    Handgun
    Shotgun
    Shrapnel
    Other missile
  Stab wound
    Knife
    Other impalement
  Iatrogenic
    Pelvic surgery
    Laparoscopy
Transanal
  Iatrogenic
    Diagnostic
      Thermometer
      Barium enema
      Endoscopy
        Colonoscopy
        Sigmoidoscopy
        Proctoscopy

Table 23-1   (*Continued*)

PENETRATING
Transanal
    Therapeutic
        Cleansing enema
        Endoscopy
            Colonoscopy
            Sigmoidoscopy
            Proctoscopy
    Sexually induced
        Anal-receptive intercourse
            Penile insertive
            Digital insertive
            Brachioreceptive ("Fist-fornication")
            Foreign body
    Other
        Impalement
        Chemical
        Pneumatic
Transperineal
    Projectiles
        Handgun
        Shotgun
        Shrapnel
        Other missile
    Stab wound
        Knife
        Other impalement
    Other
        Radiation necrosis
        Other

This type of injury may range from simple rectal perforation with minimal soft tissue injury to severe rectal impalement, characterized by transfixation by the impaling object with resultant extensive perineal trauma and multiple-organ damage.[6]

The distal rectum angulates posteriorly in relation to the anal canal. Forceful introduction of a rigid object may therefore perforate the distal rectum anteriorly. Iatrogenic injuries may occur during endoscopy, barium enema examinations, gynecologic or urologic procedures, and pelvic surgery. The injuries differ from other types of rectal trauma in that the injury is usually immediately recognized. In contrast, perforation from rectal thermometers or enema nozzles may go unnoticed until the patient becomes septic. Injuries range from minimal mucosal lacerations to full-thickness rectal perforations.

Sigmoidoscopic perforations most commonly result from using excessive force just proximal to or at the rectosigmoid junction.[7] Nelson and associates[8] reported

an incidence of perforation from rigid proctosigmoidoscopy of 0.018 percent. Endoscopic polypectomy or biopsy carries a slightly higher risk of perforation.

Injuries related to barium enema examinations have been attributed to (1) trauma from the enema tip, (2) overinflation of the balloon, (3) recent colonic instrumentation, especially if a biopsy was performed, and (4) the presence of rectal mucosal disease.[9] Retrospective reviews have found the incidence of injuries due to barium enema to be from 0.16 to 0.23 percent,[8,10] with lesions ranging from minor submucosal dissections with minimal deposition of barium, to perforation of the rectum with intra- or extraperitoneal barium extravasation. Retroperitoneal emphysema may result from rectal injury during an air contrast examination.[9,10]

The rectum is susceptible to injury during operations on adjacent structures, including the vagina, uterus, prostate, male urethra, and bladder. Predisposing conditions, such as previous surgery, infection, or irradiation, may increase the chance of inadvertent rectal injury. The reported incidence of rectal injury during radical prostatectomy ranges from 0.5 to 3.0 pecent.[11] Kozminski and associates[12] noted a 7 percent incidence of rectal injury associated with radical cystectomy when performed on patients who had not been irradiated. The rate of injury was four times greater in patients who underwent salvage cystectomy after definitive pelvic irradiation.

One of the most common causes of anorectal injury is tearing of the perineum during childbirth. Third degree lacerations involve the external anal spincter, and fourth degree lacerations extend through the rectal mucosa. The reported incidence is as high as 24 percent.[13] A midline episiotomy increases the risk of anorectal injury when compared with a mediolateral episiotomy or no episiotomy.[14]

Retained rectal foreign bodies and anorectal injuries secondary to homosexual activities, sexual asaults, and anal autoeroticism have become commonplace in contemporary society.[15] Forceful anal penetrations can cause fissures, contusions, thrombosed hemorrhoids, lacerations, and sphincter disruption.[16] Severe injuries, including rectosigmoid perforations, deep rectal lacerations, sphincter disruption, and pelvic cellulitis have resulted from the practice of fist fornication.[17,18] An impressive variety of rectal foreign bodies have been documented,[19] the majority of which are self-inserted and rarely cause significant injury.

Anal assaults account for a large proportion of cases of child sexual abuse.[20,21] Black and associates[22] found the majority of cases in their series of pediatric anorectal trauma to be due to child abuse. Out of 200 cases of alleged anal assaults occurring over a 2-year period, only 11 patients required treatment. Injuries varied from simple anal lacerations and perineal contusions to more destructive lesions: anorectal tear, rectovaginal tear, anal sphincter disruption, and rectal perforation.

Miscellaneous causes of anorectal injuries that have been reported include chemical burns,[19,23] pneumatic injuries,[24] and radiation necrosis.[25]

Diagnosis

In severe perineal trauma the diagnosis of anorectal injury may be obvious; however, internal injuries may be easily missed if careful systematic examination is not performed. The diagnostic approach is influenced by the type of injury and the condition of the patient. It is not the purpose of this chapter to discuss the management of the patient with multiple trauma, but rather to focus specifically on the evaluation and management of anorectal injuries.

The perineum is examined for any obvious signs of trauma. Digital rectal examination is necessary to assess sphincter tone, the prostatic bed in men, and the presence of blood in the rectum. Blood on the examining glove is highly specific for a colon or rectal injury and should not be confused with blood from a coexisting perianal injury. The absence of blood, however, does not exclude rectal injury, as blood has been found in digital rectal examination in only 70 to 80 pecent of patients with rectal gunshot wounds.[26,27]

Hemodynamically stable patients should undergo rigid sigmoidoscopy. The presence of blood and the location and extent of any injury are noted. Rectal contents should be evacuated through the sigmoidoscope as necessary. Positive findings, such as the presence of blood or rectal disruption, have been reported in 90 percent of rectal gunshot wounds.[26,27] Digital rectal examination and sigmoidoscopy have a combined sensitivity of 95 to 100 percent in establishing the presence of rectal injury.[27,28]

Other diagnostic tests may be required to assess other organs at risk for injury. Roentgenograms of the abdomen in the flat, upright, and decubitus positions may reveal free intraperitoneal air resulting from hollow viscus injury. Extraperitoneal rectal peforation may manifest as retroperitoneal air, which may appear as a few bubbles of pararectal air or progress to extensive retroperitoneal emphysema.[9]

Diagnostic peritoneal lavage is a sensitive test to determine the presence of intraperitoneal injuries; however, extraperitoneal injuries may be missed.

The use of barium enema for contrast studies to evaluate rectal injury is contraindicated because spillage into the peritoneal cavity may lead to severe peritonitis with associated high mortality. However, a contrast study with an iodinated water-soluble contrast agent can be safely done, and will demonstrate a full-thickness rectal perforation. The compound is quickly absorbed from the peritoneal cavity in case of spillage, and is excreted in the urine.[29]

Other studies that may be useful in patients with rectal and associated injuries include computed tomography (CT) with rectal contrast, cystourethrography, intravenous pyelography, and arteriography.[28,30,31] These studies should be performed as clincially indicated.

Treatment

The modern treatment of rectal injuries has evolved from military experience. The principles of management of rectal trauma in World War I included careful wound debridement; colostomy was reserved for extensive injuries.[2] The mortality associated with penetrating rectal injury was 45 percent. Death was due to rapidly advancing retroperitoneal sepsis. With improvements in surgical care, availability of blood transfusions, and the development of more effective antibiotic agents, the mortality decreased during World War II. In 1943, the Department of the Army directed that colostomy and retrorectal drainage were to be used in the management of rectal injuries.[32] Mortality was reduced to 23 percent. Improvements in transport time, management of shock, and antibiotic therapy lowered the comparable mortality during the Vietnam conflict to 14 percent.[33] Distal rectal washout was suggested as another component in the operative management of rectal injuries from the Vietnam War experience.

Based on this extensive military experience the current principles of management of rectal trauma include (1) closure of the rectal injury when possible, (2) diverting sigmoid colostomy, (3) cleansing of feces from the rectal stump, (4) presacral transperineal drainage, and (5) broad spectrum antibiotics.

The mortality of civilian rectal trauma in various series in the 1980s ranged from 0 to 10 percent (Table 23-2).[26-27,34-38] Civilian injuries differ from military injuries in several important aspects. Military rectal injuries (Table 23-3)[39-54] are frequently caused by high-velocity missiles and are associated with multiple organ injury. Depending on the conflict, the time from injury to definitive treatment is often relatively lengthy. Civilian injuries are usually caused by low-velocity gunshot wounds or stab wounds and the patient is rapidly transported to a specialized trauma hospital. The wider variety of etiologies associated with civilian rectal trauma precludes the universal application of standard techniques.[26]

Management of the Rectal Injury

The management of a rectal injury begins with determining the location and extent of the injury. This is depicted in algorithmic approach in Figure 23-1. Extraperitoneal injuries may not be obvious at laparotomy and may be easily overlooked. Digital rectal examination is mandatory. Rigid sigmoidoscopy should be included when possible, either in the emergency room or under anesthesia, with the patient in the modified lithotomy position. Rectal contents are evacuated through the sigmoidoscope with suction and water irrigation. All patients who are about to undergo an operation for trauma should receive preoperative broad spectrum antibiotics and tetanus prophylaxis as indicated.

At operation, the first priority is to control bleeding. Following this, temporary control of intestinal spillage can be quickly achieved with sutures or intestinal clamps. A detailed exploration of the abdominal cavity is then performed. The trajectory of the penetrating object should be determined in order to uncover unsuspected injury.[55]

Intraperitoneal rectal perforations are debrided and closed with one or two layers of interrupted, inverting sutures. There are no specific guidelines regarding wound size when contemplating primary closure versus debridement. The extent and duration of intestinal spillage, number of associated injuries, condition of the bowel wall, condition of the patient, and experience of the surgeon are important considerations. Larger wounds may not be satisfactorily closed with suture and are best managed by resection of the injured bowel, end sigmoid colostomy, and formation of a rectal pouch (Hartmann procedure).

Repair of isolated extraperitoneal rectal injuries is not necessary unless uncovered during the exposure of other structures, or if there is communication with the peritoneal cavity. Repair was recommended by Vietnam-era military surgeons.[2,33] Most civilian series recommend repair of the extraperitoneal injury when possible.[34,35,37] Others have found that many extraperitoneal injuries were not amenable to closure.[26,27] Tuggle and Huber[36] repaired only 19 of 47 rectal injuries. They found that failure to repair the rectum did not increase the morbidity or length of hospitalization. Burch and

Table 23-2 Morbidity and Mortality of Civilian Rectal Injuries*

| Author/Year | No. patients | Management, %† | | Complications, %‡ | Morbidity, % |
		Washout	Drain		
Vitale et al[34] 1983	32	10	100	16	3
Grasberger and Hirsch[35] 1983	20	100	100	40§	10
Tuggle and Huber[36] 1984	47	0	100	36	0
Mangiante et al[27] 1986	43	93	50	37 (100% with no washout)	0
Shannon et al[37] 1988	26	50	100	60 (90% with no washout)	4
Burch et al[38] 1989	100	50	100	11	4
Thomas et al[26] 1990	52	50	67	10	0

* Mechanisms of injury and methods of reporting varied considerably (see text).
† All series routinely used colostomy, and accessible rectal injuries were repaired.
‡ Complications were predominantly infections, including sepsis, abscesses, fistulae, wound infections, etc.
§ Morbidity figures given for only 8 patients.

Table 23-3   Military (Combat) Rectal Injuries

Conflict Authors	Year	No. patients	Associated injuries, %	Management, % C	W	D	Mortality, %
CIVIL WAR[39]				Observation			>90
WORLD WAR I							
Dunn and Drummond[40]	1917	6	ns	ns	ns	ns	58
American Forces[30]	1917–18	ns	ns	ns	ns	ns	45
Wallace and Cuthbert[41]	1918	21	19	Y	Y	ns	67
Drummond[42]	1919	16	50	44	ns	ns	88
WORLD WAR II							
British 8th Army[40]	1942	ns	ns	ns	ns	ns	52
Olgivie[43]	1944	47	ns	ns	ns	ns	36
Hurt[44]	1945	6	67	10	0	100	0
Imes[45]	1945	36	39	100	0	100	19
Croce et al[46]	1945	10	40	90	0	40	10
Laufman[47]	1946	35	60	97	0	97	9
Porritt[48]	1946	109	64	ns	ns	ns	45
Taylor and Thompson[49]	1948	25	48	96	0	48	20
Chunn and Hauver[50]	1955	116	59	99	ns	92	23
KOREA							
Bowers[51]	1956	ns	ns	ns	ns	ns	18
VIETNAM							
Ganchrow et al[52]	1970	30	87	100	90	90	17
Lavenson and Cohen[33]	1971	29	35	100	38	90	14
Allen[53]	1973	65	66	100	100	100	3
Armstrong et al[54]	1973	32	56	100	25	28	13

C = Colostomy.
W = Rectal washout.
D = Drainage (presacral).
ns = Not specified.
Y = Yes

associates[38] repaired 21 of 100 extraperitoneal rectal perforations, mostly injuries encountered during exposure of associated nonrectal injuries. These authors also found no correlation of closure with outcome. They recommended that a modest effort be made to identify and repair injuries near the peritoneal reflection, and to repair large lacerations not associated with significant loss of the rectal wall.

Very rarely, abdominoperineal resection is necessary to control bleeding in a severely traumatized rectum, or after destruction of the anal sphincter.[33,34,38] Getzen and associates[56] found this approach useful in successfully treating massive rectal injuries caused by explosive weapons. Five soldiers with such injuries were treated with abdominoperineal resection and all five survived; five other soldiers treated with debridement, pararectal drainage, and colostomy all died of exsanguination or sepsis.

An additional method to control pelvic bleeding secondary to rectal trauma is to pack the rectum, transanally, or the pelvis, transabdominally, with epinephrine-soaked gauze rolls or laparotomy pads. In the absence of massive tissue destruction this technique will control bleeding in most patients. The packing is removed 36 to 48 hours later, under general anesthesia.

Colostomy

Diversion of the fecal stream is considered mandatory in the management of most penetrating rectal trauma.[2,26,27,32–38,55] Colostomy is also indicated in patients with extensive soft tissue injury in the perirectal

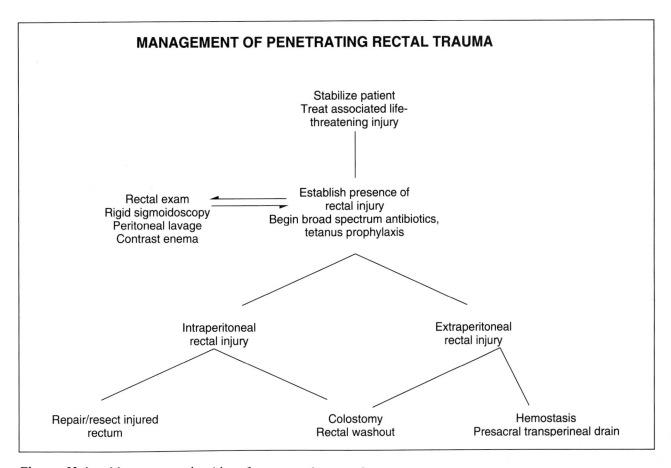

Figure 23-1.   Management algorithm for penetrating rectal trauma.

area such as from severe blunt trauma or a high-energy bullet, even in the absence of a rectal perforation.[5,26,55]

The colostomy may be fashioned as a loop, an end loop, or an end stoma (Fig. 23-2). The loop colostomy is easiest and quickest to perform and is completely diverting when properly constructed. The end-loop colostomy is another option. A loop of bowel is exteriorized and divided with a stapler. The proximal limb is matured into a colostomy, while the antimesenteric border of the distal limb is sutured to the skin. The end colostomy may be preferred because it is smaller and may develop fewer complications. The distal limb may be closed and sutured to the parietal peritoneum adjacent to the stoma, left in the subcutaneous tissue, or left open and exteriorized as a mucous fistula.[57]

Mangiante and coworkers[27] found the complication and mortality rates to be similar between loop colostomy and end colostomy with mucous fistula. The use of loop colostomy was more expedient in this series; it took 30 minutes less time to construct and 15 minutes less to close than did an end colostomy. Others have

shown no difference in complication rates between the two types of colostomies.[26,38]

Occasional reports appear in the literature on the management of rectal perforations without the creation of a colostomy.[11,12,26,58,59] For the most part these represent special selected cases with limited injury, such as iatrogenic perforations in mechanically cleansed bowels. There are no prospective randomized studies of rectal perforation managed with or without fecal diversion. Haas and Fox[59] successfully managed three patients with gunshot wounds limited to the extraperitoneal rectum without operation. Although such an approach goes against current surgical dogma, it illustrates the healing potential of such isolated injuries in carefully selected cases.

Thomas and coauthors[26] suggested the possibility of treating intraperitoneal rectal injuries as colon injuries, with primary repair as the sole treatment provided certain requirements were met: no evidence of shock, no other significant associated injury, minimal blood loss, and minimal fecal contamination. There is little support

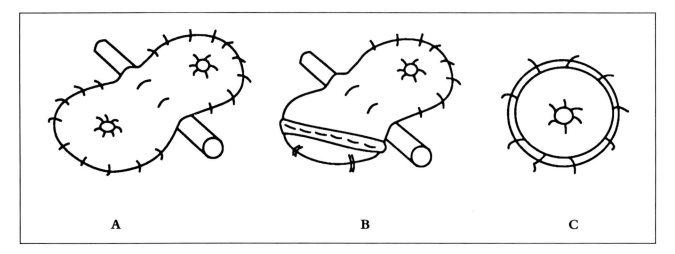

Figure 23-2. Construction of a stoma. (A) Loop colostomy. (B) End-loop colostomy. (C) End colostomy.

in the current literature for primary closure in civilian rectal trauma and, accordingly, neither the authors nor the editors endorse the routine use of this approach.

Iatrogenic injuries deserve a special comment. These are often discovered at the time of injury and are quickly repaired before significant contamination occurs. Furthermore patients may have had a mechanical bowel preparation prior to the procedure. In these selected cases, primary repair without diversion may be safely undertaken.

Morse and colleagues[11] reported nine patients who had sustained rectal injuries during urologic procedures. Two patients with transurethral rectal perforations that were recognized immediately were treated successfully with suprapubic drainage and parenteral antibiotics. Two patients with similar injuries that were initially missed required diverting colostomy. One of these patients had a septic course and eventually died 5 months later. In five other patients who had sustained rectal injuries during an open prostatectomy, the rectal injury was closed, and four of the patients were initially managed without a colostomy. Three of the four developed rectourethral fistulas, but only one subsequently required a colostomy to heal the fistula.

Kavoussi and coworkers[60] reported successfully managing a transurethral rectal perforation with transurethral catheter drainage of the bladder, manual dilatation of the anal sphincter, and parenteral antibiotics. Kozminski and associates[12] treated 9 of 12 patients who sustained rectal perforation during radical cystectomy without a diverting colostomy. Only one patient in the no-colostomy group had a postoperative rectal leak that required diversion. In addition to primary repair of the

rectal injury, this patient also underwent a sigmoid resection.

Distal Rectal Washout

Removal of stool from the traumatized rectum has been shown to reduce septic complications. Lavenson and Cohen[33] reported on 29 casualties with rectal injuries incurred during the Vietnam conflict. There were 13 complications and 4 deaths in the 18 patients who had not undergone rectal washout. In the 10 patients who had rectal washout there were no major complications and no deaths.

Civilian series have also demonstrated a decreased rate of infection with rectal washout. Mangiante and coauthors[27] reported no major intraabdominal infections when distal rectal washout was used. In the group of patients in whom rectal washout was omitted there were three major infections: an intraabdominal abscess, a pelvic abscess, and a rectal intramural abscess. Shannon and colleagues[37] retrospectively reviewed 26 patients with penetrating, extraperitoneal rectal wounds. A higher incidence of major complications was found in the no-washout versus the washout group, including pelvic abscess, 46 percent verses 8 percent; rectal fistulas, 23 percent verses 8 percent; and sepsis 15 percent verses 8 percent. The single death in this series occurred in a patient in the no-washout group who developed a pelvic abscess and succumbed to multisystem organ failure 4 weeks after injury. The benefit of distal rectal washout was greater in rectal injuries due to pelvic fracture or high-energy gunshot wounds.

Not all investigators, however, have shown benefit

from distal rectal washout.[26] Tuggle and Huber[36] performed rectal washout in only 1 of 47 patients with penetrating rectal trauma. Although 36 percent had major morbidity, no deaths were reported. Burch and associates[38] found no evidence of either benefit or harm from rectal washout when performed in 46 of 100 patients with rectal trauma.

Several reasons may account for the disparate results from rectal washout among the different series. In civilian series, most rectal injuries are due to handguns. The wounding potential of these low-velocity missiles is low compared to injuries caused by high-powered rifles. Military rifles fire a small caliber, high-velocity missile which delivers significantly more kinetic energy to its target, and when striking bone, causes a shattering secondary missile effect, resulting in a wide area of adjacent tissue damage.[2] It is also difficult to compare rectal injuries caused by extensive pelvic fractures due to blunt trauma with the numerous other mechanisms which cause rectal injury.

One could theorize that irrigating the rectum would eliminate prolonged contact of feces with the rectal injury and lessen contamination of the perirectal spaces. Irrigation may also reduce septic complications by diminishing the possibility of bacterial translocation from the gut.[37] It is important to note that although not all series demonstrated a benefit from distal rectal washout, no series reported a higher morbidity or mortality in the group of patients in whom it was performed.

Optimally, rectal washout should be done during the preoperative proctosigmoidoscopy. If this is not possible, then the washout is done at the completion of the celiotomy. Another method of washout is through irrigation of the distal colostomy limb (Fig. 23-3). With the patient in the dorsal lithotomy position, an irrigation tube is secured in the distal colostomy limb. A large bag of irrigation fluid is suspended 2 to 3 feet above the patient and the fluid is allowed to run in by gravity as rapidly as possible while the anus is kept open. It is important to keep the anus open during irrigation to avoid generating high intraluminal pressures and possibly driving contaminated fluid into perirectal tissues.[38]

Presacral Drainage

Rectal injuries are particularly susceptible to septic complications. This may be explained by the high proportion of fat in the retrorectal area, its relative avascularity,[32] and the presence of fecal contamination in the midst of traumatized tissue.

Transperineal drainage allows for dependent drainage of the presacral space (Fig. 23-4). The presacral space is dissected from within the abdomen. Several

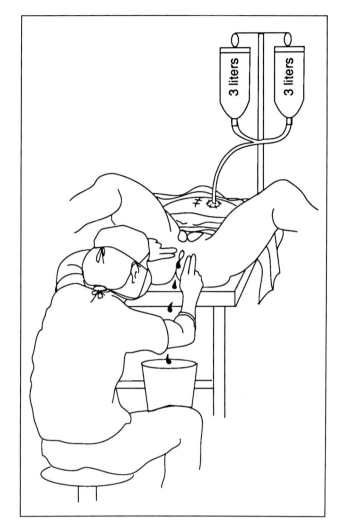

Figure 23-3.   Intraoperative distal rectal washout. Irrigation fluid is introduced through the distal colostomy limb or mucus fistula while manually keeping the anus open.

Penrose drains are left in the presacral space, extending to the level of the coccyx. After the abdomen is closed the patient is placed in lithotomy position and a transverse incision is made between the anus and the tip of the coccyx. The dissection is carried just anterior to the coccyx, through the endopelvic fascia to enter the presacral space. The distal ends of the Penrose drains are brought out through the incision and sutured to the skin. Alternatively the drains may be placed into the presacral space from the perineal incision. The drains are removed after 3 to 5 days or when discharge is minimal.

Although most civilian series continue to advocate the routine use of presacral drains in extraperitoneal rectal injuries,[32-38,55] others could not demonstrate a benefit from routine drainage.[26,27]

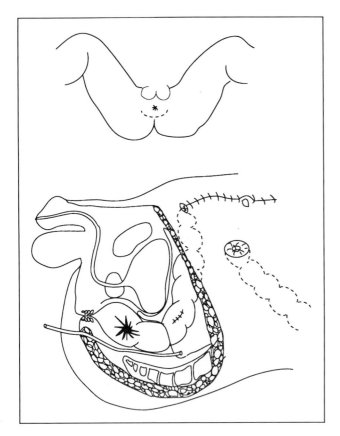

Figure 23-4.   Management principles of anorectal trauma: diverting colostomy, repaired intraperitoneal wound, open extraperitoneal wound, presacral (transperineal) drain. (*Adapted from:* Trunkey D, Hays RJ, Shires GT. Management of rectal trauma. *J Trauma.* 1989;29:1335–1340.)

Anal Injuries

Minor lacerations below the levators may be observed. Local control of bleeding is easily accomplished by cautery or suture. Minor impalements should be treated by cleansing the rectum of feces during sigmoidoscopy and by careful observation. Systemic antibiotic treatment is generally advisable and an elemental diet may be of value.[58]

The anal sphincter should be primarily repaired if the patient is medically stable, and after other associated injuries have been addressed. Delayed repair is preferred when inflammation or infection has occurred. Extensive lacerations with sphincter disruption and perforation into the rectum are managed according to the principles of treating rectal injuries with colostomy, distal rectal washout, presacral drainage, and antibiotics, with the addition of primary sphincter repair.[61] If delayed sphincteroplasty is elected, the ends of the sphincter can

be tagged with heavy nonabsorbable sutures to facilitate subsequent identification.

Meticulous hemostasis and careful anatomic reapproximation of the muscle without tension is essential in repair of sphincter injuries. The several techniques of suture placement[62–64] are addressed in more depth in Chapter 8. Broad spectrum antibiotics should be used prophylactically to prevent infection which could disrupt the repair.

Foreign Bodies

Most rectal foreign bodies do not cause severe injury. Often they can be removed in the emergency department.[65] Endoscopy should be routinely performed to assess the mucosa after removal of the object. The patient must be admitted to the hospital if perforation is suspected or if bleeding ensues. Patients with no abdominal tenderness or with only minor anorectal abrasions may be discharged.

Nehme-Kingsley and Abcarian[15] noted no severe injuries in over 50 patients who had rectal foreign bodies removed using a management protocol. They recommended routine biplanar roentgenograms of the abdomen and pelvis, in addition to digital rectal examination and anoscopy prior to extraction. All foreign bodies were extracted under direct visualization to avoid iatrogenic injury.

If the object cannot be easily removed through a lax anus, removal is done in the operating room with local or regional anesthesia for sphincter relaxation. Long grasping forceps are placed through the operating proctoscope and the object is gently manipulated out. Occasionally, mild downward pressure on the lower abdomen displaces the object distally where it can be secured by forceps. This is facilitated by placing the patient in the lithotomy position.

When the object is beyond the reach of the sigmoidoscope and there are no signs of abdominal distress or bleeding, the patient is admitted for observation.[65] The foreign body will often spontaneously pass to the rectum and become accessible within several hours.

Rigid sigmoidoscopy is done after removal of the object to assess mucosal integrity. If there is doubt whether bowel perforation has occurred, a Gastrografin® enema is obtained; barium should never be used.

If a high-lying foreign body remains impacted for 24 hours or longer, resultant bowel wall edema may prevent transanal extraction, necessitating a laparotomy.[15] Patients with documented or suspected bowel perforation should have a prompt celiotomy. If the foreign body is still present then it is guided to the rectum and extracted transanally. If this maneuver fails, the object can be extracted through a colotomy which is then exteriorized, or closed; a proximal diverting colostomy may be necessary.

Necrotizing Perineal Infections

Necrotizing perineal infections are rare complications of anorectal infections. The most common cause is a perirectal abscess, followed in frequency by genitourinary infections. These severe infections have been reported following anorectal trauma or surgery.[66] Many patients have associated debilitating diseases,[66-68] suggesting that an incompetent immune system may influence the virulence of the infection.

These infections are usually caused by mixed enteric organisms.[66-68] The presence of subcutaneous gas does not necessarily imply infection by clostridia. When the infection is primarily due to *Clostridium perfringens*, a more fulminant course is seen.[68]

Anatomically, the infection spreads through perineal fascial planes. A perirectal abscess may penetrate Colles' fascia of the perineum, with direct communication to the dartos fascia of the scrotum, Buck's fascia of the penis, and Scarpa's fascia of the abdominal wall. A supralevator infection may involve the rectovesical space or presacral space and spread extraperitoneally or retroperitoneally (Fig. 23-5).

Patients may present with nonspecific rectal symptoms, lasting days or weeks, with a sudden deterioration as the infection spreads. Clinical features may include severe systemic toxicity; perineal skin changes, such as edema, erythema, crepitus, bullae, or black spots; and an absence of frank suppuration.[66] The mainstay of therapy is early recognition and aggressive surgical debridement, aiming to remove all necrotic tissue (Fig. 23-6). Incision and drainage alone will not suffice, as the infection is always more extensive than can be appreciated by examination of the skin.

Broad spectrum antibiotics are used,[66,68,69] to include high dose penicillin for gram-positive and clostridial organisms, an aminoglycoside for gram-negative bacteria, and metronidazole or clindamycin for anaerobic organisms. A colostomy is necessary if the infection is due to rectal trauma or when the anal sphincter has been destroyed.[66,70] Some investigators advocate mandatory colostomy in necrotizing infections of anorectal origin[67]; however, others think that this procedure need not be done routinely to keep the perineum clean.[70,71] With proper bowel management, this additional procedure can often be avoided in these gravely ill patients. A suprapubic cystostomy is created when there is urethral disruption but is otherwise unnecessary.[66]

In males, the testes are usually spared, even in the presence of extensive necrosis of the scrotum, owing to their separate blood supply. To prevent desiccation, the testes should be placed in anterior, subcutaneous thigh pockets and retrieved during subsequent reconstruction of the scrotum.

Secondary debridement is usually required. In addition, daily whirlpool or Water-Pik® treatments are helpful in keeping the wounds clean. Hyperbaric oxygen therapy may be of benefit when the infections are primarily due to clostridial organisms, but should not delay or be a substitute for adequate surgical debridement.[66,68]

The mortality of necrotizing perineal infections in recent series ranged from 20 to 67 percent.[66-69,71] Improved survival is achieved by early diagnosis and prompt radical debridement.

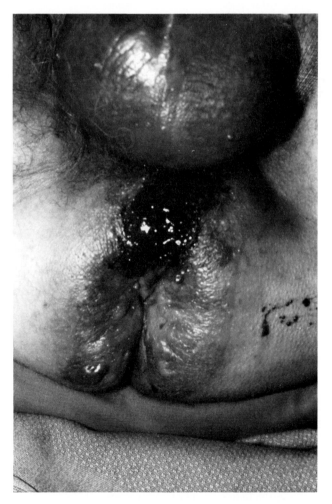

Figure 23-5. Perineal necrosis.

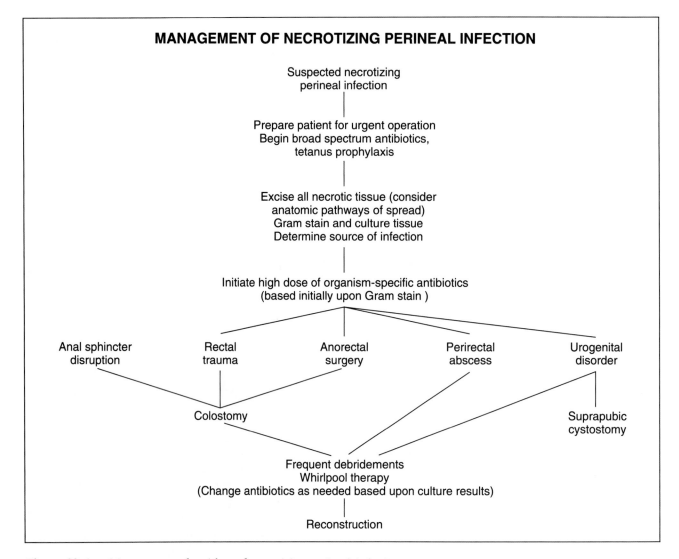

Figure 23-6.   Management algorithm of necrotizing perineal infection.

References

1. Abcarian H. Rectal trauma. *Gastroenterol Clin North Am.* 1987:16:115–123.
2. Lung JA, Turk RP, Miller RE, Eiseman B. Wounds of the rectum. *Ann Surg.* 1970;172: 985–990.
3. Kram HB, Clark SR, Mackabee JR, Melendez R, Shoemaker WC. Rectal prolapse caused by blunt abdominal trauma. *Surgery.* 1989;105:790–792.
4. Wrobleski DE, Dailey TH. Spontaneous rupture of the distal colon with evisceration of small intestine through the anus—report of two cases and review of the literature. *Dis Colon Rectum.* 1979;22: 569–572.
5. Maull KL, Sachatello CR, Ernst CB. The deep perineal laceration—an injury frequently associated with open pelvic fractures: a need for aggressive surgical management. *J Trauma.* 1977; 17:685–695.
6. Bousamra M, Guisto DF, Gervin AS. Rectal impalement. *Surg Rounds.* December 1990:55–59.
7. Goligher J. *Surgery of the Anus, Rectum and Colon,* 5th ed. London: Bailliere Tindall; 1984:1119–1129.
8. Nelson RL, Abcarian H, Prasad ML. Iatrogenic perforation of the colon and rectum. *Dis Colon Rectum.* 1982;25:305–308.
9. Tadros S, Watters JM. Retroperitoneal perforation

of the rectum during barium enema examination. *Can J Surg.* 1988;31:49–50.

10. Fry RD, Shemesh EI, Kodner IJ, Fleshman JW, Timmcke AE. Perforation of the rectum and sigmoid colon during barium enema examination. *Dis Colon Rectum.* 1989;32:759–764.

11. Morse RM, Spirnak JP, Resnick MI. Iatrogenic colon and rectal injuries associated with urological intervention-report of 14 patients. *J Urol.* 1988; 140:101–103.

12. Kozminski M, Konnak JW, Grossman HB. Management of rectal injuries during radical cystectomy. *J Urol.* 1989;142:1204–1205.

13. Thacker SB, Banta HD. Benefits and risks of episiotomy—an interpretative review of the English language literature, 1860–1980. *Obstet Gynecol Serv.* 1983;38:322–338.

14. Green JR, Soohoo SL. Factors associated with rectal injury in spontaneous deliveries. *Obstet Gynecol.* 1989;73:732–738.

15. Nehme-Kingsley A, Abcarian H. Colorectal foreign bodies—management update. *Dis Colon Rectum.* 1985;28:941–944.

16. Bush RA, Owen WF. Trauma and other noninfectious problems in homosexual men. *Med Clin North Am.* 1986;70:549–566.

17. Sohn N, Weinstein MA, Gonchar J. Social injuries of the rectum. *Am J Surg.* 1977;134:611–612.

18. Weinstein MA, Sohn N, Robbins RA. Syndrome of pelvic cellulitis following rectal sexual trauma. *Am J Gastroenterol.* 1981;75:380–381.

19. Busch DB, Starling JR. Rectal foreign bodies—case reports and a comprehensive review of world's literature. *Surgery.* 1986;100:512–520.

20. Hobbs CJ, Wynne JM. Child sexual abuse—an increasing rate of diagnosis. *Lancet.* 1987;2:837–841.

21. Muram D. Anal and perianal abnormalities in prepubertal victims of sexual abuse. *Am J Obstet Gynecol.* 1989;161:278–281.

22. Black CT, Pokorny WJ, McGill CW, Harberg FJ. Ano-rectal trauma in children. *J Pediatr Surg.* 1982; 17:501–504.

23. Foster DE, Barone JA. Rectal hydrofluoric acid exposure. *Clin Pharm.* 1989;8:516–518.

24. Weil PH. Injuries of the retroperitoneal portions of the colon and rectum. *Dis Colon Rectum.* 1983;26: 19–21.

25. Nowacki MP, Towpik E. Reconstruction of the anus, rectovaginal septum, and distal part of the vagina after postirradiation necrosis. *Dis Colon Rectum.* 1988;31:632–634.

26. Thomas DD, Levison MA, Dykstra BJ, Bender JS. Management of rectal injuries—dogma versus practice. *Am Surg.* 1990;56:507–510.

27. Mangiante EC, Graham AD, Fabian TC. Rectal gunshot wounds—management of civilian injuries. *Am Surg.* 1986;52:37–40.

28. Fallon WF, Reyna TM, Brunner RG, Crooms C, Alexander RH. Penetrating trauma to the buttock. *South Med J.* 1988;81:1236–1238.

29. Ott DJ, Gelfand DW. Gastrointestinal contrast agents—indications, uses, and risks. *JAMA.* 1983;249:2380–2384.

30. Duncan AO, Phillips TF, Scalea TM, Maltz SB, Atweh NA, Sclafani SJA. Management of transpelvic gunshot wounds. *J Trauma.* 1989;29: 1335–1340.

31. Theodorakis SP, Baffes TG. Penetrating wounds of the pelvis. *South Med J.* 1985;78:782–783.

32. Trunkey D, Hays RJ, Shires GT. Management of rectal trauma. *J Trauma.* 1973;13:411–415.

33. Lavenson GS, Cohen A. Management of rectal injuries. *Am J Surg.* 1971;122:226–229.

34. Vitale GC, Richardson JD, Flint LM. Successful management of injuries to the extraperitoneal rectum. *Am Surg.* 1983;49:159–162.

35. Grasberger RC, Hirsch EF. Rectal trauma—a retrospective analysis and guidelines for therapy. *Am J Surg.* 1983;145:795–799.

36. Tuggle D, Huber PJ. Management of rectal trauma. *Am J Surg.* 1984;148:806–808.

37. Shannon FL, Moore EE, Moore FA, McCroskey BL. Value of distal colon washout in civilian rectal trauma—reducing gut bacterial translocation. *J Trauma.* 1988;28:989–993.

38. Burch JM, Feliciano DV, Mattox KL. Colostomy and drainage for civilian rectal injuries: is that all? *Ann Surg.* 1989;209:600–611.

39. Welch CE. War wounds of the abdomen. *N Engl J Med.* 1947;237:156–194.

40. Dunn JS, Drummond H. Ulceration of the colon in the neighborhood of gunshot wounds. *Br J Surg.* 1917;5:59.

41. Wallace, Cuthbert. *War Surgery of the Abdomen.* London: J.A. Churchill, Pub; 1918.

42. Drummond H. Gunshot wounds of the large intestine and rectum with special reference to surgical treatment. *Proc R Soc M Lond.* 1919:24–34.

43. Ogilvie WH. Abdominal wounds in the Western Desert. *Surg Gynecol Obstet.* 1944;78:225–239.

44. Hurt LE. The surgical management of colon and rectal injuries in the forward areas. *Ann Surg.* 1945;122:398–407.

45. Imes PR. War surgery of the abdomen. *Surg Gynecol Obstet.* 1945;81:608–616.

46. Croce EJ, Johnson VS. The management of war injuries of the extraperitoneal rectum. *Ann Surg.* 1945;122:408–431.

47. Laufman H. The initial surgical treatment of penetrating wounds of the rectum. *Surg Gynecol Obstet.* 1946;82:219–228.

48. Porritt AE. Surgery of the abdominal wounds in 21 Army group (Jun 1944–May 1945). *Br J Surg.* 1946; 33:267–274.

49. Taylor ER, Thompson JE. The early treatment, and results thereof, of injuries of the colon and rectum. *Intl Abstracts Surg.* 1948;87:209–228.

50. Chunn CF, Hauver RV. Wounds of the colon and rectum (1,222 casualities). In: *General Surgery,* vol 2: *Surgery in World War II.* Washington, DC: Office of the Surgeon General, Dep of the Army;1953: 255–274.

51. Bowers WF. Surgical treatment in abdominal trauma: a comparison of results in war and peace. *Military Med.* 1956;1183:9–22.

52. Ganchrow MI, Lavenson GS Jr, McNamara JJ. Surgical management of traumatic injuries of the colon and rectum. *Arch Surg.* 1970;100:515–520.

53. Allen BD. Penetrating wounds of the rectum: a review of 65 cases. *Tex Med.* 1973;69:77–81.

54. Armstrong RG, Schmitt HJ Jr, Patterson LT. Combat wounds of the extraperitoneal rectum. *Surgery.* 1973;74:570–574.

55. Abcarian H, Barrett JA. Complications of surgery for trauma to colon and rectum. In: Ferrari BT, Ray JE, Gathright JB, eds. *Complications of Colon and Rectal Surgery—Prevention and Management.* Philadelphia: WB Saunders; 1985:143–155.

56. Getzen LC, Pollak EW, Wolfman EF. Abdominoperineal resection in the treatment of devascularizing rectal injuries. *Surgery.* 1977; 82:310–313.

57. Corman ML. *Colon and Rectal Surgery.* 2nd ed. Philadelphia: JB Lippincott; 1989:909–912.

58. Robertson HD, Ray JE, Ferrari BT, Gathright JB. Management of rectal trauma. *Surg Gynecol Obstet.* 1982;154:161–164.

59. Haas PA, Fox TA. Civilian injuries of the rectum and anus. *Dis Colon Rectum.* 1979;22:17–22.

60. Kavoussi L, Mikkelson D, Clayman R. Rectal perforation as a complication of urethral instrumentation. *J Urol.* 1989;142:1333–1334. Letter to the Editor.

61. Critchlow JF, Houlihan MJ, Landolt CC, Weinstein ME. Primary sphincter repair in anorectal trauma. *Dis Colon Rectum.* 1985;28:945–947.

62. Tancer ML, Lasser D, Rosenblum N. Rectovaginal fistula or perineal and anal sphincter disruption, or both, after vaginal delivery. *Surg Gynecol Obstet.* 1990;171:43–46.

63. Hambrick E. Sphincteroplasty/perineoplasty for traumatic anal sphincter injuries. In: Schrock TR, ed. *Perspectives in Colon and Rectal Surgery.* St Louis; MO: Quality Medical Publishing; 1989;vol 2:91–98.

64. Wexner SD, Marchetti F, Jagelman DG. The role of sphincterplasty for fecal incontinence reevaluated: a prospective physiological and functional review. *Dis Colon Rectum.* 1991;34:22–30.

65. Barone JE, Yee J, Nealon TF. Management of foreign bodies and trauma to the rectum. *Surg Gynecol Obstet.* 1983;156:453–457.

66. Enriquez JM, Moreno S, Devesa M, et al. Fournier's syndrome of urogenital and anorectal origin: a retrospective, comparative study. *Dis Colon Rectum.* 1987;30:33–37.

67. Barkel DC, Villalba MR. A reappraisal of surgical management in necrotizing perineal infections. *Am Surg.* 1986;52:395–397.

68. Bubrik MP, Hitchcock CR. Necrotizing anorectal and perineal infections. *Surgery.* 1979;86:655–662.

69. Huber P, Kissack AS, Simonton CT. Necrotizing soft tissue infection from rectal abscess. *Dis Colon Rectum.* 1983;26:507–511.

70. Abcarian H, Eftaiha M. Floating free-standing anus: a complication of massive anorectal infection. *Dis Colon Rectum.* 1983;26:516–521.

71. DiFalco G, Guccione C, D'Annibale A, et al. Fournier's gangrene following a perianal abscess. *Dis Colon Rectum.* 1986;29:582–585.

CHAPTER 24

ULCERATIVE PROCTITIS AND CROHN'S DISEASE: MEDICAL MANAGEMENT

Neil W. Randall

Ulcerative Proctitis

Proctitis is defined as inflammation of the mucous membrane of the rectum. It is frequently a vexing problem, as it may cause many troubling symptoms and require much medical attention. This is despite its normally benign course; relatively few individuals progress to surgery or develop carcinoma or other intestinal complications.[1,2] Patients suffering from proctitis frequently turn from one physician to another, looking for a cure for their disturbing symptoms. Many therapies have been tried to control these symptoms, and this chapter discusses these treatments.

Etiology

Some authors[3,4] view ulcerative proctitis as a milder form of ulcerative colitis because some individuals with ulcerative proctitis go on to develop more proximal spread of inflammation in the colon. Thus, a certain percentage will develop spread to the sigmoid colon (proctosigmoiditis), to the descending colon (left-sided colitis), proximal to the splenic flexure (ulcerative colitis), or through the entire colon (pancolitis). One article looked at a pediatric group to see how many developed proximal extension.[5] This retrospective chart review described 85 patients with proctosigmoiditis diagnosed before the age of 21. The mean age at the onset of bowel disease was 16, and the mean follow-up was 14.6 years. Although 42 percent of patients developed no extension of inflammation, 20 percent developed extension to the descending colon, 12 percent to the transverse colon, and 26 percent to the entire colon. In addition, 23 percent of the group underwent surgery, while only one patient developed carcinoma.

This study is somewhat weakened by the loss from follow-up of 22 percent of the patients. However, it does suggest that the rate of substantial extension is higher in patients diagnosed before the age of 21 than in older patients. It is unclear whether these data can be extrapolated to adults to say that individuals diagnosed with proctosigmoiditis at an earlier age are at higher risk of extension than individuals diagnosed at a later age.

The etiology of inflammatory bowel disease is not certain, but many suspect that ulcerative colitis and Crohn's disease are autoimmune diseases.[6] Autoantibodies to colonic epithelial cells have been described in ulcerative colitis, while additional autoantibodies against antigens expressed by enteric epithelial cells and leukocytes have been noted. Non-GI autoimmune diseases coexist more commonly than expected in patients with ulcerative colitis, but not in patients with Crohn's disease. There is no particular association between HLA phenotype and either ulcerative colitis or Crohn's disease. In both diseases, lymphocytic infiltrates are seen in the involved mucosa, and induced epithelial HLA class II antigens are expressed. Additionally, both diseases respond to corticosteroids. It is concluded that " autoimmune mechanisms are more likely to be involved in the pathogenesis of ulcerative colitis than of Crohn's disease."[6] The trigger for these diseases, if they are autoimmune disorders, remains obscure.

There has been some speculation that proctitis might be a paraneoplastic phenomenon. This is based upon one Swedish study in which 1165 patients with proctitis were reviewed.[7] The authors found a relative risk of breast and gastric carcinomas and of prostatic and other urogenital tract carcinomas of 1.3 as compared to the expected risk. An increased number of colorectal carcinomas was also seen, with a relative risk of 1.7.

Another theory is that proctitis can be an allergic disorder.[8] Investigators have examined colorectal mucosa in patients with proctocolitis; findings have included increased eosinophils, high histamine concentration, increased immunoglobulin E–containing cells,[9] and increased mast cells, some of which have degranulated. Elevated levels of circulating eosinophils have also been described. The putative allergic agent has not been described.

Symptoms

The cardinal symptom of proctitis is bright red rectal bleeding. Other common symptoms include diarrhea, mucoid discharge, abdominal pain, and tenesmus. Constipation and anorexia are less often seen. Extraintestinal manifestations of inflammatory bowel disease, including joint symptoms, skin lesions, nephrolithiasis, cholelithiasis, liver disease, and uveitis, have been described in proctitis, but they occur less commonly than with other forms of inflammatory bowel disease.

Epidemiology

Several studies have noted an increasing incidence of proctitis. One of these, a Swedish study, described 1065 patients with proctitis.[10] The male:female ratio was 1.4:1, similar to the slight male predominance found in most studies of ulcerative colitis. Urban incidence rates consistently exceeded rural rates. Peak age-specific incidence for both sexes was between 20 and 30 years old. A Scottish study of 537 patients with proctocolitis also confirmed both a striking rise in incidence and an urban predominance.[11]

Diagnosis

Older studies depended upon rigid sigmoidoscopy and barium enema for diagnosis. These two studies are complementary, since the barium enema provides an inadequate view of the rectum and sigmoid colon, while rigid sigmoidoscopy assesses only the rectum and sigmoid colon. Since the advent of fiberoptic endoscopy, diagnosis of the extent of proximal spread has been more accurate.[12] Barium enema can underestimate the extent of proximal inflammation. Typically, areas of the colon that appear radiographically normal are frequently endoscopically or histologically inflamed.[13] Therefore, flexible sigmoidoscopy has become the accepted standard for diagnosis of proctitis.

Histologic findings in proctitis are frequently non-specific. One study described the histologic features that are seen more frequently in ulcerative proctitis than in infectious colitis.[14] These features include distorted crypt architecture, villous surface abnormalities, surface erosions, crypt atrophy, increased number of round cells and neutrophils in the lamina propria, lymphoid aggregates, and neutrophils in the surface epithelium. Crypt abscesses have been demonstrated in Crohn's disease as well as in ulcerative colitis, so that alone they do not differentiate between the two types of inflammatory bowel disease. Rectal granulomata favor Crohn's disease, but they are rarely seen.

A French study described a histologic variant of ulcerative proctitis which the authors named lymphoid follicular proctitis.[15] Rectal biopsies showed well-defined, large lymphoid follicles with reactive germinal centers and preserved mantle zones, frequently with coalescence. Some crypts adjacent to the hyperplastic lymphoid follicles were displaced and appeared distorted. As compared with biopsies from ulcerative proctitis, neutrophils and eosinophils were scanty or absent in the lamina propria, whereas an increase in lymphocytes and plasma cells was seen in both types of lesions. Endoscopically, the mucosa appeared congested and granular, and no ulcers were seen. Clinically, the patients appeared to have less frequent bleeding. However, these patients did not appear to improve as readily on local corticosteroid therapy, although this was not tested in a prospective way.

Prognosis

The clinical course of proctitis is quite variable, since the extent of proximal spread over time greatly influences the course. One study followed patients with proctosigmoiditis from the time of their first attack of symptoms.[15a] Of the 99 patients who were initially included in this study, 60 had been followed for at least 5 years. Only 23 percent of patients in this study remained symptom-free after treatment of their first attack, while 17 percent of patients required some type of surgery. Patients who were younger and those who took longer to improve after their first attack had a less favorable prognosis. No presenting symptom nor histologic finding could predict the future course.

Treatment

Available therapeutic agents for proctitis are listed in Table 24-1.

Corticosteroids

Many years ago, corticosteroids were shown to be effective in the treatment of proctitis,[16] and they have

Table 24-1 Treatment Choices for Ulcerative Proctitis

CORTICOSTEROIDS
Hydrocortisone enema
Hydrocortisone foam
Prednisone, oral
Beclomethasone enema (not available in U.S.)
Budesonide enema (not available in U.S.)
Tixocortol enema (not available in U.S.)

ASA DERIVATIVES
Sulfasalazine, oral or enema (enema not available in U.S.)
5-ASA, oral
5-ASA enema
5-ASA suppository
4-ASA enema (not available in U.S.)

OTHER
Sucralfate enema (not available in U.S.)
Cromolyn, oral or enema (enema not available in U.S.)
6-mercaptopurine, oral
Short chain fatty acids enema (not available in U.S.)
Lidocaine gel
Bismuth (De-Nol) enema (not available in U.S.)
Cyclosporin enema (not available in U.S.)

been a mainstay of treatment ever since. These are preferentially given as enemas to minimize the occurrence of steroid side effects. In the United States, the most commonly used preparation contains 100 mg of hydrocortisone in a 60-ml aqueous solution (Cortenema®). In Europe, a commonly used enema contains 20 mg of prednisolone-21-phosphate (Predsol®), while another contains 5 mg of betamethasone phosphate (Betnesol®). Only rarely are oral corticosteroids used for treatment of proctitis, and then they are usually used for very short periods. This is because the long-term use of orally administered corticosteroids is associated with a high frequency of significant side effects. The relative benignity of proctitis usually precludes usage of such toxic therapy. Also, oral corticosteroids have been shown to be ineffective in preventing relapse in ulcerative colitis.[17]

The extent of spread of steroid enemas was evaluated by adding [99m]technetium sulfur colloid to an aqueous hydrocortisone enema.[18] Healthy volunteers who did not receive an evacuation enema prior to the hydrocortisone enema showed little spread of the enema from the rectum. However, healthy volunteers who did receive an evacuation enema prior to the hydrocortisone enema showed considerable spreading of the radiolabeled enema, even reaching as far as the ascending colon. Patients with inflammatory bowel disease showed spread of the enema a distance greater than or equal to the

extent of disease involvement. This study showed why corticosteroid enemas are useful in inflammatory bowel disease that extends proximal to the rectum.

The extent and consequences of absorption of corticosteroid enemas were evaluated in a British study.[19] Prednisolone-21-phosphate enemas were administered once to 8 patients with proctocolitis, and plasma prednisolone levels were measured. These proved to be 44 percent of an identical dosage given orally to 9 healthy volunteers. This showed that absorption of corticosteroid enemas does occur in inflamed mucosa, but plasma levels are lower than with oral administration. After administration of the corticosteroid enemas, plasma cortisol levels fell, suggesting suppression of endogenous adrenocorticotrophic hormone (ACTH) by prednisolone absorbed from the enemas. However, most of these patients had an appropriate rise in plasma cortisol after receiving an intramuscular injection of synthetic adrenocorticotrophic hormone, whereas the rest of the patients had a slightly blunted rise. This showed that the hypothalamic–pituitary–adrenal (HPA) axis is only mildly impaired by corticosteroid enemas, while oral corticosteroids are known to be able to completely suppress this axis. Thus, the purported advantage of corticosteroid enemas over oral corticosteroids—fewer side effects—was shown to be true.

Since some patients with proctitis have difficulty retaining an enema, corticosteroids have been placed in suspension in an inert foam base for rectal administration. A British study compared a 100-mg hydrocortisone enema with 100 mg of hydrocortisone foam used for 2 weeks by 30 patients with proctosigmoiditis.[20] Both forms of administration significantly reduced diarrhea, rectal urgency, and tenesmus, and both improved the endoscopic appearance. Significantly more patients reported subjective improvement with the foam. A significant difference was that 53 percent of patients who received the enema reported difficulty retaining the treatment, while none of the patients receiving the foam had this difficulty. The patients who received the enema had a significant improvement in histologic score, while the patients who received the foam did not. Thus, objectively the foam appeared to be as effective as the enema. Subjectively, the foam preparation was preferred.

To decrease the potential side effects from corticosteroids even further, prednisone metasulfobenzoate has been assessed.[21] Prednisolone metasulfobenzoate is a poorly absorbed corticosteroid that presumably acts at the site of application. Forty patients were treated for a 2-week period with enemas of either prednisolone-21-phosphate or prednisolone metasulfobenzoate. Similar symptomatic improvement was seen in both groups. This improvement was paralleled by similar endoscopic and histologic improvement as well. However, plasma prednisolone levels were lower after administration of prednisolone metasulfobenzoate.

Beclomethasone dipropionate is a very potent gluco-corticoid which has significant topical antiinflammatory activity when tested on the skin. It is frequently used in the treatment of asthma. This agent is well absorbed from the gastrointestinal tract, but it is rapidly metabolized in the liver to inactive compounds.[22] Several groups have investigated this agent in an enema form for the treatment of distal ulcerative colitis. One Canadian trial compared 100-ml enemas containing 0.5-mg beclomethasone dipropionate against 100-ml, 5-mg betamethasone phosphate enemas used for 2 weeks in 9 patients with distal ulcerative colitis.[23] Clinical and endoscopic improvement rates were similar between the two groups, but only betamethasone phosphate significantly suppressed plasma cortisol levels. A similar Swiss study compared the same two enemas at the same dosages as the Canadian trial.[24] In this study 16 patients with distal ulcerative colitis were treated for 20 days. Clinical, endoscopic, and histologic improvement was similar in both groups. However, only betamethasone phosphate significantly suppressed plasma cortisol levels, both at a basal state and after stimulation with synthetic ACTH. Last, a Dutch study compared 1.0-mg beclomethasone dipropionate enemas against predni-solone-21-phosphate enemas.[25] Eighteen patients with distal ulcerative colitis were treated for 4 weeks. Because the beclomethasone dipropionate enemas were not found to be as effective as the prednisolone-21-phosphate enemas, the investigators repeated the study with a higher dosage of beclomethasone.[26] Twenty-three patients with proctosigmoiditis were randomized between a 30-mg prednisolone-21-phosphate, a 2-mg beclomethasone dipropionate, or a 3-mg beclomethasone dipropionate enema used nightly for 4 weeks. Endoscopic, clinical, and histologic improvement were similar in all three groups. Fasting serum cortisol and urinary free cortisol decreased significantly in the prednisolone-21-phosphate group, while there were no changes in either beclomethasone group.

Budesonide is another potent corticosteroid that undergoes an extensive first-pass metabolism to metabolites of minimal biologic activity, thus accounting for few systemic effects. A Swedish study compared a 2-mg budesonide enema with a 31.25-mg prednisolone-21-phosphate enema used by 64 patients for 4 weeks.[27] A significantly greater number of patients who received budesonide enemas showed endoscopic, histologic, clinical, and subjective improvement. Additionally, those patients who received prednisolone-21-phosphate enemas showed significant depression of plasma cortisol levels, while no significant change was seen in those patients who received budesonide enemas.

A Dutch study compared a 2-mg budesonide enema with a 4-g 5-aminosalicylic acid (5-ASA) enema for 4 weeks in 62 patients.[28] Both drugs induced significant clinical, endoscopic, and histologic improvement. No clinical signs of corticosteroid toxicity or other side effects were seen.

Tixocortol pivalate is a nonglucocorticoid, nonmineralocorticoid corticosteroid that has been shown to be effective in the treatment of refractory proctosigmoiditis and left-sided colitis.[29] In one study, 125 such patients were treated for 3 weeks with enemas containing either 250 mg of tixocortol pivalate or 100-mg of hydrocortisone.[30] No differences in clinical and endoscopic improvement were seen between these two therapies.

Sulfasalazine

Sulfasalazine has been used for many years in the treatment of ulcerative colitis. This usage has been extended to proctitis, and orally administered sulfasalazine has been another of the mainstays of therapy for proctitis. Sulfasalazine is effective in acute ulcerative colitis[31,32] and also as maintenance therapy to decrease the frequency of recurrences.[33,34] However, sulfasalazine is associated with toxicity, intolerance, or both in 15 to 30 percent of patients taking it.[35] Dose-dependent side effects include dyspepsia, anorexia, nausea, vomiting, headache, and reversible oligospermia, while idiosyncratic side effects include fever, neutropenia, anemia, rash, pruritus, hepatitis, pancreatitis, myocarditis, and pneumonitis. Clearly, these extensive side effects have limited the usefulness of oral sulfasalazine, particularly for relatively benign disease such as proctitis.

The problem of side effects led investigators to study sulfasalazine enemas. A British group compared 3-g sulfasalazine enemas against placebo enemas used for 2 weeks by 34 patients with ulcerative colitis.[36] Clinical and endoscopic improvement was significantly better in the sulfasalazine group as compared with the placebo group and there was also a trend toward histologic improvement. The overall incidence of improvement with sulfasalazine enemas was 69 percent. No side effects were seen, even in patients with a history of sensitivity to sulfasalazine when orally administered.

Sulfasalazine suppositories were subsequently investigated.[37] Seventeen patients with intractable distal inflammatory bowel disease were treated with sulfasalazine suppositories. Fifty-nine percent of the patients had a clinical response, 12 percent had a complete endoscopic response, and 47 percent had a partial endoscopic response. Side effects included pruritus, leukopenia, and an increase in rectal discharge.

Sulfasalazine is composed of sulfapyridine linked to 5-ASA by a diazo (2 nitrogen) bond. This diazo bond is split by bacteria, largely in the colon but also partially in the terminal ileum, and sulfapyridine and 5-ASA are released. The sulfapyridine is absorbed; then acetylated, hydroxylated, and glucuronidated in the liver; and finally excreted in the urine. A small portion of 5-ASA is absorbed, acetylated, and excreted in the urine. Most of the 5-ASA, however, is passed in the feces. This led to suspicion that 5-ASA might be the active agent in sulfasalazine, whereas sulfapyridine might be necessary only for carrying the 5-ASA to the colon. In addition the sulfa moiety is the portion of the sulfasalazine to which most of the adverse side effects can be attributed. These side effects limit the use of the drug.

Azad Khan and colleagues studied 62 patients with mild or moderate clinical or endoscopic evidence of a flare of ulcerative colitis.[38] Three groups of patients each received an enema nightly for 2 weeks. The enemas contained either 2 g sulfasalazine, 1.3 g sulfapyridine, or 0.7 g 5-ASA. Clinically, sulfapyridine was significantly inferior to sulfasalazine or 5-ASA, as only 38 percent of patients improved as compared to 75 percent with sulfasalazine and 73 percent with 5-ASA. Endoscopically, sulfapyridine was also significantly inferior to sulfasalazine or 5-ASA; only 37 percent of patients improved as compared to 64 percent with sulfasalazine and 71 percent with 5-ASA. Last, there was a trend toward histologic improvement with sulfasalazine and 5-ASA as compared to sulfapyridine, although this did not reach statistical significance. These results were interpreted to mean that sulfapyridine acts as a carrier for 5-ASA and may not be involved in the mechanism of sulfasalazine in the treatment of ulcerative colitis.

A Dutch group studied 45 patients with proctitis.[39] Three groups of patients each received a suppository twice daily for 4 weeks: either 300 mg sulfapyridine, 200 mg 5-ASA, or placebo. A clinical remission was achieved in 60 percent of 5-ASA patients, as compared to only 13 percent of the sulfapyridine patients and 27 percent of the patients who received a placebo. Endoscopic resolution was seen in 60 percent of 5-ASA patients, as compared to 13 percent of the sulfapyridine patients and 27 percent of the patients who received a placebo. Both the clinical and the endoscopic results showed statistically significant improvement with 5-ASA versus sulfapyridine or placebo. These data and others confirmed the original study of Azad Khan and associates.[38,40]

These above-cited studies have led to the current focus on various forms of 5-ASA for the treatment of ulcerative colitis and proctitis. A recent article entitled "Sulphasalazine in ulcerative colitis: in memoriam?" questioned whether or not sulfasalazine still has any place in the treatment of ulcerative colitis.[41] The authors argue that sulfasalazine may still be useful, since it may have mechanisms of action other than 5-ASA. Sulfapyridine has immunomodulatory activity in rheumatoid arthritis.[42] Sulfasalazine inhibits the lipoxygenase pathway of arachadonic acid metabolism to a greater extent than 5-ASA.[43] Finally, sulfasalazine affects neutrophil and lymphocyte function more than does 5-ASA.[44] Thus, further investigation into the mechanisms of action of sulfasalazine may be warranted.

Even in light of the 5-ASA data, sulfasalazine may have a place in the treatment of left-sided colitis. In many of the 5-ASA trials discussed below, the patients continued whatever medications they were on before starting the study. However, one study had patients stop sulfasalazine if they had been taking it before beginning a 4-ASA enema trial.[45] Of the 19 patients, 12 stopped sulfasalazine before entering the trial, while 7 were not on sulfasalazine. Of the sulfasalazine patients, 62 percent deteriorated, as compared with none of the patients who had not received sulfasalazine. Of those patients who deteriorated after discontinuation of sulfasalazine, 63 percent improved when it was resumed, while the remaining 37 percent required corticosteroids to improve. The explanation for these results is unclear. It is possible that oral sulfasalazine has a mechanism of action complementary to that of topical ASA. Alternatively, enemas may not reach high enough drug levels in the descending colon, so that an oral medication might be more effective in controlling such disease.

5-Aminosalicylic Acid (5-ASA)

Enemas. The pharmacokinetics of 5-ASA enemas were investigated in a British study.[46] Seven patients were given 0.7-g 5-ASA enemas and blood and urine levels of 5-ASA and acetyl 5-ASA were measured afterwards. The mean serum level of 5-ASA was 0.1 μg/ml, whereas the mean serum level of acetyl 5-ASA was 0.3 μg/ml. These extremely low serum levels lend credence to the belief that 5-ASA acts topically, not systemically. The mean urinary excretion of 5-ASA was 1.0 mg/8 hours, while the mean urinary excretion of acetyl 5-ASA was 40.3 mg/8 hours. This confirms that most 5-ASA is acetylated before being excreted in urine. Similar results were reported by an Italian group, who also noted that urinary recovery of acetyl 5-ASA is lower in patients with active disease and is dose and volume dependent in patients in remission.[47]

Several trials have compared 5-ASA enemas with corticosteroid enemas for the treatment of distal ulcerative colitis. In an Italian study, 86 patients with mild or moderate attacks of ulcerative colitis were randomized to receive either a 4-g 5-ASA enema or a 100-mg hydrocortisone enema for 15 days.[48,49] Clinical and endoscopic remission were noted in 93 percent and 93 percent of the former group, and 57 percent and 54 percent of the latter group, respectively. Of the 5-ASA group, 77 percent showed pronounced histologic improvement as compared with only 33 percent of the hydrocortisone group. All of these differences were statistically significant. The same authors later used ^{99m}TC-labeled 5-ASA enemas to show that 5-ASA enemas invariably spread at least to the splenic flexure and sometimes even more proximally.[50]

A similar trial compared a 4-g 5-ASA enema against a 100-mg hydrocortisone enema used in 18 patients for 3 weeks.[51] These patients had continued to have active distal ulcerative colitis after at least 3 weeks of therapy with 100-mg hydrocortisone enemas. Of the former patients receiving 5-ASA, 78 percent improved clinically as compared with only 11 percent of those receiving hydrocortisone, a statistically significant difference. There were also trends favoring 5-ASA in endoscopic and histologic improvement.

A Danish study compared a 1-g 5-ASA enema against a 25-mg prednisolone enema used in 123 patients for 4 weeks.[52] Of these, 114 of them completed the study. Clinical and endoscopic improvement was noted in 79 percent and 72 percent of the 5-ASA group (of 53 patients), and 84 percent and 72 percent respectively of the prednisolone group (of 61 patients). There was no statistically significant difference in the incidence of side effects between the two treatments. It was also noted that more than half of the patients who had not improved after 2 weeks of treatment improved after two additional weeks of treatment, suggesting a possible advantage to longer treatment schedules.

A Dutch group compared a 3-g 5-ASA enema (15 patients) to a 30-mg prednisolone-21-phosphate enema (14 patients) used for 4 weeks in subjects with active proctosigmoiditis.[53] No statistically significant differences were observed in clinical, endoscopic, or histologic improvement. The authors did note that combination enemas of 5-ASA and corticosteroids are commonly used in the Netherlands, but they have not been investigated to see if they are more effective than are single-ingredient enemas.

Several studies have reported that 5-ASA enemas are effective in the treatment of proctocolitis in patients who have been unresponsive to or intolerant of all other therapies.[54-58] In one study 47 patients with left-sided colitis unresponsive to other therapies were treated with 4-g 5-ASA enemas for 3 months.[59] Eighty-three percent achieved clinical remission and an additional 4 percent showed clinical improvement. Although 25 clinical relapses occurred, 92 percent responded to retreatment.

No systemic side effects were seen, although 23 percent of patients developed anorectal side effects.

A second study randomized 153 patients with left-sided colitis to receive either 4-g 5-ASA or placebo enemas for 6 weeks.[60] Statistically significant differences favoring 5-ASA were seen in stool frequency, endoscopic appearance, and physician's assessment of disease severity. No statistically significant difference was found in the incidence or type of side effects.

Optimal dosage of 5-ASA enemas remains to be determined. A multicenter trial reported 276 patients with mild to moderate distal ulcerative colitis who were receiving no other therapy.[61] These patients received 1-g, 2-g, or 4-g 5-ASA enemas, or placebo enemas daily for 8 weeks. Clinical improvement was seen in 81 percent, 72 percent, 72 percent, and 41 percent of patients, respectively. All of the dosages were significantly better than placebo, but there were no significant differences among the three dosages of 5-ASA enemas. The incidence of side effects was negligible. The authors concluded that there were no significant dose-response differences between 1-g, 2-g, and 4-g 5-ASA enemas.

The optimal length of treatment with 5-ASA enemas has not been established. One study reviewed the course of 90 patients with left-sided colitis whose disease had been refractory to other therapy and were treated with long-term daily 4-g 5-ASA enemas.[62] At 8 and 12 weeks, 80 percent and 87 percent of patients had improved clinically, but only 29 percent and 54 percent had achieved remission, respectively. Of the 20 percent of patients who had not achieved remission by 34 weeks, 71 percent did show endoscopic improvement. This study also found that 85 percent of patients who experienced a relapse responded within 8 weeks to 5-ASA enemas.

Use of the 5-ASA enemas may be tapered either by reducing the daily dosage or by decreasing the frequency of enema administration. Relapse is common regardless of which tapering method is employed. Life-table analysis in one study showed that virtually all patients relapse with tapering.[63] In this same study, 63 percent of relapsers achieved a second remission with retreatment with full-dose 5-ASA enemas. A similar study attempted to determine what the frequency of 5-ASA enemas should be in order to prevent relapse.[64] This study ended with one patient taking no medication, eight patients using a 5-ASA enema every third night, three patients using a 5-ASA enema every other night, and three patients requiring a 5-ASA enema each evening.

Ironically, despite the fact that relapse is so common during tapering, 5-ASA enemas have been shown to be useful in maintaining remission.[65] Twenty-five patients with left-sided colitis in remission were randomized between a 1-g 5-ASA enema and a placebo enema used every day for 1 year. Although 75 percent of the 5-ASA patients stayed in remission, this was true of only 15 percent of the placebo group.

Thus, 5-ASA enemas have been shown to be effective therapy for left-sided colitis. Local side effects consist largely of perianal trauma from enema insertion, and systemic side effects have been quite unusual. There are more remissions seen after an extended duration of treatment. Relapse is frequent if therapy is discontinued, but repeat administration of 5-ASA may again induce remission. Tapering the dosage, the time interval, or both is a possible method of maintenance therapy, although the best schedule for maintenance therapy has not yet been established. These data have led many to recommend 5-ASA enemas as primary therapy for proctosigmoiditis. The results of a number of these trials are listed in Table 24–2.

Suppositories

Some patients do develop perianal irritation from enema administration, and some are unable to retain enemas. Therefore, it was proposed that 5-ASA suppositories be used for the treatment of proctitis. One study investigated 27 patients with proctitis who were randomized to receive either a 0.5-g 5-ASA suppository or a placebo suppository three times a day for 6 weeks.[66] Remission was achieved in 79 percent of 5-ASA patients, as compared with 7 percent of placebo patients. Tolerance of 5-ASA suppositories was excellent and no patients reported side effects. Radiolabeling of a 5-ASA suppository in 6 patients with inflammatory bowel disease and 6 healthy volunteers showed that the 5-ASA was confined to the rectum or distal sigmoid colon and did not spread to other organs. These results have been confirmed by other authors.[67]

An Italian study group compared two dosages of suppositories with placebo. All patients received three suppositories a day. These included either three, two, or no 500-mg 5-ASA suppositories. If the suppository contained no 5-ASA, it contained a placebo. Thus patients received a daily dosage of 5-ASA via suppository of 1.5 g, 1.0 g, or none. Clinical remission was achieved in 74 percent, 69 percent, and 39 percent, respectively. These data showed a statistically significant difference between either dosage of 5-ASA suppositories and placebo, but no difference between the two dosages of 5-ASA. No serious side effects were seen.[68]

5-ASA suppositories can be used for maintenance of remission in proctosigmoiditis. Thirty patients with proctosigmoiditis were given either a 0.4-g 5-ASA suppository or a placebo suppository twice a day for a year.[69] Ninety-two percent of the 5-ASA patients remained in remission, a significant difference over the 21 percent of placebo patients who remained in remission. No anal side effects were seen.

Finally, one interesting use for 5-ASA suppositories is for the patient with ulcerative colitis who is symptomatic from an out-of-circuit rectum.[70]

The cited studies show that 5-ASA suppositories are effective for treatment of proctitis, either for an acute attack or for maintenance of remission. The anal irritation and difficulty in retaining the medication that are seen with 5-ASA enemas are not seen with 5-ASA suppositories. However, 5-ASA suppositories have only a fair spread to the distal sigmoid colon and rarely spread more proximally, so they have little usefulness in left-sided colitis.

4-Aminosalicylic Acid (4-ASA)

4-Aminosalicylic acid (4-ASA) is also known as *para*-aminosalicylic acid (PAS). It has been used since the 1940s for the treatment of tuberculosis. It differs from 5-ASA only in the position of the amino group. 4-ASA is inexpensive and safe. It is also much more stable in

Table 24-2   Results of 5-ASA Enemas vs. Corticosteroid Enemas, %

	Clinical response	Endoscopic response	Histologic response
5-ASA			
Campieri et al[50]	93	93	77
Danish 5-ASA group[52]	78	72	. . .
Mulder et al[53]	74	73	73
CORTICOSTEROIDS			
Campieri et al[50]	57	54	33
Danish 5-ASA group[52]	84	72	. . .
Mulder et al[53]	79	86	57

aqueous solution than 5-ASA. Therefore, while experimentation into developing a stable 5-ASA enema proceeded, several investigators studied whether or not 4-ASA enemas are useful in the treatment of distal colitis. The mechanism of action of 4-ASA is unclear. It does not appear to modulate the lipoxygenase metabolites of arachidonic acid or to interact with free oxygen radicals as does 5-ASA.[71]

A British group compared 1-gm 4-ASA enemas against placebo enemas in 30 patients and 2-gm 4-ASA enemas against placebo enemas in 22 patients.[72] Patients had mild to moderate left-sided colitis, and enemas were given for 2 weeks. Combining the results from the two studies, 80 percent of the patients who received 4-ASA enemas improved clinically, significantly better than the 41 percent improvement noted in the placebo group. Endoscopic improvement was seen in 72 percent and in 30 percent, respectively. Other authors have reported clinical improvement in 83 percent of patients who received 4-ASA and in only 15 percent of patients in the placebo group.[73]

Somewhat different results were described in another study.[74] Forty-seven patients with distal ulcerative colitis were treated with either 2-g or 1-g 4-ASA enemas or placebo enemas twice a day for 2 weeks. Clinical improvement was significantly better with the 1-g 4-ASA enemas than with placebo, and there was a trend toward more clinical improvement with the 2-g 4-ASA enemas as compared with placebo. No significant differences in either endoscopic findings or side effects were noted.

An Italian group compared 4-ASA enemas with 5-ASA enemas.[75] Sixty-three patients with mild or moderate left-sided colitis received either a 2-g 4-ASA enema or a 2-g 5-ASA enema daily for 15 days. No statistically significant differences between the two groups were noted relative to clinical, endoscopic, or histologic improvement.

Tapering of 4-ASA enemas for maintenance of remission has been attempted, similarly to 5-ASA enemas. One study retrospectively assessed whether histologic inflammation predicted which patients with complete remission would symptomatically relapse during tapering.[76] No flares occurred in the 7 patients without histologic changes of acute activity. This was significantly better than the 75 percent rate of recrudescence noted in the 8 patients in whom histologic changes of acute activity had been noted.

These data show that 4-ASA enemas are better than placebo and as effective as 5-ASA enemas in the treatment of distal ulcerative colitis. The mechanism of action of 4-ASA is unclear, and it may be different than the mechanism of action of 5-ASA. 4-ASA enemas are effective as maintenance therapy after remission, and they may be tapered in the absence of histologic changes of acute activity.

Sucralfate

Sucralfate is a sulfated disaccharide complex with aluminum hydroxide. It is used for the treatment of peptic ulcer disease, and it is thought to act topically by stimulating gastric mucus secretion, epithelial cell renewal, endogenous prostaglandin production, and mucosal blood flow. Several investigators have speculated that these properties might be useful in the treatment of inflammatory lesions in the colon.

A British group compared 4-g sucralfate enemas to 20-mg prednisolone metasulfobenzoate enemas used daily for 4 weeks in 44 patients with mild to moderate distal colitis.[77] Complete resolution of rectal bleeding occurred in 28 percent of patients taking sucralfate, significantly less than 71 percent of the patients using prednisolone metasulfobenzoate. Similar differences were noted relative to histologic remission. In addition, 10 percent of the patients using sucralfate enemas developed constipation.

An Indian group used 2-g sucralfate enemas for a variety of distal colonic ulcerative lesions, including radiation proctitis, ulcerative proctitis, solitary rectal ulcer syndrome, and ulcerated polyps awaiting polypectomy.[78] All 5 patients with ulcerative proctitis had improvement in diarrhea, tenesmus, and urgency, while 4 of them had cessation of bleeding. None of the patients had any side effects.

These very preliminary investigations suggest that sucralfate enemas may be useful for the treatment of proctitis, but there is little to lead one to suspect that sucralfate will be better than current conventional therapy.

Cromolyn

Cromolyn is a mast cell stabilizer which is used in asthma. Since one theory of proctitis is that is an allergic disorder with increased mast cell degranulation, cromolyn therapy has been tried. A British group studied 30 patients with proctitis.[79] One hundred milligrams of disodium cromoglycate was taken orally three times a day and 200 mg disodium cromoglycate was given twice a day as an enema. A placebo was given orally and rectally to the other group. After 4 weeks of therapy, each group was changed to the other therapy. Fifty-four percent of patients improved clinically on disodium cromoglycate, as compared with 8 percent of patients on placebo. Patients who responded to disodium cromoglycate had significantly more eosinophils in their rectal biopsies than those who failed to respond.

Another trial compared oral regimens of 200 mg disodium cromoglycate four times a day, 500 mg sulfasalazine four times a day, and both 200 mg disodium cromoglycate and 500 mg sulfasalazine four times a day.[80] This study was carried out in 120 patients with ulcerative colitis in remission; 107 completed the study. On entering the study, 69 patients were in clinical and endoscopic remission. Of these, 44 percent of the 25 disodium cromoglycate patients had a clinical relapse, as compared with 12 percent of the sulfasalazine group (of 25 patients) and 11 percent of the 19 patients receiving both drugs. Similarly, 42 percent of the disodium cromoglycate patients had an endoscopic relapse, as compared with 13 percent of the sulfasalazine group and 11 percent of the patients who received both drugs. The patients receiving disodium cromoglycate did significantly worse in both clinical and endoscopic evaluation, but there was no difference between the patients who received sulfasalazine alone and the patients who received sulfasalazine and disodium cromoglycate. It was concluded that disodium cromoglycate was not effective for maintenance of remission in ulcerative colitis.

A double blind multicenter trial compared twice-daily 600-mg sodium cromoglycate enemas against 20-mg prednisolone-21-phosphate enemas in 70 patients with ulcerative colitis for 9 weeks.[81] Both drugs were associated with significant decreases in symptom scores, but there was a significantly greater improvement in the reduction of rectal bleeding at the 4-week checkup in the prednisolone-21-phosphate group. Both drugs caused significant endoscopic and histologic improvement, and there were no significant differences between the 2 drugs. It was also noteworthy that neither treatment significantly affected mucosal eosinophil counts.

These data are not particularly impressive, particularly when compared to the higher percentage of patients who improve on aminosalicylate therapy. Therefore, little further investigation into the effectiveness of cromolyn has proceeded.

6-Mercaptopurine

6-Mercaptopurine is a purine analog with immunosuppressive activity. It has a small, but real, teratogenic potential. Therefore, many physicians are reluctant to use it even for widespread inflammatory bowel disease. However, one study retrospectively reviewed 27 patients with intractable proctosigmoiditis who were treated with 6-mercaptopurine orally at a mean daily dosage of 50 mg.[82] Complete or moderate improvement occurred in 63 percent of patients with a mean response time of 3.8 months. Reversible leukopenia occured in 15 percent of patients. Other side effects possibly attributable to 6-mercaptopurine included herpes zoster in 7 percent of patients and nausea in 4 percent of patients.

Short Chain Fatty Acids

Short chain fatty acids, including acetate, propionate, and butyrate, have been purported to improve diversion colitis.[83] The underlying hypothesis is that the colonic epithelium in colitis may be in a state of cellular energy deficiency. A German group compared 100-mM sodium butyrate enemas versus placebo enemas twice daily for 2-week periods in 5 patients with distal colitis.[84] Endoscopic and histologic improvement was seen, but this was not significantly better than with placebo. Another small study evaluated 12 patients with left-sided colitis.[85] Twice-daily rectal irrigation with solutions containing 8 mM sodium acetate, 3 mM sodium propionate, and 4 mM sodium butyrate was given. Of the 10 patients who completed the trial, 90 percent had clinical and endoscopic improvement. Their histologic score was significantly improved, too.

Topical Anesthetics

A Swedish group has suggested that topical anesthetics may inhibit hyperactive nervous reflexes and block neuroimmune interactions in ulcerative proctitis. Ten patients with colitis were treated with 2% lignocaine gel given intrarectally three times daily for 3 weeks.[86] The total daily dose of lignocaine was 800 mg. All patients had clinical remission and endoscopic improvement. The investigators then tried using lidocaine gel in patients with proctitis.[87] Their largest study includes 100 patients with several types of ulcerative colitis.[88] In this study, 800 mg of lidocaine was administered in a gel to 28 patients with proctitis for 3 to 8 weeks. All proctitis patients clinically improved with this treatment, but 68 percent developed recurrent disease within 1 year. These investigations are clearly quite preliminary.

Bismuth

A British group studied tripotassium dicitrato bismuthate (De-Nol) enemas for the treatment of proctosigmoiditis.[89] This same agent has been used orally in the treatment of peptic ulcer disease. Eleven patients with proctosigmoiditis were treated with 480-mg tripotassium dicitrato bismuthate enemas daily for 4 weeks; 45 percent improved clinically, 82 percent improved endoscopically, and 55 percent improved histologically. The mechanism of action of bismuth is unknown, although the authors speculate that it may be related to immobilization of thiol (hydrosulfide, or −SH) groups in organisms.

Cyclosporin

Cyclosporin is an immunosuppressant that is used extensively to prevent rejection of transplanted organs. A Danish group gave hydrophilic 250-mg cyclosporin enemas daily for 2 weeks to 8 patients with colitis.[90] Clinical and endoscopic improvement was seen in 75 percent of the patients. Only 1 patient had any detectable blood level of cyclosporin, which was thought to account for the lack of side effects other than two cases of nausea.

Conclusions

During the 1980s many new treatments for proctitis have been developed.[91] Currently available preparations in the United States include 5-ASA in enema, suppository, and oral preparation. Newer corticosteroid enema preparations are being explored and show great promise, as they appear to offer less adrenal suppression. The allergic theory of proctitis is on the wane. Further advances in the treatment of proctitis will depend upon advances in understanding the etiology or etiologies of proctitis. Figure 24-1 outlines a useful therapeutic approach to ulcerative proctitis.

Crohn's Disease

Medical therapy for anorectal Crohn's disease is rather limited. Although anecdotes abound about the use of 5-ASA enemas or corticosteroid enemas for Crohn's disease, it is generally thought that these mucosal agents will not be helpful in healing a lesion that involves deeper layers of the rectum.[92] Only two drugs have been purported to be helpful for anorectal Crohn's disease, metronidazole and 6-mercaptopurine.

Metronidazole

Metronidazole has not been found to be useful in the treatment of proctitis in a controlled trial.[93] However, an uncontrolled trial of oral metronidazole at a dosage of 20 mg/kg/day in three to five doses daily was conducted

Step 1.	Hydrocortisone enema or foam
	or
	5-ASA enema or suppository
	or
	Sulfasalazine given
Step 2.	Switch to an alternative step 1 therapy
Step 3.	5-ASA given orally
Step 4.	Brief course of orally administered prednisone

Figure 24-1.   Treatment schema for ulcerative proctitis.

in 21 patients with perineal Crohn's disease.[94] All patients showed decreased drainage, erythema, and induration. Of the patients taking the drug for at least 2 months, 56 percent had complete healing, 28 percent had partial healing, and another 11 percent had decreased inflammation. Side effects were common, and these included metallic taste, dark urine, gastrointestinal upset, and peripheral neuropathy. A later study showed that peripheral neuropathy was extremely common in patients with inflammatory bowel disease who were taking metronidazole, but this side effect was usually reversible by a decrease or discontinuation of the drug.[95]

6-Mercaptopurine

6-Mercaptopurine has been suggested for treatment of many types of fistulae in Crohn's disease. One study reported on 34 patients with fistulae due to Crohn's disease who were treated with 1.5 mg/kg/day of 6-mercaptopurine for a minimum of 6 months.[96] Thirty-nine percent of patients had complete closure of their fistula, while another 26 percent improved. The mean time to respond was 3.1 months. Of 18 perirectal fistulae, 33 percent closed and 22 percent improved. Of 6 rectovaginal fistulae, 33 percent closed and 17 percent improved.

Clearly, medical treatment for anorectal Crohn's disease is quite limited. The available drugs are fairly toxic, work very slowly if at all, and are not very effective. Other agents are starting to be considered, including methotrexate, but there is no reliable medical treatment at this time.

References

1. Greenstein AJ, Sachar DB, Smith H, et al. Cancer in universal and left-sided ulcerative colitis: factors determining risk. *Gastroenterology*. 1979;77:290–294.

2. Nugent FW, Veidenheimer MC, Zuberi S, Garabedian MM, Parikh NK. Clinical course of ulcerative proctosigmoiditis. *Am J Dig Dis*. 1970;15:321–326.

3. Tytgat GNJ, Fockens P, Schotborgh RH, Hofer SOP. Proctitis. *Neth J Med*. 1990;37(suppl):S37–S42.

4. Farmer RG. Nonspecific ulcerative proctitis. *Gastroenterol Clin North Am* 1987;16:157–174.

5. Mir-Madjlessi SH, Michener WM, Farmer RG. Course and prognosis of idiopathic ulcerative proctosigmoiditis in young patients. *J Pediatr Gastroenterol Nutr*. 1986;5:570–575.

6. Snook J. Are the inflammatory bowel diseases autoimmune disorders? *Gut*. 1990;31:961–963.

7. Ekbom A, Adami HO. Ulcerative proctitis—a paramalignant phenomenon? *Gastroenterology*. 1991;100:A208. Abstract.

8. Rosekrans PCM, Meijer CJLM, Van der Wal AM, Lindeman J. Allergic proctitis, a clinical and immunopathological entity. *Gut*. 1980;21:1017–1023.

9. Heatley RV, Rhodes J, Calcraft BJ, Whitehead RH, Fifield R, Newcombe RG. Immunoglobulin E in rectal mucosa of patients with proctitis. *Lancet*. 1975;2:1010–1012.

10. Ekbom A, Helmick C, Zack M, Adami HO. Ulcerative proctitis in central Sweden 1965–1983: a population-based epidemiological study. *Dig Dis Sci*. 1991;36:97–102.

11. Sinclair TS, Brunt PW, Mowatt NAG. Nonspecific proctocolitis in Northeastern Scotland: a community study. *Gastroenterology*. 1983;85:1–11.

12. Farmer RG, Whelan G, Sivak MV. Colonoscopy in distal ulcerative colitis. *Clin Gastroenterol*. 1980;9:297–306.

13. Das KM, Morecki R, Nair P, Berkowitz JM. Idiopathic proctitis, I: the morphology of proximal colonic mucosa and its clinical significance. *Am J Dig Dis*. 1977;22:524–528.

14. Surawicz CA, Belic L. Rectal biopsy helps to distinguish acute self-limited colitis from idiopathic inflammatory bowel disease. *Gastroenterology*. 1984;86:104–113.

15. Flejou JF, Potet F, Bogomoletz WV, et al. Lymphoid follicular proctitis: a condition different from ulcerative proctitis? *Dig Dis Sci*. 1988;33:314–320.

15a. Juby LD, Long DE, Dixon MF, Axon ATR. Prognostic indicators and clinical course in proctosigmoiditis. *International Journal of Colorectal Disease*. 1990;5:177–180.

16. Truelove SC. Treatment of ulcerative colitis with local hydrocortisone. *Br Med J*. 1956;2:1267–1272.

17. Lennard-Jones JE, Misiewicz JJ, Connell AM, Baron JH, Avery Jones F. Prednisone as maintenance treatment for ulcerative colitis in remission. *Lancet*. 1965;1:188–189.

18. Jay M, Digenis GA, Foster TS, Antonow DR. Retrograde spreading of hydrocortisone enema in inflammatory bowel disease. *Dig Dis Sci*. 1986;31:139–144.

19. Lee DAH, Taylor GM, James VHT, Walker G. Plasma prednisolone levels and adrenocortical responsiveness after administration of prednisolone-21-phosphate as a retention enema. *Gut*. 1979;20:349–355.

20. Ruddell WSJ, Dickinson RJ, Dixon MF, Axon ATR. Treatment of distal ulcerative colitis (proctosigmoiditis) in relapse: comparison of hydrocortisone enemas and rectal hydrocortisone foam. *Gut*. 1980;21:885–889.

21. McIntyre PB, Macrae FA, Berghouse L, English J, Lennard-Jones JE. Therapeutic benefits from a poorly absorbed prednisolone enema in distal colitis. *Gut*. 1985;26:822–824.

22. Martin LE, Tanner RJN, Clark TJH, Cochrane GM. Absorption and metabolism of orally administered beclomethasone dipropionate. *Clin Pharmacol Ther*. 1974;15:267–275.

23. Kumana CR, Seaton T, Meghji M, Castelli M, Benson R, Sivakumaran T. Beclomethasone dipropirinate enemas for treating inflammatory bowel disease without producing Cushing's syndrome or hypothalamic pituitary adrenal supression. *Lancet*. 1982;1:579–583.

24. Bansky G, Buhler H, Stamm B, Hacki WH, Buchmann P, Muller J. Treatment of distal ulcerative colitis with beclomethasone enemas: high therapeutic efficacy without endocrine side effects. A prospective, randomized, double-blind trial. *Dis Colon Rectum*. 1987;30:288–392.

25. Van der Heide H, van den Brandt-Gradel V, Tytgat GNJ, et al. Comparison of beclomethasone dipropirinate and prednisolone 21-phosphate enemas in the treatment of ulcerative proctitis. *J Clin Gastroenterol*. 1988;10:169–172.

26. Mulder CJJ, Endert E, van der Heide H, et al. Comparison of beclomethasone dipropirinate (2

and 3 mg) and prednisolone sodium phosphate enemas (30 mg) in the treatment of ulcerative proctitis. An adrenocortical approach. *Neth J Med.* 1989;35:18–24.

27. Danielsson A, Hellers G, Lyrenas E, et al. A controlled randomized trial of budesonide versus prednisolone retention enemas in active distal ulcerative colitis. *Scand J Gastroenterol.* 1987;22:987–992.

28. Lamers C, Meijer J, Engels L, et al. Comparative study of the topically acting glucocorticosteroid budesonide and 5-aminosalicylic acid enema therapy of proctitis and proctosigmoiditis. *Gastroenterology.* 1991;100:A223. Abstract.

29. Friedman G. Tixcortol pivalate (JO 1016). *Am J Gastroenterol.* 1983;78:529–530.

30. Hanauer SB, Kirsner JB, Barrett WE. The treatment of left sided ulcerative colitis with tixocortol pivalate (TP). *Gastroenterology.* 1986;90:1449. Abstract.

31. Baron JH, Connell AM, Lennard-Jones JE, Avery Jones F. Sulphasalazine and salicylazosulphadimidine in ulcerative colitis. *Lancet.* 1962;1:1094–1096.

32. Dick AP, Grayson MJ, Carpenter RG, Petrie A. Controlled trial of sulphasalazine in the treatment of ulcerative colitis. *Gut.* 1964;5:437–442.

33. Dissanayake AS, Truelove SC. A controlled therapeutic trial of long-term maintenance treatment of ulcerative colitis with sulphasalazine (Salazopyrin). *Gut.* 1973;14:923–926.

34. Misiewicz JJ, Lennard-Jones JE, Connell AM, Baron JH, Avery Jones F. Controlled trial of sulphasalazine in maintenance therapy for ulcerative colitis. *Lancet.* 1965;1:185–188.

35. Das KM, Eastwood MA, McManus JPA, Sircus W. Adverse reactions during salicylazosulfapyridine therapy and the relation with drug metabolism and acetylator phenotype. *N Engl J Med.* 1973;289:491–495.

36. Palmer KR, Goepel JR, Holdsworth CD. Sulphasalazine retention enemas in ulcerative colitis: a double-blind trial. *Br Med J.* 1981;282:1571–1573.

37. Saibil FG. Treatment of intractable distal inflammatory bowel disease (IBD) with sulphasalazine suppositories. *Gastroenterology.* 1984;86:1227. Abstract.

38. Azad Khan AK, Piris J, Truelove SC. An experiment to determine the active therapeutic moiety of sulphasalazine. *Lancet.* 1977;2:892–895.

39. Van Hees PAM, Bakker JH, Van Tongeren JHM. Effect of sulphapyridine, 5-aminosalicylic acid, and placebo in patients with idiopathic proctitis: a study to determine the active therapeutic moiety of sulphasalazine. *Gut.* 1980;21:632–635.

40. Klotz U, Maier K, Fischer C, Heinkel K. Therapeutic efficacy of sulfasalazine and its metabolites in patients with ulcerative colitis and Crohn's disease. *N Engl J Med.* 1980;303:1499–1502.

41. Hallyar J, Bjarnason I. Sulphasalazine in ulcerative colitis: in memoriam? *Gut.* 1991;32:462–463.

42. Neumann VC, Taggart AJ, Le Gallez P, Astbury C, Hill J, Bird HA. A study to determine the active moiety of sulphasalazine in rheumatoid arthritis. *J Rheumatol.* 1986;13:285–287.

43. Nielsen ST, Beninati L, Buonato CB. Sulfasalazine and 5-aminosalicylic acid inhibit contractile leukotriene formation. *Scand J Gastroenterol.* 1988;23:272–276.

44. Comer SS, Jasin HE. In vitro immunomodulatory effects of sulfasalazine and its metabolites. *J Rheumatol.* 1988;15:580–586.

45. Ginsberg AL, Steinberg WM, Nochomovitz LE. Deterioration of left sided ulcerative colitis after withdrawal of sulfasalazine. *Gastroenterology.* 1985;88:1395. Abstract.

46. Dew MJ, Cardwell M, Kidwai NS, Evans BK, Rhodes J. 5-Aminosalicylic acid in serum and urine after administration by enema to patients with colitis. *J Pharm Pharmacol.* 1983;35:323–324.

47. Campieri M, Lanfranchi GA, Boschi S, et al. Topical administration of 5-aminosalicylic acid enemas in patients with ulcerative colitis: studies on rectal absorption and excretion. *Gut.* 1985;26:400–405.

48. Campieri M, Lanfanchi GA, Bazzocchi G, et al. Treatment of ulcerative colitis with high-dose 5-aminosalicylic acid enemas. *Lancet.* 1981;2:270–271.

49. Campieri M, Gionchetti P, Belluzzi A, et al. Efficacy of 5-aminosalicylic acid enemas versus hydrocortisone enemas in ulcerative colitis. *Dig Dis Sci.* 1987;32(suppl):67S–70S.

50. Campieri M, Lanfranchi GA, Brignola C, et al. Retrograde spread of 5-aminosalicylic acid enemas in patients with active ulcerative colitis. *Dis Colon Rectum.* 1986;29:108–110.

51. Friedman LS, Richter JM, Kirkham SE, DeMonaco HJ, May RJ. 5-Aminosalicylic acid enemas in refractory distal ulcerative colitis: a randomized, controlled trial. *Gastroenterol.* 1986;81:412–418.

52. Danish 5-ASA Group. Topical 5-aminosalicylic acid versus prednisolone in ulcerative proctosigmoiditis: a randomized, double-blind multicenter trial. *Dig Dis Sci.* 1987;32:598–602.

53. Mulder CJJ, Tytgat GNJ, Wiltink EHH, Houthoff HJ. Comparison of 5-aminosalicylic acid (3 g) and

prednisolone phosphate sodium enemas (30 mg) in the treatment of distal ulcerative colitis: a prospective, randomized, double-blind trial. *Scand J Gastroenterol.* 1988;23:1005–1008.

54. Campieri M, Lanfranchi GA, Brignola C, Bazzochi G, Minguzzi MR, Calari MT. 5-Aminosalicylic acid as rectal enema in ulcerative colitis in patients unable to take sulfasalazine. *Lancet* 1982;1:403. Letter.

55. Barber GB, Lee DE, Antonioli DA, Peppercorn MA. Refractory distal ulcerative colitis responsive to 5-aminosalicylate enemas. *Am J Gastroenterol.* 1985;80:612–614.

56. Hanauer SB, Schultz PA, Kirsner JB. Treatment of refractory proctitis with 5-ASA enemas. *Gastroenterology.* 1985;88:1412. Abstract.

57. Janssens J, Geboes K, Delanote C, Vantrappen G. 5-Amino-salicylic acid (5-ASA) enemas are effective in patients with resistent [sic] ulcerative rectosigmoiditis. *Gastroenterology.* 1983;84:1198. Abstract.

58. Sutherland LR, Martin F. 5-Aminosalicyclic acid enemas in treatment of distal ulcerative colitis and proctitis in Canada. *Dig Dis Sci.* 1987;32(suppl):64S–66S.

59. McPhee MS, Swan JT, Biddle WL, Greenberger NJ. Proctocolitis unresponsive to conventional therapy: response to 5-aminosalicylic acid enemas. *Dig Dis Sci.* 1987;32(suppl):76S–81S.

60. Sutherland LR, Martin F, Greer S, et al. 5-Aminosalicylic acid enemas in the treatment of distal ulcerative colitis, proctosigmoiditis, and proctitis. *Gastroenterology.* 1987;92:1894–1898.

61. Hanauer SB, Kane SV, Guernsey B, et al. Randomized clinical trial of mesalamine (5-ASA) enemas in distal ulcerative colitis: a dose-ranging placebo controlled study. *Gastroenterology.* 1989;96:A195. Abstract.

62. Biddle WL, Miner PB. Long-term use of mesalamine enemas to induce remission in ulcerative colitis. *Gastroenterology.* 1990;99:113–118.

63. Hanauer SB, Schultz PA. Relapse rates after successful treatment of refractory colitis with 5-ASA enemas. *Gastroenterology.* 1987;92:1424. Abstract.

64. Guarino J, Chatzinoff M, Berk T, Friedman LS. 5-Aminosalicylic acid enemas in refractory distal ulcerative colitis: long-term results. *Gastroenterol.* 1987;82:732–737.

65. Biddle WL, Greenberger NJ, Swan JT, McPhee MS, Miner PB. 5-Aminosalicylic acid enemas: effective agent in maintaining remission in left-sided ulcerative colitis. *Gastroenterology.* 1988;94:1075–1079.

66. Williams CN, Haber G, Aquino JA. Double-blind, placebo-controlled evaluation of 5-ASA suppositories in active distal proctitis and measurement of extent of spread using 99mTc-labeled 5-ASA suppositories. *Dig Dis Sci.* 1987;32(suppl):71S–75S.

67. Stein LB, Vitti RA, Knight LD, Maurer A, Siegel H, Fisher RS. Distribution of 5-ASA suppositories in left-sided inflammatory bowel disease (LSIBD). *Gastroenterology.* 1991;100:A253. Abstract.

68. Campieri M, De Franchis R, Bianchi Porro G, Ranzi T, Brunetti G, Barbara L. Mesalazine (5-aminosalicylic acid) suppositories in the treatment of ulcerative proctitis or distal proctosigmoiditis: a randomized controlled trial. *Scand J Gastroenterol.* 1990;25:663–668.

69. D'Arienzo A, Panarese A, D'Armiento FP, et al. 5-Aminosalicylic acid suppositories in the maintenance of remission in idiopathic proctitis of proctosigmoiditis: a double-blind placebo-controlled clinical trial. *Am J Gastroenterol.* 1990;85:1079–1082.

70. Mayberry JF, Balfour TW, Long RG. Inflammation in the rectal stump: the role of 5-amino salicylic acid suppositories. *J Clin Gastroenterol.* 1990;12:119–120. Letter.

71. Nielsen OH, Ahnfelt-Ronne I. 4-Aminosalicylic acid, in contrast to 5-aminosalicylic acid, has no effect on arachidonic acid metabolism in human neutrophils, or on the free radical 1,1-diphenyl-2-picrylhydrazyl. *Pharmacol Toxicol.* 1988;62:223–226.

72. Selby WS, Bennett MK, Jewel DP. Topical treatment of distal ulcerative colitis with 4-aminosalicylic acid enemas. *Digestion.* 1984;29:231–234.

73. Ginsberg AL, Beck LS, McIntosh TM, Nochomovitz LE. Treatment of left-sided ulcerative colitis with 4-aminosalicylic acid enemas: a double-blind, placebo-controlled trial. *Ann Intern Med.* 1988;108:195–199.

74. Gandolfo J, Farthing M, Powers G, Eagen K, Goldberg M, Berman P, Kaplan M. 4-Aminosalicylic acid retention enemas in treatment of distal colitis. *Dig Dis Sci.* 1987;32:700–704.

75. Campieri M, Lanfranchi GA, Bertoni F, et al. A double-bind clinical trial to compare the effects of 4-aminosalicylic acid to 5-aminosalicylic acid in topical treatment of ulcerative colitis. *Digestion.* 1984;29:204–208.

76. Goodman MW, Eberle DE, Kuchler LA, Fossum EA. Microscopic activity predicts relapse in patients with distal ulcerative colitis on 4-aminosalicylic acid enemas. *Gastroenterology.* 1988;94:A151. Abstract.

77. Riley SA, Gupta I, Mani V. A comparison of sucralfate and prednisolone enemas in the treatment

of active distal ulcerative colitis. *Scand J Gastroenterol*. 1989;24:1014–1018.

78. Kochhar R, Mehta SK, Aggarwal R, Dhar A, Patel F. Sucralfate enema in ulcerative rectosigmoid lesions. *Dis Colon Rectum*. 1990;33:49–51.

79. Heatley RV, Calcraft BJ, Rhodes J, Owen E, Evans BK. Disodium cromoglycate in the treatment of chronic proctitis. *Gut*. 1975;16:559–563.

80. Willoughby CP, Heyworth MF, Piris J, Truelove SC. Comparison of disodium cromoglycate and sulphasalazine as maintenance therapy for ulcerative colitis. *Lancet*. 1979;2:119–122.

81. Grace RH, Gent AE, Hellier MD. Comparative trial of sodium cromoglycate enemas with prednisolone enemas in the treatment of ulcerative colitis. *Gut* 1987;28:88–92.

82. Love MA, Rubin PH, Chapman ML, Present DH. 6-Mercaptopurine is effective in intractable proctosigmoiditis. *Gastroenterology*. 1991;100:A832. Abstract.

83. Harig JM, Soergel KH, Komorowski RA, Wood CM. Treatment of diversion colitis with short-chain-fatty acid irrigation. *N Engl J Med*. 1989; 320:23–28.

84. Scheppach W, Bartram P, Christl SU, Burghardt W, Kirchner T, Kasper H. Butyrate irrigation for the treatment of distal ulcerative colitis. *Gastroenterology*. 1991;100:A248. Abstract.

85. Breuer RI, Buto SK, Christ ML, Bean JA, Vernia P, Di Paulo MC, Caprilli R. Short chain fatty acids for distal ulcerative colitis. *Gastroenterology*. 1990;98:A161. Abstract.

86. Bjorck S, Ahlman H, Dahlstrom A. Lignocaine and ulcerative proctitis. *Lancet*. 1988;2:1330. Letter.

87. Bjorck S, Dahlstrom A, Ahlman H. Topical treatment of ulcerative proctitis with lidocaine. *Scand J Gastroenterol*. 1989;24:1061–1072.

88. Bjorck S, Dahlstrom A, Ahlman H. Topical treatment with lidocaine in patients with ulcerative colitis. *Gastroenterology*. 1991;100:A198. Abstract.

89. Srivastava ED, Swift GL, Wilkinson S, Williams GT, Evans BK, Rhodes J. Tripotassium dicitrato bismuthate enemas in the treatment of ulcerative proctitis. *Alimentary Pharmacol Ther*. 1990;4: 577–581.

90. Brynskov J, Freund L, Thomsen OO, Anderson CB, Rasmussen SN, Binder V. Treatment of refractory ulcerative colitis with cyclosporin enemas. *Lancet*. 1989;1:721–722. Letter.

91. Sutherland LR. Topical treatment of ulcerative colitis. *Med Clin North Am*. 1990;74:119–131.

92. Ginsberg AL. Topical salicylate therapy (4-ASA and 5-ASA enemas). *Gastroenterol Clin North Am*. 1989;18:35–42.

93. Davies PS, Rhodes J, Heatley RV, Owen E. Metronidazole in the treatment of chronic proctitis: a controlled trial. *Gut*. 1977;18:680–681.

94. Bernstein LH, Frank MS, Brandt LJ, Boley SJ. Healing of perineal Crohn's disease with metronidazole. *Gastroenterology*. 1980;79:357–365.

95. Duffy LF, Daum F, Fisher SE, et al. Peripheral neuropathy in Crohn's disease patients treated with metronidazole. *Gastroenterology*. 1985;88:681–684.

96. Korelitz BI, Present DH. Favorable effect of 6-mercaptopurine on fistulae of Crohn's disease. *Dig Dis Sci*. 1985;30:58–64.

CHAPTER 25

ANORECTAL CROHN'S DISEASE: SURGICAL MANAGEMENT

John D. Cheape,
David G. Jagelman, and
Steven D. Wexner

Crohn's disease is a chronic inflammatory disease of unknown etiology that affects a relatively young population and may involve any portion of the gastrointestinal tract. It has a tendency for exacerbation and remission and its clinical features vary. Since there is no known cure, therapy is empirical and focuses on symptoms and specific complications. These symptoms and complications can be quite debilitating and can lead to social, sexual, and employment restrictions.

Three major clinical patterns of intestinal Crohn's disease have been described: ileocolic, small-intestinal, and colonic. Bissell first described the association between anal and intestinal disease.[1] Penner and Crohn later reported perianal fistulas in several cases of regional ileitis.[2] Anal involvement may be associated with any of these patterns but occurs most commonly with colonic disease, followed by the ileocolic and small-intestinal patterns.[3,4] Exclusive anal involvement is uncommon, seen in only 5 percent of patients in one study.[5] Although anal manifestations may be the initial presentation, intestinal involvement may follow in many cases. The clinical recognition of the perianal manifestations of Crohn's disease is important but may be difficult if these are the first evidence of Crohn's disease.

Management of this disease has tended to be cautious; because of this approach many patients have been debilitated by the symptoms of fissure, abscess, and fistula. Both medical and surgical therapy play distinct roles in the relief of pain and other symptoms. Several important points must be remembered. First, sound healing may not occur in some cases because of the inherent nature of the disease. Second, these patients may have diarrhea; damage to the sphincters may exacerbate fecal soiling. Despite these problems, however, symptoms should be treated. If medical management fails, surgery has an important role in the relief of the pain, discomfort, and debilitation that these lesions can create. Medical management is discussed in detail in Chapter 24.

Incidence of Anal Involvement

The reported incidence of anal involvement in Crohn's disease varies, in part because of the definitions of anal involvement. If anal involvement is defined as the presence of fissure, fistula, or abscess, the incidence is lower than if stenosis, skin tags, and maceration are included. In the absence of sepsis, anal involvement may be relatively asymptomatic and not appreciated unless a thorough examination is performed. In addition, most studies are retrospective and do not reflect the true incidence.

Williams and colleagues[6] retrospectively reviewed anal complications in 1098 patients with Crohn's disease. Complications were defined as the presence of fissure, fistula, or abscess. In this series, 242 patients (22 percent) were found to have anal manifestations of Crohn's disease. Multiple complications occurred in 48 (20 percent) of the 242 patients. Anal involvement was more common in those patients whose primary disease was colonic in distribution (52 percent), as compared with those who had small-intestinal disease (14 percent). Bernard and associates[7] found that 45 percent of 225 patients with Crohn's disease had a fissure, abscess, or fistula. This study, however, had more patients with primary colonic disease than did the study by Williams and colleagues.[6]

The National Cooperative Crohn's Disease Study (NCCDS) also defined perianal disease as the presence of fissure, fistula, or abscess. Prior to randomization to a therapeutic study, 205 of 569 patients (36 percent) had a history of perianal disease. Seventy-nine (14 percent) had active perianal manifestations at the time of randomization and 70 (12 percent) developed perianal complications during the study. A history of perianal disease was more common in patients with colonic and ileocolic disease than in those with exclusively small-bowel involvement.[8]

Other reports in the literature cite anal involvement in 20 to 80 percent of patients with Crohn's disease.[4,5,9-11] These reports also note that patients with colonic disease have a higher incidence of anal involvement than do patients with ileal or ileocolic disease.

Clinical Manifestations

Perianal Crohn's disease may manifest itself as superficial erosions or maceration skin tags, fissure, abscess, fistulas, or anal stenosis.[12,13] The etiology of these changes is multifactorial and to a large degree idiopathic. The perianal skin may be edematous with a cyanotic discoloration. Diarrhea can lead to maceration and superficial erosions which are not necessarily specific for Crohn's disease. Secondary bacterial or fungal infection may exacerbate these conditions.[12] Large, firm, edematous skin tags are a common feature of anal Crohn's disease (Fig. 25-1). They can lead to further difficulties with anal hygiene and subsequent exacerbation of perianal irritation.[12,13] As compared with skin tags, symptomatic internal hemorrhoids are rare.[13] Fissures may be due to active anal and perianal inflammation, to diarrhea, or to idiopathic causes. These fissures tend to be large, deep ulcers with undermined edges. They may be eccentrically located in the anal canal and are often multiple. Severe pain should heighten suspicion of underlying sepsis. A chronic-appearing fissure found in a location other than anterior or posterior is characteristic of perianal Crohn's disease.[12,13] These are illustrated in Figures 12-1 and 12-7. Patients with Crohn's disease may also develop simple fissures that resemble a typical idiopathic fissure in ano; these lesions are related to the disordered bowel function of their underlying disease. This differentiation must be considered in the situation in which sphincterotomy is consid-

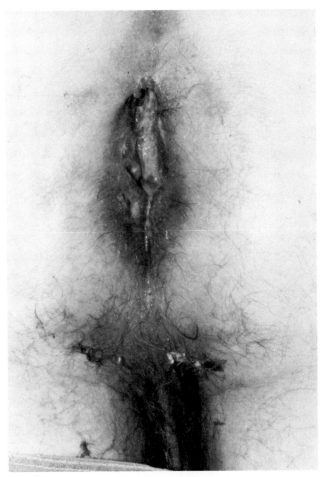

A

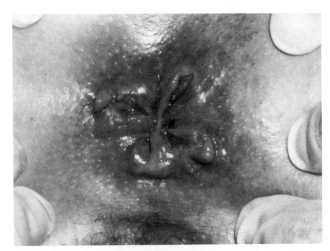

B

Figure 25-1.   (A) and (B) The typical appearance of perianal Crohn's disease. Note the large, firm edematous skin tags and multiple fissures.

ered as treatment for the pain associated with such a fissure.[12]

A mild degree of anal stenosis is frequently present in patients with Crohn's disease. It results from long-standing diarrhea, perianal sepsis, and fibrosis. Minor stenosis is usually well tolerated because the patient's stools are often semisolid or liquid. Longer, more severe strictures are often a result of previous surgery in the anal canal,[12,13] or, less often, are related to the severity of the disease process.

Anal fistulas in patients with Crohn's disease arise either from a penetrating fissure or an infected anal gland. They may resemble ordinary fistulas found in patients without Crohn's disease or may be more complicated. An indurated track extending from a cyanotic opening can often be palpated. Multiple external openings are common and may appear on the buttock, thigh, or genitalia (Fig. 25-2) Anal fistulas in Crohn's disease tend to be chronic and are sometimes painless, but painful episodes are common and usually indicate inadequate drainage of pus.[12,13] Long periods when the fistula ceases drainage may alternate with periods of exacerbations of drainage and pain. Horseshoe fistulas are particularly common and are often associated with multiple external openings. Of particular importance in female patients are rectovaginal fistulas, which can be severely symptomatic with drainage and dyspareunia. These particular fistulas may emit gas, pus, or stool into the vagina. The sepsis associated with rectovaginal fistulas may ascend along the rectovaginal septum to create severe induration.

General Concepts of Management

The primary consideration when making treatment decisions is the patient's symptoms. Despite severe perineal disease, few symptoms may exist. Patients often complain only of drainage and pruritus. When perianal pain is present, undrained sepsis should be suspected. Deep postanal space abscesses, particularly, present in this fashion.

The remainder of the gastrointestinal tract should be examined to determine the extent and severity of disease. The small intestine is most effectively studied with enteroclysis. Colonoscopy is the best method for examining the large bowel and distal ileum since small aphthous ulcers may be recognized. Contrast radiography may miss these small ulcers. Upper gastrointestinal endoscopy may be performed when indicated.[12] It is important to correlate the patient's symptoms with the findings of all the gastrointestinal investigations.

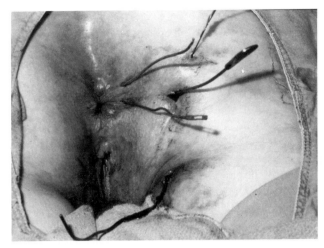

A

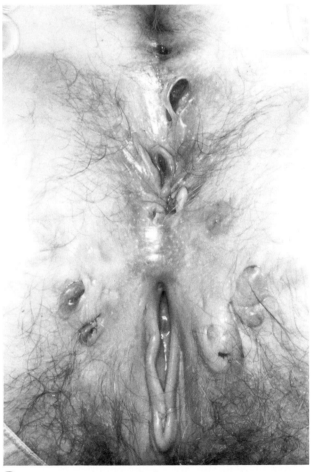

B

Figure 25-2.   (A) and (B) Multiple external fistulous openings.

Several small, retrospective studies have reported healing of anal fistulas after resection of intestinal disease.[11,14] Hellers and associates[11] found that 20 of 43 patients (47 percent) had spontaneous healing of perineal fistula after resection of intestinal disease. Seven of these patients had recurrence of anal fistulas within 2 to 5 years. Orkin and Telander[14] noted improvement of anorectal disease in 5 of 19 patients (29 percent) after intestinal resection. Buckman and associates[15] and Marks and associates,[16] however, found no evidence of improved healing after resection of proximal diseased bowel. VanDongen and Lubbers reported successful surgical treatment of fistulas in 8 of 10 patients with quiescent bowel disease.[17]

The authors and editors believe that symptomatic intestinal disease should be addressed independently of the perineal disease except in cases in which the two are obviously interrelated such as in extrasphincteric fistula. The resection of asymptomatic intestinal disease will have little impact on anorectal disease. Medical therapy of intestinal Crohn's disease, however, may have an ameliorative effect on the fistula and should be considered.

Thorough perianal, anal, and proctosigmoidoscopic examination are of utmost importance to fully assess the extent of perineal disease. If the patient is tender because of sepsis, ulcers, or skin tags these examinations can be performed under anesthesia. It is usually too painful to probe fistulous tracts without anesthesia. In addition, both internal and external apertures are often so small that the use of general anesthesia is essential.

Management

Skin Irritation

Skin irritation and maceration are usually a result of diarrhea and poor anal hygiene. Treatment should be focused on the control of diarrhea with appropriate medications and local perineal care. Warm baths after bowel movements and atraumatic cleansing of the perineal region are important points of anal hygiene in these patients.

Skin Tags

Symptomatic internal hemorrhoids are rare; large edematous skin tags are a more common feature (see Fig. 25-1) Symptoms from skin tags usually result from perianal irritation from frequent loose stools. Surgical excision of these lesions should be avoided because the

wounds may heal poorly. Treatment is conservative with warm baths and medical control of diarrhea being most helpful.

Anal Stenosis

Although mild anal stenosis is a common occurrence in perianal Crohn's disease, it seldom requires treatment (Fig. 25-3) Short segments of stenosis in the anus or lower rectum may require gentle dilatation. Longer anorectal strictures are often difficult to treat and may ultimately lead to proctectomy.

Medical Management

Most patients with perianal Crohn's disease will undergo medical therapy for the intestinal component of the disease. Prednisone and other medical agents may relieve the symptoms of the perianal abscess and fistula and some[18,19] but not all investigators have found metronidazole to be of some value.

There have been anecdotal reports that erythromycin and other antianaerobic agents relieve symptoms, but none of these antibiotics, however, has been assessed in a controlled manner. Medical management is discussed fully in Chapter 24.

Abscess and Fistula

Perianal abscesses and fistulas in patients with Crohn's disease deserve special consideration. The surgical options are outlined in Table 25-1. Patients with Crohn's disease may develop fissures and fistulas in the rectum because of disordered bowel function. Although surgical wounds created in these patients may heal normally, patients may also develop lesions of this kind through involvement of the anal and perianal tissues by Crohn's disease. The involved tissues of this latter group tend to heal slowly, and therefore extensive operations in which large open wounds are created frequently lead to complex management problems.

The goal of initial therapy is to drain any underlying sepsis and relieve pain. This goal can be achieved by making small incisions and inserting small drainage tubes such as mushroom catheters or setons (Fig. 25-4; see also Fig. 9-5). Complex fistulas may be best treated by providing long-term drainage. Asymptomatic fistulas do not require treatment. Large incisions that are long or distant from the anal verge should be avoided. As with all fistulas, therapy should be directed toward closure of the internal opening and providing adequate

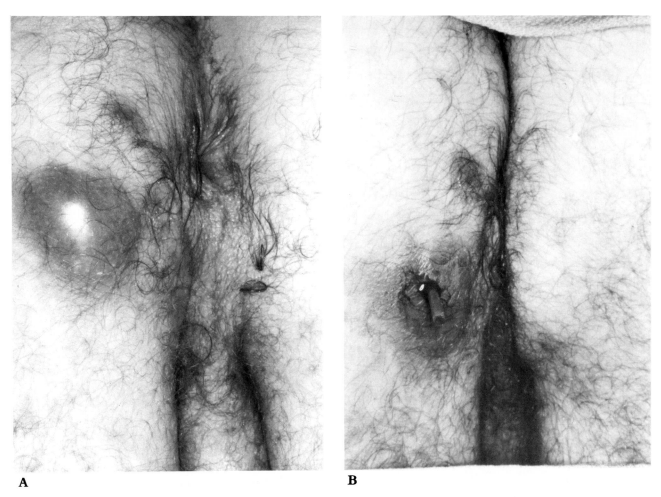

Figure 25-3. (A) and (B) Mushroom-tipped catheter drainage of an ischiorectal abscess.

Table 25-1   Surgical Management of Fistulas in Crohn's Disease*

Type of fistula	Rectal disease	Treatment	
Low, simple	None	Fistulotomy	
	Active	Medical only with or without seton	
High, complex	None	Advancement flap with catheter drain	
	Active	First	Seton
		Second	Temporary ileostomy
		Third	Proctectomy
Rectovaginal	None	Advancement flap	
	Active	Temporary ileostomy	

* Medical management may be added to each surgical option (see Chapter 24).

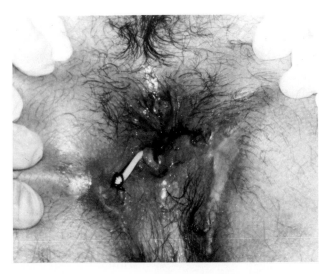

Figure 25-4.   Seton drainage of a high transsphincteric fistula.

drainage. The presence of active rectal disease must be considered.

Treatment is guided by the position and nature of the fistula. Most anal fistulas in patients with Crohn's disease are similar to the cryptoglandular anal fistulas that occur in patients without Crohn's disease. Marks and associates[16] classified the anal fistulas in their Crohn's patients using the Parks classification (Table 25-2). Rectovaginal fistula, usually a variant of a transsphincteric fistula, is discussed later in this section and also in Chapter 10, as these lesions are common in Crohn's disease and demand special attention. The modified Park's classification is illustrated in Figure 9-9.

VanDongen and Lubbers[10] reported a series of 55 patients with perianal fistulas related to Crohn's disease: 13 patients (24 percent) did not require treatment. Primary proctectomy was necessary in 5 (9 percent). Local surgery was successful in 22 (78 percent) of the 28 patients treated surgically.

Deeper abscesses in the postanal space require drainage, and this will often necessitate some division of the internal and external sphincters. Intersphincteric abscesses can be directly drained through the inter-

Table 25-2   Type of Fistulas

Low or superficial
High or intersphincteric
Transsphincteric with extension
Extrasphincteric
Suprasphincteric
Rectovaginal

sphincteric space without muscle division. When abscesses occur in areas not immediately adjacent to the anus such as the ischiorectal space, drainage should be performed through a small incision into the abscess cavity. A small mushroom catheter is placed in the cavity for continual drainage (see Fig. 9-5) With adequate drainage of the pus, the pain will resolve. The drain may be left in position for weeks or months, converting the abscess to a fistula to control pain. After a period of 4 to 6 weeks anoscopy is performed to identify the internal opening. If the internal opening cannot be identified and is healed the drain can be removed. Some surgeons inject the drain with methylene blue or peroxide to convince themselves there is no internal opening although we have not found this necessary.[20]

Although primary healing is always a concern when treating Crohn's disease, some fistulas (intersphincteric and low transsphincteric) can often be treated with fistulotomy. In a review of 47 patients who underwent surgical treatment of fistula in ano, Levien and associates[21] reported primary healing in 29 patients (62 percent); 37 patients (79 percent) either had complete healing or obtained significant improvement; 5 patients (11 percent) required proctectomy. The best results were in patients with a "classic" internal opening at the dentate line and with no rectal disease. The success or failure of fistulotomy in these patients usually relates to the presence or absence of Crohn's infiltration into the perianal tissues. At the time of fistulotomy, therefore, it is important to send biopsy material to confirm or deny the presence of such involvement. Granulomata and chronic inflammatory reaction may well be seen; this is particularly common in those patients who have blue discoloration of the perianal skin around these lesions.

Morrison and associates[22] reported the results of 35 patients operated on between 1973 and 1986 for Crohn's disease and anorectal fistulas: 29 lesions were classified as low intermuscular fistulas; 19 patients underwent primary fistulotomy and 8 had partial fistulectomy with seton insertion; 3 patients required primary proctectomy. Of the 32 patients who underwent fistulotomy 30 healed, however, 7 patients required more than one operation. One patient ultimately underwent proctectomy and one fistula recurred but was asymptomatic.

Suprasphincteric and extrasphincteric fistulas are frequently more complex and associated with significant rectal and sigmoid inflammation. The abdominal or pelvic sepsis responsible for extrasphincteric fistulas usually originates in perforated ileal or colonic Crohn's disease. The diseased bowel segments must be resected for these fistulas to heal. The sepsis may tract down behind the rectum in the presacral space or through the greater sciatic notch. The abscess may point either adjacent to the rectum behind the rectum, or even on the buttock. This latter situation occurs particularly in those cases in which the disease perforates through the sciatic notch. The aim with complex fistulas with suprasphincteric components is adequate drainage and resection of the perforated diseased segment. Drains such as mushroom-tipped catheters or noncutting Silastic setons often will allow adequate drainage and alleviate symptoms. Some cases of high transsphincteric fistula in ano may be treated by closing the internal opening using the mucosal flap advancement technique. This method is a transanal approach to elevate and advance downward a flap of mucosa and internal sphincter to recreate the dentate line. This inevitably removes the fibrosis and sepsis associated with the internal opening of the fistula and also removes the anal gland, infection of which is the originating factor in fistula in ano. This technique is particularly useful in patients who have rectovaginal fistulas; it is discussed later and in chapters 9 and 10.

The degree of rectal involvement appears to influence the success of surgical correction of these fistulas and therefore may affect clinical management. The authors and editors would be less likely to recommend a mucosal advancement flap procedure in the presence of severe active rectal inflammation. Two studies[16,23] have found the results of surgery for anal fistulas in Crohn's disease to be better when there is little or no rectal inflamation. VanDongen,[17] however, found no difference in healing.

Pritchard and colleagues from the Lahey Clinic retrospectively reviewed the outcomes of 38 patients with Crohn's disease who underwent drainage of perirectal abscesses.[24] Thirty-two percent of the patients had no prior history of anorectal Crohn's disease. There were 30 "single" abscesses and 8 "complex" horseshoe abscesses. At operation 53 percent of patients underwent incision and drainage whereas 26 percent had mushroom-tipped catheters placed. After reduction of the initial abscess, recurrences were noted in 45 percent of the catheter drainage group and in 56 percent of the group that had undergone incision and drainage alone. In addition, 31 percent of the former and 44 percent of the latter group underwent subsequent proctectomy to control perineal sepsis. The healing time of the perineal wound was longer than 6 months in 83 percent of those patients.

Williams and colleagues from the University of Minnesota assessed the outcome of 64 symptomatic fistulas in 55 patients with Crohn's disease.[25] Forty-one fistulas in 33 patients were treated by conventional fistulotomy. Thirty wounds (73 percent) healed within 3 months and 8 additional wounds within 6 months; thus 93 percent of the entire group had healed within 6 months. Two of

the three patients whose wounds remained unhealed by 12 to 18 months required proctectomy. There were no changes in continence in 26 patients; 4 had minor incontinence. Drainage setons were used to treat 16 high transsphincteric, 5 suprasphincteric, and 1 extrasphincteric fistula in 22 patients. Although 3 patients required another seton and 3 a proctectomy, 8 reported no change in continence. In most cases these changes were related to diarrhea rather than to anal disease.

Some patients with severe anorectal disease and poorly functioning anal sphincters will be candidates for primary proctectomy. Generally, these patients have a history of unsuccessful medical therapy and numerous failed attempts at surgical correction. They continue to be in pain, they continue to have drainage, and their wounds have failed to heal after fistulotomy. The majority of these patients will have severe colonic disease so that the proctectomy is usually combined with a colectomy and a permanent ileostomy. It is both a psychological and a physical injustice to the patient with an anus ravaged by Crohn's disease to attempt sphincter preservation. Similarly the patient in whom the anus is affected by only a single simple intersphincteric fistula but who has severe rectal disease may not be a candidate for fistulotomy. In this latter situation the rigid noncompliant rectum serves as a conduit rather than a reservoir. Division of any muscle might lead to fecal incontinence. Thus there are instances in which a primary proctectomy is the best alternative.

Fecal diversion alone[26,27] may be a valuable option in some patients with very severe perianal disease. Diverting the fecal stream does not eradicate the fistulas but may convert them to a totally or comparatively asymptomatic state. In patients who have very severe perianal disease with multiple fistulous openings and deep sepsis surrounding the rectum, preliminary fecal diversion or subtotal colectomy and ileostomy may be an appropriate approach. This allows the sepsis to resolve and the fistula to become asymptomatic, rendering a subsequent proctectomy to be much easier to perform. Furthermore, primary healing of the perineal wound is facilitated. Conversely, removal of a severely diseased rectum with perianal sepsis carries a greater risk of an unhealed perineal wound. Unfortunately, fecal diversion has only a temporary effect, although this may last for many months. The fistulas will reactivate after intestinal continuity is reestablished.

Another benefit of temporary ileal diversion is that the patient can become accustomed to a diverting stoma. Many patients who will not allow permanent diversion as an initial alternative are much more accepting after they experience a "trial run." In 86 patients with anorectal Crohn's disease followed at the Mayo Clinic for 10 to 40 years, the probability of avoiding

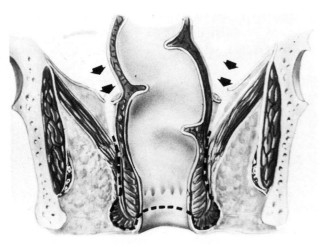

Figure 25-5. Technique of intersphincteric proctectomy.

proctectomy at 10 and 20 years was 92 to 83 percent respectively.[25]

If proctectomy is performed, the intersphincteric technique of dissection minimizes the size of the wound and greatly reduces the incidence of unhealed sinuses.[28] This technique is illustrated in Figure 25-5. As can be seen in the illustration, the procedure entails dissection in the intersphincteric plane, between the internal and external sphincters. The levators are then divided immediately adjacent to the rectum. All of the muscle layers are individually reapproximated, as is the skin.

Rectovaginal Fistula

Rectovaginal fistula is a serious complication of Crohn's disease. These fistulas rarely heal spontaneously. Management is dependent on the proximity of the fistula to the anus and on the state of the rectal disease. Small, low-lying fistulas that are relatively asymptomatic do not require surgery. Persistent purulent vaginal fecal drainage or discharge of gas via the vagina is a indication for repair of the rectal vaginal fistula. High-lying fistulas frequently require proctectomy if medical therapy cannot control symptoms.

The rectal mucosal advancement flap technique may be used for symptomatic low rectovaginal fistulas or other fistulas in which significant amounts of sphincter muscle are affected. The technique is discussed and illustrated in Chapters 9 and 10. Patients are preoperatively prepared with a mechanical bowel preparation and intravenous antibiotics. The procedure may be performed under regional or general anesthesia. After induction of anesthesia, patients are placed in the prone position with the buttocks taped laterally.[20] Initially the anoderm and

rectal submucosa are injected with a solution of epinephrine to aid hemostasis and to define the planes of dissection. A flap of anoderm, mucosa, and internal sphincter is elevated beginning just distal to the internal opening of the fistula. Dissection is carried cephalad past the firm inflammatory tissue around the fistula to a point where the submucosa is normal and the flap will easily advance over the fistulous opening. After the tract has been curetted, absorable suture is placed in the muscles to close the internal opening. The distal part of the flap where the fistula traverses is trimmed and the advancement flap is sutured to cover the defect. Rectovaginal fistulas treated in this fashion do not require a drain, but other fistula with longer tracts may require an external drain in the external opening until the flap is healed.

This method can be safely performed without fecal diversion, although in those patients who do not heal with this method or who have recurrent disease fecal diversion occasionally may be appropriate. The use of the advancement flap has been a major advance in the surgical management of patients with Crohn's disease.

Fry and Kodner have reported an 80 percent healing rate in 10 patients with Crohn's disease treated with this technique.[20] Morrison and associates reported on 12 patients with Crohn's disease and rectovaginal fistula[29]: 4 patients required primary proctectomy and 8 patients underwent repair of the fistula as four staged and four primary repairs. The primary repairs consisted of two endorectal advancement flaps and fistula excision with repair. All four of the fistulas repaired in stages recurred. Two healed after further surgery, one required proctectomy and one remained relatively asymptomatic.

Radcliffe and associates reported data on 90 patients with rectovaginal fistulas due to Crohn's disease[30]: 24 patients required no or minimal surgical procedures, 8 patients underwent fecal diversions, and 46 had proctectomy. Of these last, 12 had primary repair, 9 of which healed. Other authors have reported similar rates of success.[31-33]

An alternative technique is the transvaginal repair of rectovaginal fistula. Sher and associates[33] reported successful use of this technique in 14 of 15 patients. However, all patients had a diverting loop ileostomy performed either as a preliminary or concurrent step to fistula repair. Although this approach may be successful in certain patients, the majority of colorectal surgeons are more comfortable with the transanal approach. Furthermore the transanal approach is best undertaken with the patient in the prone jackknife position. This position permits much better assistance than does the lithotomy position used for transvaginal repair. Lastly the transvaginal repair does not address the high-pressure side of the fistula and therefore appears to require fecal diversion more often than does the transanal repair. For all of these reasons, the authors and editors prefer the transanal approach.

Conclusion

Perianal involvement can be an extremely debilitating component in Crohn's disease. Treatment should be dictated by symptoms. The presence of a fistula with minor drainage can be treated medically with prednisone or possibly by metronidazole and other antimicrobial agents. Pain is usually associated with the development of an abscess and should be treated with drainage. Drainage may either be in the form of a small mushroom catheter or a seton placed through the fistulous tract. In general a conservative approach should be used in the surgical management of patients with perianal Crohn's disease. Infiltration of Crohn's lesions into the perianal skin must be distinguished from a simple fistula occurring in a patient with Crohn's disease. Surgical intervention should be considered for patients whose disease is resistant to medical treatment and conservative drainage procedures. Surgical techniques include fistulotomy for a simple low cryptoglandular fistula and advancement flaps, setons, and mushroom-tipped catheters for more cephalad fistulae. Strong consideration should be given to fecal control

and to avoiding division of the sphincter mechanism in these patients because of the fear of incontinence.

The success of the surgical approach is impaired because of the disease process and its effect on healing. Good symptomatic relief and often complete healing of these fistulous tracts can occur with appropriately conservative surgical intervention.

Some patients with severe disease resistant to both medical and surgical therapy will require proctectomy either in a single or staged fashion to control and relieve their symptoms. Staging of the procedure with preliminary fecal diversion and secondary proctectomy may assist in ultimate perineal wound healing. Performance of a primary proctectomy in the presence of severe sepsis increases the risk of an unhealed chronically draining perineal wound. In addition, the use of an intersphincteric proctectomy result in a relatively small perineal wound. Rates of primary healing after the intersphincteric technique are generally higher than those after a more radical proctectomy.

In conclusion, a wide array of both medical and surgical options exist for the treatment of anal and perianal Crohn's disease. No one procedure is either uniformly appropriate or universally successful. Recognition of the myriad of manifestations of anal and perianal Crohn's disease and timely utilization of appropriate judiciously aggressive surgery offer the best change for success.

References

1. Bissell AD. Localized chronic ulcerative colitis. *Ann Surg*. 1934;99:957–966.
2. Penner A, Crohn BB. Perianal fistula as a complication of regional ileitis. *Ann Surg*. 1938;108:867–873.
3. Farmer RG, Hawk WA, Turnbull RB. Indications for surgery in Crohn's disease: analysis of 500 cases. *Gastroenterology*. 1976;71:245–250.
4. Farmer RG, Hawk WA, Turnbull RB. Clinical patterns in Crohn's disease: a statistical study of 615 cases. *Gastroenterology*. 1975;68:627–635.
5. Lockhart-Mummery HE. Crohn's disease: anal lesions. *Dis Colon Rectum*. 1975;18:200–202.
6. Williams DR, Coller JA, Corman ML, et al. Anal complications in Crohn's disease. *Dis Colon Rectum*. 1981;24:22–24.
7. Bernard D, Morgan S, Tasse D. Selective surgical management of Crohn's disease of the anus. *Can J Surg*. 1986;29:318–321.
8. Rankin GB, Watts HD, Melnyk CS, Kelley ML. National cooperative Crohn's disease study: extra-

intestinal manifestations and perianal complications. *Gastroenterology*. 1979;77:914–920.
9. Fielding JF. Perianal lesions in Crohn's disease. *J R Coll Surg Edinb*. 1972;17:32–37.
10. VanDongen LM, Lubbers EJC. Perianal fistulas in patients with Crohn's disease. *Arch Surg*. 1986;121:1187–1190.
11. Hellers G, Bergstrand O, Ewerth S, et al. Occurrence and outcome after primary treatment of anal fistula in Crohn's disease in pediatric Crohn's disease. *Gut*. 1980;21:525–527.
12. Cohen Z, McLeod RS. Perianal Crohn's disease. *Gastroenterol Clin North Am*. 1987;16:175–189.
13. Alexander-Williams J. Alan and perianal Crohn's disease. In: Kodner IJ, Fry RD, Poe JP, eds. *Colon, Rectal and Anal Surgery*. St. Louis: CV Mosby; 1985.
14. Orkin BA, Telander RL. The effect of intraabdominal resection on fecal diversion on perianal disease in pediatric Crohn's disease. *J Pediatr Surg*. 1985;20:343.

15. Buckman P, Keighley MRB, Allan RN, Thompson H, Alexander-Williams J. Natural history of perianal Crohn's disease: ten year follow-up. A plea for conservation. *Am J Surg*. 1980;140:642–644.

16. Marks CG, Richie JK, Lockhart-Mummery HE. Anal fistulas in Crohn's disease. *Br J Surg*. 1981; 68:525–527.

17. VanDongen LM, Lubbers EJC. Perianal fistulas in patients with Crohn's disease. *Arch Surg*. 1986; 121:1187–1190.

18. Bernstein LH, Frank MS, Brandt LJ, Boley SJ. Healing of perineal Crohn's disease with metronidazole. *Gastroenterology*. 1980;79:357.

19. Jakobovits J, Schuster MM. Metronidazole therapy for Crohn's disease and associated fistulae. *Am J Gastroenterol*. 1984;79:533.

20. Fry RD, Kodner IJ. Management of anal and perineal Crohn's disease. *Infect Surg*. 1989; June: 209–219.

21. Levien DH, Surrell J, Mazier WP. Surgical treatment of anorectal fistula in patients with Crohn's disease. *Surg Gynecol Obstet*. 1989;169:133–136.

22. Morrison JG, Gathright JB, Ray JE, et al. Surgical management of anorectal fistulas in Crohn's disease. *Dis Colon Rectum*. 1989;32:492–496.

23. Wolf BG, Culp CE, Beart RW, et al. Anorectal Crohn's disease: a long-term prospective. *Dis Colon Rectum*. 1985;28:709–711.

24. Pritchard TJ, Schoetz DJ Jr, Roberts PL, Murray JJ, Coller JA, Veidenheimer MC. Perirectal abscesses in Crohn's disease. Drainage and outcome. *Dis Colon Rectum*. 1990;33:933–937.

25. Williams JG, Rothenberger DA, Nemer FD, Goldberg SM. Fistula-in-ano in Crohn's disease. Results of aggressive surgical treatment. *Dis Colon Rectum*. 1991;34:378–384.

26. Jagelman DG, Zelas P. Loop ileostomy on the management of Crohn's colitis in the debilitated patient. *Ann Surg*. 1980;191:164.

27. Lee E. Split ileostomy in the treatment of Crohn's disease of the colon. *Ann R Coll Surg Engl*. 1975; 56:94.

28. Lyttle JA, Parks AG. Intersphincteric excision of the rectum. *Br J Surg*. 1977;64:413–416.

29. Morrison JG, Gathright JB, Ray JE, et al. Results of operation for rectovaginal fistula in Crohn's disease. *Dis Colon Rectum*. 1989;32:497–499.

30. Radcliffe AG, Richie JK, Hawley PR, et al. Anovaginal and rectovaginal fistulas in Crohn's disease. *Dis Colon Rectum*. 1988;31:94–99.

31. Fry R, Shemesh EI, Kodner IJ, et al. Techniques and results in the management of anal and perianal Crohn's disease. *Surg Gynecol Obstet*. 1989;168: 42–48.

32. Jone IT, Fazio VW, Jagelman DG. The use of transanal rectal advancement flaps in the management of fistulas involving the anorectum. *Dis Colon Rectum*. 1987;30:919–923.

33. Sher ME, Bauer JJ, Gelernt I. Surgical repair of rectovaginal fistulas in patients with Crohn's disease: transvaginal approach. *Dis Colon Rectum*. 1991;34:641–648.

CHAPTER 26

OTHER PROCTITIDES

Richard L. Whelan

Included in the varied group assembled here as "other" proctitides are conditions caused by infectious agents, radiation injury, fecal diversion, medications, and a large number whose etiology is unknown. A number of these conditions are found almost exclusively in specific patient populations such as the immunocompromised, but others are found in patients without apparent risk factors. For the most part, the symptoms produced by these varied conditions are nonspecific and include diarrhea, abdominal pain, and tenesmus. Although the majority of these conditions are medically treated, surgery is occasionally indicated. A few inflammatory conditions involve the rectum alone, but the vast majority of these diseases involve varying lengths of the colon as well. In a similar fashion, inflammatory conditions that primarily involve the colon can, at times, also extend into the rectum. Therefore, a thorough discussion of the proctitides, by necessity, must include mention of many of the colitides.

It is not possible to cover each of these conditions in depth. The more commonly seen proctitides and the more recently identified conditions have been emphasized. Where appropriate the reader is referred to other chapters in this text. For more detailed information the reader is referred to the references and to specialty textbooks in the fields of infectious disease and gastroenterology.

General Evaluation

It is helpful to have a well thought out and organized approach to the patient with proctitis or colitis. The recommended evaluation can be broken down into five parts which, for the most part, should be carried out in sequence. The evaluation should include (1) a thorough history, (2) immediate anorectal and sigmoidoscopic examination, (3) stool cultures and analysis as well as specific serologic tests, (4) complete colonic examination with biopsies if necessary, and, rarely (5) upper gastrointestinal evaluation. Most patients will not require the entire sequence of tests. For example, if the diagnosis can be established by sigmoidoscopy, then colonoscopy and upper GI evaluation would most likely not be necessary.

History

As with any medical evaluation, a thorough history is vital to narrowing the differential diagnosis. A careful GI history, including questions concerning diarrhea, constipation, blood or mucus per rectum, painful defecation, or any recent change in bowel habits, should be obtained. If diarrhea is present, it is important to determine the number of bowel movements per day. The extent and character of rectal bleeding, if present, must also be determined. Questions regarding the presence of fever, malaise, weight loss, and other constitutional symptoms should also be asked. The duration of the symptoms and a history of similar complaints or of other colorectal disorders should be established.

A history of a malignancy and its subsequent treatment may provide information vital to making the diagnosis. Previous pelvic irradiation or recent chemotherapy may well account for a patient's symptoms. A history of recent travel or of exposure to person(s) with gastrointestinal infections should be sought. A complete list of the patient's medications, including nonsteroidal antiinflammatory drugs, recent antibiotic therapy, or recent chemotherapy should be obtained since these agents can cause proctitis or colitis. Questions regarding the patient's sexual activities, especially anorectal intercourse, must be asked. Finally, immunocompromised patients should be identified because they are at risk for developing certain specific infections such as cytomegalovirus (CMV), herpes simplex virus (HSV), and cryptosporodiosis.

Anorectal and Sigmoidoscopic Evaluation

This evaluation should be carried out at the initial patient encounter. Enemas should be avoided when an infectious etiology is under consideration, as this may purge the rectum of organisms. The examination should begin with a visual inspection of the perianal area. The presence and location of fissures and fistulas should be noted. Erythema, edema, and superficial ulceration of the perianal skin may be secondary to diarrhea or they may be related to a primary pathologic process such as herpes or syphillis.

A digital examination follows inspection: tenderness, induration, or fluctuance may indicate an abscess or perirectal infection. Bidigital palpation is performed with the index finger in the anus and the thumb on the perianal skin. This is the best clinical means of localizing anorectal infection. It is important to note the sphincter tone as well as the presence of stenosis or stricture. Anorectal masses, if present, should be well characterized.

Anoscopy allows thorough evaluation of the anal canal. Internal fistulous openings, fissures, ulcerations, masses, and internal hemorrhoids should be sought. Although complex fistulous disease in a patient with persistent or recurrent diarrhea is suggestive of inflammatory bowel disease, it may also be caused by a specific infection such as amebiasis, tuberculosis, or actinomycoses.

Sigmoidoscopy should be performed as part of the initial evaluation. A bowel preparation should not be carried out as it may interfere with the collection and recovery of infectious agents. Although a rigid sigmoidoscopy will suffice, a flexible examination is preferable because sigmoiditis may exist despite the presence of normal rectal mucosa distally. If moderate to severe colitis is encountered at any point during the examination, further insertion of the endoscope should be avoided since there is a significant risk of perforation. The main goal of the sigmoidoscopic examination is to establish the presence of inflammation. Once this has been done, little is to be gained from more proximal examination of the bowel. The endoscopic findings, including the size, shape, location, and extent of all mucosal lesions should be carefully noted. Likewise, the presence of mucosal erythema, petechial hemorrhages, echymoses, erosions, ulcerations, and friable or easily bruised mucosa should be documented. Finally, mention must be made of any blood, purulence, or exudate found on examination. Cultures and other analyses can be sent from stool, mucosal biopsies, and other material recovered during endoscopy.

Stool and Blood Tests

With few exceptions, stool for culture and analysis should be routinely obtained. Routine stool cultures for enteric pathogens will detect *Salmonella typhi*, *Shigella*, and *Aeromonas hydrophelia*. In some institutions, cultures for *Campylobacter jejuni* and *Yersinia enterocolitica* must be specifically requested since they are not routinely performed. Because bacteria are intermittently shed in the stool, the detection rate from a single bacterial culture is low. For this reason, it is recommended that at least three separate specimens from different bowel movements be sent for bacterial cultures. Stool specimens for bacterial culture should be immediately placed in an appropriate transport medium that allows for room temperature storage and delayed delivery without adversely affecting the detection rate. Final results should be available 2 to 4 days after the plating of the specimens.

In patients at risk for gonococcal proctitis, an anorectal swab should be sent in a culturette for gonococcal culture. Swabs of mucopurulent discharge have a much higher yield than do blind swabs. Specimens for chlamydial culture must be obtained with a cotton-tipped metal swab and placed into specific transport media.

In the vast majority of patients it is not necessary to perform fungal cultures. Fungal anorectal infections are rare and usually occur in immunocompromised patients. The detection of fungal pathogens requires special stool cultures.

Viral stool cultures need not be routinely obtained; however, they should be obtained in immunosuppressed patients and homosexual men. In these patients, viral proctocolitis is common, most often due to herpes simplex and cytomegalovirus. Viral pathogens are most difficult to culture, and a specific transport medium must be used to deliver viral specimens. Most viral transport media must remain frozen until one half hour before the specimen is obtained. Furthermore, the transport medium must be processed or at least refrigerated within several hours of collection. Separate cultures are required for each particular virus. However, a single specimen in transport medium can be used for several cultures. Viral cultures take up to 4 weeks for final results.

Collection and culture techniques differ among laboratories. It is important to find out both the specific transport media and the collection techniques recommended by one's local laboratory.

Stool specimens for "ova and parasite" evaluation are

not cultured but are microscopically analyzed for the various parasites. Because of intermittent shedding three specimens from different bowel movements are recommended. A number of transport media are currently in use which allow for delayed transport (up to several days). A commonly used system involves polyvinyl alcohol (PVA) and a 10 percent formalin solution. Stool from a single bowel movement is placed in a container of each solution. The two containers comprise a single "specimen." Results can usually be obtained in a single day provided the analysis is carried out immediately.

Stool for *Clostridium difficile* toxin titers should be obtained from any patient with a history of current or recent antibiotic usage or chemotherapy. Where available, cultures for *C. difficile* can be helpful in establishing the diagnosis of pseudomembranous colitis.

Stool smears can also be examined for polymorphonuclear leukocytes. This information is useful since PMNs are found in the stool in certain bacterial and parasitic infections. In addition, Gram stains of rectal swabs may be used to presumptively diagnose gonorrhea. This issue is further discussed in Chapter 21.

In patients who practice anorectal intercourse a VDRL should be obtained. If appropriate, an HIV test (following informed consent) should be carried out. Other serologic tests, such as the gel diffusion precipitate test (for amebiasis), counterimmune electrophoresis, and ELISAs are also available for specific organisms.

Colonic Evaluation

If the foregoing evaluation has not led to a diagnosis or confirmed the presence of a significant proctitis or colitis then a complete colonic evaluation is indicated. Certain colitides have a predilection for the proximal colon and will be missed if only a sigmoidoscopy is performed (*C. difficile*, amebiasis, mycobacterial infections, *Yersinia enterocolitica*, etc.). Although a contrast examination of the colon is acceptable, a colonoscopy is preferred. Besides allowing a full visual mucosal inspection, endoscopy allows for tissue biopsies and sampling of the luminal fluid. The procedure should be discontinued once moderate to severe colitis is encountered because proximal examination beyond a colitic segment risks colonic injury and perforation.

Upper Gastrointestinal Evaluation

Esophagogastroduodenoscopy and an upper GI series can be helpful in the evaluation of persistent diarrhea. These are the evaluations of choice for the diagnosis of sprue and malabsorption.

Infectious Etiologies

Clostridium Difficile

C. difficile infection can cause problems ranging from mild diarrhea to severe pseudomembranous colitis with perforation and sepsis. The majority of cases are seen following antibiotic usage. The remaining cases (10 percent) include patients receiving chemotherapy, patients with inflammatory bowel disease, and a group of patients with a variety of other medical problems.[1-10] *C. difficile* has been implicated in only 20 to 40 percent of cases of antibiotic associated colitis and diarrhea.[11-13] Therefore, despite the attention focused on antibiotic-related *C. difficile* overgrowth, most antibiotic-associated diarrhea is not caused by this organism.

Almost all antibiotics—the exceptions being the aminoglycosides and vancomycin—have been associated with *C. difficile* infection.[14-16] The most commonly implicated agents are ampicillin, clindamycin, and the cephalosporins. Neither the antibiotic dosage nor the length of administration has been found to correlate with the development of *C. difficile* infection. The majority of *C. difficile* infections occur 5 to 7 days into the course of antibiotics, but 25 to 33 percent of cases present 4 to 6 weeks after cessation of the antimicrobials.[11,17,18]

It is thought that *C. difficile*, an obligate anaerobic gram-positive bacillus, colonizes the colon after the native bacterial flora has been modified by antibiotics. *C. difficile* has the capability of producing toxins, most notably toxin A (enterotoxin) and toxin B (cytotoxin), which are thought to be responsible for the diarrhea and colitis associated with infection.[19] The exact mechanism by which this occurs is unknown. Non-toxin-producing *C. difficile* has been found in 2 to 3 percent of healthy adults and in 11 percent of hospitalized patients without diarrhea.[11,17,20,21] It is not clear how the organism gains access to the gastrointestinal tract. The most likely source is the hospital environment where *C. difficile* has been found to be a common contaminant.[22]

Clinical Presentation and Physical Findings

The clinical presentation depends on the severity of disease. Diarrhea is the most common symptom and is found in 90 to 95 percent of cases.[23] The diarrhea in most cases is watery, often with abundant mucus. In 10 to 15 percent of patients diarrhea with gross or occult blood is found.[1,23] The number of bowel movements per day varies widely; 80 percent of patients have 4 to 10 movements daily.[1] Patients with mild disease may present with diarrhea alone, but most will have a low grade fever and crampy abdominal pain as well. These pa-

480   Fundamentals of Anorectal Surgery

tients may have mild direct tenderness and an otherwise unremarkable abdominal examination; however, up to 20 percent may have rebound tenderness.[18] A small percentage of patients develop fulminant colitis with high fever and severe abdominal pain.[24] Diarrhea may be absent in patients with severe disease who develop an ileus or toxic megacolon. Impressive abdominal distention may develop in these patients. Hypotension, oliguria, and other manifestations of septic shock may also be found in these profoundly ill patients.

Endoscopic and Laboratory Findings

All patients suspected of having *C. difficile* infection should be evaluated endoscopically. The mucosal findings vary with the severity of disease. In those with mild or moderate disease endoscopy most often reveals normal mucosa or nonspecific inflammatory changes.[25] In the great majority of those with severe disease examination demonstrates the classic pseudomembranes which are round, punctate yellow or whitish lesions, 2 to 5 mm in diameter (Fig. 26-1). These lesions may occur singly or in clusters.[1,18] The mucosa surrounding the lesions is usually edematous and erythematous.

The presence of pseudomembranes is not limited to those with severe colitis. In one study pseudomembranes were found in 23 percent of patients with mild disease.[1] The converse is also true; membranes may be absent in up to 30 percent of those with the most severe

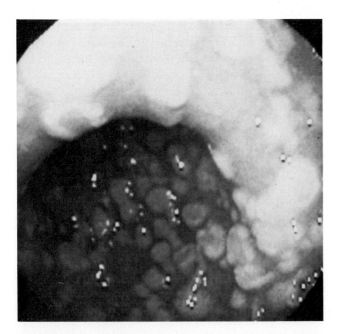

Figure 26-1. Endoscopic appearance of classic pseudomembranes of pseudomembranous colitis. (Courtesy of Jessie Eisenman, M.D., and Eli Ehrenpreis, M.D., Ft. Lauderdale, FL.)

clinical presentation. In the majority of patients membranes are present distally within reach of the rigid or flexible sigmoidoscope. A small percentage of patients will have mucosal findings limited to the right colon. This has prompted some investigators to recommend complete colonoscopy for patients suspected of having pseudomembranous colitis who are found to have a normal distal colonic examination.[26-28] Although the finding of pseudomembranes almost certainly confirms the diagnosis of pseudomembranous colitis, biopsy of these lesions is recommended to definitively establish the diagnosis.[29]

The white blood cell count (WBC) may be normal or elevated. Eighty percent of those with pseudomembranous colitis have WBCs between 10,000 and 20,000 per mm^3. Microscopic examination of stool may reveal fecal leukocytes.[30]

Currently, the most reliable laboratory tests for documenting *C. difficile* infection are the toxin assay and stool cultures. Controversy exists as to which of these techniques is more reliable. There is a very high correlation between the presence of toxin in the stool and clinical *C. difficile* disease.[31] This assay tests the ability of toxin B (cytotoxin) to induce cytopathic changes in tissue culture cells. For a test to be considered positive, not only must the toxin's cytopathic effect be observed, it must also be demonstrated that this effect is inhibited by the addition of clostridial antitoxin to the culture medium.[32] The finding of stool cultures positive for *C. difficile* also correlates highly with clinically significant infection. Isolation of *C. difficile* from feces requires a selective medium that permits the growth of this organism while inhibiting the myriad of other bacteria found in stool. Cultures, however, do not distinguish between toxin-producing and non-toxin-producing organisms. Only toxin-producing strains produce clinical disease. Therefore, a small but substantial number of false-positives are found if cultures alone are relied upon for diagnosis. The consensus is that the toxin assay is the preferred single test.[8,33,34] However, most investigators recommend that, when available, both tests be carried out.[13,18,35] In addition, as previously mentioned, if endoscopic evaluation has revealed typical mucosal lesions biopsy should be performed. Superficial necrosis with an acute inflammatory mucosal exudate is the most typical finding (Fig. 26-2).

Immunoassays have been developed in recent years to detect either *C. difficile* toxins or toxin-specific antibodies.[36] Immunoassays are rapid tests that can be completed within a few hours in most hospital laboratories. The three types of *C. difficile* immunoassays developed thus far are counterimmunoelectrophoresis (CIE), latex agglutination, and enzyme-linked immunosorbent assays (ELISAs); none has been shown to be as consistently reliable as the toxin titer assay. It remains to be

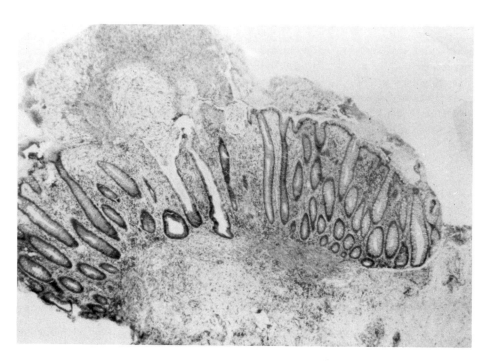

Figure 26-2. Histopathologic appearance of pseudomembranous colitis showing superficial necrosis and acute inflammatory mucosal exudate. The appearance of this exudate reveals the microscopic nature of the macroscopic pseudomembrane. (Hematoxylin and eosin, ×60.) (Courtesy of Robert Petras, M.D., Cleveland, OH.)

seen what future role these tests will have in the diagnosis of C. difficile disease.[13]

Treatment

When C. difficile infection occurs in patients receiving antibiotics, the offending antibiotic should be immediately discontinued if possible. In patients with mild disease no other specific treatment is necessary.[1,37] In these cases the diarrhea usually resolves within days. In all cases, adequate rehydration of the patient must be carried out. Bowel rest is recommended for patients with moderate or severe disease. Most authors agree that antimotility agents are contraindicated.[24] These agents have anecdotally been linked to the development of toxic megacolon when used in patients with C. difficile disease.

Empiric antimicrobial treatment should be begun if there is strong clinical and endoscopic evidence that moderate to severe infection is present.[18] Three orally administered antimicrobials have been shown to be effective against C. difficile intestinal infection: vancomycin, metronidazole, and bacitracin.[38] Vancomycin is considered by most to be the drug of choice. In most patients, a significant improvement will occur within 2 to 5 days after treatment is begun.[39,40] The recommended dosage is 0.5 to 2.0 g per day, in divided doses, for 7 to 10 days. The main drawbacks to vancomycin therapy are the high cost and the bad taste of this drug.

Metronidazole is generally well tolerated and is much less expensive than vancomycin. The recommended dosage is 1.0 to 1.5 g per day for 7 to 10 days. Metronidazole, unlike vancomycin, is absorbed rapidly from the GI tract and consequently fecal concentrations are low. Despite this, metronidazole has been shown to successfully ameliorate symptoms in 95 percent of patients following 2 days of treatment.[8] It has been reported to be as effective as vancomycin in several series.[1,41]

Bacitracin has been shown to be as effective a treatment as vancomycin when 20–25,000 units were given four times a day for 7 days.[37] Unfortunately, there is a paucity of published reports[42,43] regarding the efficacy of bacitracin in this setting.

In patients unable to take antimicrobials orally adequate delivery of drugs directed against C. difficile has been a problem. Intravenous metronidazole appears to be the most effective. Adequate fecal concentrations of metronidazole have been documented in patients with severe colitis after intravenous administration of this antimicrobial.[44]

Anion exchange resins have also been used successfully to treat C. difficile infection. Cholestyramine and colestipol, each given orally for 10 days, are thought to bind the C. difficile toxin in the lumen, thereby limiting the damage caused by the toxins. Colestipol is four times as effective as cholestyramine.[18] These agents have not proved to be as reliable as antimicrobials, and therefore it is recommended that they not be used as sole treatment except in cases of mild infection. It is also important that these resins are not given concomitantly with antibiotics since they have been shown to bind to antimicrobials in the intestinal lumen.

With adequate medical therapy surgical intervention is rarely needed. However, surgery may be necessary for patients in whom a perforation is suspected or those with toxic megacolon. Since a signficant number of patients with severe colitis have rebound tenderness without perforation a trial of initial observation and administration of appropriate antimicrobials is usually indicated.[45] When surgery is necessary subtotal colectomy with ileostomy or fecal diversion via end ileostomy and mucous fistula are the most commonly performed procedures.[24,46,47]

Relapse

Regardless of the type of treatment rendered, symptomatic recurrences are seen in 14 to 25 percent of patients. For this reason, most investigators recommend repeat toxin titers or cultures following treatment. Most suggest a second and longer course of antimicrobials for patients who have a symptomatic relapse. Some recommend a course of cholestyramine or colestipol after the antimicrobials. Recurrent infection is as responsive to antimicrobial treatment as are primary infections. Unfortunately, up to one third of patients who relapse once will have further recurrences.

Salmonella

The *Salmonella* species, of which *Salmonella typhi* is the best known, are motile gram-negative rods which can invade the small bowel and colonic mucosa and induce an enterocolitis. The organisms elaborate an endotoxin that is thought to increase the local inflammatory response in areas of invasion.[48] In most patients, the organisms penetrate the mucosa and gain access to the lymphatics from which they may invade the bloodstream.

Salmonella are widely found in animals. Transmission is usually via ingestion of contaminated food or water although spread through fecal–oral contact can also occur. Although infection can occur in any age group, children younger than 5 years have the highest incidence of infection.[49] As is the case with most orally ingested pathogenic bacteria, patients with decreased gastric acid production, altered gut motility, or altered intestinal flora are at increased risk for infection.[50,51]

Infection becomes evident within 48 hours of ingestion in the majority of patients. Symptoms include diarrhea (in most cases nonbloody), nausea and vomiting, fever, chills, colicky abdominal pain, and tenesmus. In most, the diarrhea is self-limited and resolves in less than a week. A few patients develop enteric fever, bacteremia, or localized infections. One to three percent of infected individuals go on to become chronic asymptomatic carriers.[52,53]

Sigmoidoscopy reveals hyperemia and petechiae in most patients. Ulcerations may also occur. Biopsy specimens commonly demonstrate acute inflammation, edema, superficial erosions, or microabscesses.[54] Definitive diagnosis is usually made by stool cultures. Blood cultures will detect only those with enteric fever or bacteremia. Serologic tests, to date, are not generally helpful or reliable.[49]

As mentioned, in the majority of patients the disease is self-limited, and therefore, antimicrobial therapy is not necessary. However, it is important that adequate fluid and electrolyte replacement be administered. When antimicrobials are required, chloramphenicol, ampicillin, or bactrim can be given.[55] The use of antimicrobials may prolong the period of excretion of viable organisms in the stool after resolution of symptoms. Rarely, severe bleeding, fulminant enterocolitis, or toxic megacolon may develop.[54] In these cases surgery, usually bowel resection, may be necessary.

Shigella

Shigella are virulent gram-negative rods that invade the small bowel and colonic mucosa and cause a characteristic illness known as bacillary dysentery. *Shigella* are spread via ingestion of contaminated food and water and through person-to-person contact. Although invasive, the organisms remain superficial and rarely penetrate through the mucosa.

The symptoms and physical findings vary according to the anatomic location of the infection. The *Shigella* first infect and invade the small bowel causing crampy abdominal pain, high fever, and large volumes of watery diarrhea. On examination, hyperactive bowel sounds and mild abdominal tenderness are usually found at this stage. Usually within 2 days the infection will have moved on to the colon. Colonic involvement corresponds with the development of more severe lower abdominal pain, the onset of bloody mucoid diarrhea, urgency, and tenesmus.[56] Impressive abdominal tenderness in the lower quadrants is often found at this stage. In a significant percentage of patients the clinical presentation will mimic acute appendicitis.[57]

Shigellosis should be suspected whenever an acute diarrheal illness productive of bloody mucoid stools lasts longer than 2 days. The diagnosis is made by stool culture. Most laboratories routinely culture fecal specimens for *Shigella*. Techniques for immunofluorescent antibody labeling of organisms recovered or cultured are available but are not widely used.[56] Serologic testing during the acute illness is not helpful. Blood cultures are rarely positive. Sigmoidoscopy, when performed, often reveals inflamed, ecchymotic, friable, or ulcerated mucosa.

In most cases the illness is self-limited, lasting an average of 1 week.[58] However, untreated patients shed viable organisms for up to 1 month after the resolution of symptoms. Antibiotic treatment shortens the clinical illness and limits the time of active shedding of the organisms. For these reasons, most authors recommend antibiotic treatment. *Shigella* are usually sensitive to ampicillin, tetracycline, ciprofloxacin, or trimethoprim–sulfamethoxazole.[55,58] The antibiotic of choice is double-strength trimethoprim–sulfamethoxazole given by mouth twice daily for 7 days. Alternatively, a single 1.5 g oral dose of tetracycline *or* 500 mg ampicillin given by mouth four times daily for 7 days is also an acceptable regimen. Antimotility agents are contraindicated as with most other intestinal infections. Although dehydration is common, intravenous hydration is required in only a small percentage of patients. Symptomatic patients and screened asymptomatic carriers should be treated until proven cured by repeat stool cultures.

Yersinia

Yersinia enterocolitica and *Yersinia pseudotuberculosis* are nonplague *Yersinia* that may cause an enterocolitis which, at times, is confused with appendicitis. Only recently has it been recognized that these gram-negative rods are important intestinal pathogens. Transmission occurs most commonly from ingestion of contaminated food and water. Spread as a result of direct contact with infected animals or patients can also occur.

Clinical manifestations are usually seen within 1 week of ingestion. The most common symptoms are diarrhea (usually nonbloody), abdominal pain, and fever. Significant abdominal tenderness may also be present. The presentation can be confused with appendicitis in up to 40 percent of cases, as the terminal ileum is the area most commonly infected.[59] Although the enterocolitis is usually self-limited, on occasion, toxic megacolon may develop and perforation may occur.[60-62] Septicemia with metastatic abscesses to the liver, spleen, or other organs may also occur and is usually seen in patients with associated medical problems. Interestingly, a number of nonintestinal manifestations such as polyarthritis and erythema nodosum have also been reported to occur.[60]

Stool cultures are the most reliable means of establishing the diagnosis. In many laboratories *Yersinia* cultures must be specifically requested. The use of selective medium maximizes the detection rate.[63] If laparotomy is performed, cultures of peritoneal fluid or mesenteric lymph nodes will often grow out the organism. Serologic tests for *Yersinia* are available but are not widely used. Sigmoidoscopy is not likely to be helpful, but colonoscopy may reveal inflammation in the cecum or ascending colon.

As mentioned, *Yersinia* enterocolitis is usually self-limited, although, symptoms may persist for 1 to 3 weeks.[60] As with all diarrheal illnesses, adequate hydration must be provided. It is not clear that antibiotics

should be given in all cases. Clearly, patients with septicemia should receive antibiotics. Effective antibiotics include trimethoprim–sulfamethoxazole, aminoglycosides, tetracycline, chloramphenicol, and most third-generation cephalosporins.[55,60]

Campylobacter

Campylobacter jejuni is an invasive curved, motile, non-spore-forming gram-negative rod which can infect the small bowel and colon causing an enteritis or enterocolitis.[64,65] In Great Britain and the United States *Campylobacter jejuni* infections appear to be more common than either salmonellosis or shigellosis.[66] Consumption of contaminated food or water and direct contact with infected individuals or animals are the means of transmission. Infection is seen in all age groups, but the highest incidence is found in infants.[67]

The most common symptoms are diarrhea, abdominal pain, and fever. The diarrhea may be bloody or nonbloody and varies widely in severity. Abdominal pain tends to be colicky in nature and can be localized to any part of the abdomen. It can be confused with appendicitis when right lower quadrant pain predominates. In the majority of patients the illness is self-limited; however, a small percentage go on to develop prolonged illness or complications. Toxic megacolon has been reported to occur.[68]

In most patients, microscopic examination of fecal smears reveals polymorphonuclear leukocytes and red blood cells. A presumptive diagnosis can be made if phase-contrast or dark-field microscopy of fresh fecal specimens demonstrates rapidly moving, curved, rod-shaped organisms. Similarly, Gram stains demonstrating vibrio forms are highly suggestive of *Campylobacter* infection.[64] However, stool culture is the only means of definitively establishing the diagnosis. In many laboratories stool specimens are not routinely cultured for *Campylobacter* and therefore specific requests are necessary. In most cases, sigmoidoscopy reveals a nonspecific colitis characterized by erythema and edema although apthous ulcerations may also be seen. Histologically, a nonspecific acute inflammatory infiltrate in the lamina propria with crypt abscesses, ulceration, and atrophy may be observed. Extraintestinal symptoms include arthralgias and tender hepatosplenomegaly.[69,70]

As mentioned, the illness is usually self-limited; antimotility agents should be avoided. It is not clear that antibiotic therapy is necessary for all cases.[71] However, presumptive treatment with antibiotics in very sick or high-risk patients is reasonable if *C. jejuni* is suspected after dark-field microscopy or Gram stain. This organism is usually sensitive to erythromycin, tetracycline, gentamicin, chloramphenicol, clindamycin, or ciprofloxacin.[55,64] The preferred regimen is 500 mg erythromycin given orally four times a day for 1 week. Alternatively, 500 mg tetracycline may be given orally four times a day for 1 week. Relapses occur in 5 to 10 percent of cases.

Entamoeba Histolytica

It is estimated that 10 percent of the earth's population is infested with *Entamoeba histolytica*. In the United States the carrier rate is estimated to be as high as 5 percent.[71,72] In certain subpopulations, especially immigrants and homosexual men, the infestation rate is significantly higher.[73-75] Interestingly, symptomatic disease develops in only a small percentage of carriers.[76] The disease is limited to a mild dysentery in the great majority of patients who develop symptoms. However, in a small percentage of patients fulminant amebic colitis ensues, and it is in this group that surgery may be necessary.[77-80]

The adult parasite, or trophozoite, populates the colon. Both trophozoites and an encysted form of the organism are intermittently shed in the stool. Although trophozoites quickly die outside the body, the cysts do not. Infection occurs when these cysts find their way into food or drinking water, usually via asymptomatic carriers. The ingested cysts release their trophozoites in the small bowel which then populate the colon. In general, they survive by feeding on bacteria and superficial mucosal cells. In a small percentage of patients the ameba invade the colonic wall. In 60 to 70 percent of cases a pancolitis is present; in the remaining patients infection is localized to one or several segments of colon.[81,82] The most commonly involved colonic segments, in descending order of frequency, are the cecum, the ascending colon, the rectum, and the sigmoid colon.[83-86]

The majority of symptomatic patients have mild disease manifested by diarrhea (possibly bloody) and mild abdominal pain and tenderness. Tenesmus and a mild leukocytosis may also be present. In contrast, patients with severe disease usually have frankly bloody diarrhea as well as severe abdominal pain and signficant tenderness. Fever, tachycardia, dehydration, and other evidence of systemic toxicity are also usually present.[76]

Diagnosis

The most commonly used test for diagnosing amebic colitis is the examination of stool for ameba. Motile trophozoites containing ingested red blood cells (hemocytophagia) must be demonstrated to make the diagnosis. Stool examination should be done within 20 minutes of collection if no transport medium is used. If multiple samples are submitted and special preparation of the specimens is carried out by the laboratory the

Table 26-1   Substances That Interfere With Stool Examination for Ameba

Barium sulfate
Enemas
Mineral oil
Castor oil
Bismuth
Kaolin compounds (Kaopectate, etc.)
Tetracycline
Sulfonamides
Metronidazole
Antiparasitic medications
Magnesium hydroxide antacids

detection rate can be as high as 92 percent.[72] It is important to note that there are numerous substances including cathartics and enemas which interfere with stool examination for ameba (Table 26-1). The use of these agents before endoscopy should be avoided in these patients.

A number of serologic tests can be used to diagnose amebic infection, including the indirect hemagglutination test, the indirect immunoelectrophoresis test, and an enzyme-linked immunosorbent assay (ELISA). Using these tests, antibodies or antigens can be detected in 82 to 91 percent of patients with amebic colitis. A positive test result is not necessarily indicative of acute disease since both patients with remote infection and asymptomatic carriers may test positive.[87,88]

Endoscopic evaluation of the colon should be performed. Sigmoidoscopy is sufficient for the majority of patients since distal disease is present in up to 85 percent.[89] The remaining patients will require colonoscopy to document more proximal disease. Findings vary; diffuse erythema and mild nonspecific changes may be all that is found (Fig. 26-3). The "classic" findings are round ulcerations ("flask-shaped" on microscopic section), 2 mm to 2 cm in diameter, covered with a yellow exudate and with normal-appearing mucosa between ulcers[76,88] (Fig. 26-4). The ulcer has a small mucosal opening with a wider base in the submucosa or muscularis propria. Biopsies of the ulcer margins should be obtained for pathology. Examination of endoscopically obtained stool and mucus samples for trophozoites will document amebic infection in up to 85 percent of cases.[72,76,89]

Treatment

The specific treatment chosen for intestinal amebiasis depends on the severity of disease. Metronidazole is the treatment of choice for most patients because it is the

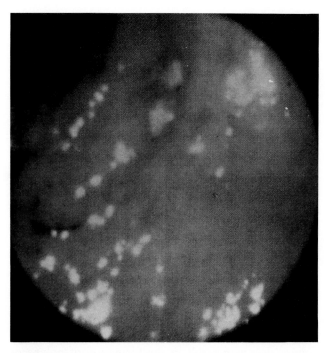

Figure 26-3. Endoscopic view of nonspecific ulcerations of *Entamoeba histolytica*.

only orally administered drug that provides amebicidal concentrations both systemically and in the bowel lumen. The usual course is 750 mg given orally twice a day for 10 days. Intravenous metronidazole does not provide amebicidal levels in the intestinal lumen. Patients with severe colitis who cannot tolerate oral agents must be given intramuscular dehydroemetine di-

hydrochloride or emetine hydrochloride; these are the only parenterally administered drugs that provide adequate tissue and luminal drug concentrations. Adverse cardiac effects are often associated with both of these agents; frequent electrocardiograms are advisable during a course of treatment. Oral metronidazole should be substituted for these drugs as soon as possible.[76,90,91] It is important to note that a course of iodoquinol, 650 mg given orally three times a day for 3 weeks, is necessary after completion of primary therapy, regardless of the drug used, to ensure full eradication of amebic cysts from the colonic lumen.[76,90] Asymptomatic carriers need receive only oral diiodohydroxyquine, 650 mg given orally three times a day for 3 weeks.[92]

Fulminant Colitis

In 3 to 11 percent of symptomatic patients fulminant colitis develops and most often results in perforation requiring surgery.[77-80,93,94] In this setting, toxic dilatation of the colon may be present.[95-98] The correct diagnosis is rarely made preoperatively. Most authorities agree that segmental or total abdominal colectomy with diverting ileostomy or colostomy is necessary, but this opinion is controversial. The involved colon is most often friable and grossly necrotic with numerous perforations.[76,88,95,99] Primary anastomosis should not be attempted in these gravely ill patients. Despite such operative treatment, the mortality of fulminant disease ranges from 66 to 83 percent.[88,94,99]

It is recommended that intravenous metronidazole be given preoperatively to patients in whom the diagnosis

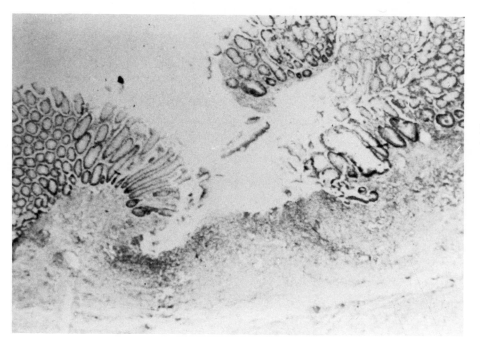

Figure 26-4. "Classic" flask-shaped ulcer noted on histopathologic examination of amebic ulcer. (Hematoxylin and eosin, ×60.) (Reprinted with permission from Corman ML, ed. *Colon and Rectal Surgery.* 2nd ed. Philadelphia: JB Lippincott; 1992.)

of fulminant colitis is being entertained. It is hoped that empiric preoperative antiamebic therapy may improve the results of surgical treatment.

It has been proposed that bacterial synergism is necessary in order for fulminant amebic colitis to develop.[76,88,100] For this reason, some investigators recommend instituting broad spectrum antibiotics in addition to antiamebic agents for fulminant disease.[88]

Ameboma

An inflammatory mass known as an ameboma may develop and can be difficult to distinguish from a carcinoma. These lesions have a fibrous outer wall and contain hyperplastic lymphatic tissue, acute inflammatory cells, trophozoites, and necrotic debris.[83,86,87] These granulomatous lesions may cause an acute inflammatory or a chronic fibrous stricture (Fig. 26-5). They rarely cause complete obstruction. Rarely, significant hemorrhage may occur or the ameboma may act as the leading edge of an intussusception.

The most common location for amebomas is the cecum, followed by the sigmoid colon. These lesions may present as a right lower quadrant mass and be confused with an appendiceal abscess. Amebomas are usually found on barium enema or endoscopy. In the absence of perforation or complete obstruction these lesions should be treated nonoperatively as the great majority will resolve with appropriate amebicidal therapy.[76,87] Those that do not resolve must be reevaluated and biopsied so as not to overlook a neoplasm. Al-

though quite rare, anorectal abscesses and fistulas have been reported to occur.[83,86]

Schistosoma

Schistosomiasis is caused by the trematodes *Schistosoma mansoni*, *S. japonicum*, and *S. haematobium*. All three species can cause rectal and colonic disease although the latter organism has a predilection for the bladder. The adult worms, which reside in the bloodstream, lay their eggs in the mesenteric or vesicular venules. The eggs secrete proteolytic enzymes which allow them to erode through the mesentery and into the bowel wall. Many traverse the full thickness of the bowel wall and enter the lumen.[101] Symptoms referrable to acute colonic involvement include abdominal pain, diarrhea, and rectal bleeding.

Chronic colonic schistosomiasis may predispose to adenocarcinoma, as dysplasia has been noted in a high percentage of such patients.[102] In addition, eggs trapped in the bowel wall can incite a severe inflammatory response that may result in the formation of polyps or strictures. These lesions, found most often in the rectosigmoid, can bleed or obstruct.[103] Finally rectal prolapse and anorectal fistula have also been reported to occur.[101,104,105]

Diagnosis is usually established by identifying the eggs of these trematodes in stool specimens. Endoscopy may reveal a friable, erythematous, and granular mucosa with punctate hemorrhages and superficial ulcerations. Proctoscopic biopsy may be diagnostic since

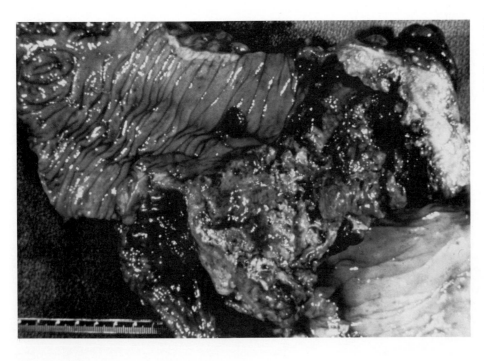

Figure 26-5. Gross appearance of an obstructing colonic ameboma. Note resemblance to malignant neoplasia.

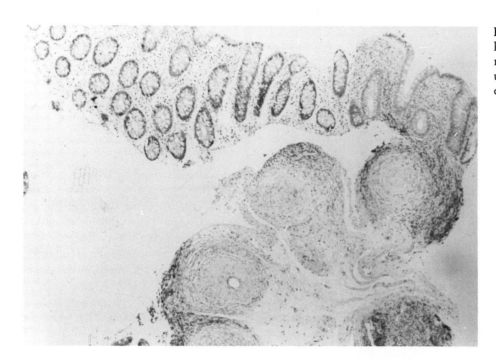

Figure 26-6. Histopathologic appearance of intramural schistosomial granulomata. (Hematoxylin and eosin, ×60.)

eggs from all three species can often be identified in the mucosa and submucosa of rectal biopsy specimens (Fig. 26-6). The drug of choice for all species is praziquantel.[101,103,106]

Large or symptomatic polyps may require colonoscopic removal.[107] Those patients with clinically significant colonic stricture will most likely require resection.[104] Patients with acute bowel obstruction will also require surgery. Proximal diversion should be strongly considered whenever primary anastomosis is performed since high anastomotic leakage rates have been reported.[108] If possible, patients scheduled to undergo surgery should receive full preoperative praziquantel treatment.

Trypanasoma Cruzi (Chagas' Disease)

Trypanasoma cruzi is a protozoan that causes an illness in humans referred to as Chagas' disease. Humans are most often infected by insects of the subfamily Triatominae. The acute phase of the disease lasts 2 to 4 months. The chronic phase of the illness follows and persists for the patient's lifetime. The gastrointestinal manifestations of this disease, mainly megacolon and megaesophagus, usually become evident many years after the acute infection.[109] The most commonly involved segments of bowel are the sigmoid colon and rectum.[110] Intestinal dilatation is thought to result from the destruction of the autonomic nerve plexuses of the intestinal wall that occurs during the acute phase of infection. Microscopically, significant but not complete

destruction of Auerbach's myenteric and Meissner's submucosal plexuses are found.[111]

The most common presenting symptoms are progressive constipation and obstipation. Sigmoid volvulus occurs in 10 to 27 percent of patients with megacolon.[112,113] Contrast enema usually reveals a markedly dilated sigmoid colon and rectum (Fig. 26-7). A complement fixation test, known as the Machado–Guerreiro test, can confirm the diagnosis in the chronic stage.[109,110]

Controversy exists as to the best operation for Chagasic megacolon. Most agree that rectosigmoid resection is necessary. If more proximal colon is dilated, that too should be resected. A variety of different techniques can be used to restore distal continuity including low colorectal anastomosis, coloanal anastomoses, or a modified two-stage Duhamel procedure.[110,111] Dehiscence has been a significant problem with all techniques involving immediate anastomosis. This has led many to recommend two- or three-stage procedures.[110,113,114] Currently, the most popular technique is the modified two-stage Duhamel procedure.[110] This is discussed in Chapter 3.

Other Parasites

Although there are a great number of other intestinal parasites, relatively few involve the rectum. Trichuriasis can, on rare occasions, result in rectal prolapse. This infection is caused by the "whipworm" *Trichuris trichiura* and most often causes diarrhea. The adult worms

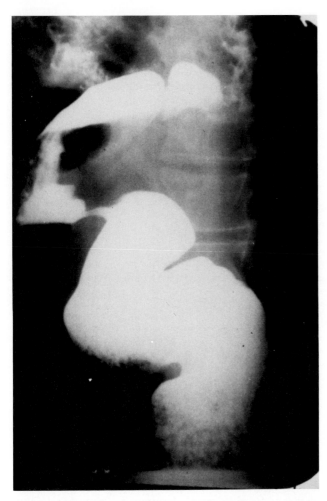

Figure 26-7. Barium enema: marked dilatation of the sigmoid colon and rectum, typical findings in Chagas' disease. Note abrupt transition to normal-diameter sigmoid colon.

usually reside in the transverse and descending colon, but in rare instances, large numbers of worms migrate to the rectum. The bulk of the worms in the rectum causes tenesmus which leads to excessive straining. Rectal prolapse may ultimately occur. The prolapse will resolve with proper medical therapy and does not require surgical intervention. Mebendazole is the treatment of choice.[115,116]

Balantidiasis, caused by the ciliate *Balantidium coli*, can lead to clinical and endoscopic findings similar to those seen with amebiasis. Crampy abdominal pain and diarrhea (with or without blood) are the predominant symptoms in the small percentage of carriers who develop clinical disease. Endoscopically, ulcerated lesions with raised margins, similar to the "flask-shaped" ulcers of amebiasis, are often found in the rectum or colon of symptomatic patients. The diagnosis is most often es-

tablished via stool analysis. Tetracylcine, iodoquinol, or metronidazole are all effective treatments.[117,118]

Noninfectious Etiologies
Diversion Colitis

Diversion colitis was first described by Glotzer and coworkers in 1981.[119] It is found in the out-of-circuit colon or rectum of patients in whom diverting stomas have been constructed. The nonexcluded proximal colon is normal in patients with this disease. Reestablishment of intestinal continuity results in full resolution of the inflammatory changes found in the distal bowel.

Little was known about the pathophysiology of this condition until recently. Attempts to identify an infectious or toxic etiologic agent have been unsuccessful. There are strong preliminary data to suggest that a deficiency of short chain fatty acids (SCFAs) in the excluded colon may be the cause of this disorder.[120] SCFAs are the by-products of bacterial fermentation of carbohydrates in the colonic lumen. They have been shown to be the preferred energy source of colonic mucosal cells.[121] Harig and associates demonstrated that the levels of SCFAs in the diverted colon are negligible and that daily irrigation with SCFA solutions in patients with diversion colitis resulted in significant endoscopic and microscopic abatement of the colitis.[120]

A recent prospective study found endoscopic evidence of colitis in 93 percent of patients with diversions.[122] The vast majority of these patients (92 percent) had mild to moderate colitis. Only 8 percent had endoscopic findings consistent with severe colitis. Although two retrospective studies have reported significant symptoms in 33 to 38 percent of patients with colitis, the prospective study mentioned above found that only 5 percent of patients were symptomatic.[122-124] Symptoms, when present, include rectal bleeding, frequent mucous discharge, and tenesmus.[125,126]

In most patients the colitis is discovered on routine endoscopic examination performed prior to colostomy closure. An air contrast barium enema, if performed, may reveal numerous mucosal nodules in the diverted bowel.[127] The colitis is usually found in the rectum and may extend into the more proximal diverted colon. However, rectal sparing has been reported.[128] The endoscopic and histologic findings are nonspecific and are listed in Table 26-2.[122,129-131] The inflammatory changes are confined to the mucosa and the lamina propria[131] (Fig. 26-8). In only one study were biopsies of both the in-circuit (proximal) and diverted large

Table 26-2 Endoscopic and Histologic Findings in Diversion Colitis

ENDOSCOPIC FINDINGS
Erythema (usually focal)
Contact irritation
Pale sessile polypoid lesions (nodularity)
Edema
Petechiae
Superficial ulcerations/erosions

HISTOLOGIC FINDINGS
Chronic inflammation
Acute inflammation
Lymphoid nodules/follicles
Epithelial degeneration/superficial ulceration
Crypt abcess
Glandular atrophy

bowel peformed.[122] Despite a normal endoscopic appearance, biopsies of the in-circuit colon demonstrated the same nonspecific mild histologic abnormalities found in the diverted segments with colitis.

In all reported cases, when the colostomy or ileostomy has been closed the colitis has quickly resolved.[132] It must be stressed that there is no need to treat asymptomatic patients found to have diversion colitis. However, the rare patient with significant symptoms can be treated with SCFA irrigations.[120,132] In patients in whom closure is not possible the colitic changes have been noted to persist for many years.[119,122,125,131] In one instance, a paraplegic patient who was not a candidate for closure came to proctectomy because of severe symptomatic diversion colitis.[131]

There is little justification to support an extensive evaluation prior to closure of the colostomy or ileostomy. Establishing the diagnosis of either inflammatory bowel disease or an infectious colitis would lead to a postponement of surgery. However, the chance of finding either disorder in an asymptomatic patient is exceedingly small.[122] Therefore, routine preoperative investigation is not recommended. However, the few patients who are either symptomatic or have a history of colitis should undergo a full evaluation.

Collagenous Colitis

Collagenous colitis is a rare condition that is characterized by profuse watery diarrhea often associated with abdominal cramps. Biopsies of the colon and rectum reveal a markedly thickened subepithelial band of collagen that may be responsible for the diarrhea.[133-135]

The etiology of collagenous colitis is unknown. The consensus of opinion is that the most likely cause of the diarrhea is the thickened collagen layer itself which impedes the mucosal absorption of water and electrolytes.[135-137]

Collagenous colitis most commonly occurs in women. Although it has been reported to occur in patients in their twenties, the majority of patients present in their late forties or fifties. Most patients have had symptoms for at least 2 years at the time of diagnosis.[134] As mentioned, the most common symptoms are watery, nonbloody diarrhea and intermittent abdominal cramping. Other reported symptoms include nausea, flatulence, and incontinence. The frequency and number of bowel movements varies considerably from patient to patient, ranging from 3 to 20 movements per day. In severe cases significant weight loss may occur.

Contrast studies of the colon are usually normal. A variety of nonspecific endoscopic findings have been reported: edema, hyperemia, pallor, and friability.[138-140] Many patients, however, have a normal mucosal examination.[136,141-144] Since the diagnosis is established histologically, rectal and colonic biopsies must be taken in all patients at risk, regardless of the mucosal appearance.

As mentioned, biopsies reveal an abnormally thickened subepithelial collagen layer. It has been established that the maximal thickness of this layer in control populations ranges from 4.6 microns to 6.9 microns.[145,146] The thickness of this layer (Fig. 26-9) in those with collagenous colitis ranges from 10 to 60 microns. This subepithelial thickening can be either pancolonic or patchy in distribution.[136,141-143] Other histologic findings include (1) focal areas of epithelial degeneration or erosion, (2) flattening of the surface epithelium, and (3) increased numbers of lymphocytes and plasma cells in the lamina propria.[134]

The natural history of collagenous colitis is highly variable. Symptoms may persist for years or spontaneously resolve.[147,148] In this latter group relapses may occur months or years later. Partial or complete resolution of the histologic findings has been documented during quiescent periods in some patients, whereas in others, the histologic changes persist despite fluctuations in clinical symptoms.

To date, there have been no controlled trials testing the efficacy of any of the therapeutic agents that have been suggested for the treatment of collagenous colitis. Drugs that have been used include sulfasalazine, mepacrine hydrochloride, systemic corticosteroids, corticosteroid enemas, bismuth subsalicylate, and narcotic-containing medications.[137,140-142,148,149] None of these agents has been consistently successful. Because spontaneous remissions do occur, it is difficult to judge the

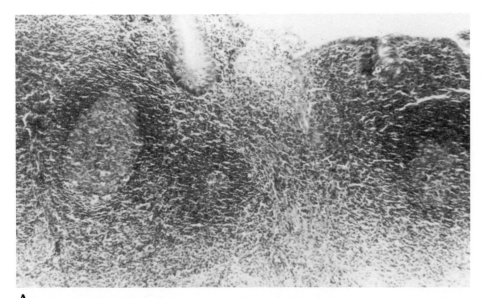

A

Figure 26-8. (A) Diversion colitis. Note the lymphoid aggregates limited to the mucosa with scattered cryptitis. (B) and (C) An uncommon case of diversion proctitis together with mucosal ulcerative colitis. Note the lymphoid aggregates and coexistent crypt abscesses. (Hematoxylin and eosin: Figs. A and B—×135; Fig. C—×60.) (Courtesy of Robert Petras, M.D., Cleveland, OH.

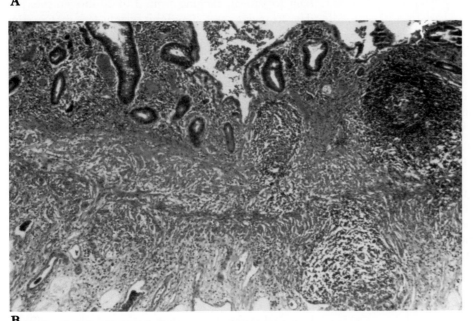

B

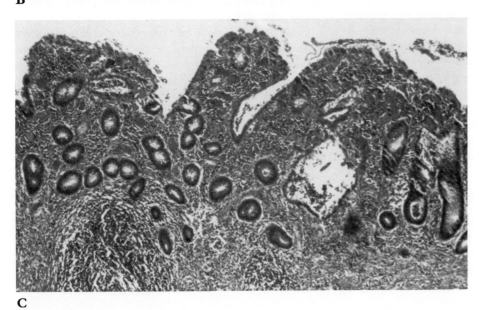

C

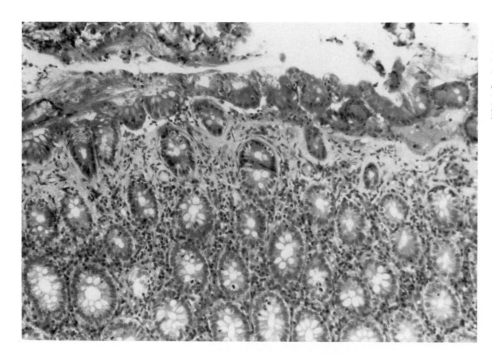

Figure 26-9. Thickening of the subepithelial collagen layer noted in collagenous colitis. (Hematoxylin and eosin, ×135.) (Courtesy of Robert Petras, M.D., Cleveland, OH.)

significance of individual case reports attributing resolution to a specific medication. There appears to be no role for surgery in the treatment of this disorder.

Colitis Cystica Profunda

Colitis cystica profunda is a benign inflammatory condition that demonstrates a number of clinical and histologic findings commonly seen in patients with the solitary rectal ulcer syndrome (see later discussion). Like the latter, this condition is often associated with defecatory disorders. In addition, the diagnosis is based on histologic findings. Although a diffuse form of this condition has been described, in the vast majority of cases the process is localized to a focal area of the rectum. Patients most often present with complaints of rectal bleeding, tenesmus, and mucous discharge. A history of constipation, straining at stool, or a sensation of incomplete evacuation can often be elicited. Examination, on occasion, may demonstrate complete rectal prolapse. Defecography, if performed, may reveal internal rectal prolapse, puborectalis dysfunction, or some other pelvic floor disorder.[150,151]

Endoscopy may reveal erythema, edema, polypoid lesions, contact irritation, or ulcerations. These findings are usually limited to a portion of the anterior rectal wall less than 3 cm in diameter.[150] Deep biopsy reveals the characteristic submucosal cysts which can be mistaken for malignant glands.[152,153] (Fig. 26-10). These mucin-containing cysts are located beneath the muscularis mucosae and are usually lined with benign-appearing epithelial cells. Other histologic findings include fibro-

muscular obliteration of the lamina propria and a prominent muscularis mucosae.[150,151] These latter changes are also found in patients with solitary rectal ulcer syndrome.

The natural history of colitis cystica profunda varies considerably. Symptoms and findings may persist for years or may resolve spontaneously; recurrences are not uncommon. If a full-thickness rectal prolapse is present, operative correction of the prolapse is indicated. Stuart reported resolution of rectal inflammation in 78 percent of patients thus treated.[154] However, if prolapse is not present a trial of medical treatment is initially indicated.

The mainstay of medical management is the regulation of bowel habits. This includes alterations in diet, the administration of fiber supplements, and avoidance of straining. For patients who are found to have anismus or the nonrelaxing puborectalis syndrome, biofeedback training may be of benefit. Medications, including corticosteroids and sulfasalazine, are not effective. If medical management is unsuccessful, transanal excision of the area in question can be carried out. Resolution of symptoms is reported to occur in up to 79 percent of patients following local excision.[151]

Medication-Related Colitis

A number of medications have been anecdotally associated with proctitis or colitis[155-165] (Table 26-3). Although this medication-related side effect is exceedingly rare it should be considered in patients with unexplained proctitis or colitis. In the majority of reported cases, the patients have had no prior history of colitis.

The symptoms and endoscopic findings usually resolve shortly after the offending medication is stopped. Interestingly, in patients with a history of inflammatory bowel disease, certain medications have been associated with reactivation of the colitis. This is further discussed in chapters 24 and 25.

Numerous nonsteroidal antiinflammatory drugs, (NSAIDs), including ibuprofen, naproxen, and meclomen, have been reported to cause proctitis and left-sided colitis.[155-158] The resulting diarrhea is most often bloody. The mechanism of injury is not clear although it has been suggested that the inhibition of prostaglandin or of prostaglandin synthesis may play a role.[157,158] NSAIDs have also been associated with relapses of ulcerative colitis.[159,160]

Intramuscular gold therapy for rheumatoid arthritis has been associated with colitis and enteritis in 21 cases.[162] Spontaneous perforation occurred in 10 per-

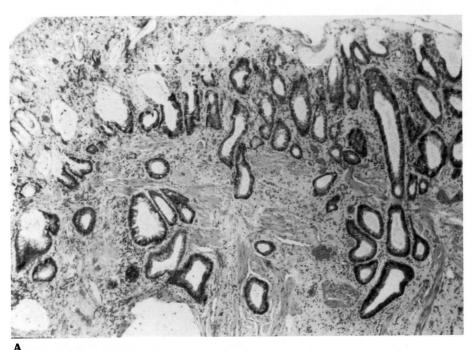

A

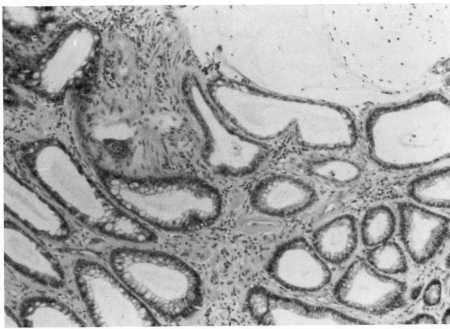
B

Figure 26-10.   (A) and (B) Histopathologic appearance of the characteristic submucosal cysts found in colitis cystica profunda. Note also the dissecting pools of mucus and the fibromuscular obliteration of the lamina propria. (Hematoxylin and eosin: Fig. A—×135; Fig. B—×190.) (Courtesy of Robert Petras, M.D., Cleveland, OH.)

Table 26-3   Medication-related Proctitis

Medication	Clinical Setting, Findings
Mefenamic acid (Ponstan)	Short-term or chronic use; diarrhea, hematochezia, proctitis or colitis
Meclofenemate sodium (Meclomen)	Crampy abdominal pain, bloody diarrhea; segmental ascending colitis
Flufenamic acid	Short-term or chronic use; bloody diarrhea, left-sided colitis
Naproxen	Short-term use; bloody diarrhea, left-sided colitis
Ibuprofen	Short-term use; diarrhea, proctitis
Indomethacin (suppositories)	Dose-related; proctitis, diarrhea
Salicylate (aspirin)	Presumed allergic reaction; proctocolitis
Amitriptyline	Overdose; nonocclusive ischemic colitis (gangrene of colon)
Chlorpromazine	Short course; nonocculsive ischemic colitis
Gold (intramuscular)	Watery diarrhea, pancolitis, crypt abscesses and nonspecific inflammation; often associated enteritis
Isotretinoin (synthetic vitamin A analog)	Short-term use; diarrhea, proctosigmoiditis, apthous ulcers, nonspecific acute inflammation; also associated with onset or exacerbations of IBD

cent of these patients and 29 percent died as a result of the colitis. Disodium cromoglycate may be useful in the treatment of these patients.[162,163]

Soap Colitis

There have been numerous reports of colitis and proctitis being caused by soap-containing enemas.[166-171] In a survey of 2000 patients, approximately one third reported deranged or altered bowel function following soapsuds enemas.[169] Reported symptoms range from watery diarrhea to serosanguinous or frankly bloody stools which develop 3 hours to 12 hours following administration of the soap enema.[167,169,170] The condition may follow a single enema or a series of enemas.[166,167] Endoscopic examination may reveal mild erythema and edema or hemorrhagic, ulcerated, and friable mucosa.[166,167,170] Mucosal findings have been reported to extend as far as the transverse colon.[166,170] The colonic symptoms and findings usually resolve without specific treatment 1 to 4 weeks after cessation of the enemas.

The etiology of this colitis is unknown. Both hard and soft soaps have been implicated. It is possible that the fatty acids found in soaps may play a role.[172,173] Fatty acids are converted to hydroxy fatty acids by colonic bacteria in the colon.[174] Both fatty acids and hydroxy fatty acids have been shown to inhibit colonic absorption of water and electrolytes.[172,173,175] Assiduous avoidance of soap-containing enemas obviates the potential for this complication.

Solitary Rectal Ulcer Syndrome

The solitary rectal ulcer syndrome is a benign anorectal condition that has recently received much attention and is thought to be the result of abnormal defecatory patterns. The majority of patients present with nonspecific symptoms such as rectal bleeding, abdominal or anorectal pain, diarrhea, and mucous discharge.[176-179] In addition, complaints concerning constipation, excessive straining at stool, a sensation of incomplete evacuation, or rectal prolapse can often be elicited from these patients.[180] This syndrome is more commonly seen in young adults and is somewhat more prevalent among women.[176]

Characteristically, a solitary ulceration of the anterior rectal wall is found 4 to 12 cm from the anal verge with a surrounding ring of erythematous mucosa (Fig. 26-11). However, ulcerations may be numerous, located posteriorly, or absent altogether.[177,179] A focal area of reddened, granular, friable mucosa may be all that is found. It may be difficult or impossible to distinguish this condition from a nonspecific proctitis on the basis of proctoscopic appearance alone. Definitive diagnosis requires biopsy and is based on characteristic histopathologic findings. The most common findings are fibrous obliteration of the lamina propria, hypertrophy of the muscularis mucosae with extension of smooth muscle fibers into the lamina propria, and regenerative changes in epithelial crypt architecture.[178,179] These changes are often indistinguishable from those seen in colitis cystia profunda (see Fig. 26-10).

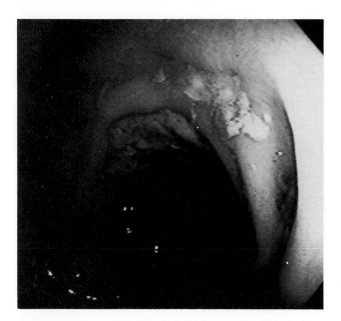

Figure 26-11. Endoscopic appearance of a solitary rectal ulcer. (Courtesy of Jessie Eisenman, M.D., and Eli Ehrenpreis, M.D., Ft. Lauderdale, FL.)

A significant proportion of patients with solitary rectal ulcer syndrome have been demonstrated to have rectal prolapse.[179-183] Although complete rectal prolapse may be found, internal intussusception (hidden or occult prolapse) is more often associated with solitary ulcers. The nonrelaxing puborectalis syndrome, the descending perineum syndrome, and simple rectal mucosal prolapse may also be seen in conjunction with the SRUS.[181,182] These associated conditions may be responsible for many of the evacuation-related symptoms found in patients with this disorder.

Digital examination may reveal focal induration of the rectal wall above the anorectal sphincter. Proctosigmoidoscopy will most often reveal the mucosal findings already described. These lesions can easily be confused with a rectal tumor and therefore biopsy is necessary.[177] Evaluation of the more proximal colon is recommended to exclude neoplasms, diffuse colitis, and synchronous ulcerations. Other causes of anorectal ulceration must be excluded.

Rectal prolapse may be demonstrable if the patient is examined while squatting and straining. Fig. 26-12 shows prolapse of rectal mucosa on which a solitary rectal ulcer rests. Alternatively, with a proctoscope in place, the prolapsing rectal wall may be visualized while the patient strains. Defecography is the best means of confirming the diagnosis.[182] Defecography may also demonstrate the nonrelaxing puborectalis syndrome or the descending perineum syndrome.[180,181] This is discussed in Chapter 6 and 25.

The best treatment for solitary rectal ulcer syndrome remains unclear. If a documented full-thickness prolapse is present, a surgical procedure to correct the prolapse seems reasonable. Unfortunately, such operations have not been universally successful.[178,184,185]

The indication for surgery in patients without prolapse is even less clear. Results of a number of operations have been generally disappointing and inconclusive. The results of direct suturing of the ulcer have been poor. Local excision, either alone or in conjunction with hemorrhoidectomy, has been followed by recurrence rates of 50 to 70 percent.[178,186-189]

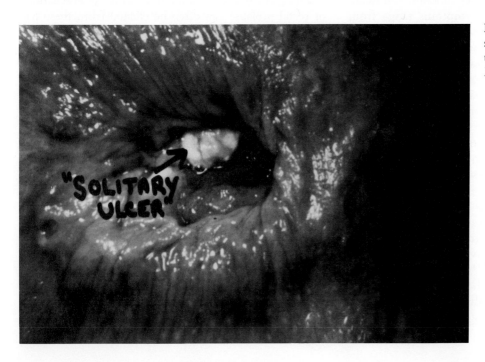

Figure 26-12. Prolapsing solitary rectal ulcer. (Courtesy of Irwin R. Berman, M.D., Brunswick, GA.)

Several investigators have reported significant clinical improvement with medical treatment alone.[177,184,186] Medical treatment includes dietary manipulations and the administration of stool bulking agents in an effort to regulate bowel habits. Rectal digitalization and avoidance of straining are also recommended. Topical corticosteroids and oral azulfidine have also been tried, but results have been generally poor.[178,186] More recently, however, sucralfate retention enemas have been shown successful in achieving macroscopic healing and symptomatic relief.[190] When a specific defecatory syndrome is identified, treatment directed toward that condition is warranted. Examples include biofeedback for nonrelaxing puborectalis syndrome and pelvic strengthening exercises for patients with descending perineum syndrome. Because the results of surgery have been poor, a trial of medical management seems warranted before a surgical approach is considered.[177,179]

References

1. Talbot RW, Walker RC, Beart RW Jr. Changing epidemiology, diagnosis, and treatment of *Clostridium difficile* toxin-associated colitis. *Br J Surg.* 1986;73:457–460.

2. Church JM, Fazio VW. A role for colonic stasis in the pathogenesis of disease related to *Clostridium difficile. Dis Colon Rectum.* 1986;29:804–809.

3. Rampling A, Warren RE, Berry PJ, et al. Atypical *Clostridium difficile* colitis in neutropenic patients. *Lancet.* 1982;2:162–163.

4. Silva J, Fekety R, Werk C, et al. Inciting and etiologic agents of colitis. *Rev Infect Dis.* 1984;6 (suppl 1):S214–S221.

5. Fainstein V, Bodey GP, Fekety R. Relapsing pseudomembranous colitis associated with cancer chemotherapy. *J Infect Dis.* 1981;143:865.

6. Wald A, Mendelow H, Bartlett JG. Non-antibiotic associated pseudomembranous colitis due to toxin producing clostridia. *Ann Intern Med.* 1980;92:798.

7. Moskovitz M, Bartlett JG. Recurrent pseudomembranous colitis unassociated with prior antibiotic therapy. *Arch Intern Med.* 1981;141:663.

8. Pothoulakis H, Triadafilopoulos G, LaMont JT. Antibiotic-associated colitis. *Comp Ther.* 1985;11:68–73.

9. Trinka YM, LaMont JT. Association of *Clostridium difficile* toxin with symptomatic relapse of chronic inflammatory bowel disease. *Gastroenterology.* 1981;80:693.

10. Bolton RP, Sheriff RJ, Read AE. *Clostridium difficile* associated with diarrhea: a role in inflammatory bowel disease? *Lancet.* 1980;1:383.

11. Bartlett JG. Antibiotic-associated pseudomembranous colitis. *Rev Infect Dis.* 1979;1:530–539.

12. Lishman AH, Al-Jumaila IJ, Record CO. Spectrum of antibiotic-associated diarrhoea. *Gut.* 1981;22:34.

13. Rolfe RD. Diagnosis of *Clostridium difficile*–associated intestinal disease. *Crit Rev Clin Lab Sci.* 1986;24:235–265.

14. Ruff D, Jaffe J, London R, Candio J. Pseudomembranous colitis following low dose trimethoprim-sulfamethoxazole. *J Urol.* 1985;134:1218–1219.

15. Bailey RR, Walker RJ, Cook HB. Ceftriaxone-induced colitis. *N Z Med J.* 1985;98:969. Letter.

16. Block BS, Mercer LJ, Ismail MA, Moawed AH. *Clostridium difficile*–associated diarrhea follows perioperative prophylaxis with cefoxitin. *Am J Obstet Gynecol.* 1985;153:835–838.

17. George WL, Rolfe RD, Sutter VL, Fineegold SM. Diarrhea and colitis associated with antimicrobial therapy in man and animals. *Am J Clin Nutr.* 1979;32:251.

18. Amin NM. Antibiotic-associated pseudomembranous colitis. *Am Fam Physician.* 1985;31:115–120.

19. Wilkins TD. Role of *Clostridium difficile* toxins in disease. *Gastroenterology.* 1987;93:389–390.

20. Aronsson B, Mollby R, Nord CE. Antimicrobial agents and *Clostridium difficile* in acute enteric disease: epidemiologic data from Sweden. *J Infect Dis.* 1985;151:476–481.

21. Viscidi R, Willey S, Bartlett JG. Isolation rates and toxigenic potential of *Clostridium difficile* isolates from various populations. *Gastroenterology.* 1981;81:5.

22. Fekety R, Kim K-H, Brown D, et al. Epidemiology of antibiotic-associated colitis. Isolation of *Clostridium difficile* from the hospital environment. *Am J Med.* 1981;70:906–908.

23. Tedesco FJ. Pseudomembranous colitis: pathogenesis and therapy. *Med Clin North Am.* 1982;66:655–664.

24. Van Ness MM, Cattau EL Jr. Fulminant colitis complicating antibiotic-associated pseudomembranous colitis: case report and review of the clinical manifestations and treatment. *Am J Gastroenterol.* 1987;82:374–377.

25. Gebhard RL, Gerding DN, Olson MM, et al. Clinical and endoscopic findings in patients early in the course of *Clostridium difficile*–associated

pseudomembranous colitis. *Am J Med.* 1985; 78:45–48.

26. Tedesco FJ. Antibiotic associated pseudomembranous colitis with negative proctosigmoidoscopy examination. *Gastroenterology.* 1979;77:295–297.

27. Burbige EJ, Radigan JJ. Antibiotic-associated colitis with normal appearing rectum. *Dis Colon Rectum.* 1981;24:198–200.

28. Russo A, Cirino E, Sanfilippo G, et al. Ampicillin associated colitis. *Endoscopy.* 1980;12:97–99.

29. Sumner WH, Tedesco FJ. Rectal biopsy in clindamycin-associated colitis: an analysis of 23 cases. *Arch Pathol.* 1975;99:237.

30. Burdon DW; Borriello SP, ed. *Spectrum of Disease in Antibiotic Associated Diarrhoea and Colitis.* Boston: Martinus Nijhoff; 1984:10.

31. Holst E, Halin I, Mardh PA. Recovery of *Clostridium difficile* from children. *Scand J Infect Dis.* 1981;13:41.

32. George WL, Rolfe RD, Finegold SM. *Clostridium difficile* and its cytotoxin in feces of patients with antimicrobial agent–associated diarrhea and miscellaneous conditions. *J Clin Microbiol.* 1982; 15:1049.

33. Aronsson B, Mollby R, Nord CE. Diagnosis and epidemiology of *C. difficile* enterocolitis in Sweden. *J Antimicrob Chemother.* 1984;14(suppl):85.

34. Bartlett JG. *Clostridium difficile* and cytotoxin in feces of patients with antimicrobial agent–associated colitis: comment on the report by W.L. George et al. *Infect Immunol.* 1982;10:208.

35. Lashner BA, Todorczuk J, Sahm DF, Hanauer SB. *Clostridium difficile* culture-positive toxin-negative diarrhea. *Am J Gastroenterol.* 1986;81:940–943.

36. Burdon DW, George RH, Mogg GAG, et al. Fecal toxin and severity of antibiotic-associated pseudomembranous colitis. *J Clin Pathol.* 1981; 34:548.

37. Young GP, Ward PB, Bayley N, et al. Antibiotic associated colitis due to *Clostridium difficile:* double blind comparison of vancomycin with Bacitracin. *Gastroenterology.* 1985;89:1038–1045.

38. Fekety R, Silva J, Browne RA, et al. Clindamycin-induced colitis. *Am J Clin Nutr.* 1979;32:244–250.

39. Bartlett JG. Treatment of *Clostridium* colitis. *Gastroenterology.* 1985;89:1192–1195.

40. McClain WJ, Sylvia LM, Baciewicz AM. Antibiotic-associated colitis. *Infect Surg.* July 1986: 401–411.

41. Teasley DG, Olson MM, Gebhard RL, et al. Prospective randomized trial of metronidazole versus vancomycin for *Clostridium difficile*–associated diarrhoea and colitis. *Lancet.* 1983;2:1043–1046.

42. Tedesco F, Markham R, Gurwith M, et al. Oral vancomycin for antibiotic-associated pseudomembranous colitis. *Lancet.* 1978;2:226–228.

43. AMA Drug Evaluations. 4th ed. Chicago:AMA Press; 1980:1301.

44. Bolton RP, Culshaw MA. Faecal metronidazole concentrations during oral and intravenous therapy for antibiotic associated colitis due to *Clostridium difficile.* Gut. 1986;27:1169–1172.

45. Corman ML. *Colon and Rectal Surgery.* Philadelphia: JP Lippincott; 1984:737.

46. Jackson BT, Amders CJ. Idiopathic pseudomembranous colitis successfully treated by surgical excision. *Br J Surg.* 1972;59:154–156.

47. Boyd WC, DenBesten L. Subtotal colectomy for refractory pseudomembranous enterocolitis. *JAMA.* 1976;235:181.

48. Hornick RB, Greisman S. On the pathogenesis of typhoid fever. *Arch Intern Med.* 1978;138:357.

49. Hook EW. *Salmonella* speces. In: Mandell GL, Douglas RG, Bennett JE, ed. *Principles and Practices of Infectious Diseases.* New York: Churchill Livingstone; 1990:1700–1716.

50. Hook EW. Salmonellosis: certain factors influencing the interaction of *Salmonella* and the human host. *Bull N Y Acad Med.* 1961;37:499.

51. Waddell WR, Kunz LJ. Association of *Salmonella* enteritis with operations on the stomach. *N Engl J Med.* 1956;255:555.

52. Hoffman TA, Ruiz CJ, Counts GW, et al. Waterborne typhoid fever in Dade County, Florida: clinical and therapeutic evaluations of 105 bacteremic patients. *Am J Med.* 1975;59:481.

53. Kaye D. Merselis JG, Connolly CS, et al. Treatment of chronic carriers of *Salmonella typhosa* with ampicillin. *Ann N Y Acad Sci.* 1967;145:429.

54. Mandal BK, Mani V. Colonic involvement in salmonellosis. *Lancet.* 1976;1:887.

55. Abramowicz M, ed. The choice of antimicrobial drugs. *Med Lett.* 1988;30:33–40.

56. Dupont HL. *Shigella* species (bacillary dysentery). In: Mandell GL, Douglas RG, Bennett JE, ed. *Principles and Practices of Infectious Diseases.* 3rd ed. New York: Churchill Livingstone; 1990: 1716–1722.

57. Corman ML. *Colon and Rectal Surgery.* 2nd ed. Philadelphia: JB Lippincott; 1989: 992.

58. Gorbach SL. Infectious diarrhea. In: Sleisinger MH, Fordtran JS, ed. *Gastrointestinal Disease: Pathophysiology, Diagnosis, and Management.* 4th ed. Philadelphia: WB Saunders; 1989:1199–1203.

59. Vantrappen G, Agg HO, Ponette E, et al. *Yersinia* enteritis and enterocolitis: gastroenterological aspects. *Gastroenterology.* 1977;72:220–227.

60. Butler T. Yersinia species. In: Mandell GL, Douglas RG, Bennett JE, eds. *Principles and Practices of Infectious Diseases*. 3rd ed. New York: Churchill Livingstone;1990: 1754–1756.
61. Rabinovitz M, Stremple JF, et al: *Yersinia enterocolitica* infection complicated by intestinal perforation. *Arch Intern Med*. 1987;147:1662–1663.
62. Stuart RC, Leahy AL, Cafferkey MT, Stephens RE. *Yersinia enterocolitica* infection and toxic megacolon. *Br J Surg*. 1986;73:590.
63. Simmonds SD, Noble MA, Freeman HJ. Gastrointestinal features of culture-positive *Yersinia enterocolitica* infection. *Gastroenterology*. 1987; 92:112–117.
64. Blaser MJ. *Campylobacter* species. In: Mandell GL, Douglas RG, Bennett JE, eds. *Principles and Practices of Infectious Diseases*. 3rd ed. New York: Churchill Livingstone; 1990:1649–1658.
65. Lambert ME, Schofield PF, Ironside AG, Mandal BK. *Campylobacter* colitis. *Br Med J*. 1979;1: 857–859.
66. Blaser MJ, Wells JG, Feldman RA, et al. *Campylobacter* enteritis in the United States. A multicenter study. *Ann Intern Med*. 1983;98:360.
67. Riley LW, Finch MJ. Results of the first year of national surveillance of *Campylobacter* infections in the United States. *J Infect Dis*. 1985;151:956.
68. McKinley MJ, Taylor M, Sangree MH. Toxic megacolon with *Campylobacter* colitis. *Conn Med*. 1980;44:496.
69. Blaser MJ, LaForce FM, Wilson WA, et al. Reservoirs for human campylobacteriosis. *J Infect Dis*. 1980;141;665–669.
70. Guerrant RL, Lahita RG, Winn WC, et al. Campylobacteriosis in man: pathogenic mechanisms and review of 91 bloodstream infections. *Am J Med*. 1978;65:584–592.
71. Anders BJ, Lauer BA, et al. Double-blind placebo controlled trial of erythromycin for treatment of *Campylobacter* enteritis. *Lancet*. 1982;1:131.
72. Walsh JA. Problems in recognition and diagnosis of amebiasis: estimation of the global magnitude of morbidity and mortality. *Rev Infect Dis*. 1986 8(2):228–238.
73. Simmons RL, Howard RJ. Surgical infectious diseases. New York: Appleton-Century-Crofts; 1982:959.
74. Schmerin MJ, Gelston A, Jones TC. Amebiasis. An increasing problem among homosexuals in New York City. *JAMA*. 1977;238:1386–1387.
75. Robilotti JN. The gay bowel syndrome. A review of colonic and rectal conditions in 200 male homosexuals. *Am J Gastroenterol*. 1977;67:478–484.
76. Brooks JL, Kozarek RM, Amebic colitis: prevent-

77. Pelaez M, Villazon A, Sieres Zaraboso R. Amebic perforation of the colon. *Dis Colon Rectum*. 1966;9:356–362.
78. Chen WJ, Chen KM, Lin M. Colon perforation in amebiasis. *Arch Surg*. 1971;103:676–680.
79. Clark HC. Distribution and complications of amebic lesions found in 186 post-mortem examinations. *Am J Trop Med Hyg*. 1925;5:157–171.
80. Adams EB, MacLeod IN. Invasive amebiasis. *Medicine*. 1977;56:315–323.
81. Kean B, Gilmore H, Van Stone W. Fatal amebiasis: report of 148 cases from the Armed Forces Institute of Pathology. *Ann Intern Med*. 1956;44:831–843.
82. Clark HC. Distribution and complications of amebic lesions found in 186 postmortem examinations. *Am J Trop Med*. 1925;5:157–171.
83. Nevin RW. The surgical aspects of intestinal amoebiasis. *Ann R Coll Surg Eng*. 1947; 29:69–84.
84. D'Antoni JS. Amebic and bacillary colitis in New Orleans area; preliminary report. *Am J Trop Med*. 1942;22:319–324.
85. Cutler D, Avendano E, Maldonado P, et al. Necrotizing amoebic colitis. *Am J Gastroenterol*. 1974;62:345–355.
86. Hawe P. The surgical aspect of intestinal amebiasis. *Surg Gynecol Obstet*. 1945;81:387–404.
87. Patterson M, Schoppe LE. The presentation of amoebiasis. *Med Clin North Am*. 1982;66(3): 689–705.
88. Ellyson JH, Bezmalinovic Z, Parks SN, Lewis FR. Necrotizing amebic colitis: a frequently fatal complication. *Am J Surg*. 1986;152:21–26.
89. Corman ML. *Colon and Rectal Surgery*. 2nd ed. Philadelphia: JB Lippincott; 1989:999–1004.
90. Abramowicz M, ed. Drugs for parasitic infections. *Med Lett*. 1990;32(814):23–24.
91. *AMA Drug Evaluations*. 4th ed. Chicago, Ill: American Medical Association; 1980:1402.
92. Peppercorn MA. Enteric infections in homosexual men with AIDS. *Contemp Gastroenterol*. 1989;2:23–32.
93. Stein D, Bank S. Surgery in amoebic colitis. *Gut*. 1970;11:941–946.
94. Eggleston FC, Verghese M, Handa AK. Amoebic perforation of the bowel: experiences with 26 cases. *Br J Surg*. 1978;65:748–751.
95. Wig D, Talwar BL, Bushnurmath SR. Toxic dilatation complicating fulminant amoebic colitis. *Br J Surg*. 1981;68:135–136.
96. Faegenburg D, Chiat H, Mandel PR, Rose ST.

Toxic megacolon in amebic colitis. Report of a case. *Am J Roentgenol.* 1967;99:74–76.

97. Wruble LD, Duckworth JK, Duke DD, Rothschild JA. Toxic dilatation of the colon in a case of amebiasis. *N Engl J Med.* 1966;285:926–928.

98. Greenstein AJ, Greenstein RJ, Sachar DB. Toxic dilatation in amebic colitis: successful treatment without colectomy. *Am J Surg.* 1980;139:456–458.

99. Shukla VK, Roy SK, Vaidya MP, Mehrotra ML. Fulminant amebic colitis. *Dis Colon Rectum.* 1986;29:398–401.

100. Krogstad DJ, Spencer HC, Healy GR. Current concepts in parasitology. Amebiasis. *N Engl J Med.* 1978;298:262–265.

101. Owen RL. Parasitic diseases. In: Slesinger MH, Fordtran JS, eds. *Gastrointestinal Disease: Pathophysiology, Diagnosis, and Management.* 4th ed. Philadelphia: WB Saunders; 1989:1182–1186.

102. Katz M, Despommier DD, Gwadz RW. *Parasitic Diseases.* 2nd ed. New York: Springer-Verlag; 1989:96–108.

103. Mig-Chai C, Chi-Yuan C, Fu-Pan W, et al. Colorectal cancer and schistosomiasis. *Lancet.* 1981;1:971–973.

104. Goligher J. *Surgery of the Anus, Rectum, and Colon.* 5th ed. London: Bailliere Tindall; 1984:1024.

105. Corman ML. *Colon and Rectal Surgery.* 2nd ed. Philadelphia: JB Lippincott; 1989:1007–1009.

106. Abramowicz M, ed. Drugs for parasitic infections. *Med Lett.* 1988;30:15–22.

107. Bessa SM, Helmy I, El-kharadly Y. Colorectal schistosomiasis: endoscopic polypectomy. *Dis Col Rectum.* 1983;26:772–774.

108. Bessa SM, Helmy I, Mekky F, Hamam SM. Colorectal schistosomiasis: clinicopathologic study and management. *Dis Colon Rectum.* 1979;22:390–395.

109. Earlam RJ. Gastrointestinal aspects of Chagas' disease. *Dig Dis.* 1972;17:559–571.

110. Goligher J. *Surgery of the Anus, Rectum, and Colon.* 5th ed. London: Balliere Tindall; 1984:335–345.

111. Lazaro da Silva A, Tafuri WL. Megcolon surgery. *Int Surg.* 1975;60:402–404.

112. Habr Gama A, Haddad J, Simonsen O, et al. Volvulus of the sigmoid colon in Brazil: a report of 230 cases. *Dis Colon Rectum.* 1976;19:314–320.

113. Ferreira-Santos R. Megacolon and megarectum in Chagas' disease. *Proc R Soc Med.* 1961;54:1047.

114. Haddad J. Treatment of acquired megacolon by retrorectal lowering of the colon with a perineal colostomy: modified Duhamel operation. *Dis Colon Rectum.* 1969;12:46.

115. Corman ML. *Colon and Rectal Surgery.* 2nd ed. Philadelphia: JB Lippincott; 1989:1013.

116. Katz M, Despommier DD, Gwadz RW. *Parasitic Diseases.* 2nd ed. New York: Springer-Verlag; 1989:6–10.

117. Corman ML. *Colon and Rectal Surgery.* 2nd ed. Philadelphia: JB Lippincott; 1989:1004–1005.

118. Katz M, Despommier DD, Gwadz RW. *Parasitic Diseases.* 2nd ed. New York: Springer-Verlag; 1989:143–146.

119. Glotzer DJ, Glick ME, Goldman H. Proctitis and colitis following diversion of the fecal stream. *Gastroenterology.* 1981;80:438–441.

120. Harig JM, Soergel KH, Komorowski RA, Wood CM. Treatment of diversion colitis with short-chain-fatty acid irrigation. *N Engl J Med.* 1989;320:23–28.

121. Roediger WE. Role of anaerobic bacteria in the metabolic welfare of the colonic mucosa in man. *Gut.* 1980;21:793–798.

122. Abramson D, Hashmi H, Whelan RL. Diversion colitis: a prospective study. *Am Surg.* In press.

123. Ma CK, Gottlieb C, Haas PA. Diversion colitis: a clinicopathologic study of 21 cases. *Hum Pathol.* 1990;21:429–436.

124. Haas PA, Fox TA, Szilagy EJ. Endoscopic examination of the colon and rectum distal to a colostomy. *Am J Gastroenterol.* 1990;85:850–854.

125. Ona FV, Boger JN. Rectal bleeding due to diversion colitis. *Am J Gastroenterol.* 1985;80:40–41.

126. Bories C, Miazza B, Galian A, et al. Idiopathic chronic watery diarrhea from excluded rectosigmoid with goblet cell hyperplasia cures by restoration of large bowel continuity. *Dig Dis Sci.* 1986;31:769–772.

127. Lechner RL, Frank F, Jantsch H, et al. Lymphoid follicular hyperplasia in excluded colonic segments: a radiologic sign of diversion colitis. *Radiology.* 1990;176:135–136.

128. Lusk LB, Reichen J, Levine JS. Apthous ulceration in diversion colitis: clinical implications. *Gastroenterology.* 1984;87:1171–1173.

129. Bosshardt RT, Abel MD. Proctitis following fecal diversion. *Dis Colon Rectum.* 1984;27:605–607.

130. Korelitz BI, Cheskin LH, Sohn N, Sommers SC. Proctitis after fecal diversion in Crohn's disease and its elimination with reanastomosis: implications and surgical management. *Gastroenterology.* 1984;87:710–713.

131. Murray FE, O'Brien MJ, Birkett DH, Kemmedy SM, LaMont JS. Diversion colitis: pathologic finding in a resected sigmoid colon and rectum. *Gastroenterology.* 1987;93:1404–1408.

132. Komorowski RA. Histologic spectrum of diversion colitis. *Am J Surg Path.* 1990;14:548–554.

133. Lindstrom CG. "Collagenous colitis" with watery diarrhea: a new entity? *Pathol Eur.* 1976;11:87–89.

134. Guarda LA, Nelson RS, Stroehlein JR, Korinek JK, Raymond AK. Collagenous colitis. *Am J Clin Pathol*. 1983;80:503–507. Case Reports.

135. Bamford MJ, Matz LR, Armstrong JA, Harris ARC. Collagenous colitis: a case report and review of the literature. *Pathology*. 1982;14:481–484.

136. Danzi JT, McDonald TJ, King J. Collagenous colitis. *Am J Gastroenterol*. 1988;83:83–85.

137. Salt WB II, Llaneza PP. Collagenous colitis: a cause of chronic diarrhea diagnosed only by biopsy of normal appearing colonic mucosa. *Gastrointest Endosc*. 1986;32:421–423.

138. Coverlizza S, Ferrari A, Scevola F, et al. Clinicopathological features of collagenous colitis: case report and literature review. *Am J Gastroenterol*. 1986;81:1098–1103.

139. Teglbjaerg PS, Thaysen EH, Jensen HH. Development of collagenous colitis in sequential biopsy specimens. *Gastroenterology*. 1984;87:703–709.

140. Rokkas T, Filipe MI, Sladen GE. Collagenous colitis with rapid response to sulphasalazine. *Postgrad Med*. 1988;64:74–76.

141. Weidner N, Smith J, Pattee B. Sulfasalazine in treatment of collagenous colitis. *Am J Med*. 1984;77:162–166.

142. Farah DA, Mills PR, Lee FD, McLay A, Russell RI. Collagenous colitis: possible response to sulfasalazine and local steroid therapy. *Gastroenterology*. 1985;88:792–797.

143. Jessurun J, Yardley JH, Lee EL, et al. Microscopic and collagenous colitis: different names for the same condition? *Gastroenterology*. 1986;91:1583–1584.

144. Eckstein RP, Dowsett JF, Riley JW. Collagenous enterocolitis: a case of collagenous colitis with involvement of small intestine. *Am J Gastroenterol*. 1988;83:767–771.

145. Bogomoletz WV, Adnet JJ, Birembaut P, et al. Collagenous colitis: an unrecognized entity. *Gut*. 1980;21:164–168.

146. Van den Oord JJ, Geboes K, Desmet VJ. Collagenous colitis: an abnormal collagen table? Two cases and review of the literature. *Am J Gastroenterol*. 1982;77:377–381.

147. Debongnie JC, DeGalocsy C, Caholessur MO, Haot J. Collagenous colitis: a transient condition? Report of two cases. *Dis Colon Rectum*. 1984;27:672–676.

148. Kingham JGC, Levison DA, Morson BC, Dawson AM. Collagenous colitis. *Gut*. Case Report. 1986;27:570–577.

149. Girard DE, Keefe EB. Therapy for collagenous colitis. *Ann Int Med*. 1987;106:909. Letter.

150. Levin DS. "Solitary" rectal ulcer syndrome: are "solitary" rectal ulcer syndrome and "localized" colitis cystica profunda analagous syndromes caused by rectal prolapse. *Gastroenterology*. 1987;92:243–253.

151. Nelson H, Pemberton JH. Solitary rectal ulcer. In: Fazio VW, ed. *Current Therapy in Colon and Rectal Surgery*. Toronto: BC Decker; 1990:98–102.

152. Schein M, Veller M, Decker GAG. Colitis cystica profunda simulating rectal carcinoma. *S Afr Med J*. 1987;72:289–290.

153. Walker JP, Wiener I, Rowe EB. Colitis cystiica profunda: diagnosis and management. *South Med J*. 1986;79:1167–1170.

154. Stuart M. Proctitis cystica profunda—incidence, etiology, and treatment. *Dis Colon Rectum*. 1984;27:153–156.

155. Hall RI, Petty AH, Cobden I, Lendrum R. Enteritis and colitis associated with mefenamic acid. *Br Med J*. 1983;287(6400):1182.

156. Doman DB, Goldberg HJ. A Case of meclofenemate sodium-induced colitis. *Am J Gastroenterol*. 1986;81(12):1220–1221.

157. O'Brien WM, Bagby GF. Rare adverse reactions to nonsteroidal anti-inflammatory drugs. *J Rheumatol*. 1985;12(3):562–567.

158. Ravi S, Keat AC, Keat ECB. Colitis caused by non-steroidal anti-inflammatory drugs. *Postgrad Med J*. 1986;62:(730):773–776.

159. Walt RP, Hawkey CJ, Langman MJS. Colitis associated with non-steroidal anti-inflammatory agents. *B Med J*. 1984;288:238.

160. Rampton DS, Sladen GE. Relapse of ulcerative proctocolitis during treatment with anti-inflammatory drugs. *Postgrad Med J*. 1980;57:297.

161. Rutherford D, Stockdill G, Hamer-Hodges DW, Ferguson A. Proctocolitis induced by salicylate. *Br Med J*. 1984;288(6419):794. Letter.

162. McCormick PA, O'Donoghue D, Lemass B. Gold induced colitis: case report and literature review. *Ir Med J*. 1985;78:17–18.

163. Martin DM, Goldman JA, Gilliam J, Nasrallah SM. Gold induced eosinophilic enterocolitis: response to oral cromolyn sodium. *Gastroenterology*. 1981;80:1567–1570.

164. Gollock JM, Thomson JPS. Ischaemic colitis associated with psychotropic drugs. *Postgrad Med J*. 1984;60:564–565.

165. Martin P, Manley PN, Depew WT, Blakeman JM. Isotretinoin-associated proctosigmoiditis. *Gastroenterology*. 1987;93(3):606–609.

166. Orchard JL, Lawson R. Severe colitis induced by soap enemas. *South Med J*. 1986;79:1459–1469.

167. Pike BF, Phillipi PJ, Lawson EH. Soap colitis. *N Engl J Med*. 1971;285:217–218.

168. Toffler RB, Barry JM. Colonic mucosal slough following detergent enemas. *Am J Gastrenterol.* 1972;58:638–640.

169. Hicks ES. Observation regarding enemas. *Can Med Assoc J.* 1944;51:358–359.

170. Barker CS. Acute colitis resulting from soapsuds enema. *Can Med Assoc J.* 1945;52:285.

171. Kirchner SG, Buckspan GS, O'Neill JA et al. Detergent enemas: a cause of caustic colitis. *Pediatr Radiol.* 1977;6:141–146.

172. Binder HJ. Fecal fatty acids—mediators of diarrhea? *Gastroenterology.* 1973;65:847–850. Editorial.

173. Ammon HV, Phillips SF. Inhibition of colonic water and electrolyte absorbtion by fatty acids in man. *Gastroenterology.* 1973;65:744–749.

174. Thomas PJ. Identification of some enteric bacteria which convert oleic acid to hydroxystearic acid in vitro. *Gastroenterology.* 1972;62:430–435.

175. Bright-Asare P, Binder HJ. Stimulation of colonic secretion of water and electrolytes by hydroxy fatty acids. *Gastroenterology.* 1973;64:81–88.

176. Henry MM, Swash M. Coloproctology and the pelvic floor. London: Butterworths; 1985:284.

177. Britto E, Borges AM, Path MRC, et al. Solitary rectal ulcer syndrome: twenty cases seen at an oncology center. *Dis Colon Rectum.* 1987;30:381–385.

178. Niv Y, Bat L. Solitary rectal ulcer syndrome—clinical, endoscopic, and histological spectrum. *Am J Gastrenterol.* 1986;81:486–491.

179. Levine DS. "Solitary" rectal ulcer syndrome: are "solitary" rectal ulcer syndrome and "localized" colitis cystica profunda analogous syndromes caused by rectal prolapse? *Gastrenterol.* 1987; 92:243–253.

180. Goei R, Baeten C, Janevski B, van Engelshoven J. The solitary rectal ulcer syndrome: diagnosis with defecography. *AJR.* 1987;149:933–936.

181. Womack NR, Williams NS, Holmfield JH, Morrison JF. Anorectal function in the solitary rectal ulcer syndrome. *Dis Colon Rectum.* 1987;30: 319–323.

182. Kuijpers HC, Schreve RH, ten Cate Hoedmakers H. Diagnosis of functional disorders of defecation causing the solitary rectal ulcer syndrome. *Dis Colon Rectum.* 1984;27:507–512.

183. Womack NR, Williams NS, Holmfield JHM, Morrison JFB. Pressure and prolapse—the cause of solitary rectal ulceration. *Gut.* 1987;28: 1228–1233.

184. Keighley MRB, Shouler P. Clinical and manometric features of the solitary rectal ulcer syndrome. *Dis Colon Rectum.* 1984;27:507–512.

185. White CM, Findlay JM, Price JJ. The occult rectal prolapse syndrome *Br J Surg.* 1980;67:528–530.

186. Ford MJ, Anderson JR, Gilmour HM, et al. Clinical spectrum of "solitary ulcer" of the rectum. *Gastroenterology.* 1983;84:1533–1540.

187. Kennedy DK, Hughes ESR, Masterton JP. The natural history of benign ulcer of the rectum. *Surg Gynecol Obstet.* 1977;144:718–720.

188. Madigan MR, Morson BC. Solitary ulcer of the rectum. *Gut.* 1969;10:871–881.

189. Jalan KN, Brunt PW, Maclean N. Benign solitary ulcer of the rectum—a report of 5 cases. *Scand J. Gastroenterol.* 1970;5:143–147.

190. Zargar SA, Khuroo MS, Mahajan R. Sucrafate retention enemas in solitary rectal ulcer. *Dis Colon Rectum.* 1991;34:455–457.

INDEX

Page numbers followed by the letter "f" indicate figures; those followed by "t" indicate tables.

501